HOME
HEALTH
CARE
NURSING

Second Edition

HOME
HEALTH
CARE
NURSING

IDA M. MARTINSON, RN, PhD, FAAN,
Professor,
Department of Family Health Care Nursing,
School of Nursing,
University of California, San Francisco,
San Francisco, California

ANN G. WIDMER, MA, EdD,
Dean and Professor,
School of Management,
Department of Health and Social Services,
Concordia University,
Portland, Oregon

CARMEN J. PORTILLO, RN, PhD, FAAN,
Associate Professor,
School of Nursing,
Department of Community Health Systems,
University of California, San Francisco,
San Francisco, California

W.B. SAUNDERS COMPANY
An Imprint of Elsevier Science
Philadelphia   London   New York   St. Louis   Sydney   Toronto

W.B. SAUNDERS COMPANY
An Imprint of Elsevier Science

The Curtis Center
Independence Square West
Philadelphia, Pennsylvania 19106

Vice President/Publishing Director, Nursing: Sally Schrefer
Senior Editor: Loren S. Wilson
Senior Developmental Editor: Michele D. Hayden
Production Manager: Pat Joiner
Production Editor: Gena Magouirk
Designer: Mark A. Oberkrom

NOTICE:
Pharmacology is an ever-changing field. Standard safety precautions must be followed, but as new research and clinical experience broaden our knowledge, changes in treatment and drug therapy may become necessary or appropriate. Readers are advised to check the most current product information provided by the manufacturer of each drug to be administered to verify the recommended dose, the method and duration of administration, and contraindications. It is the responsibility of the treating appropriately-licensed health care provider, relying on experience and knowledge of the patient, to determine dosages and the best treatment for each individual patient. Neither the Publisher nor the editor assume any liability for any injury and/or damage to persons or property arising from this publication.

Library of Congress Cataloging-in-Publication Data

Home health care nursing / [edited by] Ida M. Martinson, Ann G. Widmer, Carmen J. Portillo.—2nd ed.

p.   cm.

Includes bibliographical references and index.

ISBN 0-7216-7766-5 (pbk)

1. Home nursing. I. Martinson, Ida Marie   II. Widmer, Ann.   III. Portillo, Carmen J.

RT61.H67 2002   610.73—dc21

                                                    2001057695

HOME HEALTH CARE NURSING

Printed in the United States of America

Last digit is the print number: 9   8   7   6   5   4   3   2   1

Contributors

Mila Ann Aroskar, RN, EdD, FAAN
Associate Professor Emeritus,
Center for Bioethics,
University of Minnesota,
Minneapolis, Minnesota

David Arthur, RN, PhD
Associate Professor,
Department of Nursing and Health Science,
Hong Kong Polytechnic University,
Hung Hom, Kowloon, Hong Kong

Violet H. Barkauskas, RN, PhD, FAAN
Associate Professor,
School of Nursing,
University of Michigan,
Ann Arbor, Michigan

Lowanna S. Binkley, RN, MS, CNN
Thousand Oaks, California

Maria G. Boosalis, PhD, MPH, RD
Associate Professor, Clinical Nutrition,
University of Kentucky,
Lexington, Kentucky

Kathryn H. Bowles, RN, PhD
Assistant Professor,
School of Nursing,
University of Pennsylvania;
Director of Nursing Research,
VNA of Greater Philadelphia,
Philadelphia, Pennsylvania

Katherine Camacho Carr, PhD, ARNP, CNM, FACNM
Instructor,
State University of New York,
Downstate Midwifery Education Program;
Instructor,
Philadelphia University,
Graduate Midwifery Program;
Nurse-Midwife,
Highline Midwifery and Women's Health,
Seattle, Washington

Linda Chafetz, RN, DNSc
Associate Professor,
Department of Community Health Systems,
School of Nursing,
University of California, San Francisco,
San Francisco, California

†Marsha H. Cohen, RN, DNS, CFNP
San Francisco, California

Roberta M. Conti, RN, PhD, FAAN
Coordinator,
Nursing Administration Graduate Program,
College of Nursing and Health Sciences,
George Mason University,
Fairfax, Virginia

Glen Doyle, EdD, MSN, GCS, GNP
Professor, Gerontology,
College of Health and Human Services,
California State University-Fresno,
Fresno, California

---

†Deceased.

v

Ellen D'Errico, MSN, PHN
Assistant Professor,
School of Nursing,
Loma Linda University,
Loma Linda, California

Barbara Germino, RN, PhD
Professor,
School of Nursing,
University of North Carolina at Chapel Hill,
Chapel Hill, North Carolina

Philip M. Gold, MD, MACP
Professor,
Chief, Department of Pulmonary
   and Critical Care Medicine,
Loma Linda University School of Medicine,
Loma Linda, California

Brian K. Goodroad, PhD(c), RN, ACRN
Assistant Professor;
Director of Advanced Practice Nursing,
School of Nursing,
Metropolitan State University,
St. Paul, Minnesota

Donna M. Guyot, RN-C, MS, MA, ANP
Nevada County Behavioral Health
   Department,
Nevada City, California

Tony Hilton, RN, MPH
Clinical Nurse Specialist,
Loma Linda University Medical Center,
Loma Linda, California

Bonnie Huiskes, MSN, FNP
Nurse Practitioner,
Cardiomyopathy Program,
Loma Linda University Medical Center,
Loma Linda, California

Marjorie Jamieson, RN, MS, FAAN
Executive Director,
Living at Home, Block Nurse Program, Inc.,
St. Paul, Minnesota

Patricia Jones, RN, PhD, FAAN
Professor,
School of Nursing,
Loma Linda University,
Loma Linda, California

Raija Kuisma, PhD, MSc, PT
Assistant Professor,
Department of Rehabilitation Sciences,
Hong Kong Polytechnic University,
Hung Hom, Kowloon, Hong Kong

Claudia K.Y. Lai, RN, MN, CS
Assistant Professor,
Department of Nursing and Health
   Sciences,
Hong Kong Polytechnic University,
Hung Hom, Kowloon, Hong Kong

Sandra MacKay, RN, PhD
Professor,
San Francisco State University,
San Francisco, California

David W. K. Man, PhD, MSc
Assistant Professor,
Department of Rehabilitation Sciences,
Hong Kong Polytechnic University,
Hung Hom, Kowloon, Hong Kong

Tina M. Marrelli, RN, MSN, MA,C
Marrelli and Associates, Inc.,
Englewood, Florida

Jeannee Parker Martin, RN, MPH
President and Co-owner,
The Corridor Group, Inc.,
San Francisco, California

Karen S. Martin, RN, MSN, FAAN
Health Care Consultant,
Martin Associates,
Omaha, Nebraska

Eleanor McClelland, RN, PhD, MPH
Associate Professor,
College of Nursing;
Director, Undergraduate Academic
   Advising/Mentor Program;
Adjunct Associate Director,
University of Iowa,
Community Home Care, Inc.,
Iowa City, Iowa

Helen Miramontes, RN, MS, FAAN
Clinical Professor, Emeritus,
School of Nursing,
University of California, San Francisco,
San Francisco, California

Leslie Jean Neal, RN,C, PhD, CRRN
Assistant Professor,
Marymount University,
Arlington, Virginia

Gretchen M. Oliver, RN, MSN,
Private Holistic Nurse Practitioner,
San Francisco, California

Pamela Kees Parlocha, RN, DNSc
Professor,
Department of Nursing and Health
   Sciences,
California State University Hayward,
Hayward, California

Ronald M. Perkin, MD
Pediatric Intensive Care Unit,
Loma Linda University Medical Center,
Loma Linda, California

Susan A. Pfettscher, RN, DNSc
Associate Professor,
Department of Nursing,
California State University, Bakersfield,
Bakersfield, California

Karen L. Schumacher, RN, PhD
Assistant Professor,
School of Nursing,
University of Pennsylvania,
Philadelphia, Pennsylvania

Juliann G. Sebastian, RN, PhD, MSN
Assistant Dean for Advanced-Practice,
   Nursing;
Director of Graduate Studies,
College of Nursing,
University of Kentucky,
Lexington, Kentucky

Janet Sit, PhD, MHA, RN
Assistant Professor,
Department of Nursing and Health
   Sciences,
Hong Kong Polytechnic University,
Hung Hom, Kowloon, Hong Kong

Mary P. Tarbox, RN, EdD
Professor and Chair,
Department of Nursing,
Mount Mercy College,
Cedar Rapids, Iowa

Jo Ann Wegmann, RN, PhD
Professor,
Division of Nursing,
California State University,
Carson, California

Betty Winslow, RN, PhD
Associate Professor,
School of Nursing,
Loma Linda University,
Loma Linda, California

Tammy Young, RN, MSN, FNP
Family Nurse Practitioner,
Redlands, California

Joyce V. Zerwekh, RN, EdD
Professor of Nursing,
College of Nursing,
Florida Atlantic University,
Boca Raton, Florida

Reviewers

Margaret M. Anderson, EdD, RN,C, CNAA
Associate Professor and Chair,
Department of Nursing and Health
  Professions,
Northern Kentucky University,
Highland Heights, Kentucky

Charlotte F. Armbruster, MS, RN, CS
Faculty Associate,
College of Nursing,
Arizona State University,
Tempe, Arizona

Laura E. Basile, RNC, MSN, FNP
Associate Professor,
School of Nursing,
San Diego City College;
Family Nurse Practitioner,
San Diego, California

Lasca Beck, RN, MS
Nursing Liaison,
ASU West College of Nursing;
Clinical Associate Professor,
College of Nursing,
Arizona State University—West,
Phoenix, Arizona

Barbara Brillhart, RN, PhD, CRRN, FNP-C
Associate Professor,
College of Nursing,
Arizona State University,
Tempe, Arizona

Judy C. Campbell, RN, DNS
Assistant Professor,
School of Nursing,
Ball State University,
Muncie, Indiana

Judith Conway, MS, CS, ET, APRN
Hartford Hospital,
Hartford, Connecticut

Cynthia Fryhling Corbett, PhD, RN,C
Assistant Professor,
Intercollegiate Center of Nursing,
College of Nursing,
Washington State University,
Spokane, Washington

Ellen L. Davel, RN, MSN, EdD
Coordinator,
Associate Degree Nursing Program,
College of DuPage,
Glen Ellyn, Illinois

Jane L. Derby, RN, MSN, CPNP
Instructor,
San Angelo Community Medical Center;
West Texas Medical Associates,
San Angelo, Texas

Deborah L. Evers, MSN, RN
Educator,
Mercy Hospital School of Nursing;
Mercy Home Care,
Pittsburgh, Pennsylvania

Linda Graham
Professor,
School of Nursing,
Indiana University/Purdue University,
Fort Wayne, Indiana

Marcia Hackman, RN, MSN
Nursing Instructor,
School of Nursing,
Regis University,
Denver, Colorado

Sheila Q. Hartung, RN,C, MSN
Assistant Professor,
Bloomsburg University,
Bloomsburg, Pennsylvania;
Doctoral Candidate,
Barry University,
Miami Shores, Florida

Marian Yavorka Jobe, RN, MS, MSN
Instructor,
Mercy Hospital School of Nursing,
Pittsburgh, Pennsylvania

Karen J. Karner, EdD, RN, CS
Professor and Chair,
Department of Nursing,
East Stroudsburg University;
Clinical Specialist in Gerontological
    Nursing,
East Stroudsburg, Pennsylvania

JoAnn Clements Kauss, RN, MSN
Faculty,
Mercy Hospital School of Nursing,
Pittsburgh, Pennsylvania

Martha Ann Kokinda, RN, PhD
Associate Professor,
Department of Nursing,
College Misericordia,
Dallas, Pennsylvania

Janet A. Lohan, RN, PhD
Assistant Professor,
Intercollegiate Center of Nursing,
College of Nursing,
Washington State University,
Spokane, Washington

Carol O. Long, RN, PhD
Assistant Professor,
College of Nursing,
Arizona State University,
Tempe, Arizona

Rebecca Lynn, MSN, CRNP
Family Nurse Practitioner,
Campbell-Philbin Medical Associates,
Pittsburgh, Pennsylvania

Charlotte Harrison Mackey, RN, MSN
Assistant Professor, Nursing,
West Chester University,
St. Davids, Pennsylvania

Leslie J. Neal, RN,C, PhD, CRRN
Burke, Virginia

Cecelia G. Orme, RN,C, MSN
Assistant Professor, Nursing,
Chesapeake College,
Easton, Maryland

Jean A. Roolf, RN, MSN
Nurse Educator,
Mercy Hospital School of Nursing,
Pittsburgh, Pennsylvania

Anne W. Ryan, RN,C, MSN, MPH
Associate Professor, Nursing,
MGW Nursing Program,
Chesapeake College,
Easton, Maryland

Robin G. Seal-Whitlock, RN, BSN, MSN
Assistant Professor, Nursing,
Anne Arundel Community College,
Arnold, Maryland

Stephen M. Setter, PharmD, CGP, DUM
Assistant Professor, Pharmacy Practice,
College of Pharmacy and Elder Services,
Washington State University,
Spokane, Washington

Cheryl Aubin Smith, RN, MSN
Clinical Instructor,
College of Nursing,
Arizona State University;
Staff Nurse,
Odyssey Degnita Hospice,
Tempe, Arizona

Linda Sue Smith, RN, DSN
Rogers, Arkansas

Roselena Thorpe, RN, PhD
Professor and Department Chairperson,
Community College of Allegheny County,
Allegheny Campus,
Pittsburgh, Pennsylvania

Julie L. Townsend, RN, CMS, FNP
Family Nurse Practitioner,
Urgent Care Associates,
Tucson, Arizona

Deborah A. Wendt, RN, PhD
Associate Professor of Nursing,
College of Mount St. Joseph,
Cincinnati, Ohio

Dolores Wright, RN, MS, DNSc
Associate Professor,
School of Nursing,
Loma Linda University,
Loma Linda, California

Preface

A unique and significant field has developed in nursing practice. Home health care is ever more urgently on the national health agenda for both consumers and providers. In this spirit we offer *Home Health Care Nursing* as a comprehensive and authoritative text for nurses working in this dynamic field. This text is appropriate for professional nurses, both in clinical practice and in management positions. It will also serve as a text for nursing students. Nurses whose previous experience has been in hospitals or long-term settings will find the book an in-depth introduction to home care.

We have included both administrative and clinical content in the book. We believe that home health care professionals responsible for providing quality care need to understand the basic concepts of the total home health care system. Clinicians need to understand the impact of reimbursement and discharge planning issues on their practices, just as administrators require knowledge of therapies, levels of care, and community services to understand how services can be planned and delivered in ways that are both cost effective and beneficial to clients. This text's value is based in the concept that older, more ill, and more diverse clients are stretching our capabilities to create significant teaching and support systems.

We are committed to the increasingly complex role of the home health care nurse as an essential part of our health care delivery system and have attempted to present the state of the art in home health care nursing practice.

ORGANIZATION AND CONTENT

Part I, "Home Health Care Nursing and the Health Care System," provides an industry, organizational, and financial framework for the book. The first chapter by Widmer, "The Continuum of Care: Partners in Acute and Chronic Care," describes the currently available services that assist the client and family to make such transitions as hospital-to-home and acute-to-chronic care. A new chapter, "Case Management and Home Health Care," by Conti, presents case management as the major practice strategy used throughout the health care system. A thorough discussion of its process and value to home care is included. In discussing "Discharge Planning: Home Health Care Considerations," McClelland and Tarbox take a client-centered approach to continuity of care. They argue for basing continuity of care on the needs of the client rather than on the goals of the provider and offer a model for achieving continuity. Their model reflects the complexity of giving care to clients whose needs change significantly over time. They make a strong case for including home health care agencies in the comprehensive planning and delivery of care to the client.

In the chapter "Nurse-Directed System of Care for Families," Martinson and Jamieson describe nurse-directed systems of care that serve families' health care needs. Alternatives include the related services, the types of professional staff needed, information regarding regulations and funding, and the relationship between the model and the home care field as a whole. The chapter by Martin on "Managed Care", new to this edition, addresses the structure, advantages, and potential challenges to home health care within a managed-care system. Payor- and provider-based organizations are defined, and their financial incentives are outlined with implications for home care. The final chapter by Marrelli, "Reimbursement in Home Care," discusses the complex reimbursement process for home care and the home health care nurse's role in this process. This chapter addresses the dominant role Medicare plays in setting the standards for home care services.

Part II, "Nursing Competencies in Home Health Care," begins with "Family Assessment in Home Care," by Widmer and Martinson. Included are the characteristics that differentiate assessment in home health care from assessment in the acute-care setting. Focusing on those assessment measurements needed for holistic-care planning, the chapter offers both a conceptual framework for understanding family caregiving and actual assessment techniques. "Skills in Family Teaching," by Arthur, follows. It covers those subjects relevant to teaching clients and families how to care for themselves. It begins with learning theory and moves through discussions of assessment, planning, implementation, and evaluation. Teaching strategies and social and cultural influences on the learning environment are included.

Nursing diagnoses in home health care nursing is the subject of the chapter, "Use of the Omaha System," by Martin and Bowles. They describe the work of the Visiting Nurses Association of Omaha in developing a problem-classification scheme out of the experience of a community-based nursing agency. In her chapter, "Symptom Control and Medication Management," Wegmann discusses symptom control with specific emphasis on pain management. While control of pain is essential if home care is to be possible for the client, controlling symptoms, such as incontinence, and treatment side effects, such as nausea and vomiting, are also important. The chapter addresses the concomitant psychosocial problems of illness that can complicate symptom control. Neal, Kuisma, Sit, and Man, in their chapter "Rehabilitation in the Home," describe the place of rehabilitation services in the home care setting. They describe the various levels of rehabilitation available for home care, common treatment approaches, and the rehabilitation team. This chapter includes predischarge assessment and therapeutic adaptation among the important issues associated with rehabilitation in the home.

Sebastian and Boosalis, in "Nutritional Aspects of Home Health Care," discuss the nutritional needs of children, adults, and the elderly. They include an assessment tool and discuss the specific data needed in the assessment of clients with specific acute and chronic conditions. Another new chapter, Guyot and Oliver's "Complementary Therapies," presents those therapies that complement or add to another approach. This dynamic field includes principles from India, naturopathy, herbalism, indigenous peoples, and others. These are well reflected by the holistic nursing movement and represent valuable care options.

Given the steadily expanding demand and projected demographics, the home care industry will increasingly face and must cope with issues involving ethnic diversity. An important new chapter on "Cultural Competence in Home Care," by Portillo, focuses on the knowledge and specific ingredients needed to provide a more culturally competent outcome. Home care must plan and implement strategies to handle the growing challenges of cultural diversity among its client population.

Part III, "Home Care Throughout the Life Cycle," includes topics relevant to generational issues. Carr's chapter, "Home Care of the New Family," introduces this section on care throughout the generations. Her chapter provides a valuable discussion of postpartum assessment and support following hospital discharge. Through sensitivity to cultural needs and individuality, techniques that enable the mother and family to care for themselves, to promote health, and to prevent complications are presented. "Home Care of Children," by Cohen and Martinson, offers an up-to-date guide to pediatric home care for the often intense care and supervision of extremely ill and technology-dependent children. It includes, among many other issues, sibling responses, family and community support, finances, home care plans, and family training.

The elderly may see health as an integrated concept that involves functional independence and provides a positive sense of well-being and social support, rather than just the absence of disease. The chapter "Home Health Care of the Elderly," by Lai, deals with clinical and relational aspects of maintaining older people at home and focuses on care that addresses their strengths, rather than merely focusing on dysfunction and disabilities. "Home Care of the Dying," by Zerwekh, discusses American attitudes surrounding death, the pathophysiology and nursing process when death is imminent, the goals of palliative care, and self-care for the hospice nurse. The care system that enables a client to die at home and the accompanying spiritual, financial, and emotional support of caregivers are addressed.

Part IV, "Clients with Specific Disorders," comprises chapters that give in-depth information on a number of disorders most commonly seen in the home care setting: pulmonary disorders, cancer, HIV/AIDS, stroke, Alzheimer's disease and related disorders (ADRD), cardiac disorders, and renal, genitourinary, and psychiatric disorders. The first chapter in this section, "Pulmonary Compromise in Home Care," by Hilton, Young, Gold, and Perkin, includes an overview of pulmonary anatomy and physiology. Assessment, including physical, emotional, and environmental concerns, is discussed, and there is a thorough discussion of medication, oxygen, and therapies. The next chapter, "Cancer," by Germino and Martinson, provides an epidemiological introduction, followed by a conceptual framework for working with clients and their families. The plan for home care encompasses nutritional support, chemotherapy, symptom management, and emotional support.

"Stroke," by MacKay, introduces this disease as the leading cause of long-term disability among adults in the United States. The physiological aspects of completed and progressive strokes are enhanced by discussion of assessment before discharge and the care that logically follows. The special needs of wheelchair and bedridden clients, as well as psychosocial and cultural aspects of stroke, are included in "Care of Clients with Alzheimer's Disease and Related Disorders," by D'Errico, Winslow, and Jones. This chapter informs the reader on aspects of Alzheimer's disease from etiology to impact of the disease. A staging approach to home management includes the differing needs of early-, middle-, and late-stage clients. Common, as well as difficult, issues such as sexual aggression, catastrophic reactions, and resistance are covered.

Chronic heart failure, its history, epidemiology, and pathophysiology open the new chapter, "Heart Failure and Home Care." Treatment, medications, and the essential home care interventions are outlined. Home care clinical pathways are emphasized as essential to all phases of the disease, including remissions and maintenance.

"Renal and Genitourinary Disorders," by Pfettscher and Binkley, addresses the special needs and problems associated with kidney disease and life-long therapies clients must undergo. A comprehensive discussion includes acute and chronic renal failure along with end-stage disease, put into a framework of total systemic impact. A discussion of dialysis and transplantation completes the chapter. "HIV/AIDS and the Home Care Client," by Miramontes and Goodroad, begins with a discussion of the pathogenesis of HIV by stages of the infection. This is fol-

lowed by medication treatments and guidelines. A substantial portion of this chapter deals with adherence issues and methods for increasing adherence.

The final chapter in section IV is "Psychiatric Home Care Nursing," a new addition by Parlocha and Chafetz, that targets problems specific to mental disorders. An overview of the evolution of psychiatric home care services and a description of the most prevalent psychiatric problems in home care populations are followed by a section on the role of the nurse in home care interventions.

Part V, "Professional Challenges in Home Health Care Nursing," addresses four key issues that affect the professional growth of both the individual home health care nurse and the entire home health care nursing subspecialty. These issues are ethics, burnout, advanced-practice nursing, and research.

Aroskar's chapter, "Home Care: The Ethical Challenges," presents an overview of ethical questions and concerns in home care agencies. She offers a case study and a framework for ethical decision-making that include ethical values, principles, and relevant legal policies and precedents. Widmer, in "Stress and Burnout in the Home Health Care Professional," then outlines the physical, emotional, psychological, and social factors that contribute to burnout among home health care nurses. Self-concept and personal motivations for becoming a health care professional are explored, along with external factors, such as work-site and administrative frustrations. The new chapter, "Advanced-Practice Nursing in Home Care," by Schumacher and Portillo, is dedicated to addressing a new way of thinking on providing care to clients. The need for highly skilled providers who have advanced clinical expertise has become essential in home care. Complex cases are appropriate examples whereby advanced-practice nurses can impact care by reducing the number of visits and reducing the overall cost of care.

The book concludes with the Barkauskas' chapter, "Research in Home Care," which emphasizes the need for research in the home health setting and increases the reader's ability to critically appraise research studies and to design and generate research that is of value to home health care.

Ida M. Martinson
Ann G. Widmer
Carmen J. Portillo

Contents

HOME HEALTH CARE NURSING

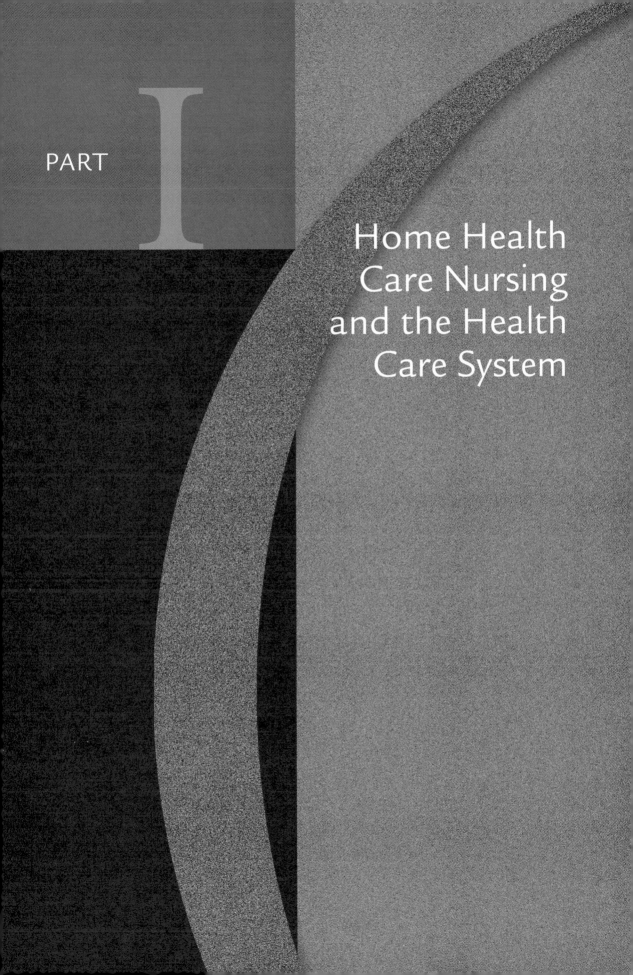

PART I

Home Health
Care Nursing
and the Health
Care System

1

The Continuum of Care
Partners in Acute and Chronic Care

Ann G. Widmer

Home health care can precede or follow acute care in the institutional setting. It can follow convalescent care in a long-term care facility or be used in combination with outpatient care or in conjunction with respite care. Home health care can include or coordinate with a program of hospice care. This chapter points out the large areas of overlap between the systems of health care and the possibilities and interdependence each system offers a particular client in an integrated delivery system.

Development of successful models of integration of acute-care and chronic-care services has long been a goal for researchers and practitioners according to Brown (1999). The Centers for Medicare and Medicaid Services (CMS) and the states have demonstrated new approaches to integrating these two systems for Medicare beneficiaries. With passage of the Balanced Budget Act of 1997 and the rate increases of the Benefits Improvement and Protection Act (BIPA) enacted in December, 2000, there has been interest in alternative organizational approaches for acute care. Programs such as PACE, the *Program of All Inclusive Care for the Elderly* pioneered by ON LOK Senior Health Services in San Francisco, have demonstrated the potential effectiveness of integrated acute and long-term care (Hansen, 1999).

One of the reasons behind the many care levels and systems is the changed nature of disease. Continuity of care is essential to health care delivery and entitles every client to case management that assesses his or her physical, emotional, and medical-nursing needs (Judge, 1995). With the advent of immunization programs and antibiotics, the improvements in nutrition and sanitation, and the ever-lengthening average life span, health care problems have shifted from infectious diseases to chronic illnesses. Heart disease, cancer, stroke, and AIDS have replaced typhoid and smallpox as high-incidence problems. These leading diseases often necessitate both acute and chronic care on a cyclical basis for individuals. Care needs to be provided over a period of years rather than weeks. Clients need aggressive therapies to control the disease process and convalescence and rehabilitation to stabilize and achieve the greatest degree of health possible. This transition from one type of care to another may occur many times for a client. In 1995, the Department of Veterans Affairs reorganized its facilities into 22 geographically based health care networks that link medical centers, clinics, and nursing homes (Charns, 1997). Their goals are to provide higher quality care, improve access to care, and increase consistency and efficiency in the delivery of care (*New England Journal of Medicine,* 1999).

Another reason for the development of alternative systems of care is the incentive to save health care dollars. In this era of cost containment, there is general approval of system overlap, which allows choice by both client and provider of the option that provides the most appropriate care at the least expense (Ford, 1996). Efficient coordination and high-quality transitional services can speed discharges from hospitals and nursing homes, prevent inappropriate admissions to institutions, and use acute-care services more successfully. Cross-training hospital nurses to provide home health care for discharged clients has been shown to lead to a decrease in readmission (Donlevy, 1996). In other programs, multidisciplinary teams of home health care and inpatient caregivers have reduced admissions from 12% to 3% (Lumsdon, 1994a). In these cases, cost effectiveness can be practiced to the best possible advantage. Meaningful cost effectiveness focuses on the alternative that either incurs the least cost for a given result or provides the highest-quality result for a given cost over a lifetime. Finally, the delivery, financing, and organizational structures are changing. Hospitals are increasingly joining with other hospitals and hospital networks into horizontally integrated regional, and even national, systems (Barber, 1998). Mergers, acquisitions, alliances, and consolidations are creating new systems and structures that comprise acute and subacute, ambulatory, long-term, and home health care services. In 1996, 55% of America's hospitals were in some type of alliance (Luke, Olden, 1995). It should be noted that legally merging multiple entities into a corporate structure does not ensure that the culture and practice of integration of care will occur (Anderson, 1998).

Finally, the ability of the client to move among the health care systems allows combining the maximal level of care with the highest level of independence. Modern consumers of health care are better educated and more informed in health matters, and, to a large extent, participatory in their treatment plan. They are often interested in, and take responsibility for, their therapies. Available choices that restore the client to the highest level of independence possibly minimize the dangers of over-care and learned dependency.

In the following sections we will look at the partners in this care continuum. These include hospitals, long-term care facilities, and home health care. Additional providers are discussed in Chapter 5.

ROLE OF THE ACUTE-CARE FACILITY: THE HOSPITAL
Historical Purposes and Functions

The role of the hospital in modern health services is a pivotal one. Historically the hospital has not been as important as it is today and initially served simply to house the ill poor and to protect the community from the contagiously sick. In the nineteenth century it was largely a welfare institution. There was little medical reason for a client to enter a hospital. Most who went to the physician for care expected the medical treatment and surgery to take place in the office or in the home. Physicians kept track of their seriously ill clients with frequent home visits (Sultz, Young, 2001).

With the development of scientific medicine and medical technology, the hospital changed radically. Modern surgery and anesthesiology, the aseptic delivery room, the incubator for premature infants, and the standby equipment for emergency treatment have equipped hospitals with an array of electronic, radiological, biochemical, and other diagnostic techniques for the detection and treatment of diseases. The teaching hospital is the principal setting for educational programs in medicine, nursing, x ray and laboratory technology, medical-social work, hospital administration, pharmacology, and dentistry. Most recently hospitals have served as community centers for the neighborhood—a role to which they are still learning to adjust.

The hospital industry is complex and diverse. Hospitals can be classified generally in one of three ways: according to length of stay, type of service provided, or ownership. In terms of length of stay, the most common type of hospital is the short-stay hospital. There are also long-term hospitals, most of which are chronic disease, psychiatric, or tuberculosis institutions. Hospitals also differ by the type of service they provide. General hospitals offer a wide range of medical and surgical services; specialty hospitals, on the other hand, may serve specific client groups such as children or women. They may focus on medical specialties, such as eye, ear, nose, and throat. Hospitals can also be classified according to form of ownership; some are government or publicly owned, and others are privately operated for profit (proprietary).

The most significant trend during the 1980s and 1990s has been the acquisition of a substantial number of hospitals by large investor-owned corporations to form multiunit, for-profit hospital systems. During the 1990s the United States also experienced an increase in the types of corporate for-profit care providers and insurers. Hospitals have become increasingly competitive and, as a result, have begun to specialize, market, and monitor productivity like other businesses (Lee, Estes, 1997).

There has also been a recent proliferation of hospital-based home health care agencies that has increased opportunities to integrate these systems. Strategically integrating hospital and home health care services is done to improve profitability. Maintaining clients in the hospital when the option for in-system home health care is available is not perceived as cost-effective use of resources. Hospital-based teams identify alternatives to extended hospital stays, and redesigned treatment plans are implemented from which clients and families can benefit if appropriate services are coordinated (Rumberg, 1994).

Client Characteristics

The hospital is the logical site of delivery for many of the advanced services made possible by medical technology and has provided unparalleled potential for altering the course of disease. The system is primarily curative. In 1996 five diagnostic categories, according to the National Center for Health Statistics, accounted for more than a million of the 30.5 million discharges from short-stay, nonfederal hospitals. These were heart disease, child delivery, malignant neoplasms, pneumonia, and psychoses (Graves, 1998).

Diagnosis-specific length of stay has been declining as a function of both medical progress and cost containment. In the 1950s physicians often prescribed a 4- to 8-week hospital stay for a myocardial infarction. This decreased to 2 weeks in the 1970s, and in the 1990s averaged 8.1 days (Kovner, 1995). By 1996 the average hospital length of stay had fallen to 5.2 days with geographical variation (Graves, 1998). For many other medical conditions, clients have moved from inpatient to outpatient settings.

There are also social determinants of hospitalization. Being separated or divorced, being elderly, having comprehensive insurance, or living at a distance from regular care increases an individual's chance of being hospitalized (Kovner, 1995). People 65 years of age and older now account for 38% of all discharges (Graves, 1998).

Care-giving Characteristics

In the hospital setting the client is generally dependent in a variety of ways. Since he or she is acutely ill, he or she may lack the strength and stamina to make decisions and carry them through. He or she may also be selectively dependent because it is not unusual to relinquish control in times when energy levels are low. It should be mentioned that paternalistic family control or domestic abuses may cause clients to select hospitals over home as a place of treatment (Ruddick, 1994). Chief executive officers are also opting for the peacefulness of the hospital, where the benefit, it appears, lies chiefly in being removed from the everyday, familiar scene, where every object is apt to remind the invalid of some duty undone

or business needing attention (*Journal of the American Medical Association,* 1996).

The environment and routine of the hospital may actually reward dependency. The client who is compliant and passive adjusts to the scheduled interventions and confinement with greater ease than one who wants to be involved in decision making. Isolation also impacts those who are immunosuppressed and confined in isolation rooms (Rigor, 1997). While hospitals attempt to keep clients informed, often the information is explanation of procedures and is for the purpose of obtaining consent. Caregiving, while often excellent, sometimes includes a less sensitive or sympathetic attitude toward those with long-term complications, terminal illnesses, and debilitation in aging (Rigor, 1997).

Since the therapies and technology involved in acute care are extremely sophisticated, they are the main focus of activity for the client. The client will be constantly monitored and seen daily by a physician. Most efforts center in the immediate task of cure.

Advantages and Disadvantages of Hospital Care

The hospital is the resource and organizational center of the delivery of acute-care services, the training of health care personnel, and the pursuit of health-related research. There are advantages in the size and sophistication of the facility and in the gathering of professional expertise and resources under one roof. Physicians find this centralization of services and clients to be a convenient way to manage client care. It is often the most cost-effective way to provide complex, expensive, high-tech diagnostic and treatment procedures. Compliance advantage exists in the controlled quality of the environment. Hospitals manifest a more detached efficiency and control for some of the variables found in the home setting, where a client has more control. At its best, the hospital provides the most modern health care interventions followed by high-quality client-family education and discharge planning.

Disadvantages of the hospital setting include depersonalization of care and a tendency to create over-dependency in the client. Although attempts are made to provide a supportive environment, it is difficult to integrate family caregivers into the actual daily schedule. Clients therefore are sometimes lonely, isolated, and not motivated to recover. Historically, measures of hospital quality have been limited to mortality rates and medically related outcomes; more recently in the competitive marketing environment, outcomes such as staff courtesy, food preparation, and family support services are also measured. We will see in the next section that while the functions and purposes of the long-term care facility are quite different, some of these same disadvantages are present.

ROLE OF THE CHRONIC-CARE FACILITY: THE NURSING HOME
Historical Purposes and Functions

The concept of the "nursing home" has evolved from several models. At the turn of the century, the infirm and elderly who did not have families to care for them were often housed in public or county homes for the aged or in boarding houses. Quality of care in these "homes" was largely dependent on the skill and compassion of the managers and caregivers. There was no formal licensing or regulatory credentialing. Most homes were considered adequate if they provided decent food, personal care, and the basic amenities. Almost none provided nursing, psychiatric, or social care, and they accounted for very little of the care given.

Today the term *nursing home* is broadly applied by the public to many types of facilities. The two categories of long-term care institutions that are directly defined by their federal and state financing are skilled nursing facilities (SNFs) and intermediate care facilities (ICFs). These categories are usually referred to as *levels of care.*

SNFs provide nursing service on a 24-hour basis for clients. Registered nurses and licensed certified nursing assistants provide services prescribed by the client's physician. Emphasis is on medical nursing care, with restorative, physical, occupational, and other therapies also provided. This type of facility is eligible to participate in both Medicare and Medicaid programs. ICFs provide regular medical, nursing, social, and rehabilitative services, in addition to room and board, for people not able to live independently.

ICFs are for clients requiring less intensive nursing care than provided by SNFs. This type of facility may elect to participate in the Medicaid program. It should be noted that there are differ-

ences in the way these definitions are applied from state to state. For the purpose of the following descriptions, the National Center for Health Sciences' definition of *nursing home* refers to a facility certified by either Medicare or Medicaid as a skilled or intermediate care facility (National Center for Health Statistics, 1997).

Client Characteristics

In the most recent survey there were 16,000 facilities certified as skilled or intermediate care facilities by Medicare, Medicaid, or both (National Center for Health Statistics, 1997). The results of this survey indicate that nursing home clients were predominately women 75 years of age or older. A total of 42.3% were 75 to 84 years of age and 40.2% were 85 years of age and over. This elderly nursing home population is 89.5% white, 92.1% non-Hispanic, and 66% widowed. When those who are divorced, separated, or never married are included, the percentage climbs to 82.6% without a spouse.

A high percentage of clients require help with multiple activities of daily living (ADLs). Some 74.6% cited need with at least three ADLs. Bathing, eating, and continence help were the most frequently cited areas of need. Table 1-1 provides more specific information on the functional activities for which assistance was received.

Family Characteristics

A number of family demographic trends also must be considered when attempting to understand why families are ultimately placing relatives in nursing facilities. A lower birth rate and increasing life expectancy have combined to bring about a situation in which there may be more people in need of care than there are caregivers in a family. The geographical spread of families and the increase in the number of women working outside the home have decreased the traditional female population available at home to provide care. Finally, as the population is becoming older at the onset of frailty and illness, so are the caregivers. The potential caregiving child of an elderly person in his or her late 80s may herself be a woman of 60 (Bulter, 1998). There are many reasons that families choose to institutionalize relatives: family members have already cared for the client at home as long as they were able, caregivers themselves are chronically ill, and care-

Table 1-1 National Nursing Home Survey	
Functional Status	Both Sexes Number
Total	1,385,400
Received Assistance with the Following ADLs	**Percent**
Bathing or showering	96.3
Dressing	86.6
Eating	45.1
Transferring in or out of bed/chair	23.8
Using toilet room	57.8
Received Assistance with Number of ADLs	**Percent**
0	3.1
1	8.5
2	13.8
3	33.1
4	32.9
5	8.6
Received Assistance with the Following ADLs	**Percent**
Care of personal possessions	77.6
Managing money	69.2
Securing personal items	76.8
Using telephone	69.2
Received Assistance with Number of ADLs	**Percent**
0	13.7
1	6.1
2	13.0
3	5.4
4	60.9

From *An overview of nursing homes and their current residents,* Hyattsville, Md, 1997, National Center for Health Statistics.

givers have been burdened with the care throughout their adult lives. They may feel that at age 65 or 66 they deserve some freedom to enjoy life before they, too, become debilitated (Bulter, 1998). It is not surprising that many families, at least at the end of the caregiving cycle, turn to an institution for help (Freedman, 1996).

Description of and Programs in Nursing Homes

The goal of nursing home care is to keep clients functioning more independently than in acute care. The client is encouraged to remain in as active a social and physical role as possible. Care should be related to rehabilitation, restoration, or at least maintenance of the client's well-being. Care, if comprehensive, addresses the often multiple physical and emotional problems of a client through a variety of on-site and contracted support services. Examples include, but are not limited to, services such as dental, home health, hospice, medical, mental health, nursing, nutrition, occupational therapy, personal care, physical therapy, podiatry, medications, social services, sheltered employment, speech or hearing therapy, special education, transportation, vocational rehabilitation, equipment, and others (National Centers for Health Statistics, 1997). Social activities implemented by a trained activities coordinator include such events as birthday parties, celebrations of various holidays, religious and musical events, and trips outside the facility for those who are able to participate.

ADVANTAGES AND DISADVANTAGES OF NURSING HOME CARE

There are many advantages to providing rehabilitation and continuing care for clients in a facility. Other family members do not suffer inconveniences, especially when living quarters are crowded or when caregivers themselves have physical limitations. Institutional care may be less expensive and, in some cases, may be the only way to have certain services reimbursed. The client's illness may be difficult to monitor in the home, and in a facility, staff can provide 24-hour coverage. This is particularly true when the client exhibits severe personality disorders that cannot be handled or tolerated by family. Physicians are sometimes more confident that consistent care and client compliance are present when the client is in a facility. Good nursing homes also provide an advantage in the types of available activities and socialization opportunities for the client. It must be remembered that nursing homes also provide an indispensable service to people who do not have family or even homes of their own in which care could be provided.

The disadvantages of nursing home care have been catalogued many times and are often applied incorrectly to both poor and excellent homes. Nursing homes have been characterized as depressing environments, imposing the worst features of institutional care on those least able to resist. The incentives of policies, cost saving, and organization have sometimes caused such outcomes in clients as dependency, depersonalization, and low self-esteem. They can create geographic and social distance from family and cultural milieu. Loneliness, desexualization, and infantilization can also occur.

Individual control and personal decision making on the part of nursing home clients have been shown to decrease because of a phenomenon called *learned helplessness* (Stanford, 1995). According to this theory, when a person believes that his or her actions no longer gain a response or make any difference in the actions of others, he or she stops attempting to influence events. Depression and an inability to make choices often accompany learned helplessness (Stanford, 1995).

The institution's policies and routine caregiving may do nothing to prevent this phenomenon and may even promote it. The numerous activities and therapies outlined in the facility's marketing materials may exist only as occasional volunteer or contracted adjunct services. Clients with strong family advocates may receive attention to such needs as denture repair, prescription updates, or nutritional awareness, but those without advocates to call attention to their problems often fade into the shadows.

Care is provided by a widely diverse group of caregivers, causing some clients to be isolated by culture and language. Preferences surrounding eating, personal care, family values, and support are complicated by experiences associated with color, age cohort, religion, or nationality (Stanford, 1995). The task is to help staff in these homes become more sensitive to individual client needs.

ASSISTED LIVING

It should be noted that many care environments are discussed in Chapter 4. Assisted living, however, has become an integral component of long-term care and often even a partner with nursing homes. This form of residential care is 1 of 30 types of congregate living facilities that serve a predominately elderly population and go by such different names as *personal care homes, homes for the aged, residential care facilities, shelter care homes, adult care homes, family care homes,* and *community residential facilities* (Hawes, 1999). The assisted living industry provides 24-hour individualized assistance to meet clients' needs. It has rapidly developed into a combination of housing, health services, and assistance with the activities of daily living in an individual home or facility with many apartment units. Assisted living is also provided in some states in homes for five or fewer clients. In this setting, called *adult foster care,* one of the caregivers (or a caregiving family) may live on premise. In successful placements, clients maintain higher levels of personal autonomy than is possible in large, long-term care settings (Tinsley, 1996). Pressure to reduce Medicaid expenditures on nursing homes has increased support of assisted living programs that are paid for privately. Reimbursement for these services varies from state to state. Some states have forms of assisted living that are licensed as types of home health care; in other states, operations of assisted living complexes cannot deliver hands-on personal care or nursing services themselves but can help clients access services from certified home health care agencies. Oregon, by funding assisted living through Medicaid and Supplemental Social Security Income, has maintained a model program for low-income people who would otherwise be in more expensive nursing homes (Bulter, 1998).

Advantages and Disadvantages

State-of-the-art assisted living facilities are most often constructed in a residential model and provide clients with a private room and bath and freedom to use a living room and kitchenette. Such individualized space provides a comfortable homelike setting. Since construction of such residential space is less costly than that of a nursing home, operators can share these construction cost savings through lower monthly fees for clients (Tinsley, 1996). To compete with the assisted living industry, nursing homes are also evolving into more marketable homelike environments with gardens, libraries, and private areas (Kruczek, 1997).

A lack of laws and policies at the national level allows for state-by-state variations in the quality of assisted living facilities and care. Government payments for assisted living remain limited, but some state or local governments provide subsidies to low-income persons; some states have the option to use Medicaid funds for services to low-income, frail elderly. Private health insurance programs are increasingly covering assisted living care. The care in assisted living has been estimated to cost between 20% and 30% less than nursing home care. Consequently, nursing homes are constructing or acquiring assisted living facilities and maintaining clients at that level of care (Pallarito, 1996).

ROLE OF HOME HEALTH CARE
Historical Purposes and Functions

In 1883 Lillian Wald established the first organized home nursing service in the United States as part of the Henry Street Settlement services to New York City's poor. All clients who could be were cared for at home, and those for whom hospitalization was helpful were hospitalized. The Metropolitan Life Insurance Company covered home health care for its policyholders in New York City in 1909. In 1912 the Red Cross pioneered a visiting nurse service in which nurses in rural areas independently provided services to the sick, well-baby care services, and school nursing. County health departments adopted this plan and employed nurses to provide home health care.

During World War II, physicians began to stop their home visits, and visiting nurse associations grew rapidly to fill the need for home health care. Most home health care was delivered by voluntary visiting nurse agencies. Nursing was the main service offered, but some homemaker and home health aide services were also available. Rural home health care developed innovative solutions in many communities without physicians and extensive facilities.

Today home health care can be defined as the provision of services, education, and setting for the purpose of maintaining or restoring a client's maximum level of health, function, and comfort. The key to achieving these goals is to integrate all services available in the health care and community systems.

The Growth of Home Health and Hospice Care

The home health care agency benefit under the Medicare program was established by Congress in 1966 to provide less expensive supplemental care to acute inpatient care. Medicare provides benefits for individuals 65 years of age and older who are covered by Social Security. Because of the rapid growth in the use of home health care, this benefit has been one of the most rapidly expanding. From 1990 to 1996, Medicare spending on home health care grew from $3.9 to $17.3 billion (*Caring*, 1998). In response to these rapidly expanding costs, the Balance Budget Act (BBA) of 1997 modified the home health care benefit by capping the amount it will pay per beneficiary. After years of above-average growth in the home health care Medicaid expenditures, health care costs were slowed by the BBA (Harris, 1999) then increased slightly in 2000 by the BIPA. Medicare reimbursement, previously paid pursuant to a cost-based system, then transitioned to both reduced per-visit limits and an annual per-beneficiary limit on visits. While Chapter 6 discusses these issues in detail, by current estimates, home health care agencies have experienced on average over 30% revenue cuts under the new system (Harris, 1999). These cost-saving practices have affected, and will continue to affect, the continuity of health care. Since October 1, 1999, this interim payment system has been replaced with a prospective payment system and has resulted in significant classes of Medicare beneficiaries that previously had been served under the home health care benefit being eliminated from home health care rolls (*Caring*, 1998). Home health care companies are facing a changing environment. The year 1998 will be remembered by the home health care industry as "The Year of IPS" (Interim Payment System). January 2000 saw significant profit loss for agencies. Cuts in Medicare have made the strenuous work of nurses and nursing aides even more demanding as agencies have made up for reduced income by requiring workers to deliver more care in less time (Rimer, 2000). Almost every state is grappling with a shortage in home health care aides. This topic is covered more thoroughly in Chapter 6.

Home health care has, however, become appealing to managed-care companies in their effort to provide high-quality, cost-effective health services for other than financial reasons. In an effort to gain managed care contracts, home health care services are consolidating or forming alliances. These new alignments can result in the increase of offered services and geographic coverage that managed care organizations require (Lumsdon, 1994b).

From the hospital's perspective, home health care is essentially an after-care service. Home health care actually includes much more than this, being both a total support program for the homebound and a maintenance program to ensure wellness and rehabilitation. Today, as was discussed in the previous section on hospitals, hospital "walls" are really nonexistent, and services, high technology, and complex care modalities are realities of home health care. There are frequent opportunities to use many of the same resources, therapists, skilled nurses, and capable management professionals that exist within the hospital, and, in some cases, staff are integrated. There are more and more equipment and expertise available to assist home health care clients. The technology available ranges from blood glucose monitoring to in-home intensive care units with ventilators, central venous lines, and long-distance telemetry for the acutely ill (Hoye, 1997).

The hospital-based home health care program requires a sophisticated management and financial system. The management expertise necessary to effectively handle the essential divisions of home health care in a noninstitutional setting is not always well developed in the hospital. Expertise in managing pharmaceutical supplies, housekeeping, home nursing care, diet and nutrition, social services, family counseling, and community support is sometimes not present in hospitals.

Another challenge facing hospital-based home health care departments is the education of medical and hospital staff to the range and comprehensiveness of home health care. Some physicians may still lack an understanding of, and confidence in, the range and quality of home health care services. Since professional medical standards, like other health standards, are client centered, physicians will resist using home health care if they do not have confidence in it.

Lack of understanding leads to reluctance to turn clients over to what is erroneously perceived as maintenance or housekeeping rather than

solid nursing care. To increase accuracy and attitudes regarding home health care, the AMA has developed 10 competencies/goals for a home health care curriculum and some medical schools have incorporated home health care into their curricula (Spratt, 1997).

Client Characteristics

The 1996 National Survey and a subsequent survey in 1998 revealed that two thirds of home health care and over half of hospice care clients were female. Of the home care clients, 72% were 65 years of age or older, 65% were white, 35% were widowed, and 65% were married. Of the hospice clients, 78% were over 65 years of age, 84% were white, 32% were widowed, and 44% were married (Haupt, 1998).

Information on the diagnosis of home health and hospice care clients collected through the National Home and Hospice Care Survey in 1996 showed an average of 3.0 diagnoses per home health care client. The most common primary diagnosis was a disease of the circulatory system. Other frequent diagnoses were diseases of the respiratory system, injury and poisoning, diabetes mellitus, and musculoskeletal system diseases (Haupt, 1998). The most common primary diagnosis (58%) in hospices was malignant neoplasms (Haupt, 1998). Hospices have, in the last 2 years, reached a turning point in the AIDS struggle. There has been a dramatic decline in the number of AIDS deaths (Lui, 1999). The Centers for Disease Control and Prevention reports that those living with HIV are living longer because of refinements in treatment, especially combination therapy with several antiviral agents, use of complementary therapies, wider use of drugs that prevent secondary infections, and the introduction of protease inhibitors (Fairfield, 1998). Chapter 21 addresses these areas in detail.

AIDS statistics between 1994 and 1998 show a 54% reduction in serious HIV-related illness and a 40% reduction in the death rate (Armstrong, 1999; Kogan, 1998). This has changed the care continuum for AIDS clients substantially (Houts, 1998). In current programs, clients receive intermittent acute care, sometimes live in transition residences for 3 to 4 months while they learn elaborate medication schedules and healthy diets, or live in their own family homes where a home health care agency can be used as appropriate (*The Oregonian,* 1997).

Characteristics of Successful Home Health Care

Caregiving is more often successful when the caregiving circumstances meet the following criteria: (1) there is a caregiver at home or available when needed, willing to be of assistance, and capable of being trained; (2) the caregiver is not an individual at high risk for fatigue, emotional instability, or illness; (3) the client's physical home environment is such that daily care can be given; (4) the emotional environment is conducive to rehabilitative efforts; and (5) it is the client's choice to be home. Chapter 7 describes numerous issues that face family caregivers. For the majority, when the caregiving criteria are met, it is possible for the home health care client to be more satisfied and take an active role in decision making about care and the home environment.

Advantages and Disadvantages to Clients Receiving Home Health Care

When the client is not able to do some degree of self-care and when family members or friends are not involved, care may fail. Often, assumptions are made about the availability of community and turn out to be false because access criteria and geographic barriers may exist. Family and other support systems may be too committed and ultimately "burn out" rather than admit to what they consider to be defeat by asking for more help. Sometimes the home environment is unhealthy or unsafe. Situations arise in which abuse has occurred, prescription drugs have been stolen by family members, or patients have been left alone over a weekend and discovered only after a tragedy has occurred. Physicians have sometimes seen their house calls as lacking in technical support, time-consuming, poorly reimbursed, and a duplication of home nursing effort. Some physicians will not see home health care clients unless they are brought to their offices (Keenan, 1992). Nurses have sometimes had difficulty maintaining the medical communication with physicians necessary to update care plans.

Most health care professionals agree, however, that when the criteria for home health care are met, home health care's advantages far outweigh its disadvantages. While anecdotal evidence on home health care client satisfaction is abundant, a number of researchers have documented through survey and observation the advantages of home health care over institutional care (Connochie, 1997). Home health care can provide the company of a client's family, a less restrictive and more familiar environment, greater personal choice and dignity, greater client participation, and a retention of usefulness. It can enable the patient to preserve activities, relationships with pets, and religious and ethical customs. Care, food, and schedules can be individually tailored to the client's taste, and more effective client learning and motivation can take place. A confused or mildly demented client may be far more functional in his or her own home than in any new environment where he or she has lost the ability to process new sensations and information.

Hospice programs provide some of the most successful home health care. Clients receiving hospice care in the home setting have access to a number of support services, including client and family services, care and bereavement services, advocacy services, and pain-management programs that have an impact on the spiritual, psychological, social, and physical aspects of pain (Head, 1997). Hospice programs have not only provided high-quality terminal care but have also elevated the standards of quality, particularly in pain and symptom control, for all health care providers.

SUMMARY

In the past, the U.S. health care system has used discrete settings and providers, each providing defined types and levels of care. Structures (facilities and programs) were closely associated with specific levels of care. For example, hospitals cared for those with acute illnesses, nursing homes cared for medically stable individuals with significant physical or psychosocial disabilities, and home health care provided after-acute care and low-need personal care. Clients were transferred among sites, and providers developed predictable niches. At the beginning of the twenty-first century, many services are provided at multiple settings; care may be a set of levels and processes rather than programs and places. Providers do many of the same things but to varying degrees; thus it is possible to base reimbursement on care provided rather than on the provider's characteristics. In a managed care environment, it is cost effective to define a client's problems and seek the best combination of services for defining and managing the cause (diagnosis) and consequence (function) (Levenson, 1996). Broad and flexible benefits and services can support alternative care plans and contribute to reduced use of institutional care (Brown, 1999).

This chapter has highlighted the need for and evolution of a total health care system, an integrated delivery system (IDS) that is responsive to client needs, characteristics, and circumstances. Of the categories discussed—hospital, long-term care, and home health care—none is perfect in every situation. The focus should be on decreasing fragmentation and redundancy. Each has advantages and disadvantages inherent to its purposes and method of delivery. Health care professionals need to understand the strengths and weaknesses of each and to counsel clients wisely in their selection of care providers. In addition, both professionals and the system itself need to integrate various levels of care and support choices of clients, families, and individual caregivers. When nurses, physicians, social workers, therapists, and aides participate in care planning and provision of services and direct and coordinate the provision of care delivered by other caregivers, an IDS can be excellent. The challenge of the twenty-first century is to integrate and redistribute resources so that they reach the client in the most appropriate and cost-effective models.

REFERENCES

Anderson S: How healthcare organizations can achieve true integration, *Journal of the Healthcare Financial Management Association* 52(2):31-34, 1998.

An overview of nursing homes and their current residents, Hyattsville, Md, 1997, National Center for Health Statistics.

Armstrong G et al: Trends in infectious disease mortality in the United States during the 20th century, *Journal of the American Medical Association* 281:61-66, 1999.

Barber J et al: Evolution of an integrated health system, *Journal of Healthcare Management* 43(4):359-377, 1998.

Brown TE: Integration of acute and chronic care: Lessons learned from South Carolina, *Generations* 23:15-20, 1999.

Bulter RN: *Aging and mental health,* ed 5, Needham Heights, Mass, 1998, Allyn & Bacon.

Charns MP: Organization design of integrated delivery systems, *Hospital and Health Services Administration* 42(3):411-432, 1997.

Connochie KM et al: Ensuring high-quality alternatives while ending pediatric care as we know it, *Archives of Pediatrics and Adolescent Medicine* 151(4):341, 1997.

Donlevy JA, Pietruck BL: The connection delivery model: Care across the continuum, *Nursing Management* 27(5):34, 1996.

Editorial, *Caring* 17(8):10-16, 1998.

Editorial, *New England Journal of Medicine* 340(1):52-53, 1999.

Fairfield KM et al: Patterns of use, expenditures, and perceived efficacy of complementary and alternative therapies in HIV infected patients, *Archives of Internal Medicine* 158:2257-2264, 1998.

Ford D: Beginning of an integrated delivery system, *Nursing Homes* 45:53, 1996.

Freedman VA: Family structure and risk of nursing home admission, *The Journals of Gerontology, Series B* 51(2):561-569, 1996.

Graves EJ, Owings MF: *Summary: National hospital discharge survey,* Pub No 301, Hyattsville, Md, 1998, National Center for Health Statistics.

Hansen JC: Practical lessons for delivering integrated services in a changing environment, *Generations* 23:22-28, 1999.

Harris G: *Home health care, an industry in turmoil, but with promise down the road,* 1999, Salomon Smith Barney, Equity Research.

Haupt BJ: *An overview of home health and hospice care patients: 1996 National Home and Hospice Care Survey,* Pub No 297, 1998.

Hawes C: A key piece of the integration puzzle: Managing the chronic care needs of the frail elderly in residential care settings, *Generations* 23:51-55, 1999.

Head B: An overview of hospice home care. In Spratt JS et al: *Home health care,* Delray Beach, Fla, 1997, GR/St. Lucie Press.

Houts PS: *American College of Physicians: Home care guide for HIV and AIDS,* Philadelphia, 1998.

Hoye RE, Dalton MT: Systems approach needed for home health care. In Spratt JS et al: *Home health care,* Delray Beach, Fla, 1997, GR/St. Lucie Press.

Judge KM: Case management, *Independent Living Provider* 10(2):28, 1995.

Keenan JM et al: A national survey of the home visiting practice and attitudes of family physicians and internists, *Archives of Internal Medicine* 152(10):2025-2032, 1992.

Kogan RJ: Do drugs cost too much? Consider the alternatives, *Wall Street Journal,* December 14, 1998.

Kovner AR: *Hospitals: Jonas's care delivery in the United States,* ed 5, 1995, Springer.

Kruczek T: Making residents feel "at home" in the nursing home, *Nursing Homes,* 46(3):31, 1997.

Lee PR, Estes DL: *The nation's health,* ed 5, Sudbury, Mass, 1997, Jones & Bartlett.

Levenson SA: Innovations in long-term care: Levels of care, *Generations* 20(4):69, 1996.

Lui C: Housing crisis is seen among poor with HIV, *Los Angeles Times,* 1999.

Lumsdon K: Does the continuum ever end? *Hospitals and Health Networks* 68(22):38, 1994a.

Lumsdon K: Home care prepares to catch wave of managed care, networking, *Hospitals and Health Networks* 68(7):58, 1994b.

Luke RO, Olden P: Foundations of market restructuring: Local hospital cluster and HMO infiltration, *Medical Interface* 8(9):71-75, 1995.

Pallarito K: Assisted living leads growth, *Modern Healthcare* 26(21):996, 1996.

Rigor BM: Pain control in home care. In Spratt JS: *Home Health Care,* Delray Beach, Fla, 1997, GR/St. Lucie Press.

Rimer S: Home health aides for elderly in short supply, *The New York Times,* 2000.

Ruddick W: Transforming homes and hospitals, *The Hastings Center Report* 24(5):11, 1994.

Rumberg JM, Gerard M: Strategically integrating hospital/home care services for improved profitability, *Physician Executive* 20(11):25, 1994.

Spratt JS et al: A physician's perspective. In Spratt JS et al: *Home health care,* Delray Beach, Fla, 1997, GR/St. Lucie Press.

Stanford EP, Schmidt MG: The changing face of nursing home residents: Meeting their diverse needs, *Generations* 19(4):20, 1995.

Sultz HA, Young KM: *Health care USA,* ed 3, Gaithersburg, Md, 2001, Aspen.

The hospital hotel, *Journal of the American Medical Association* 275(4):324, 1996.

The Oregonian: AIDS hospice will serve life, not death, Portland, Ore, 1997, Associated Press.

Tinsley R: Sizing up assisted living, *Nursing Homes* 45(4):9, 1996.

2 Case Management and Home Health Care

Roberta M. Conti

Case management is the major practice strategy being used throughout health care delivery systems and is one of the most rapidly evolving professional roles within the health care professions.

Today's health care market focuses on efficiency and effectiveness, resource management, and treatment of the delivery system as a business. These mandates have resulted from two significant paradigm shifts. First, fiscal constraints have resulted in a shift from fee-for-service payment and professional autonomy to a corporate focus on the bottom line, with decisions based primarily on financial considerations. It is, in essence, a shift from professional to managerial values, evidenced by such things as greater oversight and regulation of use and increases in the number and types of alternatives to expensive acute hospital care. This shift emphasizes effectiveness, outcomes, and accountability, with desired clinical, functional, and financial outcomes being specified. Managed care has emerged as an important umbrella strategy for this corporate-focused paradigm shift. Critical elements in a managed care system include an efficient system of triage and referral, smooth transitions from one level or site of care to another, and a full range of providers.

The second major paradigm shift occurring in health care delivery is a change from a curative approach to one emphasizing prevention at all levels. Such a strategy has the obvious benefit of avoiding costly acute care. In addition, research on preventive-care delivery has consistently demonstrated its cost efficiency when compared with acute-care delivery, with the majority of studies finding that up to $4 in acute-care costs are saved for every $1 of preventive-care costs.

The implication of these two marketplace-driven shifts in health care organization and delivery and in the priorities of the health care system will be that the community will serve as the locale for the increased percentage of service delivery. This will result in a shift from fragmented to coordinated patterns of care that are based on interdisciplinary teamwork and a better match of provider expertise with client needs. This means a move away from discipline-specific autonomy to a more open model of knowledge sharing and appreciation for the theories, perspectives, and values of others. A strategic alliance of home health care and case management is a logical outgrowth of these changes. As such, case management is posited as the major practice strategy for meeting managed care's mandate of a health care delivery system designed to manage cost, quality, and access to health care (Kongstvedt, 1996).

CASE MANAGEMENT

Case management is defined as a process that uses the integration of managerial and clinical knowledge and skills by a case manager who interacts within a "service network to provide needed services in a supportive, effective, efficient, and cost-effective manner" (Weil, Karls, 1985). *Service effectiveness* means purchasing or providing for the client the service or material resource that is absolutely right for the situation because results are what is being purchased. An example of this would be the purchase of efficient and effective neurorehabilitation services for a client with a traumatic brain injury. Results are clearly delineated by expected outcomes that include the ability to solve problems, make decisions, and articulate thoughts, thus acknowledging service efficiency. Both service effectiveness and service efficiency directly correlate with cost effectiveness over time. For example, if a client with a traumatic brain injury caused by stroke, aneurysm, tumor, or car accident is enabled to relearn risk-free environment functioning and live safely, socially, and productively in society, then the desired quality of life and long-term, cost-effective outcomes have been achieved.

Many traditional home health care agencies use nurses as case managers to coordinate care provided by multiple disciplines of professionals within the agency. In this model of case-management practice, the case manager is responsible for determining client care needs but is not responsible for evaluating these needs against financial resources or for holding accountable the other participating disciplines for the time, amount, and quality of service delivery. The case manager's primary responsibility in this model is to document the precise skilled care required and provided so that the agency will be reimbursed appropriately for its services.

With the advent of managed care, home health care agency nurses now also communicate, plan, and justify service delivery with external case managers (Gookin, 1996). In this scenario, the external case manager is responsible for developing a results-driven program of services and material resources; coordinating delivery, time, and placement; overseeing the individual allocation of clinical and financial resources for each home health care client; monitoring timely progress of results; and holding the home health care nurse and case manager accountable for purchased results while at the same time documenting the details and progress of the purchased services for the payor. As a result, home care nurses and nurse case managers may be two of several discipline-specific professionals providing home care to a client. The external case manager tracks outcomes from these multiple disciplines and holds each accountable for meeting predetermined goals.

CASE-MANAGER ROLES

Establishing role clarity for case managers is critical to the effectiveness of case-manager practice. In every case-management system, there needs to be a clear understanding across the organization as to the role set required to achieve desired client and program outcomes. That same understand-

ing must be conveyed externally to all stakeholders participating in the case-management program. Controversy regarding the case manager's role focuses on whether the role should be restricted to coordinating, monitoring, and expediting care delivered by others or include being a direct caregiver. This controversy can be attributed to factors such as the number and variety of models of case management, variety of target populations, differing home care organizational structures, diversity of program goals, lack of consistency found in role behaviors of case managers, and absence of an established program of formal education to prepare practitioners for this role.

The descriptive and research literatures of nursing, health care, and sociology demonstrate a number of recurring themes and proposed topologies that attempt to label and categorize the roles of case managers. Roles most frequently mentioned include problem solver, advocate, broker, planner, community organizer, boundary spanner, service monitor, record keeper, evaluator, consultant, collaborator, coordinator, counselor, and expediter. Unfortunately, little empirical evidence exists to substantiate these role sets. Exceptions to this include the work by Conti (1993, 1996) and Yeager (1997). Conti (1993, 1996) used content analysis of ethnographic interviews and detailed quantitative analyses of responses to written survey questions derived from interview content to identify the role behaviors and roles of nurse case managers practicing under the Broker model of case management—the one most frequently used in the health insurance industry. This work led to the identification of 16 distinct nurse case manager roles under this practice model. The roles identified were public relator, educator, expediter, monitor, problem solver, explainer, negotiator, planner, communicator, contactor, recommender, broker, researcher, assessor, documenter, and coordinator. The findings demonstrated that the nurse case manager's role is a complex one requiring both managerial and clinical expert-level competencies.

Yeager (1997) used Conti's survey tool (1993) in a study examining role behaviors of nurses practicing in a variety of practice models and across a range of settings. Using a random-sample technique, she surveyed 100 members of the Individual Case Management Association (ICMA). Participants resided in Delaware, Maryland,

Virginia, Pennsylvania, and the District of Columbia, and all possessed the Association's case manager certification. Findings from analysis of survey responses by participants ($N = 55$) validated all 16 roles previously identified by Conti (1993), with some variation noted in the frequency of performance of specific behaviors, attributable to the diversity of models and practice settings of respondents.

Managerial Work of Case Managers

Effective case-management practice requires an integration of both managerial and clinical knowledge. It is within the context, application, and implementation of managerial knowledge and the role performance of individual case managers that the components of the process are implemented. To become reality, this implementation enables the marketplace-driven foci of efficiency and effectiveness, resource management, and treatment of the delivery system as a business.

The content and processes of managerial work have changed over time, in concert with the evolution of management theories and of management as a science. Mintzberg (1973) suggested that the history of science is a chronology of humans' attempts to precisely describe the world and then use the description to systematically improve it. The work of Frederick Taylor, acknowledged as the father of scientific management, provides a classic example of the application of Mintzberg's perspective. However, it is Mintzberg's research that has provided the major theoretical foundation for the phenomenon called *managerial work*. While completing his Ph.D. in management at MIT, he developed the contingency theory of managerial work, which proposed that four sets of variables influence the managerial role requirements and characteristics. The first of these, termed *environmental variables*, includes a host of internal and external environmental factors such as culture, the nature of the industry, and the characteristics of the organization itself. Job variables, the second set, encompass features such as workflow orientation and level of specialization. Personal factors, such as the manager's personality, values and beliefs, and preferred style of interacting, comprise the third set. Finally, there are situational variables,

time-related factors such as changes in work processes, social norms, and the manager's education and practical experience in the job. Collectively, these sets of influencing variables have an impact on the preferences, competencies, and, ultimately, performance of the 10 managerial roles identified by Mintzberg (1973). The contingency theory of managerial work and its attendant 10 managerial roles significantly advanced understanding of the interrelationship of managerial knowledge, skills, and roles and, as such, promoted managerial role clarity.

Mintzberg (1973) organized the 10 roles into three categories: those that are concerned primarily with *interpersonal relationships,* those that deal primarily with the *transfer of information,* and those that essentially involve *decision making.* The interpersonal roles comprise the roles of figurehead, leader, and liaison. The figurehead represents symbolic obligations, some of which are inspirational in nature. The leader defines the vision and tone in which work will be accomplished, whereas the liaison focuses on network and relationship building across organizations. The informational roles include those of monitor, disseminator, and spokesperson. The monitor focuses on seeking and gathering information for purposes of determining problems and opportunities. The disseminator provides both factual and value-based information to assist decision making. The spokesperson provides information to the external environment. The decision-making roles encompass entrepreneur, disturbance handler, resource allocator, and negotiator. The entrepreneur searches the internal environment for opportunities to improve practice and bring about essential change. The disturbance handler appropriately acts on the unanticipated activities and behaviors negatively impacting performance. The resource allocator role concerns itself with the distribution of human and material resources and the associated consequential decisions. Within the context of the negotiator role is the authority to commit resources.

Conceptually, these 10 roles provide a valuable perspective from which to view the managerial aspects of the case-manager role. These roles provide a framework for the managerial practice behaviors of the case-manager role and provide direction on how a case manager can interact with his or her environment, focus attention, communicate, and make decisions.

Clinical Work of Case Managers

Case-management practice also includes the enactment of a variety of clinically focused behaviors, including identifying the client, performing individual assessment, setting goals and planning resource allocation, facilitating and coordinating linkages to needed services, providing direct and indirect interventions, monitoring the progress of the client, reassessing service delivery, providing quality management, advocating for both the client and the service providers, and consistently evaluating services delivered and the outcomes of the case-management process. Depending on the client's identified needs, these case-management functions can be undertaken in any sequence because the practice is not necessarily linear or sequential.

The assessment process is the primary means through which case management is individualized. Assessment and reassessment of the client are the very essence of the case manager's clinical practice and are performed in cooperation and deliberation with the client, appropriate family members, and friends. The assessment, in the context of the marketplace-driven foci, needs to be holistic with a vision for the care continuum. It often will include the professional evaluations and recommendations from other disciplines as sought by the case manager through collaboration with the multidisciplinary team and client. This information provides the framework and documentation for disclosure of the client's needs.

Moxley (1989) formulated an exemplary framework for identifying the components of a macrostructure of case-management assessment. This model is presented for its value-added context in a managed-care environment. It is comprehensive and can assist in decision making that must be offered to the client with respect to the care continuum. A comprehensive assessment that will indicate which needs the client can fulfill, which needs the client's social network can fulfill, and which needs must be attended to by the provision of services or material resources requires the following four areas to be addressed: (1) identification of unmet needs such as income, shelter, employment, health, mental health, in-

terpersonal relationships, activities of daily living, transportation, and education; (2) the client's physical, cognitive, emotional, and behavioral functioning; (3) the client's social support systems, both structural and interactional; and (4) the availability, adequacy, appropriateness, acceptability, and accessibility of professional services.

New cost-effective delivery systems in home health care practice do not result in case management being episodic or restricted to a single practice setting. Case management can occur across the spectrum of life and the care continuum. Community nurse case-management models such as the professional nurse case-management model of Carondelet Hospital and Health Center in Arizona and Winchester Medical Center in Virginia are exemplary nursing models with a focus far beyond homebound and skilled care needs, the two criteria for traditional fee-for-service medical models for home health care services. These holistic nursing models focus on high-risk populations in their respective communities who need stability in health, wellness, and quality of life.

STATE OF THE ART: CASE-MANAGEMENT PRACTICE TODAY

Applebaum and Wilson (1988) note that we have learned many lessons about case-management practice. For example, chronically disabled individuals with severe disabilities have received care in their homes without negative effects on their functioning, health status, and longevity. Second, even with the considerable expansion of home care services, family members continue to be key caregivers. Third, we have acknowledged the significance of assessing consumers across a wide range of dimensions to ensure that the agreed-on plan meets their needs. Fourth, we have learned that when given a choice, consumers want to receive services in their homes and that enactment of this choice increases consumers' perceived quality of life. Fifth, we have been able to determine the level and volume of services that consumers need to function effectively in the community, along with the cost of case-management services. Finally, we have learned how long-term care delivery needs can vary, based on fluctuations in the condition of the client.

Home Health Care

The previously discussed health care paradigm shifts have impelled hospitals and home health care providers to seize opportunities to be responsive to the need for alternatives to very expensive institutional care. The advent of the community as the premier locus of health care service delivery has resulted in examination and implementation of new home health care delivery systems and system components designed around effectiveness, outcomes, and accountability.

Paralleling the rapid growth of case management is the home health care revolution. The annual number of nurse visits per client jumped 40% between 1992 and 1997, with an annual 10% growth rate predicted through the year 2002 (*AHA News,* 1997).

Whether it is moving clients sooner and with greater frequency from acute care facilities into the home or whether it is managing health care in the home and avoiding costly hospital admissions, home health care, coupled with the practice strategy of case management, has the potential to provide coordinated care in a way that is both economical and humane.

Home care is care specified in relation to a particular kind of place. For a case manager, awareness of place is essential for the ethical practice of case management (Liaschenko, 1996). Although managed care is the catalyst for the strategic practice of case management, the implications of entry into a client's private domain cannot be ignored. Case managers should approach entry into a client's home as though they were guests with permission or an invitation. Historical constructs of case management practice were based on the value of the individual and the right of the individual to be given options for decision making as opposed to the traditional practice of health care providers making the decisions. These values permeate the present-day practice of case management.

Home care is defined as any kind of health care, personal care, or assistance with independent living given to functionally impaired, disabled, or ill persons in their own homes. Some posit that home care also includes a wide range of community services, such as delivered meals, adult day care, and transportation. Kane et al (1994) note that home care is a kind of gray zone

of health and human services because it includes both acute care and personal care services usually associated with long-term care. As a social service, it draws on the talents of a multidisciplinary cast of professionals and paraprofessionals and runs the gamut from highly technical, health-related service to a social service with broad, general goals.

Home Health Care Delivery System Redesign

There is little doubt that the current health care environment is changing the way professionals work with clients and among themselves in home care. The organizational paradigm shift is from multidisciplinary to interdisciplinary in the provision of care. Until recently, multiple disciplines worked in isolation providing care. Now, however, with today's consumers demanding quality in managed-care environments, a systems-approach design that achieves ongoing interaction, integration, and cooperation among participating disciplines is paramount and catalyzes the shift to interdisciplinary care.

In the new home care delivery system, client care also must be characterized by attributes such as coherence and congruity and must ensure open communications among providers, vendors, and clients. Home care agencies that are responsive to these challenges will create an organizational environment that fosters a strategic approach to planning and management of health care delivery systems.

As a partner in the care continuum, home care agencies will find adaptability, flexibility, and responsiveness to be essential elements of twenty-first-century organizational architecture. Organizational architecture encompasses all the "various systems, structures, management processes, technologies, and strategies that make up the 'modus operandi' of the organization" (Nadler et al, 1992). Incorporating case management as a health care delivery strategy in home care is one example of an organizational architecture redesign. Themes of integration and interaction will permeate these new architectures, with teams of professionals and nonprofessionals being the norm at all levels. Teams will have great latitude in problem solving and decision making regarding the necessary human and material resources required to provide quality, cost-effective care. Such a form of architecture moves an organization away from segmented care and toward integrated care and results in employees who understand the broad, strategic components of home care practice and who can demonstrate a wide range of knowledge and skills. In such a care delivery system redesign, the appropriate focus of both internal and external case managers is one that achieves desired outcomes in a cost-effective manner.

CASE STUDY

The following case study demonstrates the potential complexity of client movement along the care continuum and provides an example of the necessity for integration of clinical and managerial work by the case manager.

The health care plan participant was a 51-year-old married female, 5'1" tall and weighing 190 pounds. For the past 4 years, the client had numerous health problems including intraabdominal sepsis and adult respiratory distress syndrome (ARDS), which resulted in three colon resections. Case management began when the client underwent an emergency exploratory laparotomy at a small rural hospital. Findings included a stricture of a prior colonic anastomosis site and intraabdominal sepsis. After surgery, the client received numerous intravenous antibiotics as well as hyperalimentation but did not demonstrate desired improvement. By the fourteenth postoperative day, she was weak, was demonstrating spiking fevers, and had two open and draining areas in the abdominal incision.

The case manager concluded that the client was in a serious and unstable medical state and that her level of illness and care requirements might be beyond the scope of capability of the rural hospital. The case manager contacted the client's husband and daughter (a licensed practical nurse) and discussed these observations, concerns, potential options for treatment, and the decisions regarding actions needed. Critical responsibilities included counseling and coaching the husband and daughter regarding possible medical outcomes, talking with the client about transfer to a medical center (nearest being 50 miles away), talking with the surgeon about transfer, keeping the payor informed of the client's status, maintaining vigilance over the client's condition, coordinating decisions, disseminating information, advocating for the client and the payor, negotiating roles, defining parameters of necessary medical care, and initiating commitment of resources.

Within 24 hours, the client was transported by ambulance to a nearby medical center. The surgeon and medical staff determined there was leakage at the

anastomosis site and promptly arranged for surgery. The client underwent an ileostomy and colostomy to save the remaining large and small intestines. After surgery, she was transferred to an intensive care unit, where she remained for 29 days, during which time she underwent numerous additional surgeries to deal with fistulas and abdominal abscesses.

On accepting the case, the case manager's initial goals were the following:

1. *Arrange for transfer to a local medical center to leverage the availability of advanced medical practice and specialists and appropriate technology*
2. *Ensure provision of all necessary and appropriate care at the center*
3. *Use medical center resources for teaching family members to care for the ileostomy and colostomy*
4. *Determine durable medical equipment necessary for home care*
5. *Document requirements for home health care*
6. *Identify and coordinate among providers to deliver care services such as medical supply delivery and management of hyperalimentation in the home*

After 2 months of hospitalization at the medical center, the client was discharged to home. She had an open abdominal wound 1½ inches deep and approximately 6 inches wide. This open area was the site of a fistula from the small bowel and required constant suctioning by a pump and dressing changes three times each day. On each side of the open wound was a stoma that required skin care and appliance application. A total of 2 L of hyperalimentation per day was provided via a Groshong catheter, with an expectation of the client needing this nutritional support for approximately 1 year. Oral intake was limited to liquids that responded to the client's need to taste food. No nutritional value was derived because of its immediate flow after ingestion into the open wound. The client was able to use a walker to ambulate short distances but was still too weak to perform activities of daily living (ADLs) herself.

Continued

Family assessment revealed a stable, intact family consisting of a devoted husband, a son, and a daughter who was a licensed practical nurse and a single parent. The client's prolonged illness had been stressful on the family. The daughter provided the case manager with enough clues for the case manager to determine that her support in care would be limited because of her single-parent status and need to maintain full-time employment. The husband also had to maintain his job as an electrician at a major regional airport; however, he was willing to arrange his work schedule to be with his wife when other caregivers were not available. All of these factors, including the 100 miles round-trip from her home to the medical center, were taken into consideration when options were discussed for addressing problems. This was a blue-collar working family who lived in a post–World War II bungalow in rural America, 90 miles from the nearest source of durable medical equipment. Fortunately, there was a home health care agency in their community. Within a few days of the client's returning home, the husband demonstrated correct procedures for dressing changes, skin care, and hyperalimentation management.

The following are examples of clinical and managerial case manager activities:

1. *Intervened on behalf of the client and the payor to arrange for hyperalimentation service and negotiated for free nursing care to be provided by the service as well as provision of a small refrigerator for solution storage*
2. *Negotiated with a provider source 90 miles away to deliver medical supplies on a timely basis. Arranged for supplies to be provided by a local hospital in the case of emergency*
3. *Made arrangements to obtain a high-power suction pump from a provider in another state and negotiated a 20% discount on the monthly rate*
4. *Coordinated planning with the local home health care agency for provision of an average*

of 4 hours per day of care by a nurse practitioner at a 20% discount on the prevailing rate
5. *Coordinated with a durable medical equipment source to deliver an electric bed to the home before the client's arrival home*
6. *Monitored the client's situation and the adequacy of services provided and disseminated information to physicians, providers, and the payor as appropriate*
7. *Observed the direct care provided to the client by the family and other health care personnel and provided guidance and feedback as appropriate*
8. *Maintained documentation of all care decisions and medical care activities*
9. *Established a system of care delivery with the client, family, and providers. The system included monitoring medical supply inventory, designating role responsibilities, monitoring care measures, and assuming accountability for outcomes*

After 10 months of home health care services, services from other sources, and several brief inpatient stays for the treatment of acute medical problems, this client achieved closure of her abdominal wound and elimination of the ostomies, attained full ability to self-perform ADLs, and resumed a limited oral nutrition regimen. The case manager achieved a case-life cost savings of $195,553.23.

This case study demonstrates how a variety of home health care services were organized and provided over an extended period of time using an internal home health care nurse and an external case manager. The successes in client health status and in cost savings can be attributed to implementation of a holistic and proactive care delivery program that used multiple disciplines of caregivers, family members, a knowledgeable and supportive physician team, and the caring and assistance of a host of friends and neighbors in the client's community.

SUMMARY

The efficacy, effectiveness, and efficiency of case-management practice depend on attainment of role clarity by nurses performing as case managers and by the organizations that employ them. Such clarity is especially important because case management is increasingly integrated within the

care continuum. Acknowledgment and in-depth examination of the processes and outcomes associated with the practice of both clinical and managerial work in case management could result in significant strides in role clarity and actualization.

The practice of case management in home health care offers new and exciting opportunities for case-manager role development. Perhaps most important, it offers a genuinely viable means for successfully addressing current and future challenges to the task of delivering efficient and clinically and fiscally effective health care in a dynamic, paradigm-shifting care-services delivery industry.

REFERENCES

AHA News 33(6):1997.

Applebaum R, Wilson N: Training needs for providing case management for the long-term client: Lessons from the national channeling demonstration, *The Gerontologist* 28(2):9, 1988.

Conti RM: *Role behaviors of nurse case managers,* doctoral dissertation, Fairfax, Va, 1993, Mason University.

Conti RM: Nurse case manager roles: Implications for practice and education, *Nursing Administration Quarterly* 21:67-80, 1996.

Gookin LB: Minding our business: Partnering for success, *Home Care Provider* 1(2):47, 1996.

Kane RA et al: Perspectives on home care quality, *Health Care Financing Review* 16(1):69-90, 1994.

Kongstvedt PR: *The managed care handbook,* ed 3, Gaithersburg, Md, 1996, Aspen.

Liaschenko J: Home is different: On place and ethics, *Home Care Provider* 1(1):49, 1996.

Mintzberg H: *The nature of managerial work,* New York, 1973, Harper & Row.

Moxley DP: *The practice of case management,* London, 1989, Sage.

Nadler D, Gerstein M, Shaw R: *Organizational architecture,* 1992, Jossey-Bass.

ADDITIONAL READINGS

Anthony W et al: Clinical case update: The chronically mentally ill. Case management: More than a response to a dysfunctional system, *Community Mental Health Journal* 24(3):9, 1988.

Brault GL, Kissinger LD: Case management: Ambiguous at best, *Journal of Pediatric Health* 5(4), 1991.

Burdett AD: Pinpointing the counselor's role in rehabilitation, *Journal of Rehabilitation* 26, 1960.

Cassil A: Home-health costs could drive provider cuts, *AHA News* 33(6), 1997.

Desimone BS: The case for case management, *Continuing Care* 1988.

Dinerman M: Managing the maze: Case management and service delivery, *Administration in Social Work* 16(1):17, 1992.

Kane R: Case management: Ethical pitfalls on the road to high quality managed care, *Quality Review Bulletin* 14(5):161-166, 1988.

Kemp B: The case management model of human service delivery, *Annual Review of Rehabilitation* 2:212-238, 1981.

Redford LJ: Case management, *Journal of Case Management* 1(1):5-8, 1992.

Rubin A: Is case management effective for people with serious illness? A research review, *Health and Social Work* 17(2):138-150, 1992.

Surles R et al: Case management: Strategy for systems change, *Health Affairs* 11(1):151-163, 1992.

Yordi CL: Case management in the social health maintenance organization demonstration, *Health Care Financing Review* (suppl):1988.

3

Discharge Planning
Home Health Care Considerations

Eleanor McClelland and Mary P. Tarbox

*D*ischarge planning, a key component of the broader concept of continuity of care, frequently refers to the return of a client to the previous provider for ongoing care (McClelland, Kelly, Buckwalter, 1985; McEwen, 1998; Stackhouse, 1998). This somewhat narrow definition has evolved as a result of competition among care providers and is related to economic constraints in reimbursement for health care. The current focus is on control of a market segment rather than on actions of the nurse and other health care professionals to facilitate continuity of care. This chapter addresses the primary considerations of the goals of the client, not those of the provider. Continuity of care may be ensured by coordinating care that may involve arrangement for 24-hour care, or transition of services from one agency, institution, or individual to another (Humphrey, 1998; Humphrey, Milone-Nuzzo, 1996; McClelland, Kelly, Buckwalter, 1985; Urbanic, McKeehan, 1985). This coordination reflects a client-centered direction to continuity of care with health care services taking on a more holistic approach to best serve clients while giving providers the opportunity to plan needs-based services. As an integral option within the health care delivery system, discharge to home health care plays a major role.

A review of the discharge planning literature reveals a definition that is summarized as follows: astute assessment, planning, and referral to prepare and fully communicate plans for moving a client from one level of care to another within the health care delivery system or to the client's own care without assistance of others (Anderson, Helms, 1995; Klainberg et al, 1998; Lowenstein, Hoff, 1994; Iowa Intervention Project, 1996; Mefford, 1996). Discharge planning ideally considers the client, the professional orientation of the care providers, the organization of services to manage care, and the specific practice skills of caregivers. Optimal client outcomes, quality control, and organizational stability can be achieved only when there is an appropriate blend of these considerations. This chapter demonstrates that organizational, environmental, and individual factors must be considered for discharge planning to optimize home care.

CLIENT CONSIDERATIONS

There are several identified client contributions that relate to an ideal care continuum that are important to consider. First, the client's rights to reasonable continuity of care are those described in the "Patient's Bill of Rights" (American Hospital Association, 1992). Initially this referred to clients in accredited hospitals; however, the American Nurses Association's *Policy Statement on Continuity of Care* (American Nurses Association, 1986a; Reif, Martin, 1995) extends this right to all clients.

Second, matching client needs and preferences to the appropriate care modality is another consideration. This has become more complex as a result of prospective payment enforcement, incorporating ambulatory and in-home services as potential care options for health care providers. The interpretation of options available is based on congruency between client and professional interpretation of needs. This implies the necessity for collaboration and boundary crossing that may challenge the current competitive market place. This means that the provider needs to weigh the ethical responsibilities of providing a human service for the social good and the more pragmatic approach of providing a service for the economic good (Klainberg et al, 1998; Little, 1985).

More recently, discharge planning activities

have been formalized through case-management plans (Huber, 1996; Zander, 1988, 1994). These are frequently initiated during a hospital stay. The case manager's role, often assumed by a nurse, encompasses responsibility for specific client outcomes during the client's hospital stay. Care plans contributed by various disciplines are integrated into single case-management plans called *critical paths*. The critical path becomes a guidance document for a common plan that may be individualized to manage a specific client's care. The discharge planning goals are essential to a client's critical path.

A third consideration relates to maximizing the independence of clients and their significant others. Recognition of a client's capabilities for independence should result from initial and on-going assessment of his or her health-related needs. Client limitations may be minimized when planning is designed as a positive activity incorporating client preferences (Clemen-Stone, McGuire, Eigsti, 1998; Reichelt, Newcomb, 1980).

Collaboration of health professionals with client involvement in care is essential. The aim of collaboration is to avoid duplication, fragmentation, and contradictory efforts that confuse the client and the client's family members. In addition to client considerations related to an ideal care continuum, there are professional considerations to take into account.

PROFESSIONAL CONSIDERATIONS

Discharge planning, as an important element of the care continuum, requires that the practitioner maintain both client and professional orientations regardless of setting. This means that while there are acknowledged economic pressures and bureaucratic expectations, it is necessary to have an open communication system designed not only to permit, but also to encourage, collaboration across multiple boundaries.

HEALTH CARE PROVIDER ROLES

The recognition of various roles assumed by health care providers acknowledges various loyalties: the inherent loyalties to their employing organizations, loyalties to the advancement of their profession through informed practice, and loyalties to the client. Research findings validate that all three loyalties are evident among nurses (Corwin, 1960; Davis, 1972; Kelly, 1987; Kramer,

1968), and there is potential for conflict among these loyalties. The care provider, regardless of such conflicts, is obliged to maintain client and professional orientations for the goal of continuity of care to be achieved.

Because discharge planning moves a client from one health care delivery setting to another, the demand for continuity of care can be met only by the cooperative efforts of all parties involved. The client who is discharged from an inpatient setting to home depends on the cooperation of professional care providers for services that will most effectively and efficiently meet the identified needs of that client. Outcome measures have become the focus of planning and intervention by health care professionals who provide discharge to home care and must meet guidelines for reimbursement. The emphasis on communication, collaboration, cooperation, and care must be acknowledged to ensure continuity of care in discharge to home care.

Discharge planning for home care is a point on the care continuum that must be flexible to accommodate the evolving needs of the client. Once discharged from inpatient care to the home, the client needs may change; the expectations of the client and the care providers may change; and the availability of resources—human, material, and financial—always fluctuates. It is clear therefore that the facilitation of a smooth transition from institution to home and continuity of care is possible only through the partnership of professionals, paraprofessionals, support persons, and the client and the client's family.

A partnership ensures the relationship between individuals in which the individuals pool their resources to achieve a determined goal. The provisions for determining responsibilities for the proportions of profit and loss may sound like informal business terms, but the home care providers and the client must establish a relationship that aspires toward profitable outcome measures and works to minimize the loss of the client's function, health, and resources.

Partners in home care delivery are many and varied, so the needs of the client and family must be determined through the cooperative efforts of partners in institutional care and partners in home care through discharge planning. Partners who provide care in this transition may be identified as professional or technical. Professional partners are driven by their practice, which is based on standards determined through scientific theory and research developments (Humphrey, Milone-Nizzo, 1996). Professionals are licensed or certified care providers with specific qualifications for their roles (e.g., physical therapists, occupational therapists, and recreational therapists). Technical partners are those whose care is product driven and most often support the plans and actions of professional partners (e.g., medical equipment technicians, oxygen suppliers, and others). The client and family are partners with the most to gain or lose in health care delivery and must have an equal or greater share in all related activities. The co-operation and collaboration of partners are essential to successful health care delivery, which is determined by the positive measure of predetermined outcomes.

The partnership of providers in the transition of client care from institution to home, or home to another service, is most successful when coordinated by a skilled professional with the knowledge and experience to work with all interested parties. The literature related to discharge planning and home care indicates that the professional nurse, sometimes designated as the liaison nurse from the home health care agency, is most suited to fill that role, although in many institutions, medical-social workers are responsible for discharge planning (Christopher, Toughill, 1997; Harris, Krimker, 1997; Kelly, 1987; Kluka, 1997; Lowenstein, Hoff, 1994). The nurse who is most effective in the role of coordinator is the one who recognizes the importance of the knowledge of services in the acute care setting as a necessary component of the overall knowledge base of services available both in institutions and in home health care.

Skills in assessment, communication, and documentation that focus on transitions are essential to the unique practice of the nurse coordinating discharge planning to home health care. Effective coordination of the care provided in the transition partnership should include specialized skills in areas such as knowledge of financial coverage, provision of direct care in the home environment, coordination of services of multilayered providers, referrals to the necessary services, case conferences with families and partners in care, supervision of paraprofessionals of all skill levels, continuity of care in an ever-changing environment, and client advocacy in a setting where services may be determined and directed by payors rather than by diagnoses and identified client needs (Humphrey, Milone-Nuzzo, 1996; Lowenstein, Hoff, 1994; Perry, Potter, 1997). Client education directed toward self-care must become an essential role of the nurse in coordinating discharge planning.

The home care nurse, as the coordinating partner, must be able to work with other professional partners such as physicians, physical therapists (PTs), occupational therapists (OTs), speech therapists (STs), recreational therapists (RTs), social workers, dietitians, and other nurses. Paraprofessionals such as home care aides and homemaker aides are essential to meeting the daily needs of clients, yet demand specific supervisory skills of the nurse. The agency staff provides necessary support and ensures that health care delivery can continue. Technical staff may work directly with a client, but the nurse-coordinator must know about the services and equipment provided and may be responsible for coordinating care. Through all the varied skills and services provided by these partners, the nurse-coordinator must also focus on the client and family and ensure their optimal functioning as partners in the delivery of the desired and available home care.

The nurses involved in discharge planning from institutional care to home health care play specific roles in health care delivery. The nurse in the institution must be prepared to facilitate effective discharge planning, and the home health care nurse must assume the role of coordinator to provide continuity of care. Each nurse must work within the parameters defined by their agencies and by each client's unique situation and needs.

ORGANIZATIONAL CONSIDERATIONS

For optimal client care to occur as a result of collaboration among health care providers from different settings, the organizations represented must possess certain qualities. For example, the philosophy or mission of the organization must reflect care for the client in the context of the client's needs. Resulting programs and policies should give evidence of being consistent with that philosophy. The support of management of the organization is critical to successful implementation.

Another organizational consideration relates to the discharge planning model the organization selects for implementation. Often, physicians, rather than nurses, initiate discharge of the client. The primary nurses responsible for discharge planning must follow through with a plan based on considerable knowledge of resources and payor regulations. If discharge planners are solely responsible for discharge planning based on referrals to intervene with specific clients, this model is dependent on adequate orientation of providers regarding discharge planners' roles and timeliness of service.

Finally, a contractual model, which is an arrangement between institutions and community provider organizations, may be in place. This model requires staff orientation across boundaries and availability of coordinators in a timely manner. The strength in this model relates to open communication.

While each model has benefits and constraints, these constraints are greatly reduced when there is administrative support and resource availability. Adequate resources in settings other than hospitals has become a major factor in discharge planning. Decreased hospitalizations and reduced length of stays have resulted in the "quicker and sicker" label that is applied to many clients.

CASE MANAGEMENT AND MANAGED CARE

During the 1990s, the health care delivery system underwent extraordinary scrutiny in an effort to control the escalating costs of health care delivery. As a result of that examination, both internal and external factors associated with health care delivery have changed or are undergoing very rapid changes. Providers involved in the discharge of clients from institutional care to home health care have felt the impact of such changes and have begun to consider the elements of case management and managed care as they have af-

fected health care delivery at these points on the care continuum.

Case management, which may have a new title, is a role performed by the nurse. It is a well-established role of the nurse in the coordination of care for a client who is moving from one level of care to another. Discharge planning nurses are case managers who perform as "catalysts and facilitators responsible for coordinating high-quality care in a time-effective, cost-effective manner across the continuum of health care" (More, Mandell, 1997). Case managers are usually internal to an organization and are part of the established structure that oversees the implementation of services to clients associated with that organization. Nurse case managers possess specific skills not only in providing client care, but also in coordinating care and working with the reimbursement system of the organization. As a coordinator and partner in providing health care and ensuring appropriate discharge planning, the nurse case manager recognizes the specific needs of the client and works with the established services of the agency to ensure cost-effective, high-quality care.

Managed care is a system of overseeing health care delivery to clients from a perspective that is external to the agency providing care. Third-party payors usually administer managed care programs directed specifically at cost containment. Health maintenance organizations (HMOs), preferred provider organizations (PPOs), and physician-hospital organizations (PHOs) are all within the scope of managed care. These programs use a mechanism called *managed competition* to obtain and maintain business in an effort to control the costs of health care and enhance productivity of the services (More, Mandell, 1997). Insurance companies and government third-party payors are most often the players in managed care.

The effect of managed care is evident in the rapid, substantial changes in both institutional and home health care. Discharge planning has become particularly important in the assessment of client needs and the appropriate, cost-effective plan for health care delivery outside the institution. The care providers must be attuned to the influence of internal and external forces that have a direct impact on the quality and cost effectiveness of client care services.

PRACTICE CONSIDERATIONS

The ideal discharge plan begins with the client's initial exposure to the preadmission procedure in the physician's office or to the institution during an unplanned admission. When discharge planning begins at either of these points, it is more effectively facilitated throughout the client's experience. A model that has been developed for balancing current health care realities with the ideals of a care continuum (Figure 3-1) (Kelly, 1987) reflects some aspects of discharge planning omitted from the literature. For example, the model identifies a variety of possible entry points for discharge planning to occur other than an acute care, 24-hour institutional setting. The model also depicts the potential for entry into the health care system at any point on the care continuum. In addition, movement through the care continuum may be multidirectional. Because the client's care needs may change in intensity, this movement is accompanied by appropriate setting changes.

This model encompasses inherent variables often assumed or implied in various definitions and conceptual frameworks for discharge planning, but not often noted in practice. Skills in discharge planning, whether the client is discharged from an institution or from home health care, require that the nurse use the nursing process effectively at each phase and that the client be involved whenever possible. Specific components

of the nursing process in discharge planning are assessment, nursing diagnosis, planning, implementation, and evaluation.

Assessment

Unique assessment skills go beyond physical and psychosocial factors to include assessment of specific teaching needs, environmental aspects, client and family perceptions of needs, high-risk needs, and consideration of financial needs, copayment, managed care parameters, and types of facilities available. These are essential components for referral to necessary professionals and services. Consultation with the client, the family, and other health care providers becomes part of the comprehensive assessment for discharge planning.

Clients pose unique problems in the discharge planning of nurses and other professional staff. The literature on discharge planning and home health care is replete with descriptions of specialty teams that are formed to confront the unique needs of elderly clients, children, postpartum mothers, mental health clients, and clients with specific diseases or injuries.* Each special population requires some unique skills on the part of the nurses involved, and attention to those skills is essential. Further assessment has been mandated for Medicare beneficiaries as defined by the Outcome and Assessment Information Set (OASIS), used to determine the

---

*Deal, 1994; Harris, 1999; Johndrow, 1999; Mathews-Flint, Lucas, 1999; McEwen, 1998; Shaughnessy et al, 1998; Sperling, 1998a; Stackhouse, 1998; Stanhope, Lancaster, 1996; Twohy, Reif, 1997; Weis, Mathers, Schank, 1997.

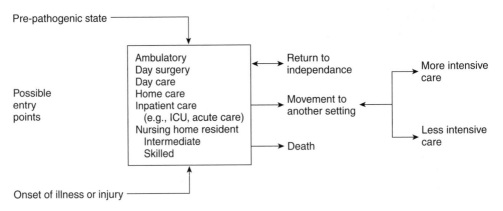

Fig. 3-1 Illness-wellness continuum through discharge planning. *(From Kelly K:* Discharge planner role: Factors related to bureaucratic professional and service conceptions, *unpublished doctoral dissertation, Iowa City, 1987, University of Iowa.)*

effectiveness of interventions and to document outcomes (Sperling, 1998b).

Nursing Diagnosis

The data collected from a thorough assessment that considers special needs of specific populations may be clustered according to the theoretical format of the institution or agency to assist in the identification of specific problems. Whether identifying patterns, hierarchical needs, or body systems, the analysis of the assessment data will lead to nursing diagnoses that may be associated with discharge planning (Box 3-1).

In the transition of a client from one agency to another, the complete and accurate statement of the nursing diagnosis is essential to the effective communication of needs to be addressed by the receiving agency. As more documentation systems become computerized, there is more emphasis on the standardization of diagnosis statements, and the systems that use the nursing diagnosis statements depend on accuracy and appropriateness of diagnoses.

Planning

Planning begins with the recognition that a problem, which needs the attention of the agencies involved with the client, exists. Setting priorities mutual to client and agencies is essential to the beginning of planning, which will continue to involve the actual writing of client-centered goals or outcomes. Identifying expected, measurable

---

Box 3-1 Nursing Diagnoses Associated with Discharge Planning

Adjustments, impaired
Anxiety
Caregiver role strain
Family process, altered
Fatigue
Fear
Home maintenance management, impaired
Injury, risk for
Knowledge deficit
Management of therapeutic regimen, ineffective
Relocation stress syndrome
Self-care deficit

From *Iowa Intervention Project,* 1997, North American Nursing Diagnosis Association.

---

outcomes and communicating those outcomes are essential not only to the success of the client's involvement with the agency but also to the allocation of resources and reimbursement based on the achievement of those outcomes. The nurse must identify outcomes that address the nursing diagnosis yet recognize prevention, problem resolution, and ongoing care strategies. The ability to communicate the identified priorities and outcomes is also important to the documentation and communication requirements of discharge planning for continuity of care (Anderson, Helms, 1995).

Implementation

The nurse coordinating the discharge plan must begin before the client's discharge from the institution to the home. It is conceivable as well that the discharge plan may facilitate the transition of the client from home to institution. The implementation skills of the nurse are seen in two phases: interventions and documentation.

Discharge planning interventions reflect the strategies specific to the identified nursing diagnoses and to the achievement of identified client-centered outcomes. The specific activities associated with the strategies will be unique to the client and family, will be performed by the appropriate provider or partner, and will reflect the established standards of care. Current efforts to standardize the language of nursing interventions (Iowa Interventions Project [McCloskey, 1996]) reveal specific interventions and activities associated with discharge planning. The Nursing Interventions Classification (NIC) has been linked with nursing diagnoses (North American Nursing Diagnosis Association [NANDA]) and the Omaha Systems problems. As addressed on the following pages, the NIC interventions have also been linked with a standardized language for measuring outcomes as in the Nursing Outcomes Classification (NOC) (Johnson, Maas, 1997). Many additional interventions that may be used in discharge planning are identified but will be just as important in the nursing care associated with all aspects of home health care and ensuring continuity of home care.

Through the work of expert nurses in the area of discharge planning and home care, the activities associated with the interventions of discharge planning and referral (Iowa Intervention Project, 1996) have been identified and

Table 3-1 Discharge Planning and Referral	
Discharge Planning	Referral
DEFINITION	
Preparation for moving a patient from one level of care to another within or outside the current health care agency.	Arrangement for services by another care provider or agency
ACTIVITIES	
Assist patient/family/significant others to prepare for discharge	Perform ongoing monitoring to determine the need for referral
Collaborate with the physician, patient/family/significant others, and other health team members in planning for continuity of health care	Identify preference of patient/family/significant others for referral agency
Coordinate efforts of different health care providers to ensure a timely discharge	Identify health care providers' recommendation for referral, as needed
Identify patient's and primary caregiver's understanding of knowledge or skills required after discharge	Identify nursing/health care required
Identify patient teaching needed for post-discharge care	Determine whether appropriate supportive care is available in the home/community
Monitor readiness for discharge	Determine whether rehabilitation services are available for use in the home
Communicate patient's discharge plans, as appropriate	Evaluate strengths and weaknesses of family/significant others for responsibility of care
Document patient's discharge plans on chart	Evaluate accessibility of environmental needs for the patient in home/community
Formulate a maintenance plan for post-discharge follow-up	Determine appropriate equipment for use after discharge, as necessary
Assist patient/family/significant others in planning for the supportive environment necessary to provide the patient's post-hospital care	Determine patient's financial resources for payment to another provider
Develop a plan that considers the health care, social, and financial needs of the patient	Arrange for appropriate home care services, as needed
Arrange for post-discharge evaluation, as appropriate	Encourage an assessment visit by receiving agency or other care provider, as appropriate
Encourage self-care, as appropriate	Contact appropriate agency/health care provider
Arrange discharge to next level of care	Complete appropriate written referral
Arrange for caregiver support, as appropriate	Arrange mode of transportation
Discuss financial resources, if arrangements for health care are needed after discharge	Discuss patient's plan of care with next health care provider
Coordinate referrals relevant to linkages among health care providers	

From McCloskey JC, Bulechek GM, eds: *Nursing interventions classification (NIC),* St Louis, 1996, Mosby.

documented (Table 3-1). The nurse selects activities according to the unique needs of the client as delineated in the expected outcomes. Each professional nurse is responsible for the selection, implementation, and documentation of the specific activities used with individual clients.

Documentation of the interventions of discharge planning and referral, for example, and the associated activities may be facilitated very effectively by the use of the NIC system in client records, especially those that are computerized. The specific agency requirements will be most important, however, in determining the specific requirements for documentation. The emphasis on documentation for reimbursement purposes is apparent in all aspects of discharge in home care and is essential to the continuity of care.

Evaluation

The expected outcome measures are examined in this phase in response to two questions:

1. Did the client meet the expected outcomes?
2. Did the nursing interventions influence the client's ability to meet those outcomes?

The measures of achievement in meeting outcomes are essential to answering these questions. Such measurements may occur at any time during the discharge planning process. Periodic evaluation provides formative data related to health care delivery as an ongoing process. Summative data (e.g., rates of hospital readmissions or complications), collected at the conclusion of care, allow the nurse to determine that the care provided was effective, that discharge is appropriate, and that adequate planning has occurred for the client. Client satisfaction may also be evaluated at this time.

A thorough evaluation will identify strengths and weaknesses in the care plan. Outcomes may have been achieved or may be modified on the basis of the evaluation. Extenuating circumstances or variances may be identified, or unknown variables may emerge as influential in the achievement of outcomes.

The Iowa Outcomes Project (1997) is currently refining work on the NOC, which is a standardized language used to describe client outcomes that are responsive to nursing interventions. The outcomes identified are specific

---

| Box 3-2 | Relocation Stress Syndrome |

DEFINITION

Physiological and/or psychosocial disturbances as a result of transfer from one environment to another.

SUGGESTED OUTCOMES

Child adaptation to hospitalization
Coping
Psychosocial adjustment: life change
Quality of life

ADDITIONAL ASSOCIATED OUTCOMES

Caregiver adaptation to patient
Institutionalization
Caregiver home care readiness
Grief resolution
Social support

From Iowa Outcomes Project: *Nursing outcomes classification (NOC)*, St Louis, 1997, Mosby.

---

indicators that can be used to measure the effectiveness of nursing interventions. Linkages that assist nurses in the use of outcome measures have been identified between NANDA nursing diagnoses and outcomes (Johnson, Maas, 1997). Although the linkages are helpful, it remains the responsibility of the professional nurse to make the judgments necessary to select specific client outcomes. An example of the outcomes that may be useful in discharge planning provides the suggested outcomes for the nursing diagnosis of relocation stress syndrome (Box 3-2). Specific outcome indicators that are associated with the suggested outcome of quality of life are illustrated in Table 3-2 (Maas, 1997).

The nurse coordinating care must also coordinate the evaluation to ensure that necessary data are obtained and analyzed and that results are appropriately dispersed. Use of the evaluation data will be determined by the health care agency and the funding sources.

The following case study describes a situation in which the home health care nurse uses knowledge of discharge planning and linkages of diagnoses to interventions to outcomes to address the specific needs of the client.

Table 3-2 Quality of Life

DEFINITION: An individual's expressed satisfaction with current life circumstances

Quality of Life	Extremely Compromised 1	Substantially Compromised 2	Moderately Compromised 3	Mildly Compromised 4	Not Compromised 5
INDICATORS					
Satisfaction with health status	1	2	3	4	5
Satisfaction with social circumstances	1	2	3	4	5
Satisfaction with environmental circumstances	1	2	3	4	5
Satisfaction with economic status	1	2	3	4	5
Satisfaction with education level	1	2	3	4	5
Satisfaction with occupation level	1	2	3	4	5
Satisfaction with close relationships	1	2	3	4	5
Satisfaction with achievement of life goals	1	2	3	4	5
Satisfaction with coping ability	1	2	3	4	5
Satisfaction with self-concept	1	2	3	4	5
Satisfaction with pervasive mood	1	2	3	4	5
Other	1	2	3	4	5
_____ Specify	1	2	3	4	5

From Iowa Outcomes Project: *Nursing outcomes classification (NOC)*, St Louis, 1997, Mosby.

CASE STUDY

NANDA Diagnosis: Relocation stress syndrome related to physiological or psychosocial disturbances as a result of transfer from one environment to another.

Mrs. G., a 77-year-old widow, had been living alone in a small apartment until she fell while bathing. She was hospitalized with a left hip fracture that required total hip replacement and a postoperative stay of 6 days. On discharge, Mrs. G. moved to the home of her daughter and son-in-law, both of whom work full-time and have two teenage children at home. Mrs. G.'s daughter is taking 2 weeks of vacation to care for Mrs. G. and is very eager to learn from the home health care nurse about the assistance she can provide for her mother. Mrs. G. has never needed the assistance of anyone else to care for her. She feels she is putting a burden on her daughter and her family and feels quite isolated from her neighbors and friends from the apartment complex where she lives. In addition to the discomfort and dependence related to the surgery, Mrs. G. also fears that she may never be able to live alone again. As the home health care nurse works with Mrs. G. and her family, she identifies the nursing diagnosis of relocation stress syndrome. Therefore it is evident that interventions that assist with coping and hope enhancement are as important as pain management and exercise therapy. Collaboration with the physician and physical therapists will enhance home care for Mrs. G., as will consultation with her family and friends. Discharge from the home health care service will be facilitated by the ability of family and friends to support Mrs. G. in her care without exacerbating her feelings of dependence and loneliness. Her quality of life becomes the outcome as linked to the diagnoses and as measured by such indicators as satisfaction with her health status and social circumstances.

Use of the nursing process is essential to effective continuous health care delivery for the client who is to be discharged. The problem-solving characteristics of nurses are common to other professionals and en-hance communication among the partners in care. Reimbursement is enhanced by accurate and adequate planning and documentation as facilitated by the nursing process. Assessment of continuing care needs may result in determination of client readiness for discharge from home care.

DISCHARGE FROM HOME HEALTH CARE

Humphrey and Milone-Nuzzo (1996) outlined some standard criteria for discharging a client from home care. These criteria have been met when the client has done the following:

1. *Achieved goals as initially designated*
2. *Ceased needing skilled nursing care or therapy*
3. *Become hospitalized with an uncertain return-home date*
4. *Refused continuation of service at home*
5. *Relocated outside the agency's service area*
6. *Developed a need for services not available from the agency*
7. *Developed care needs that exceed the agency's resources to provide the care, so client is referred elsewhere*
8. *Developed a home situation that is unsafe, precluding the adequacy of intermittent care to meet needs*
9. *Died*

Application of the standard criteria should be consistent with agency policies and address the appropriate rationale for the discharge criteria. At the time of discharge from home care, documentation in the client's record should state the reason for discharge, summarize the care given, and describe the way goals were achieved and the client's status at the time of discharge. This information is communicated to the client's physician as well as to any other agency or agencies when the client is transferred to another care setting, such as a long-term care facility. Some agencies have developed an interagency communication form to assist in this process.

FUTURE CONSIDERATIONS
A Current Look at Discharge Planning

What factors have contributed to the current attention to discharge planning, especially to the home care setting? Recent literature (Kelly, McClelland, Daly, 1992; Naylor, 1990; Naylor et al, 1999) highlights discharge planning as an intervention readily suited to address health care access, quality, and cost. These three issues are feasible outcomes of effective discharge planning but imply the need for continuity of care across a variety of settings and development of new discharge planning strategies (Kelly, McClelland, Daly, 1992; Naylor et al, 1999).

HEALTH CARE DELIVERY COST FACTORS

The cost of health care delivery continues to receive considerable attention. The challenge for health care providers relates to controlling costs while meeting client needs and satisfaction. With the initiation of a prospective payment system (PPS) in hospitals, diagnosis related groups (DRGs) (Rogers et al, 1990) served to hasten the hospital discharges of clients with higher acuity levels than before. The increase in the aging population of the United States continues to increase the numbers of persons receiving, or eligible to receive, Medicare. Discharge planning has also received greater attention from Medicare-certified institutions based on the Joint Commission on Accreditation of Healthcare Organizations (JCAHO) (Indiana Association for Home Care, Inc., 1997).

Bull (1988) investigated the influence of DRGs on health care delivery in several hospitals in the Midwest. Her findings suggested that DRGs had a critical influence on discharge planning. Medicare clients were considered high risk for discharge planning and needed screening to determine their postdischarge needs. Nurses and social workers collaborated with physicians, family members, and others in developing discharge plans. Some concerns were expressed by staff nurses regarding the earlier discharges of sicker clients and the client's abilities to manage their care at home.

Interestingly, DRGs were found to facilitate implementation of the American Nurses Association *Standards of Practice* (1973), which outline the need for client participation in the areas of goal setting and health promotion, maintenance, and restoration. The family expectation then was not only being informed of the discharge date but also actively developing plans for discharge. Bull (1988) also reported that financial considerations related to follow-up posed some conflict for discharge planners who recognized that while Medicare covered 100% of the cost of therapy provided in the home and only 80% when provided on an outpatient basis, hospital-based physicians expected clients to return to the institution's outpatient facilities because it was convenient for the provider and because it generated revenue for the institution.

While many of the predominately aging population are hospitalized with chronic debilitating conditions such as congestive heart failure, cancer, and chronic obstructive lung disease, the challenge for discharge planning relates to the client's level of dependency and to social support systems, caregiving resources, and financial resources. Discharge to home care since the implementation of DRGs has resulted in a shift in the care provided by home care agency staff. Home care clients with greater acuity levels require that home care agency staff be ready to provide care for sicker clients. This affects not only professional staff, but also clients and family members who now must learn to use technology and carry out procedures independently when the nurse is not present. Family involvement in care may be viewed as a plus, until the degree of stress that family caregivers may experience is considered. This stress may result ultimately in rehospitalization or nursing home placement (Bull, 1988). Home care, which inherently may be a good choice, should be planned only when thorough planning for the transition of care is implemented. Transition of care is not automatic, and the hospital discharge planners cannot do it all.

Continued collaboration among key health care providers, caregivers, and the client is essential. Linkages among various levels of care to facilitate coordination provide a good basis for success. Nurses play a major role in assessing the needs and abilities of clients and families to plan continuing care needs.

DOCUMENTATION AND COMMUNICATION FOR REIMBURSEMENT FOR HOME HEALTH CARE

The beginnings of home care, with its roots in visiting nursing services, can be traced to the late 1800s in the United States. These services usually were developed to meet the needs of the poor at the time increased numbers of immigrants settled in the United States (Humphrey, Milone-Nuzzo, 1996). In the early part of the twentieth century, home nursing services were provided to policyholders with Metropolitan Life Insurance Company. These services, offered initially by contracts with existing nursing agencies, soon developed as insurance company–based agencies. Hamilton (1992) describes this change as an example of "how since the early 1900s other groups have tried to be in control." Subsequently, World

War II brought changes in medical care, with fewer home visits made by physicians. Medical care delivery was concentrated in physicians' offices and hospitals. Home health care was provided primarily by nurses. In this period, visiting nurse associations were established throughout the nation with health and illness care offered to the poor in their homes, with acute care services based in hospitals (Humphrey, Milone-Nuzzo, 1996).

In the 1980s, changes in home care coincided with increasing attention to hospital costs and the implementation of DRGs. Implementation of DRGs resulted in reduced length of hospital stays, calling for an increased need for home care services. Previously, Medicare and Medicaid programs, along with private insurance agencies and other third-party payors who covered home health care services, offered reduced reimbursement for hospitalizations, thus promoting the increased need for home care services.

With increased discharges to home care services came the accompanying shift for reimbursement. Documentation of services for reimbursement, as well as continuity of care, continues to be a critical element for the home care nurse when clients are discharged to home care. Thus emphasis on continuity of care and quality of care has led to mandated measures of outcomes as evident in the development and implementation of OASIS.

Payment for home care is an important reimbursement issue. Reimbursement for home care may come from various sources, although many home care services are still not reimbursable by third-party payors. Usual reimbursement sources include the following: Medicare, a national health insurance program for persons over 65 years of age and those under 65 years of age who are disabled; Medicaid, a federally assisted state program for public assistance to those who are needy and low-income; commercial insurance companies; indigent care, which is free to clients, or subsidized care; and miscellaneous other payment sources, including private pay. It is likely that discharge to home care will continue to increase with shorter hospital stays and client needs for continued care in a more cost-effective environment.

Changes in the U.S. health care system in the last decade of the twentieth century resulted in a transformation of health care in the United States (Pew Health Professions Commission, 1995). Managed care and the increased numbers of home care clients have been major outcomes of reduced hospital stays. It is likely that the trend toward a greater focus on managed care, care delivered outside the hospital setting, and providers' competition for clients will continue in the twenty-first century. Changes in the home care industry, standardized data collection, and other changes in Medicare reimbursement practices are contributing factors in this trend.

Community health nurses, as key health care professionals, can be expected to fill the roles of care managers through client care management and multidisciplinary collaboration. The following definition of *case management,* "a health care delivery process whose goals are to provide quality health care, decrease fragmentation, enhance clients' quality of life, and contain costs" (American Nurses Association, 1986b), is applicable to the anticipated continued increase in discharges to home care.

The greater emphasis on the case-management role and provision of care, which has a more global, holistic focus, has implications for preparing new nurses as well as for retooling nurses already in the workforce of the health care delivery system. The majority of these nurses may not have a community health background or may have practiced exclusively in an acute care setting. The need for better prepared nurse caregivers in the home care setting calls for attention to preparation of new nurses and to career development.

IMPLICATIONS FOR EDUCATION

Historically, hospitals have been basic education practice sites as well as primary employers for nurses until recent trends of shorter inpatient stays. As the traditional source of referrals for discharge of clients to home and community, hospitals have been the focus of concerns regarding discharge planning. With the increasing acuity of clients' conditions (Aiken, 1996) and fewer inpatient days, nurses must have greater comprehensive knowledge of discharge planning. Although trend data show an increasing level of acuity of condition of inpatients (Aiken, 1996), the likelihood remains that the production of new nurse graduates may not be appropriate to meet the demands for client care. Discharge planning remains an essential component of inpatient care but becomes even more important in assessing continuity of the increasingly complicated care in the home and community. Therefore appropriately prepared nursing graduates are essential.

What is known about client-care needs in this changing health care system has implications for ensuring the quality of the discharge planning component of client care. There is an imbalance in nursing education, with insufficient graduates to meet future needs of clients (Aiken, 1996). Many of those already in community or home health care settings are prepared with less than a baccalaureate degree. Many of these nurses are minimally equipped to practice in the community, home health care, care management, or discharge planning roles. The bachelor's degree is considered the appropriate level of preparation for the nurse who will coordinate and provide home care (Aiken, 1996).

The challenge for nursing leadership includes developing new educational models that prepare greater numbers of new graduates at the bachelor's level to deliver quality client care in community settings. This could mean rethinking the contributions of community college linkages to baccalaureate nursing educational institutions and teaching hospitals and focusing on redirecting federal nursing education funds to support baccalaureate and graduate education. Formerly, Medicare nonphysician education funding was theoretically designed to finance hospital-based nursing education, and funds were directed to the hospitals. These funding policies have not changed despite the shift from training nurses and allied health personnel in hospitals to preparing them in educational institutions. Nursing students no longer contribute the labor source for client care, as once was the case. This opens a window of opportunity for influencing Congress regarding these funds while the Medicare program is under scrutiny. Until there is a sufficient pool of baccalaureate-level nurses prepared to practice in the community, efforts should be directed toward assisting those already in practice to become prepared for delivering care in community or home care arenas. The following section describes an example of one continuing nursing education program developed for this purpose.

REDESIGNING CAREER FOR HOME HEALTH CARE NURSING PRACTICE

An identified need for career development for traditional acute care nurses and employers moving into the expanding home health care field led one major university's nursing continuing education department to make some changes (Kelly, 1996). An intensive continuing education program was designed to provide the foundation for employment in home health care nursing. This consisted of a three-phase, workshop/preceptorship of more than 70 hours, which provided insights and experiences to prepare nurses for staff orientation programs provided by their home care organization employers. This unique continuing education offering was built on nurses' biomedical knowledge and experiences in a controlled delivery setting with the content focused on the philosophies, structures, and processes of home care as related to financing issues, principles of community and family health, and interdisciplinary collaboration that frame effective delivery of home health care. The primary purpose of this workshop was to provide registered nurses with the basic content and clinical opportunities that define home care nursing practice, including home care considerations for discharge planning and the systems in which it is practiced (Kelly, 1996). The nurses with no prior home health care background who completed the workshop would be prepared to become productive home health care staff members after orientation to a specific agency.

TECHNOLOGICAL RESOURCES: IMPLICATIONS FOR PREPARATION IN DISCHARGE PLANNING

For successful discharge planning, it is imperative that the nurse's knowledge base be upgraded and updated to meet the ever-changing needs of clients and agencies. Resource demands are evident from a variety of providers in the current age of technology and make the task of remaining current appear insurmountable. Ongoing efforts in professional development are essential and take the form of formal and informal activities. Informal offerings through self-directed learning are available in the professional literature; by consultation with other professionals; through attendance at workshops, distance education, and conferences; and through the use of electronic information such as the internet (Gee, 1997a, 1997b). Formal offerings for professional development include education for credit at the undergraduate or graduate levels, organized continuing education offerings, and staff development efforts to prepare practitioners for new roles and new directions in established roles. Standardized nursing languages, linkages among languages, minimum data sets, and OASIS requirements further illustrate the need for technological skills and knowledge for the home health care nurse.

SUMMARY

This chapter has addressed the broad elements of continuity of care that encompass effective discharge planning factors related to the home care setting. Current and future considerations are incorporated as related to the U.S. health care delivery system (USHCDS). The changes in the USHCDS compel the nursing profession to examine the role of the nurse coordinating discharge not only in the acute setting but also in the multiple services of home health care. Changes in organizations, environments, skills, and technology demand that nurses examine their current abilities and seek additional knowledge and skills. Educational programs must prepare new practitioners to meet current service requirements and to know that ongoing professional development is expected.

Discharge planning is no longer only the prerogative of the institution-based nurse coordinating referrals to community agencies, but now extends beyond the hospital to the community and all the services found in that environment. As with so many roles in the USHCDS, the nurse coordinating discharge planning must be knowledgeable, flexible, cost-effective, and politically astute and must have a sense of humor!

REFERENCES

Aiken L: Understanding nursing's role in hospital restructuring, *MAIN Dimensions* 17(3):9, 1996.

American Hospital Association: *Patient's bill of rights,* Catalog No 1157759, Washington, DC, 1992, The Association.

American Nurses Association: *Standards of practice,* Washington, DC, 1973, The Association.

American Nurses Association: *Policy statement on continuity of care,* Washington, DC, 1986a, The Association.

American Nurses Association: *Council on community health nursing,* Washington, DC, 1986b, The Association.

Anderson MA, Helms LB: Communication between continuing care organizations, *Research in Nursing and Health* 18(1):49-57, 1995.

Bull M: Influence of diagnoses-related group on discharge planning, professional practice, and patient care, *Journal of Professional Nursing* 4(6):415-421, 1988.

Christopher MS, Toughill E: Nurses: Community actualizers, *Home Healthcare Nurse* 15(10):744-745, 1997.

Clemen-Stone S, McGuire S, Eigsti D: *Comprehensive community health nursing,* ed 5, St Louis, 1998, Mosby.

Corwin RG: *Role conception and mobility aspirations: A study in the formation and transformation of bureaucratic professional and humanitarian nursing identities,* unpublished doctoral dissertation, Bloomington, 1960, University of Minnesota.

Davis CK: *Anticipatory socialization: The effect on role conception, role deprivations, and adaptive strategies on graduating student nurses,* unpublished doctoral dissertation, Ann Arbor, Mich, 1972, Syracuse University.

Deal LW: The effectiveness of community health nursing interventions: A literature review, *Public Health Nursing* 11(5):315-323, 1994.

Gee P: The internet—A home care nursing clinical resource. I. *Home Healthcare Nurse* 15(2):115-120, 1997a.

Gee P: The internet—A home care nursing clinical resource. II. *Home Healthcare Nurse* 15(3):175-180, 1997b.

Hamilton D: Research and reform: Community nursing and the Framingham Tuberculosis Project, 1914-1923, *Nursing Research* 41(1):8-13, 1992.

Harris MD: Ten DRG's that can affect home care referrals, *Home Healthcare Nurse* 17(2):127-129, 1999.

Harris M, Krimker R: The medical social worker: Member of the home healthcare team, *Home Healthcare Nurse* 15(5):327-328, 1997.

Huber D: *Leadership and nursing care management,* Philadelphia, 1996, WB Saunders.

Humphrey C: *Home care nursing handbook,* ed 3, Gaithersburg, Md, 1998, Aspen.

Humphrey CJ, Milone-Nuzzo P: *Orientation to home care nursing,* Gaithersburg, Md, 1996, Aspen.

Indiana Association for Home Care, Inc. (on-line), 1997.

Johndrow PD: Phlebotomy techniques in the home, *Home Healthcare Nurse* 17(4):246-250, 1999.

Johnson M, Maas M, eds: *Nursing outcomes classification (NOC),* St Louis, 1997, Mosby.

Kelly K: *Discharge planner role: Factors related to bureaucratic professional and service conceptions,* unpublished doctoral dissertation, Iowa City, 1987, University of Iowa.

Kelly K: *Redesigning your career: Preparing for the specialty of home health nursing practice,* program brochure, Iowa City, Sept-Nov 1996, The University of Iowa College of Nursing Continuing Education On Campus and Outreach Programs.

Kelly K, McClelland E, Daly J: Discharge planning. In Bulechek G, McCloskey J, eds: *Nursing interventions essential nursing treatments,* ed 2, Philadelphia, 1992, WB Saunders.

Klainberg MB et al: *Community health nursing: An alliance for health,* New York, 1998, McGraw-Hill.

Kluka M: Fifteen common errors to avoid when completing a skilled home care referral, *Home Healthcare Nurse* 15(11):793-795, 1997.

Kramer M: Role models, role conceptions and role deprivation, *Nursing Research* 17(2):115-120, 1968.

Little AD: *The health care system in the mid 1990s,* Washington, DC, 1985, Health Insurance Association of America.

Lowenstein A, Hoff PS: Discharge planning: A study of nursing staff involvement, *Journal of Nursing Administration* 24(4):45-50, 1994.

Mathews-Flint LJ, Lucas LJ: Telecommunication relay services: Linking nurses to patients with communication disorders, *Home Healthcare Nurse* 17(5):300-306, 1999.

McClelland E, Kelly K, Buckwalter KC, eds: *Continuity of care: Advancing the concept of discharge planning,* New York, 1985, Grune & Stratton.

McCloskey JC, Bulechek GM, eds: *Nursing interventions classification (NIC),* ed 2, St Louis, 1996, Mosby.

McEwen M: *Community-based nursing: An introduction,* Philadelphia, 1998, WB Saunders.

Mefford J: Discharge planning, *Pathways Newsletter,* (on-line) winter 1996.

More P, Mandell S: *Case management: An evolving practice,* New York, 1997, McGraw-Hill.

Naylor M: Comprehensive discharge planning for hospitalized elderly: A pilot study, *Nursing Research* 39(3):156-161, 1990.

Naylor M et al: Comprehensive discharge planning and home follow-up of hospitalized elders: A randomized clinical trial, *Journal of American Medical Association* 281(7):613-620, 1999.

North American Nursing Diagnosis Association (NANDA): *Nursing diagnoses: Definitions and classification, 1997-1998,* Philadelphia, 1996, The Association.

Perry AG, Potter PA: *Clinical nursing skills and techniques,* ed 4, St Louis, 1997, Mosby.

Pew Health Professions Commission: *Critical challenges: Revitalizing the health professions for the twenty-first century,* report 3, Washington, DC, 1995, The Commission.

Reichelt P, Newcomb J: Organizational factors in discharge planning, *Journal of Nursing Administration* 10(12):36-42, 1980.

Reif L, Martin K: *Nurses and consumers: Partners in assuring quality care in home,* Pub No CH-49, Washington, DC, 1995, American Nurses Association.

Rogers W et al: Quality of care before and after implementation of the DRG-based prospective payment system, *Journal of the American Medical Association* 264(15):1989-1994, 1990.

Shaughnessy P: *Medicare's Oasis: Standardized outcome and assessment information set for home health care,* Center for Health Services and Policy Research OASIS-B1, June 1998.

Sperling RL: Continuity of care between home care and the emergency room, *Home Healthcare Nurse* 16(9):633-634, 1998a.

Sperling RL: What's this OASIS, anyway? Outcome and assessment information set, *Home Healthcare Nurse* 16(6):373-374, 1998b.

Stackhouse JC: *Into the community: Nursing in ambulatory and home care,* Philadelphia, 1998, JB Lippincott.

Stanhope M, Lancaster J: *Community health nursing: Promoting health of aggregates, families and individuals,* ed 4, St Louis, 1996, Mosby.

Twohy KM, Reif L: What do public health nurses really do during prenatal home appointments? *Public Health Nursing* 14(6):324-331, 1997.

Urbanic B, McKeehan K: Foreword. In McClelland E, Kelly K, Buckwalter KC, eds: *Continuity of care: Advancing the concept of discharge planning,* San Diego, 1985, Grune & Stratton.

Weis D, Mathers R, Schank MJ: Health care delivery in faith communities: The parish nursing model, *Public Health Nursing* 14(6):368-372, 1997.

Zander K: Nursing care management: Strategic management of cost and quality outcomes, *Journal of Nursing Administration* 18(5):23-30, 1988.

Zander K: Nursing and case management: To control or elaborate. In McCloskey J, Grace H, eds: *Current issues in nursing,* ed 4, St Louis, 1994, Mosby.

4 Nurse-Directed System of Care for Families

Ida M. Martinson and Marjorie Jamieson

Historically the family served five major functions: (1) to achieve economic survival, (2) to provide protection, (3) to pass on values and religion, (4) to educate the young, and (5) to confer status. As social institutions have taken on many of these functions, the family of today is expected to provide for the relational needs of its members. Some of these needs include fostering love, intimacy, self-acceptance, and individuation; nurturing, caring; giving and being given to; sharing the joys of posterity; and providing support through adversity.

Given the dramatic shifts in health care today, what roles do families have in relationship to health care providers? To what extent can families assist in providing health care to their members?

There has been a dramatic shift, for example, in the cause of both mortality and morbidity: from infectious diseases (in the past) to chronic conditions such as cancer, heart disease, stroke, and diabetes (now). The primary goal of care also is changing, from curing acute disease to helping individuals remain as independent as possible with the highest level of functioning. Chronic disease care is more complex than acute disease care and must be provided for longer periods of time (Goforth, 2000).

Chronic illnesses have not developed at the same rate among all racial groups, and recent evidence shows that the racial gap is spreading across all domains of health and is not related to health-risk behaviors. Consequently, more attention needs to be given to the health of local communities (Hayward et al, 2000).

The recent work by Badger and Collins-Joyce (2000) stresses the relationships among depression, which usually accompanies chronic disease, and physical health impairment, psychosocial resources, and functional ability. Depressed older adults had increased physical health problems that involved more sick days and hospitalizations. There was a lack of effect of depression on functional ability.

Their work also suggests nursing interventions that would be useful for family members in the community, including old and new technologies (Badger, Collins-Joyce, 2000). Health-promotion programs have been useful for participants in reducing their health-risk factors (Gold, Anderson, Serxner, 2000). Computers are being used to help not only the individual elderly person in the home but also the informal caregivers as well as the professionals. Computer resources can play a vital role in the future for the elderly in the home (Alexty, 2000; Durtschi, 2001).

The expanding roles of nurses today find them in a variety of settings in which they must deal with family health. Nurses now have opportunities to assist families through direct client interventions and consultations. Emphasis has shifted from the old model of nursing as only client care in a hospital setting to modern examples of highly educated professionals assisting in every aspect of family health. Health promotion as well as client advocacy is often included in today's health care delivery. Reutter (1984) noted that literature often neglects the health care function of the family. Though there has been some shifting of the paradigm, much of generic nursing education continues to depend on individual models rather than on systems models with clinical experiences still confined to hospital settings.

Nursing needs to find ways in which to work with families and to conceptualize the assessment of the family unit pursuant to the promotion of family health. One assessment tool is Orem's self-care framework (1983). Although the guidelines focus on the individual because of Orem's appreciation of the family's role in individual development, the guidelines may be adapted to assess the family unit. Reutter (1984) has also contributed to this field with her work in community health nursing. She developed a family assessment guide that categorizes the traits of healthy families versus those aspects not usually addressed in family literature.

PREP

Stewart and Archbold (1998) have developed PREP, which stands for preparation, enrichment, and predictability. The basic principles of preparation, enrichment, and predictability were used in the models of alternative systems of care. Stewart and Archbold have given words to the thinking process and doing process that are basic to providing professional home nursing under the models of both the block nurse program and the home care for the dying child. The first goal of PREP is to increase the family's skill and preparedness for family care because researchers learned that preparedness was associated with lower levels of most aspects of caregiver role strain. The second goal of PREP is to strengthen mutuality and increase the rewards of caregiving by enriching family care for both the caregiver and the client. Mutuality and meaningful rewards are associated with lower levels of caregiver strain. The third goal of PREP is to increase the predictability of family caregiving, especially when the family is unstable. There are lower levels of caregiver role strain when the caregiving situation is predictable.

In addition to the three goals, PREP has five interrelated principles that guide the nurse in goal attainment. The five principles deal with family care assessment, family focus, cooperation, multiple intervention strategies, and detection of problematic transitions in family care.

Family care assessment must be done systematically to identify family strengths and family care issues known to be associated with caregiver role strain, such as lack of skill and unpreparedness for specific care activities, low enrichment, low mutuality, unpredictability in the care routine, and caregiver and client health problems including the client health conditions that triggered the home care referral. The families decide on the issues to work on.

In assessments of family care, nurses must integrate and synthesize their knowledge from several disciplines. It is essential that they defend those aspects of family health care that call for nursing interventions. Assessment often includes (1) environmental data, which examine basic living conditions (both physical and sociological), (2) family structure, which identifies communication patterns, values, role relationships, and decision making; (3) family functioning that focuses on self-care requirements by making a thorough investigation of how individual family members' needs are met through the family unit; (4) family functioning that illustrates adaptability to change (by collecting data on adjustments to life events), and (5) family perceptions of health situations to open further elaboration and development. A skillful home care nurse will find innovative ways to explore family health care needs and engage family members in a commitment to optimal care.

Family focus requires the cooperative efforts of involved family members. At times, uninvolved but interested family members are engaged in some aspects of care.

Cooperating to blend family and nursing knowledge facilitates the resolution of family care problems. Family involvement in generating strategies to solve problems will more likely lead to success than the imposition of strategies by nurses or other health care providers. Multiple intervention strategies tailored to the family are used until the family care problem is resolved. Interventions are tailored to the cultural characteristics and preferences of the client and family. Detecting problematic transitions in family care over time is essential. Transitions occur for many reasons such as illness, death, or level of support available to the family.

There are 2 components of the PREP program: the PREP Advice Line (PAL) and the Keep In Touch (KIT) system. The PAL is available 24 hours a day, 7 days a week, and is staffed by nurses. These PREP nurses have access to the care plans for all families via computer and are able to give appropriate advice for most inquiries. KIT is a system of PREP nurse–initiated telephone assessments that are used to monitor families. This regular telephone outreach system allows a nurse to stay apprised of the family care situation between in-home visits.

Stewart and Archbold (1998) believe that families have local knowledge that is essential to good outcomes. Families have unique needs, and the home care nurse has knowledge and skills based on research and experience across many family care situations; this type of knowledge is called *cosmopolitan knowledge.* These two knowledge bases, local and cosmopolitan, are powerful and can make the difference in home health care.

This chapter will describe several nurse-directed systems of care that serve families' health care needs, including (1) the block nurse program for the elderly in a metropolitan area, followed by brief references to several related programs; (2) the home care program for children with cancer serving both urban and rural areas and covering several states, followed by an update of hospice care for children; (3) adult foster care; (4) adult day care; (5) community services; (6) conservatorships; (7) informal support systems. A description of the development of each program will be shared, followed by delineation of the level of care each program provides, the population it serves, its services, its professional staff, its regulations, its funding, and its relationship to home health care in general.

BLOCK NURSE PROGRAM

Across the nation, whether in large cities or small rural communities, a better system for delivering affordable health and long-term care services for the elderly is needed. Ideally, this "better" system would enable seniors to live with dignity in the familiar surroundings of their own homes, escaping the cost and anxiety of unnecessary or premature clinic, hospital, or nursing home care.

America has tended to look to experts, systems, agencies, organizations, and technology for answers about how to care for the aging. However, a novel idea, started in Minnesota, began with the premise that answers are in the community, where natural relationships and interdependencies are operative. Local people often depend on neighbors to provide informational, social, and support services. Why not couple them with the plethora of professional services in the community for elderly neighbors who otherwise might be admitted to nursing home and hospitals?

The ability of a family, surrogate family, and neighbors to meet the chronic care and social needs of its own elderly can play a major role in providing caregiving assistance to elderly persons (Faison, Faria, Frank, 1999). This combination is able to organize and support what resources the family has and supplement these with a mix of services and supports from the neighborhood that the family alone cannot provide. Such assistance is possible through careful planning and by following a series of steps. The steps are used to determine community-identified needs, develop common goals, develop a working partnership among key players in the community, form a community health advocate committee, recruit advocates, develop training for advocates, promote the program, involve health professional students whenever possible, and develop an evaluation process that involves continuous feedback and improvement (Maurana, Rodney, 2000).

The block nurse program (BNP) is an outstanding example of this process. The BNP, started in 1982 by nurses and residents of a community in St. Paul, Minnesota, assists in the development of a social network in local neighborhoods and communities. Mitchell and Trickett (1983) identified the following components of a social network: intensity, durability, multidimensionality, directness or reciprocity, relationship density, dispension, frequency, and homogeneity.

The initial site in St. Anthony Park was designed for elderly residents in the area by a group of neighborhood residents, with home care services provided by professionals and volunteers living in the neighborhood. There are approximately 700 people 65 years of age or older in this geographically discrete area. There are approximately 40 registered nurses, 6 churches, and a small business community serving a population of approximately 7000. The BNP's services range from health promotion and maintenance to highly skilled clinical services. In addition, arrangement of nutritional, financial, social, and transportation services is available. As care manager, the block nurse provides or finds services, many volunteered by neighbors, that keep people 65 years of age and over in their own homes and communities.

The first client was accepted into the program in July, 1982, after a development period of 6 months. In the first 4 years, the program served over 100 clients in their homes. The average monthly client load for each nurse was 14 to 18 clients. An average of 3 to 4 registered nurses, along with 2 block companions (combined home health aide and homemakers), were supplemented by volunteers living in the community who had been oriented to programs such as the Befrienders and Peer Counselors. The Befrienders are volunteers from the churches who agree to provide friendship, take the client shopping, and so forth. Peer counselors are recruited by the social worker and nurses to provide more specialized psychological services. Both Befrienders and Peer Counselors are trained volunteers.

The primary block nurse is vital in relationship to direct services to patients and is key to the program's success and cost effectiveness. In addition to client services, the primary block nurse is responsible for record keeping, care management, gatekeeping, resource coordination, and supervision of the block companions and volunteers. Block nurses and block companions, all of whom live in the community, are employees of a home health care agency with whom each BNP community board contracts. This arrangement provides clinical supervision and access to entitlements.

Each community BNP is managed by a board of directors composed of residents of each respective community. Appointment of the program director and volunteer coordinator is the responsibility of the board.

Funding for the St. Anthony Park BNP comes from three sources and typifies most programs. Approximately half of its funding is from contributions generated by fund raising and grants. In addition, one fourth comes from payments by clients or their family members according to a sliding-fee scale based on ability to pay. A combination of Medicare, Medicaid, state grants, private insurance, and other entitlements provides the remaining one fourth.

The BNP expands the services provided by public health, home health care, and visiting nurse associations, primarily because of volunteer activities and community engagement that provide all sorts of resources including in-kind support, secretarial services, church-collected commodes and wheelchairs, and social activities such as community residents taking homebound clients ice fishing, school children visiting with birthday cakes, high school students addressing Christmas cards, and trained volunteers dealing with grief and loss.

An external evaluation of the pilot site in St. Anthony Park found the following:
1. As many as 85% of clients would be forced to enter nursing homes without the BNP.
2. The total cost of care is at least 24% less than the minimum cost of a nursing home.
3. Fees for block nurse and block companion visits were lower than other programs surveyed because no minimum number of hours per visit was required.

In 1986 the BNP merged with the Living At Home Program and changed its name to the Living At Home/Block Nurse Program (LAH/BNP). A nonprofit, 501 (C) (3) (tax exempt) corporation was formed to provide technical assistance for new programs around the state. The effectiveness of the program has generated more programs across the nation; there are about 50 LAH/BNPs, both urban and rural, across the United States and in other countries.

From July 1, 1995 to June 31, 1996, 14 of the Minnesota programs volunteered 31,500 hours and kept 315 people out of nursing homes for 2195 months at a savings of $3,609,000. Thousands of dollars were saved for Medicare, insurance, and other financing programs because of the care management and service integration provided by nurses in the homes of clients.

The LAH/BNP, Inc., applied for, and became, a national demonstration site for the federal Health Care Financing Administration (HCFA; now the Centers for Medicare and Medicaid Services [CMS]) Community Nursing Organization (CNO) demonstration in 1992, along with three other sites across the country. In this demonstration, nurses authorize and manage Medicare Part A home health care services and Part B nonphysician services through capitation at full financial risk. The CNO has been successful and under the capitated rate is able to provide services usually not paid for by Medicare but without which enrollees would access more expensive acute care services. Nurses, families, and communities together are demonstrating how to keep seniors at home, where they want to be.

In 1997 the LAH/BNP, Inc., board of directors established a new entity, the Elderberry Institute, to extend and support replication of the program nationwide. To assist the initiative, an Elderberry Institute internet site has been created at www.elderberry.org. The purpose of this web site is to facilitate more efficient support and communication among current programs and to give information and technical support to communities wishing to establish programs.

ADDITIONAL NURSING PROGRAMS

There are additional nation-wide programs that have been developed, such as the Parish Nurse Program and the Program of All-inclusive Care for the Elderly (PACE). The Parish Nurse Program uses nurses in the church to assist other members of the congregation (Solari-Twadell, McDermott, 1998; Palmer, 2001).

As an advocate, the parish nurse may accompany the elder to his or her doctor and translate the diagnosis into what the client can understand as well as help him or her through the maze of the health care system. Community education programs have included breast cancer awareness, cardiopulmonary resuscitation, prostate cancer, and living wills (Palmer, 2001).

PACE is a comprehensive long-term medical, nursing, and social service and receives monthly capitation payments from Medicare and Medicaid for clients eligible for nursing homes. This program was developed originally by On Lok Senior Health Services in San Francisco's Chinatown in the late 1970s (Rich, 1999). Other nursing centers, such as the Lundeen Community Nursing Center model, are grounded in a philosophy that promotes health and primary prevention. The model requires an interdisciplinary provider team and relies on professional nurses to integrate the essential elements of nursing, primary medical care, public health, and social services (Lundeen, 1993; 1999).

In rural areas, there are challenges for the rapidly aging population. The University of North Dakota Nursing Center has addressed these challenges by educating nursing students to care for rural individuals, families, and communities through faculty demonstration of the practice of nursing. In a 2-year period, 440 individuals in rural families received nursing case-management services from this center. Another 1500 to 2200 people took part in health education sessions, and close to 1000 health screenings were conducted annually through the nursing center (Henly et al, 1998; Oermann, Harris, Dammeyer, 2001). All clients indicated that having a nurse teach them about their illness, medications, and treatments was very important. Information about the illness and health promotion, as well as the opportunity to call a nurse with questions after the visit, were significantly more important to clients with lower incomes (Oermann, Harris, Dammeyer, 2001). A nurse-managed senior health clinic was established using a nursing framework (Bear, Burnell, Covell, 1997). A primary health care model was used to develop a community-based, nurse-managed health care center (Hatcher, Scarinzi, Kreider, 1998).

Halls and Highley (1987) wrote that their experience suggests that the absence of nursing assistance to a family member with chronic disability or disease results in premature institutionalization, whereas nursing assistance to those individuals needing care prolongs the ability of the family to assist the client.

In 1993, home health care was provided to about 1.4 million persons per day by 7000 home health care agencies. Three quarters of home health care clients were 65 years of age and over, and almost 20% were 85 years of age and older. Two thirds of home health care clients were women.

According to Giampaoli (2000) women have longer life expectancies than men in the circumstances of cardiovascular disease, cancer, and dementia. Part of this increase is due to women having a higher prevalence of nonfatal chronic conditions, lower muscle strength, and lower bone density along with higher rates of sedentary behavior and obesity (Leveille, Resnick, Balfour, 2000).

Among the home health care clients in 1993, almost one half of the admission diagnoses were for the following six conditions (Wunderlich, Sloan, Davis, 1996):

- Diseases of the heart and hypertension (17%)
- Injury and poisoning (9%)
- Diabetes (7%)
- Cerebrovascular diseases (6%)
- Cancer (6%)
- Respiratory diseases (6%)

All of these are chronic conditions except for injury and poisoning. Later chapters will discuss these chronic conditions.

Hospitals now serve only very sick clients requiring highly complex care. Nursing homes also serve clients with serious disabilities and with rehabilitative and other subacute care needs (Ingold et al, 2000). Over 34.7% of clients had at least one day of inappropriate hospitalization, including 9.2% (18 clients) whose hospital admission and entire stay was reviewed as inappropriate. Most of the inappropriate days were due to delays in discharge (87.1%). Univariate analysis revealed that subjects with inappropriate days were most likely living alone and were more impaired in basic and instrumental activities of daily living (Ingold et al, 2000). The rest of the population will increasingly receive care in outpatient units, home- and community-based settings, and assisted living facilities (Wunderlich, 1996).

HOME CARE FOR THE CHILD

There is a national movement under way to provide home care for children who traditionally had been hospitalized. These include children with newly diagnosed diabetes and children with feeding tubes. Children newly diagnosed with diabetes were randomly assigned to traditional inpatient care or to home care. The results of a follow-up 24 months later suggested that using home care to reduce hospital stays for children with newly diagnosed type 1 diabetes improved the children's health outcomes without significantly increasing social costs (Dougherty, Soderstrom, Schiffrin, 1998). Early intervention services in the home for children from birth through 3 years of age have been developed (Pokorni, 1997). Children with both gastrostomy tubes and jejunal feeding tubes are now being cared for at home (Gebus, 1997).

There is now increased interest in providing a homelike atmosphere for dying children in hospitals. Hospices all over the country are more and more willing to care for dying children. There is, however, still reluctance in some major hospital centers to make referrals to home care and hospice agencies. Historically, the development of home care for dying children was nurse directed and used physicians as consultants in a system of care.

In 1972, Dr. Ida Martinson provided home care to a family who had a child dying of cancer. With 24-hour-a-day, 7-day-a-week, on-call support, the parents cared for their son until his death at home. In a pilot study followed over the next 4 years in which 8 other families received this nursing intervention, 5 of the children died at home instead of being admitted to the hospital for the final days of life. A 4-year major study showed that over a 2-year period, 58 families with a dying child participated in this home care program, and 80% of the children of the participating families died at home instead of in the hospital.

In each of the families participating in the studies, the dying child had indicated, either directly or indirectly, the desire to remain at home, and the parents were willing to honor that wish. A contributing cause for this preference may have been that the child had experienced frustration in the hospital setting. Separation of a child from family and home environment during a crisis such as the process leading to death was stressful. During hospitalization, the child and the family had limited control over what happened to them. With home care, the parents had an opportunity for direct care of their dying child, thereby maintaining their normal parental roles.

Families who participated in the studies were from a wide variety of social, economic, and educational backgrounds. The parents ranged from 20 to 59 years of age; the majority were in their 30s, and most of them had completed high school. The children's ages ranged from 5 weeks to 17 years at the time of referral. The time span from diagnosis to death of the child ranged from 1 month to 6 years 2 months.

In addition to perceiving their children's desire for home care, families also needed to recognize that home care was a possible alternative for their children. The parents especially needed to recognize their own abilities to care for their children.

All children who participated were no longer responsive to cure-oriented treatment; there was no realistic hope of recovery, and all effective drugs and treatment protocols had been tried. These programs provided the option of home, rather than the hospital, as the place of death for the children.

The nurses were on call 24 hours a day, 7 days a week and made home visits whenever the families desired. The physicians functioned as consultants to the nurses and to the families, sharing medical background of the children with the home care nurses. All medications were made available through cooperation with the children's physicians so that medications that were no longer effective, such as pain-control drugs, could be changed as needed.

It was important that the roles of the home care nurses were clear to the families and others involved in the care. While the nurses were the primary providers for the families and acted as parent advocates, facilitators, and coordinators of care, the families provided most of the care to meet the children's needs. Families managed well if they were given guidance by the nurses and assurance that they were doing what was necessary for the children's comfort.

Because special equipment was sometimes necessary for the children's particular needs, the nurses needed to know what resources were available in the community. This specialized equipment required special servicing from expert technical help. Parents had no difficulty in the maintenance of this equipment.

Control of pain is also an essential component of home care. Studies indicate that pain can be controlled as well at home as in the hospital when the increase in pain is anticipated and planned for. Nurses found it more helpful to have parameters for dosages of drugs than single dosage recommendations. Oral drugs to control pain and anxiety were preferable to injections as long as vomiting was not a problem. The home care nurses also guided parents by suggesting procedures such as keeping written records of medications given and the responses of the children, by suggesting comfort measures such as the use of a wheelchair or a flotation pad or foods that might be best tolerated by the children, and by teaching suctioning, gavaging, giving injections, administering oxygen, and monitoring intravenous lines. The nurses encouraged parents to maintain family environments and schedules of activities that were as normal as possible.

The home care nurses needed to provide consistent support to the families by calling or visiting regularly to answer questions and advise on specific problems. The families needed to know how to reach the nurses at all times. In addition to office and home numbers, beepers and a system of back-up nurses were used. Availability of the nurses at all times was a reassurance to parents.

Assistance at the time of death and follow-up after death of the children were integral parts of the home care program. The nurses often assisted families in notifying the physicians; contacting mortuaries, coroners, or medical examiners; calling clergy; and aiding in plans for the funerals.

The program was funded by the National Cancer Institute and the grant paid for the necessary nursing services. At that time reimbursement was made only for direct nursing care and did not cover the nurses' time spent teaching parents to provide care. Over time, insurance companies have come to cover the costs of such duties. At present, regardless of where families live in the United States, they should have access to hospice services for their dying children. Reimbursement for such services may still be a problem in some parts of the United States. Families need to check with their insurance companies and may be able to negotiate the coverage of home health care instead of hospital care for their dying children. Home care for dying children is an option for most parents in the United States (Martinson, 1995, 1996). Home care for children with both acute and chronic illnesses will continue to grow in the future.

Nursing continues to shift its focus to the family as a unit and searches for ways to strengthen family life and to meet relational and affective needs. Nurses working with families have the opportunity to contribute to this growing effort by synthesizing what is known about family structure and to function with what is currently understood about optimal health care.

ADULT FOSTER CARE
Population Served

While the majority of older adults remain in their own homes throughout their entire lives, many elderly need housing that provides a barrier-free environment and physical or mental support. Even those elderly who are still able to provide their own personal care often find that the difficulties they face in maintaining a home, shopping, and paying bills are not worth the advantages of staying in their own homes. Some move to easier-to-maintain housing and a variety of alternative living arrangements. Separate individual units and apartments exist for adults who still function independently and can afford the cost. Other living arrangements with private living units provide services, including meals, transportation, housekeeping, social activities, and security monitoring.

Personal-care homes have become more popular because in some ways they provide home care in small group settings. This type of home is called, in various geographical regions, *adult foster care, board and care,* or *residential care.* (*Residential care* is defined differently in various states.)

Regulations

Shared-living homes, another type of living arrangement, operate under regulations that vary from state to state, and some states still have few regulations. Those that provide some assistance with daily care are usually licensed or certified by county departments of social services. Most must meet basic building and safety codes. The level of care provided, the cost, and the educational levels of the caregivers vary greatly, and on-site visits, dialogue, and a care-plan contract with the provider are essential before selecting a living arrangement (Kleh, 1981).

Services Provided

The concept of the adult foster care home is not a new one. In ancient communities, certain homes and families were designated to take in the aged and frail who could no longer live alone. Today, adult foster care homes may provide for a small number (five or less) of adults. They offer room and board and services that "assist the resident in activities of daily living, such as assistance with bathing, dressing, grooming, eating, medication management, or recreation" (Oregon Senate Bill 519, 1985). However, shorter hospital stays and clients being discharged in sicker conditions are leading to more sophisticated levels of home health care and adult foster care (The Provider, 1985).

Staffing

Although quality and range of services are not equal among homes, many homes are supervised by registered nurses, maintain good family communications, and provide superior nutrition, personal care, and activities in a homelike setting (Sparks et al, 1986). As originally conceived, they may not provide skilled nursing, but many arrange home health care nurse visits for patients who need this level of care. Clients may be able to bring along pets, help prepare meals, and enjoy being with a larger group of residents and staff.

Selecting an Adult Foster Care Home

Important considerations when selecting an adult foster care home or residential care home are the competence and responsibility of the owner(s) and the degree to which care is monitored. Supervision will probably be consistent when an owner-provider is on the premises daily. Training levels of other staff should be assessed as appropriate for the level of care required by the clients.

Clients and families should make an effort to find a home that provides an appropriate balance of care and independence. It is vitally important to select a home that matches the service needs of the client. Families should discuss the philosophy of care in the home and the level of training and geriatric knowledge of those who are providing the daily care.

The benefits of group living include companionship and security. Clients may take part in the daily activities of the household and retain some degree of independence while receiving dependable, 24-hour assistance.

Costs

Very little of the cost of this care is reimbursable. Monthly costs range from $500 to more than $4000. For clients who have adequate income and who live in an urban area, finding such housing is possible, but for those with low incomes and minimum savings, finding comfortable and secure housing can be difficult.

Adult foster care homes are not always the client's first choice. Moving from his or her own home is often a compromise to meet a client's personal needs. It is important, therefore, to make sure that enough is gained by moving a client to compensate for the losses in environment familiarity, pride in ownership, and memories.

ADULT DAY CARE
Services

While many types of adult day care have been instituted in recent years, some model their programs after the goals set in 1972 by Hawaii, which became the first state to enact legislation on day care for the elderly. Hawaii's goals can be summarized as follows:

- To keep welfare-dependent individuals out of institutionalization as long as possible
- To provide social contact and enrichment experiences

- To make the burdens lighter for the younger family, adult children who work, and other caregivers
- To provide a nutritional program and pleasant surroundings for elderly who would be very much alone
- To provide transportation in some form for travel to medical clinics, dentists' and doctors' offices, therapists, and adult education classes; for recreational trips; and to and from the day care center (Aging, 1986).

Adult day care may provide a client a reasonable alternative, at least for a while, to moving from home. This is a definite advantage to a frail or elderly person to whom "home" may be the last bastion of reality and competence. Moving can be far more than a physical act. To stay in his or her own home means to hold on to selfhood and to maintain identity, autonomy, and control. Thus clients who are unable to do simple personal and household chores or unable to remember how to take medications properly may be relieved of such duties on a daily basis and still stay at home.

Adult day care centers can be housed in community program facilities, hospitals, long-term care facilities, or senior centers; examples exist of both for-profit and not-for-profit models. Many depend on community support to subsidize fees. Others, in hospitals and long-term care facilities, justify the necessary financial outlay by providing referrals to the parent facility. The first year of funding for the Abilene, Texas, Day Care Center included substantial funding from the Department of Public Welfare (more than 70%), grants from the Moody and the Hagg Foundations, and community donations (Smith, 1981).

The Department of Veterans Affairs (VA) participated in a 3-year project to study alternatives to nursing home care. Several VA hospitals have started adult day–health care centers, where functionally disabled veterans can receive health care and restorative therapies in a congregate setting. Veterans attend 2 to 3 days per week, 6 hours per day. In 1986, model programs existed in North Little Rock, Arkansas; Portland, Oregon; Miami Beach, Florida; and Minneapolis, Minnesota. Such combined social and health care services may differ from community social settings by including monitoring and provision of long-term care services. Even recreational activities focus on improving physical health and functional abilities. Library books are displayed, as is a daily bowl of fruit. Contacts with younger people and contributions to others are maintained in some programs through pairings with elementary school students or oral history projects. Students generally perform well in their roles. In some instances, students have been able to develop meaningful relationships with patients with whom facility staff had been unsuccessful for years (Thralow, Watson, 1974).

Nearly all adult day care programs provide therapeutic diets during the noon meal and activities to increase functional ability, social interaction, adaptive behavior, and alertness. Activities include physical and speech therapy, health screening, toileting, bathing, and personal care. In some communities, services have been volunteered by physicians, dentists, podiatrists, nurses, clergy, and other professionals.

Benefits

Day programs also exist that will accept or take exclusively people with various levels of dementia. One of the greatest benefits of day care is respite for family caregivers, who often bear the burden of daily care for a spouse or relative with a long-term illness, such as Alzheimer's disease. Another benefit can be continuing friendships and support among families who bring relatives for care. Many programs offer family support groups, workshops, and materials. In a few instances, day care center staff have become advocates for families as they attempt to deal with the health care and public assistance systems.

Costs

Adult day care offers an extremely valuable piece in the puzzle of providing appropriate care for the frail and elderly. It provides a viable alternative to nursing care and assistance to families who want to stay involved in providing care but cannot do it alone. A compelling argument in favor of day care can also be stated in financial terms. Most programs charge $15 to $20 per day—far less than inpatient care.

Use

Although there are notable successful programs, adult day care is underused in most communities. Adult care providers suspect family dynamics play an important role in the lack of interest. "Children often can't see themselves delivering an elderly parent to day care" (McDermott, 1986). It may be easier to hire a visiting home aide than to dress a frail person and get him or her out of the house, particularly if the caregiver is trying to get to work also. Programs with a van to pick up and return clients may have a real advantage over those that cannot offer this service. Other family members may not recognize their need for respite or feel guilty about it, since the relative is not totally disabled. Elders who have not been out socially for a while may complain about the prospect of going to the center out of fear or discomfort, and families often capitulate to their demands to stay home. This is unfortunate because most clients are quickly won over by the personal warmth of staff, arts and crafts, social meals, and opportunities for trips and events with security.

ASSISTED LIVING

Although there is no universal definition of *assisted living,* it is a popular and fast-growing long-term care phenomenon across the United States as the aging population insists on more options and as governments look for alternatives to nursing homes—the most expensive form of care for senior citizens. It is clear that the percentage of older people who use home health care is growing while nursing home use is declining (Wolfe, 2001).

New models of assisted living continue to form. For example, during the 2001 legislative session in Minnesota, a bill that will provide state grants to local governments for constructing assisted living apartments as publicly owned housing was passed in the Senate and referred to the Finance Committee. Rents could be no more than 30% of a resident's income, and a local match would be required (Anderson, 2001).

The U.S. Bureau of Census estimates that approximately 6.5 million people 65 years of age and over currently need assistance with their activities of daily living (ADLs). That number is predicted to double by 2020 (Minnesota Health & Housing Alliance, 1999).

Although the federal government does not regulate assisted living facilities, most states have detailed regulations. For example, in Minnesota,

assisted living providers that offer personal care and similar health-related services have specific requirements for registered nurses whenever nursing or delegated nursing services are being performed in assisted living settings. When such services are being provided, the home care regulations require that the registered nurses conduct regular assessments of clients, develop and keep an up-to-date appropriate service plan, orient each unlicensed staff person to each client before that staff person provides any care, and regularly monitor the care and the unlicensed staff that provides it (Anderson, 2000).

The number of assisted living programs rises as the elderly choose to have assistance with ADLs in a less hospital-like setting. This has resulted in less growth for skilled nursing homes (Adler, 1999). According to one report the expense for a resident in assisted living institutions is $45 to $50 per day (Moore, 1999)—cheaper than nursing home care.

COMMUNITY SERVICES

There are probably as many varieties of community-based visitation, support, and service programs as there are communities in the United States. Some are highly organized and well funded; others are loosely knit groups of self-directed volunteers.

Categories of Services

Services may be sponsored by churches or synagogues, senior or health centers, fraternal or social groups, businesses, city councils, or other community-based programs. They frequently are nonprofit, have a core professional staff, and rely heavily on volunteers and donations. Services offered may include the following:

- Emergency assistance with food, clothing, or shelter
- Dental care, podiatry, exercise, and nutrition
- Day care, which may or may not include medical care or counseling
- Consumer protection
- Alcohol and drug programs
- Home-delivered or on-site meals
- Handicapped services or equipment
- Homemaking and home repair
- Legal and financial services
- Mental health services

- Transportation
- Volunteer opportunities
- Recreation-education centers
- Support groups (cancer, heart disease, Alzheimer's, widows/widowers)
- Co-ops
- Counseling services
- Respite care

Accessing Community-Based Services

The challenge for home health care professionals is in helping their clients to access community-based services. While choices of programs may be relatively straightforward in smaller communities, the array of programs in a large metropolitan area is often mind-boggling.

Some community-originated programs serve special needs or geographic areas. For example, both the block nurse program and On Lok Services are limited nationally. Also, most of the major disease organizations have materials and services that they will provide at the client's request.

Financial and Guardianship Issues

Confusion and diminished mental capacity in elderly clients can affect their ability to manage their own affairs. There are, however, legal options to ensure that the basic needs of an incapacitated client are met and that physical or financial abuse does not occur.

Two forms of protective intervention procedures the court can establish are conservatorship and guardianship. The court appoints a conservator or guardian who is answerable to it and to the client. "The terms may seem similar, but the two types of authorization differ from each other in legal meaning, in the amount of protection afforded, and in the degree of self-determination and personal liberty for the protected person" (Trabosh, 1986). A *conservator* acts as a trustee of the financial affairs of the client, managing assets and providing for his or her financial support. A *guardian* protects or "guards" an incapacitated client, assuming full care and custody for him or her, much as a parent for a child, and making all personal care decisions. A guardian can manage funds up to a total of $10,000 in income and assets if a conservator has not been appointed.

Conservatorship   A conservatorship is the least restrictive legal protection for an individual client. It is appropriate when an elderly client appears to be unable to deal appropriately with money. Such things as not paying bills, writing inappropriate checks, or giving away money but refusing to spend it on food and living conditions may indicate that an elderly client needs someone to manage his or her finances. Exploitation by family members who want to use the elderly client's finances for themselves or who neglect the client's care to conserve money for future inheritance are other situations in which a conservatorship may be appropriate. A conservator also might be appropriate when there are no relatives and the client is alone.

The conservator takes possession of all property of substantial value that the protected client has and acts in his or her best interests. The conservator works closely with an attorney and with specialists in investments, real estate, and other fields to ensure that all transactions are properly conducted to sustain or increase the protected client's assets. The conservator needs to establish trust and a rapport with the client. The conservator also needs to understand the client's needs and wants to be certain that present or future living arrangements meet those needs (Trabosh, 1986).

The duties of a conservator can include paying bills, investing money for the best and safest return, and working to ensure there is sufficient money to provide for the present and future needs of the protected client. Conservatorships also can involve far more complicated situations. A conservator is authorized to repair, lease, buy, or sell property; run or liquidate a business; pay, collect, or contest claims for or against the protected client; borrow money to protect the client's assets; pay money for the support of those who are dependent on the protected client; make charitable contributions on the client's behalf; and perform other financial transactions that are necessary for the protected client (Trabosh, 1986).

A conservator is bonded. Accurate records are made and kept of each transaction he or she performs on behalf of the protected client. These are presented annually to the court for review and approval, and they also may be reviewed by family members and by the protected client. This accountability factor is an important safeguarding difference between a conservatorship and a power of attorney, which is a written statement by an individual giving another person authority to act for him or her in financial transactions and business (Trabosh, 1986).

Guardianship   Since guardianship permits another person to determine what is best for the protected client and to assume control over all facets of his or her life, the court tries to verify that guardianship is necessary before establishing it. The court appoints an objective third person to visit the elderly client to determine if guardianship is needed. The court visitor also contacts the proposed guardian to find out if he or she is qualified and understands the importance of the role of guardian (Trabosh, 1986).

While guardianship is a drastic measure for the elderly adult client, it may be the only option for a client made helpless by stroke, mental illness, or disease. The client may be completely unable to make decisions for himself or herself, and a court-appointed guardian may be necessary to decide what living arrangement would be best for the client.

Far too often, guardianship is considered necessary because it is the only legal option people know about. The less restrictive conservatorship, which permits retention of self-determination for personal needs, may be more desirable for the elderly client who still can function on some levels.

Whichever legal method is used to ensure that the basic needs of the elderly client are met, the human element plays a major role. Conservators or guardians must get to know their charges as they are at present, appreciate them, care for them, visit often, and be concerned for their welfare. Abuse in any living arrangement can be detected only by frequent, unannounced visits. Situations also can change rapidly in an elderly client's physical and mental health, and these often can be better observed by an objective person who is not present daily. Professional conservators and guardians specifically trained in, or with experience in, law or accounting may be available for a reasonable cost.

Informal Support Systems

There is a whole network of informal (volunteer, not affiliated with a program or agency) support care providers available for most clients. They are the family members, trusted friends and neigh-

bors, people the client has helped, community or church volunteers, people at the grocery store or drugstore who know the client, former colleagues—the list is different for everyone (Blues, Zerwekh, 1984). Often these people are willing to help or stop by and visit but do not know the client's needs.

Caregivers should encourage the client to make a list of people he or she used to see or know, particularly those he or she has helped in times of need. These people should be informed that the client might like visitors, an outing, or an errand. Perhaps some of them will be grateful for the chance to help out.

The home health care professional can be essential in prioritizing and screening prospective programs so that those with criteria matching client needs and qualifications can be recommended. The Good Neighbor Project was a collaborative effort between the Visiting Nurse Association/Hospice and the Allen Temple Baptist Church in San Francisco. After training, 68 volunteers donated more than 10,000 service hours to 55 elderly African-American clients (Brown-Hunter, Price 1998). These volunteers took the clients shopping and to the physician's office and provided friendship.

SUMMARY

Nurse-directed systems of care can be provided in a variety of settings and especially in the home. While having a range of options available is a decided advantage for the client and his or her family, careful and informed decision making about these options is essential to appropriate care. This requires accurate information about patient and family needs for the formulation of realistic parameters for both program and family participation.

REFERENCES

Adler S: The CLTC 50-plus, *Contemporary Longterm Care* 22(4):36-38, 40, 43-48, 1999.

Alexty E: Computers and caregiving: Reaching out and redesigning interventions for homebound older adults and caregivers, *Holistic Nursing Practice* 14(4):60-66, 2000.

Anderson P, ed: *Monday Mailing: news from the Minnesota Health and Housing Alliance,* 2550 University Ave. West, Suite 350S, St Paul, MN 55114-1902; telephone 1-800-462-5368.

Badger TA, Collins-Joyce P: Depression, psychosocial resources, and functional ability in older adults, *Clinical Nursing Research* 9(3):238-255, 2000.

Bear M, Burnell M, Covell M: Using a nursing framework to establish a nurse-managed senior health clinic, *Journal of Community Health Nursing* 14(4):225-235, 1997.

Blues A, Zerwekh J: *Hospice and palliative nursing care,* New York, 1984, Grune & Stratton.

Brown-Hunter M, Price L: The Good Neighbor Project: volunteerism and the elderly African-American patient with cancer, *Geriatric Nursing* 19(3):139-141, 1998.

Buijs R, Olson J: Parish nurses influencing determinants of health, *Journal of Community Health Nursing* 18(1):13-23, 2001.

Department of Health and Human Services: *Aging* (2150216), Washington DC, 1986.

Dougherty G, Soderstrom L, Schiffrin A: An economic evaluation of home care for children with newly diagnosed diabetes, *Medical Care* 36(4):586-598, 1998.

Durtschi A: Three patients' tele-home care experiences, *Home Healthcare Nurse* 19(1):9-11, 2001.

Editorial: Where is assisted living headed? *Contemporary Long Term Care* ••:••, 1999.

Faison KJ, Faria SH, Frank D: Caregivers of chronically ill elderly: Perceived burden, *Journal of Community Health Nursing* 16(4):243-253, 1999.

Gebus VC: Home care of the infant or child requiring tube feeding. In Ahmann E, ed: *Home care for the high risk infant,* ed 2, Gaithersburg, Md, 1997, Aspen.

Giampaoli S: Epidemiology of major age-related diseases in women compared to men, *Aging* 12(2):93-102, 2000.

Goforth L: Paying the piper: The crisis in chronic care, *Home Health Care Services Quarterly* 18(3):1-21, 2000.

Gold DB, Anderson DR, Serxner SA: Impact of a telephone-based intervention on the reduction of health risks, *American Journal of Health Promotion* 15(2):97-106, 2000.

Halls M, Highley B: Adult day health care. In Gilliss C et al, eds: *Family nursing,* New York, 1987, Appleton-Century-Crofts.

Hatcher P, Scarinzi G, Kreider M: Primary health care: a primary health care model for a community-based/nurse managed health center, *Nursing Health Care Perspective* 19(1):12-19, 1998.

Hayward MD et al: The significance of socioeconomic status in explaining the racial gap in chronic health conditions, *American Sociological Review* 65(6):910-930, 2000.

Henly S et al: Innovative perspectives on health services for vulnerable rural populations, *Family Community Health* 21(1):22-31, 1998.

Ingold B et al: Characteristics associated with inappropriate hospital use in elderly patients admitted to a general internal medicine service, *Aging* 12(6):430-438, 2000.

Kleh J: Community and medical resources. In O'Hara et al, eds: *Eldercare,* New York, 1981, Grune & Stratton.

Leveille SG, Resnick H, Balfour J: Gender differences in disability: evidence and underlying reasons, *Aging* 12(2):106-111, 2000.

Lundeen S: Comprehensive, collaborative, coordinated, community-based care: A community nursing center model, *Journal of Family Community Health* 16(2):59-67, 1993.

Lundeen S: An alternative paradigm for promoting health in communities: The Lundeen Community Nursing Center model, *Family Community Health* 21(4):15-28, 1999.

Martinson I: Improving care of dying children, *Western Journal of Medicine,* 163(3):258-262, 1995.

Martinson I: An international perspective on palliative care for children, *Journal of Palliative Care* 12(3):13-15, 1996a.

Martinson I: Pediatric hospice nursing. In Fitzpatrick J, Stevenson J, eds: *Annual review of nursing research,* vol 14, New York, 1996b, Springer.

Maurana C, Rodney M: Strategies for developing a successful community health advocate program, *Community Health* 23(1):40-49, 2000.

McDermott J: Day care for the elderly overlooked, *Oregonian* (Section C) January 1986.

Mitchell RE, Trickett EJ: Social networks as mediators of social support, *Community Mental Health Journal* 16:27-44, 1983.

Moore J: Fiscal exercise, *Contemporary Long Term Care* 22(8):25-26, 1999.

Oermann M, Harris C, Dammeyer J: Teaching by the nurse: how important is it to patients? *Applied Nursing Research* 14(1):11-17, 2001.

Oregon Senate Bill 519, 1985, Committee on Human Resources.

Orem DE: The self care deficit theory of nursing: A general theory. In Clements I, Roberts S, eds: *Family nursing,* New York, 1983, John Wiley.

Palmer J: Parish nursing: connecting faith & health, *Reflections on Nursing Leadership* 27(1):17-19, 2001.

Pokorni J: Promoting the overall development of infants and young children receiving home health services, *Pediatric Nursing* 23(2):187-190, 1997.

Reutter L: Family health assessment: An integrated approach, *Journal of Advanced Nursing* 9:391-399, July 1984.

Rich M: The PACE model: Prescription and impressions of the capitated model of long-term care of the elderly, *The Care Management Journal* 1(1):62-70, 1999.

Smith BK: *Adult day care—extended family,* Austin, Tex, 1981, Haag Foundation.

Solari-Twadell P, McDermott M: *Parish nursing,* Thousand Oaks, Calif, 1998, Sage Publications.

Stewart B, Archbold P: Putting families in the driver's seat: Linking family and home health nursing care, *The Third International Home Care Nursing Conference Proceedings,* Seoul, Korea, 1998.

The Provider, Richmond Va, 1985, National Association Residential Care Facilities.

Thralow U, Watson CG: Remotivation for geriatric patients using elementary school students, *The American Journal of Occupational Therapy* 28(8):469-473, 1974.

Trabosh V: A legal solution for the financial and guardianship issues for the elderly, *Institute for Health Care Economics Quarterly Review* 2:10-20, 1986.

Wolfe W: How best to care for the elderly? *Star Tribune,* Jan 18, 2001

Wunderlich G, Sloan F, Davis C, eds: *Nursing staff in hospitals & nursing homes,* Washington DC, 1996, National Academy Press.

5 Managed Care

Jeannee Parker Martin

Manage (to direct, control, or handle; to administer or regulate; to contrive or arrange)
Care (to have or show regard, interest, or concern as respecting some person, thing, or event) (Funk, Wagnalls, 1980)

"Managed care is a system of health care which places limits and restrictions on the use of services for purposes of creating efficiencies or reducing costs" (Hoss, Eklund, 1994). Although once a term reserved to describe the utilization and payment methodologies of just a few health insurance providers, *managed care* now encompasses all public and private payor groups. Client care is directed, controlled, or otherwise arranged in nearly every segment of health care delivery. In fact, it is unusual to have full access to health care without some arrangement through a payor organization. As this concept has evolved, managed care has grown to include not only payment for health care services, but also the manner in which care is administered and delivered. Key elements of the administration, payment methods, and delivery of managed care are described in this chapter.

EVOLUTION OF MANAGED CARE, 1863 TO 1999 (SMITH, 1994; BALDNOR, 1994)
Late Nineteenth Century

Elementary forms of the managed-care concept emerged in the late 1800s. It is in the late 1900s, however, that the term *managed care* began to describe sophisticated administrative, clinical, and payment systems for health care delivery in both the public and private sectors.

A century ago, case-management services delivered by public health nurses focused on access to care by the poor. This rudimentary approach to managed care touched merely on clinical care issues. There was no apparent need to focus on controlling use or costs of care delivery. Rather, there was a desire to make care available to the poor and working classes, since health care at the time was paid out-of-pocket by individuals.

Nurses were instrumental in this early adaptation of managed care delivery. Few other providers showed the same interest or compassion in caring for the poor. None better illustrated this interest than the early work of visiting nurse associations throughout the United States. These nursing organizations were formed to help manage access to care by the poor in large cities, such as Boston, New York, and San Francisco.

Post–World War I

Health cooperatives and health plans in the post–World War I era formed the first organizational structures for managed care delivery. The Group Health Association and Kaiser-Permanente Medical Group are examples of early organized health care. By the early 1950s, attention began to focus on quality care delivery with the inception of the Joint Commission on Accreditation of Healthcare Organizations (JCAHO, originally known as the Joint Commission on Accreditation of Hospitals). With this early focus on access, cost, and quality, the foundation for today's managed care plans was created.

Late Twentieth Century to Early Twenty-First Century

At present, most Americans have access to care through public or private insurance companies, and most receive managed care. The poor and elderly have limited access to health care services provided through two federally mandated programs: Medicaid for the poor and Medicare for the elderly. From their introduction in 1965 until 1983, these programs reimbursed health care providers on a fee-for-service basis. As private insurance companies formed, they followed the payment methodologies of the public payors. Fee-for-service programs allow providers to bill public and private insurance programs for each unit of service provided.

In fee-for-service payment programs, health care providers have indirect incentives to increase units of service so that they can receive more reimbursement. For example, if a client has a catastrophic or chronic illness, the health care provider may keep the client in the hospital longer, provide more laboratory tests, and offer more clinic-based services. If more invasive procedures are performed in the physician's office, the physician receives more reimbursement for these fee-for-service procedures. In the home care setting, the provider may render more nursing or home health aide visits. Since fee-for-service payment programs do not generally encourage utilization management (UM), the costs of care delivery quickly increase.

In response to rising health care costs in the fee-for-service environment, Medicare adopted a new payment system for hospitals, known as the diagnostic related group (DRG) program in 1983. The program established payment rates for diagnostic groups regardless of the services provided, length of hospital stay, or ancillary service needed by the client. Largely as a result of the DRG program, private payors responded with fervor by introducing managed care.

Since the early 1980s, private insurance payors have tried various formulas to impact the pricing of care delivery and to manage utilization efforts to contain rising health care costs. Since the 1990s, attempts have also been made to affect the quality of health care through outcomes management. To establish outcomes-management criteria, the Medicare program has adopted OASIS (Outcomes Assessment and Information Set) standards for intermittent home health care and JCAHO has implemented ORYX (not an acronym). More than 100 years after rudimentary beginnings, the managed care triad—access, quality, and cost—is complete. (Refer to Appendix A for more information.)

ADMINISTRATION OF MANAGED-CARE SERVICES
Insurance Case Managers

As catastrophic diseases such as acquired immune deficiency syndrome (AIDS) and Alzheimer's disease proliferated during the 1980s, private insurance companies negotiated directly with individual health care providers to tailor insurance payments for individual clients. Through insurance case managers, this labor-intensive effort helped ensure access to care for clients who had complex and costly illnesses in settings appropriate to their needs. More important, it helped private insurance payors manage the price of care through direct negotiations and in apparent collaboration with the health care provider. Insurance case managers began to wield authority to determine how much, and where, care would be delivered. It became apparent, though, that individual negotiations were impossible for millions of insured clients nationwide.

Managed-Care Organizations

With their origins dating back to the late 1800s, thousands of formal managed-care organizations (MCOs) exist today. Despite a federally mandated Medicare program that first embraced the managed-care concept with the inception of DRGs in 1983, publicly funded programs lag far behind private insurance companies in the implementation of cutting-edge programs. In fact, publicly funded programs, mired in legislative and regulatory issues, have taken more than 15 years to prepare for the implementation of a prospective payment system (PPS) for the Medicare home health program. In contrast, during this same period, private insurance companies have forged ahead to ensure access, cost, and quality to their members/enrollees, including programs for Medicare-eligible patients (Medicare senior risk programs). The Centers for Medicare and Medicaid Services (CMS) (formerly the Health Care Financing Administration, [HCFA]), which administers the Medicare program, pays managed-care organizations directly for these senior risk programs.

Generally, MCOs can be described as one of two types of organizations: payor-based organizations and provider-based organizations. Payor-based organizations include health maintenance organizations (HMOs), preferred provider organizations (PPOs), third-party administrators (TPAs), self-insured employers, and worker compensation administrators. Provider-based organizations include health systems, hospitals, physician groups, home care organizations, and other alternative-site service providers (Coleman, 1993; Hoss, Ekland, 1994; Smith, 1994).

Payor-Based Organizations

There are several types of payor-based organizations, but two are the most prominent: HMOs and PPOs. In 1997 there were 461 HMOs with more than 70 million enrollees and 1035 PPOs with more than 89 million eligible employees in the United States (Hoechst, 1998).

HMOs "An HMO is an organized system of health care that accepts responsibility to deliver an agreed upon set of comprehensive and coordinated health services to a group of voluntarily enrolled persons in exchange for an agreed upon fixed periodic payment" (Coleman, 1993). The HMO combines responsibility for financing and service delivery in one organization. It assumes the full risk of providing services, regardless of the extent of services required. HMOs are regulated by state and federal laws and are voluntarily monitored by the National Committee for Quality Assurance (NCQA). Structures of HMOs differ, however, and are dictated by the HMOs' primary sponsors (e.g., hospitals, physician groups, private insurance companies, businesses, labor organizations). There are five general structures for HMOs*:

- Staff Model HMO: The staff model HMO delivers health care services through physicians who are full-time employees of the HMO. The HMO, rather than the physicians, is at full risk for the costs of care delivery. Physicians in a staff model HMO care only for clients in the HMO. Kaiser Permanente is the nation's oldest example of a staff model HMO.
- Group Model HMO: The group model HMO contracts with an independent multi-specialty group of physicians to serve HMO clients. The physicians are employees of the group practice, not of the HMO. The HMO negotiates the payment rates with the physician group on a capitated or reduced fee-for-service amount. Physicians in a group model HMO may care for clients in other HMOs or clients whose care is paid for under other insurance plans.
- Network Model HMO: The network model HMO contracts with two or more independent groups of physicians to provide health services. A network is predominately organized around physician group practices, although some network members may be in solo practice. The HMO negotiates the payment rates to the physician group on a capitated or reduced fee-for-service amount. Physicians in a network model HMO may care for clients in other HMOs or clients whose care is paid for under other insurance plans.
- Independent Practice Association (IPA) Model HMO: This is the predominate HMO model and has one or more of the following characteristics:
  - The HMO contracts directly with physicians in independent practices.
  - The HMO contracts with one or more associations of physicians in independent practices.
  - The HMO contracts with one or more multi-specialty group practices.
  - The plan is predominately organized around solo and small group fee-for-service practices.
- Hybrid or Mixed Model HMO: This model is a mixture of a staff and group model HMO, a staff and IPA model HMO, or a group and IPA model HMO. These HMOs are able to serve extensive geographic areas, yet may have more complicated contracting and risk-sharing agreements.

It will be difficult to discern distinct HMO models as providers and payors attempt to meet the diverse needs of physically and socially complex client situations.

PPOs A PPO is an organization that contracts with a group or network of providers. The PPO negotiates discounted rates in exchange for provider services and increased volumes of business to the provider. The PPO member/enrollee may use participating or nonparticipating (nonpar) PPO providers; however, when using nonpar providers, the member/enrollee will have increased out-of-pocket expenses.

---

*From Coleman J: *The Managed Care Workbook: How to get started on the never ending road to managed care,* Overland Park, Kan, 1993, Corridor Media.

Other MCOs In addition to HMOs and PPOs, there are several other managed care payor-type organizations. TPAs are service bureau companies that specialize in managing the benefits package of self-insured companies. TPAs do not provide services, nor do they establish the benefits provided. Rather, TPAs discuss benefits with members/enrollees, review claims, and pay claims for self-insured companies. Self-insured companies typically are large employers who assume full risk of health care delivery for their employees. A self-insured company usually contracts directly with external providers to manage and deliver care to their clients. In essence, a self-insured company will pay a hospital, physician, or home care provider directly or through the TPA.

Provider-Based Organizations

Provider-based organizations provide service directly and assume the financial risk of service delivery. Provider-based organizations are hospitals, physician groups, home care providers, and other alternate-site providers who contract with payors directly and share risk for the cost of service delivery.

PAYMENT FOR MANAGED-CARE SERVICES

To understand the payment arrangements for managed-care services, it is imperative to understand the financial risks and economic incentives that are the driving forces of MCOs.

Financial Risks

The goal of MCOs is to keep costs lower than the premiums collected. If the costs of providing health care services are higher than the premiums collected, the MCO will experience financial loss. The MCO must apply tight controls over the management and delivery of care to ensure that costs are controlled. Therefore it is reasonable that MCOs desire a limited yet comprehensive spectrum of providers to encompass their provider panel, including physicians, hospitals, skilled nursing facilities, home care organizations, hospices, and other alternate-site providers and facilities. The MCOs limit the number of providers to facilitate control of the costs and quality of the provider panel. In addition, limiting the number of providers also helps ensure that each provider benefits from maximizing client referrals and physician productivity.

Because inadequate financial analyses have been undertaken to understand the total costs of care delivery (using different entry points into the health care system), diverse intervention methodologies, and diverse provider settings, there are no conclusive data that truly guide payor organizations or providers in their care delivery decisions. Rather, anecdotal information and a few empirical studies suggest that alternative-site care delivery is less costly than inpatient facility care. It can only be assumed that this should be true in most circumstances, other than certain catastrophic diseases (i.e., AIDS, Alzheimer's) that might be managed more cost-effectively in long-term care facilities. Until more conclusive studies are completed, it will be difficult to determine how the total cost of care is impacted by inpatient and alternate-site services, including all pharmaceuticals, home medical equipment, and other ancillary products.

Financial Incentives

MCOs must tightly control utilization and cost of care delivery to ensure that revenues from premiums exceed expenses each month. Depending on the specific payment arrangement, physicians, hospitals, and other providers may benefit through distributions of excess revenue and increasingly coordinated care delivery.

Payment methods There are various payment methods that shift financial risks and benefits between payors and providers. The most common payment methods follow:

1. Fee-for-service. The provider is paid a fee for each service or product rendered. This fee-for-service payment method is typically based on the usual and customary rates (UCRs) set by the insurance company for a specific service or product. The provider will not receive more than the UCR and may receive a fraction of the UCR, depending on payor payment policies. Hence, the provider may lose money if the provider's charges exceed the UCR. Other providers may be paid on a lower-of-costs-or-charges (LCC) basis, with a payment limit established by the payor.

2. Discounted fee-for-service: Outside publicly funded programs, discounted fee-for-service payment is the most common payment method at present. The payor and provider negotiate a specific discounted fee for services and are often bound by a contract between the payor and provider. The fee may be a dis-

counted rate from the UCR or another negotiated fee based on payor demands. Under a discounted fee-for-service arrangement, the provider assumes little risk for the care delivery costs, although there may be financial liability if the negotiated rates do not cover the provider's own costs of care delivery. This payment method spans all health care provider types, and its rate setting is highly dependent on the sophistication of the payor and provider environment.

3. DRGs: The hospital provider is paid based on the Medicare client's DRG. The provider receives this fixed payment regardless of the client's length of stay or treatment. DRGs were implemented exclusively for hospitals, although DRG-like payment rates for other providers have been implemented. The Medicare home health PPS program, implemented in October 2000, takes into account disease-specific categories as one element of the payment methodology.

4. Capitation: The provider is paid a fixed monthly fee for each member of the MCO, also known as a per-member per-month payment (pmpm). Regardless of use levels, the amount is based on the total number or a portion of the total number of members enrolled in the MCO rather than quantity or length of service required by an individual member. Although the provider may negotiate with the MCO based on age, sex, and disease history of the MCO members, the provider will ultimately accept a fixed pmpm. The provider assumes financial risk for the services it delivers but does not generally share financial risk for total costs of care delivery with the MCO.

5. Risk sharing arrangements: The provider shares a portion of the financial risk with the payor. The payor pays the provider on a pmpm basis and withholds a certain amount of reimbursement. The amount withheld is known as the *withhold*. This withhold is then distributed to the provider if certain preestablished financial goals are achieved. Such goals relate to hospital length of stay, utilization patterns by specific providers, use of ancillary services, and physician productivity as measured against other physicians participating in the plan. Withholds are distributed to the provider on an annual or other periodic basis.

6. Per diem: The provider is paid a fixed amount for each day the client receives care. There may be separate per-diem rates for different types of service rendered (e.g., medical, surgical, pediatric, maternity) or the per-diem rate may be all encompassing (all services and products rendered). This payment method is common for ancillary service providers such as pharmacy infusion and hospice.

7. Per episode: The provider is paid a fixed amount based on an episode of illness that may span different provider types over a period of time and include multiple admissions. This is considered one of the most promising, albeit most challenging, payment methods. This payment method is part of the Medicare home health PPS program. Under PPS, the provider is paid for an episode of illness that spans a predetermined number of days and is not related to the number of admissions to home care.

8. Per case: The provider is paid a fixed amount based on an admission category regardless of the quantity or type of services. The provider is paid for each admission of the client. This payment method is rarely used because appropriate rates are difficult to establish.

Other payment methods have been tried, and new payment methods will undoubtedly be developed in the future. It is likely that any new payment method will combine elements of those listed as more studies clarify the risks and benefits of certain methods and minimize the financial risks to both payors and providers. Figure 5-1 illustrates the general level of risks associated with different payment methods.

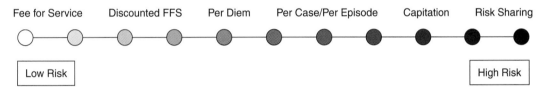

Fig. 5-1   Payment approaches and associated levels of risk. *(From Coleman J:* The managed care workbook: How to get started on the never ending road to managed care, *Overland Park, Kan, 1993, Corridor Media.)*

DELIVERY OF MANAGED-CARE SERVICES AND IMPLICATIONS FOR HOME CARE

Since 1965, Medicare has been the predominate payor of home care providers—intermittent home health care, hospice, and durable medical equipment providers. Despite the economic benefits of the Medicare cost-based, fee-for-service payment system, some home care providers took risks to be on the leading edge of health care delivery in their service areas. These pioneers recognized the need to collaborate with payors and other health care providers to help control access, cost, and quality of care delivery. These home care providers blazed the trail in the following areas:

1. Understanding what MCOs need from home care providers and what services they are willing to pay for
2. Understanding the direct and indirect costs of doing business (delivering home care services)
3. Implementing contract negotiation techniques to procure managed care contracts and capture market share
4. Implementing case-management programs that work with, not against, MCO representatives
5. Implementing disease-state management programs that complement other health care providers in the MCO care delivery continuum
6. Understanding that the relationship must be a "win-win" relationship for it to succeed and that such a "win-win" relationship requires compromise on both sides of the bargaining table

Understanding What MCOs Need and Want

Over the course of a few years, industry experts went from advising home care providers to approach every MCO in their service area to advising them to proceed with caution in their contracting activities. Once considered the only way a home care provider could survive, some contractual arrangements proved fatal, causing organizations to close because of low payment rates.

It is imperative that home care providers understand what the MCO needs and wants before approaching the organization for a contract. It is also imperative that they understand what the MCO is willing to pay for before entering into contract negotiations. MCOs generally need two critical elements from a provider:

- The ability to help control costs of care delivery to their members
- The ability to enhance or expand their network of providers in service capacity and geographic coverage

MCOs also want other elements to complement their service package:

- Comprehensive continuum of care delivery
- Disease state management programs
- Utilization review and UM
- Centralized billing and financial management for a network or system of provider organizations
- Negotiated and discounted payment rates, particularly discounted fee-for-service and capitation
- State licensure (when applicable), Medicare certification, and accreditation by JCAHO or Community Health Accreditation Program (CHAP)

Home care providers able to address both the needs and wants of MCOs will find themselves in the best negotiating position. Home care providers who offer seamless and comprehensive home care service and product lines; who have centralized administrative functions, such as intake and referral, billing, quality management, and performance improvement; who have implemented sophisticated client-management techniques in UM, disease-state management and specialty programs, and outcomes measurements; *and* who cover broad regional service areas will find themselves in an enviable position with MCOs. These home care providers will able to position themselves as desirable partners with MCOs *if* their costs of care delivery are low and will strengthen the overall financial position of the MCO.

MCOs now commonly understand the importance of home care delivery on the care delivery spectrum. Since the majority of services are provided by hospitals and physicians, MCOs still may focus little attention on negotiating contract rates with home care providers. Instead they may include home care as an add-on to an existing hospital contract or physician group contract. If the home care provider aggressively educates the hospital or physician group contracting department, their sponsors will be better prepared to negotiate appropriate payment terms into the contract language. If the home care provider fails to educate the contract negotiators in the benefits and costs of home care service delivery, the payment rates may be ill fated and harm the financial position of the home care provider.

Understanding Direct and Indirect Costs of Doing Business

Home care providers historically have failed to document and understand their costs of doing business. Providers are ill prepared to negotiate reasonable contract rates if they do not evaluate their costs of doing business relative to services being contracted. Questions the home care provider must answer before beginning contract negotiations include the following:

- What is the payor composition by client discharged from the home care provider?
- What is the total (direct plus indirect) cost of care by discharge?
- What is the total (direct plus indirect) cost of care by top 10 diagnoses by discharge?
- What is the total (direct plus indirect) cost of an intermittent home care visit by payor group?
- What is the total (direct plus indirect) cost of an intermittent home care visit by discipline?
- What are the actual administrative and indirect costs of each of the above items?
- What are the actual clinical care and direct costs of each of the above items?
- Are the home care provider's top 10 diagnoses consistent with the top 10 diagnoses served by the MCO?
- Does the home care provider have, or can it develop, disease-specialty programs to complement the diagnoses served by the MCO?
- Based on the above analysis, what payment rates will the home care provider accept for services delivered to MCO clients?

Implementing Contract Negotiation Techniques

The most difficult component of contracting is negotiating the arrangement that meets the needs of the MCO as well as the needs of the home care provider. The home care provider must be able to influence the MCO decision to use it as the preferred or exclusive home care

provider. If a discounted fee-for-service arrangement is desirable, a preferred-provider arrangement may be easier to negotiate. If the home care provider is hoping for an exclusive arrangement, it may be necessary to assume more financial risk through a capitation agreement or through a risk-sharing agreement with the MCO. In either case, the home care provider must understand the nuances of the MCO to negotiate the best terms. By answering the following questions about the MCO, the home care provider will be able to negotiate a contract that helps it procure a relationship and capture market share:

- What type of MCO is it negotiating with (i.e., HMO, PPO, staff model) and who owns the organization? Is it for-profit or not-for-profit?
- What is the service area the MCO covers and how much of the service area will the home care provider be expected to cover?
- What are the specific populations served (i.e., payor groups, members, ages, diseases)?
- Who are the participating hospitals and physician groups? What is the composition of physicians by primary care and specialty care?
- Has the MCO contracted with other home care providers? What payment methods has it used (i.e., fee-for-service, capitation) and what rates did it negotiate?
- How does the MCO control utilization and costs of care delivery?

Implementing Case-Management Programs

The home care provider must illustrate its ability to manage utilization and deliver care effectively and efficiently to clients. Home care nurses represent the foundation of case management, dating back to the late 1800s. It is through skilled intervention and understanding of the physical, psychological, and social demands on clients that nurses remain at the helm of case management.

Managed-care representatives must be educated on the body of knowledge and skill level of home care nurses to anticipate the needs of the client and to intervene at the appropriate times. By using interdisciplinary teams, home care nurse case managers are able to facilitate intervention by other disciplines to address the rehabilitative, custodial, and psychosocial needs of clients. The home care provider must develop rapport with the managed-care representatives to ensure that home care nurse case managers guide and manage care delivery. In this way, home care nurses can effectively manage client outcomes to positively impact the costs of care, rather than be driven by decisions of less knowledgeable managed-care representatives.

Implementing Disease-State Management Programs

Perhaps the most fundamental way home care providers can complement the services of other health care providers is through aggressive development of disease-state management programs. Home care providers are experienced in providing specialty services, but these are rarely sophisticated disease-management programs with advanced practice nurses. Existing specialty programs should be enhanced to create an interdisciplinary team approach guided by advanced practice nurses. These programs should encompass standardized clinical processes that can be tailored to meet the nuances of a specific client and standardized policies that allow home care nurses the authority and autonomy to work closely with other health care providers. Together, providers along the care delivery continuum can develop a plan of care that addresses the client's physical needs in an appropriate care setting and that allows for change in the course of care without extensive reauthorization but with accountability and management of client outcomes to control costs and utilization.

Understanding that the Relationship Must Be "Win-Win"

The most important element of any relationship is to ensure that it is a "win-win" situation for the parties involved. The benefits to the home care provider and to the MCO must outweigh the risks of entering into a relationship. Neither party can feel that it is unjustly compromised. The home care provider should not assume that the MCO understands the full scope of its potential to manage cases, to reduce and control costs, to expand service delivery, and to broaden the scope of services provided by the MCO. A "win-win" situation requires education and compromise on both sides of the bargaining table. The resulting contractual relationship will serve the needs of clients, payors, and providers.

SUMMARY

Managed care has evolved over the past century into sophisticated health care management systems, including administrative, clinical, and payment components. It now encompasses insurance programs in both the public and private sectors and more complex requirements for measuring client outcomes to justify care delivery.

Home care providers are central to care delivery along a continuum of health care services and play an essential role in helping MCOs control costs. By being better informed about their costs of doing business, by preparing thoroughly for contract negotiations, and by developing progressive disease-management programs, home care providers can influence MCOs in service-delivery decisions.

Managed care is neither a wave of the future nor a thing of the past. Rather, all care is managed with increasingly equal attention to access, cost, and quality of delivery. Under the rubric that care be provided in the most efficient and cost-effective manner to all persons, home care providers can assist with sophisticated interventions at home and collaborate with other health care providers to manage care for clients along a continuum of care.

REFERENCES*

Baldor RA: *Managed care made simple,* Cambridge, Mass, 1994, Blackwell.

Coleman J: *The managed care workbook: How to get started on the never ending road to managed care,* Overland Park, Kan, 1993, Corridor Media.

Funk & Wagnalls new comprehensive international dictionary of the English language, New York, 1980, JG Ferguson Publishing.

Hoechst Marion Roussel Managed Care Digest Series 1998: *HMO-PPO/Medicare/Medicaid Digest, Institutional Digest, Integrated Health System Digest, Medical Group Practice Digest,* Kansas City, Mo, 1998, Hoechst Marion Roussel.

Hoss S, Eklund K, ed: *Managed care guide,* Beaverton, Ore, 1994, Mosby.

Smith N: Managed care. In Harris MD, ed: *Handbook of home health care administration,* Gaithersburg, Md, 1994, Aspen.

*All Corridor Media references and excerpts are used with permission. Similarities to the text of the *Managed Care Workbook* are intentional and have been made with permission. Jeannee Parker Martin is the president and co-owner of The Corridor Group, Inc.

Growth and Development of Managed Care (Baldnor, 1994)

- 1863 Case management was defined through social work systems to coordinate public human services and conserve public funds.
- 1900 Case management started as a part of public health nursing.
- 1929 A rural farmers' cooperative health plan was established in Oklahoma.
- 1929 Two California physicians entered into a prepaid contract to provide comprehensive health care to 2000 water company employees.
- 1937 The Group Health Association (GHA) was founded in Washington.
- 1942 The Kaiser Permanente medical care program was established to provide health care to employees of Kaiser steel and ship building companies.
- 1945 After World War II, necessary community services were extended to discharged psychiatric clients.
- 1947 The Health Insurance Plan of Greater New York was begun.
- 1950s Employee assistance programs (EAPs) were started as an occupational health service for alcoholics.
- 1950 The Hill-Burton Act created a number of community-based regional medical centers.
- 1951 The Joint Commission on the Accreditation of Healthcare Organizations (JCAHO) (originally known as the Joint Commission on Accreditation of Hospitals) was formed.
- 1954 One of the first Independent Practice Association (IPA) plans was started in California.
- 1963 Community mental health center programs were initiated.
- 1965 Medical Assistance (Medicaid) was established by the federal government to provide health care services to the poor.
- 1965 Medicare was established by the federal government to ensure health care access for the elderly.
- 1965 The Older Americans Act was passed to provide federal funding support for older Americans and the development of the Administration on Aging.
- 1970s Workers' compensation case management was begun.
- 1973 Congress passed the HMO Act to encourage third-party payors to increase control of medical care delivery and enable managed care plans to increase in numbers and to expand enrollments.
- 1974 The Nixon administration attempted to control costs by freezing physician fees.
- 1974 The Employee Retirement Income Security Act (ERISA) allowed self-funded insurance plans to avoid paying premium taxes and to avoid compliance with state-mandated benefits, even though these costs were necessary for insurance companies and managed care plans. It also required that plans and companies provide an explanation of benefits (EOB) statement in the event that a claim was denied and to inform the individual of his or her right to appeal.
- 1979 Seventeen utilization review companies were operating for disability and medical-surgical cases.
- 1979 The National Committee for Quality Assurance (NCQA) was founded by the Group Health Association (GHA) of America and the American Managed Care and Review Association.
- Early 1980s Telephone utilization review for clients with psychiatric and substance abuse diagnoses was started.
- Early 1980s Preferred provider organizations (PPOs) began to develop.
- 1981 The Omnibus Budget Reconciliation Act (OBRA) was passed to encourage community-based alternatives to institutional placement to provide care to the elderly.

- 1982 The Tax Equity and Fiscal Responsibility Act (TEFRA) was created to control Medicare costs.
- 1983 Diagnostic related groups (DRGs) were used as a means for TEFRA control of medical-surgical diagnoses.
- 1985 The Consolidated Omnibus Budget Reconciliation Act (COBRA) was passed to require employers to offer continued health insurance coverage for a defined period of time after the group health insurance had been terminated.
- 1986-1992 Managed behavioral health care companies were carved out of traditional insurance plans, now known commonly as *indemnity medical-surgical plans.*
- 1989 The Physician Payment Review Commission was created to implement legislation that introduced a resource-based fee schedule that limited the amount physicians could charge clients above the fee schedule and volume performance standards.
- 1993 The Health Security Act (HR 3600) was enacted to provide the security of a comprehensive health benefit plan to all Americans that could never be taken away.
- 1994 The Medicare Choice Act was passed to allow Medicare-eligible beneficiaries the choice of traditional Medicare benefit plans or enrollment in an integrated health plan.
- 1996 Congress considered parity for behavioral health programs by carving them back into medical-surgical plans.
- 1998 to present Industry consolidation of managed care companies is occurring through mergers and acquisitions to achieve economies of scale and reduce redundant costs.

Managed-Care Definitions (Coleman, 1993)

- Access Fee: A charge to payors so that their covered persons can use the services of a PPO or HMO provider network. The access fee is basically a network rental fee—that is, the insurance carrier, employer, third-party administrator (TPA), or another payor pays the PPO (or HMO) a monthly fee so that their covered person can use the services in the network. The access fee usually ranges from $2 to $4 per policy holder (subscriber, covered life) or 1% to 3% of the monthly premium. In exchange for the access fee, the PPO (or HMO) maintains the provider network, reviews claims, preprocesses claims for carriers, conducts promotions, and provides marketing and other administrative services. Sometimes the access fee contains a fee for conducting utilization review (UR) and preadmission certification service for the payor. Most of the time the UR fee is charged separately. The UR fee can range from $1.00 to $2.25 depending on the scope of service negotiated by the PPO (or HMO) and the payor.
- Accountable Health Plans (accountable health partnerships [AHPs]): Under the "managed competition" concept, providers and insurance companies would form AHPs, similar to health maintenance organizations (HMOs), preferred provider organizations (PPOs), and other managed care organizations (MCOs). AHPs would compete by offering high-quality and cost-effective health care. They would be offered to different population and enrollment groups through health insurance purchasing cooperatives (HIPCs).
- Adverse Selection: The tendency of less favorable insurance risks to seek medical insurance coverage. The health plan is selected by persons who are less healthy than others enrolled in the plan and require more health services. This increases the financial risk and costs to the health plan.

- Ambulatory Care: Health services delivered on an outpatient basis. This includes physician office visits, services at surgicenters, and outpatient diagnostic/imaging centers. It does not include care in the home or in any facility that requires an overnight stay.
- Authorization: Approval for care, such as hospital admission, diagnostic tests, and referrals to specialists. Authorization may or may not be approval for payment. Preauthorization is usually required before covered services are rendered by both HMO and PPO providers. The definition and meaning will vary by health plan.
- Capitation: A per-member monthly payment to a provider for a specific medical care service (or services) paid in advance of the services being rendered. The per-member per-month (pmpm) payment to a provider is based on actuarial projections of medical use based on the use and cost experience of the population being served. The capitation rate can be adjusted for the age and sex of the members covered and other factors. The capitation payment is a fixed, predetermined payment that the provider accepts as payment in full for a specified time (month), regardless of how many times a member uses the service.
- Carrier: An insurance company that agrees to underwrite the risk of providing certain types of medical coverage and service to a group.
- Case Management: The process whereby a health care professional manages the medical and ancillary services required by a client (member/enrollee) that has a catastrophic illness or injury when the costs of such an illness or injury are extremely high. Medical case-management and catastrophic case-management services can be provided by the health plan, an independent provider group, or an insurance carrier.

- Coinsurance: The percentage of the cost of medical services paid by the client. This is characteristic of indemnity insurance plans and PPO plans. HMOs typically do not use coinsurance but use copayments. The coinsurance rates vary from 10% to 20%, or to as much as 50% of the cost, depending on the cost of the services and whether or not the client uses HMO or PPO providers. Generally, the coinsurance is applied after a deductible is paid by the client.
- Community Rating: A method of rating in which the monthly premium rates charged by insurance providers are based on actuarially determined costs of covering a community. When community rates are used, purchasers of the service pay the same premium as other purchasers in the same community group or rating category. Community rating provides uniform premium rates instead of premium rates for a specific employer or purchaser. Many different approaches are used by HMOs and carriers in applying the principles of community rating.
- Comprehensive Medical Plans (CMPs): A form of prepaid medical care. Under the Medicare TEFRA regulations, a CMP is an alternative delivery system other than a federally qualified HMO. Like their HMO counterparts, CMPs enroll Medicare beneficiaries and are at risk for providing services.
- Concurrent (Extended Stay) Review: A review of an inpatient case by a health professional to determine if the client's stay in an inpatient facility or treatment program should be continued based on medical necessity criteria established by the health plan. The review is performed concurrent to the provision of services.
- Copayment: A nominal fee charged to HMO members at the time medical care services are rendered by a provider. The copayment is the member's share of the cost. Copayments are usually charged for physician office visits ($5, $10, or $15 per visit), outpatient prescriptions ($5, $10, $15 per prescription), and inpatient care services ($100, $200, or $250 per client day).
- Deductible: A fixed dollar amount that a client must pay before health benefits are paid for by the health insurance program. Most indemnity plans have a $100, $200, or $500 deductible.

The indemnity plan pays some or all of the costs after the deductible.
- Dependent: A client who is enrolled in a managed care organization (HMO or PPO) through a subscriber.
- Exclusive Provider Organization (EPO): A form of PPO whereby a member must use the services of the EPO provider's panel. In most EPOs, the member is locked into the PPO network. The EPO provides full or more extensive coverage when the member uses a panel provider. If the member elects not to use an EPO provider, the EPO usually offers limited or no coverage for the services received. Some EPOs require their members to select a primary care physician (PCP), as do HMOs, and require them to visit their PCP before they use providers other than their PCP. Some HMOs offer an EPO in conjunction with their regular HMO plan. EPOs, by design, restrict consumer choices more than PPOs. The EPO was originally conceived as a triple-option plan whereby an indemnity carrier could offer a PPO, an EPO, and a regular indemnity plan.
- Fee-For-Service (FFS): The traditional form of reimbursement to providers that is based on a predetermined fee schedule for the services rendered. Fee-for-service payments are usually based on the usual and reasonable fees charged by physicians for a specific community or geographic area. The service fees for physician services and office procedures and tests are based on physician specialties and are paid at a specified level up to a maximum allowable amount. FFS reimbursement is used by conventional indemnity carriers.
- Gatekeeper: The most popular form of gatekeeping by an HMO or PPO is by the member's PCP. The role of the gatekeeper is to screen members/enrollees seeking medical care and effectively eliminate unnecessary referrals to specialists and for inpatient admissions. PCP gatekeepers are responsible for providing or arranging for all medical care services needed to treat a member's illness and to keep him or her healthy.

As a PCP, the physician coordinates and authorizes all medically necessary services—laboratory studies, diagnostic tests, referrals to specialty physicians, referrals to ancillary providers, and hospitalizations. In most HMOs, if a member obtains services of a specialist or inpatient facility without prior approval (or authorization) from his or her PCP, the member is responsible for paying the costs of these services. HMOs and PPOs also use other gatekeepers to manage access and use of services. These include emergency room nurses, triage nurses, physician assistants, nurse practitioners, and care managers for catastrophic case management.

- Health Alliance (See HIPC)
- Health Insurance Purchasing Cooperative (HIPC): Under the "managed competition" concept, all persons except those employed by large businesses would obtain their health insurance through HIPCs. Each HIPC would offer approved accountable health plans (AHPs). The HIPC would act as the buyer or agent of record to the populations and businesses enrolled in the HIPC. These buyers, which would be not-for-profit organizations chartered by the states, would have an assigned geographic territory. The HIPCs would offer different HMOs, PPOs, and indemnity plans that have been approved as AHPs to its enrollees. The HIPCs would provide enrollees with comprehensive data on each of the AHPs, including price, quality, and enrollee satisfaction. The HIPCs would also provide hospital services and be directed by a board that is representative of the types of enrollees that have joined. The role of the HIPCs is not yet clearly defined.
- Health Maintenance Organization (HMO): An organized system of health care that accepts the responsibility for, or otherwise assumes the delivery of, an agreed on set of comprehensive health maintenance and treatment services for a voluntarily enrolled group of persons in a geographic area. It is reimbursed with a pre-negotiated and fixed periodic payment made by, or on behalf of, each person or family unit enrolled in the plan. HMOs were initially seen as alternatives to the traditional fee-for-service health insurance and medical care system. Basically, HMOs combine the principles of insurance with a care delivery system in which members are locked into the plan's provider network for a specified time (usually 1 year) in exchange for a monthly premium. For the HMO member, it usually means reduced out-of-pocket costs (i.e., no deductible) and nominal copayments for physician office visits, prescription drugs, and hospitalization. HMOs can take several organizational forms: staff, group, network, IPA, hybrid, and point-of-service.
  - Staff Model HMO: An HMO that delivers health care services through physicians who are full-time employees of the HMO. The staff model HMO is the purest form of managed care. In a staff model HMO, physicians are entirely devoted to health care delivery on a prepaid basis. Its physicians are compensated on a salary basis, not on the units of services provided. Staff model HMOs own and operate the medical center from which services are provided and coordinated by staff physicians. This form of HMO is considered to be the most cost-efficient because of the tight internal controls placed on the use of resources and the ability to channel business to a limited number of staff physicians, hospitals, and contracting providers and because of the economies of providing the services in-house. Everyone in a staff model works for the same entity, so it is easy to use a team approach to provide health care services.
  - Group Model HMO: An HMO that primarily contracts with one independent multi-specialty group practice to provide services to its HMO members. The physician group, which is usually dedicated to providing services to HMO members, provides few or no services to fee-for-service clients. The physician group is paid on a capitation basis to provide a specific set of services. The physician group, for example, can be capitated for all physician services (primary care and specialty care), as well as for hospital and other ancillary services. The number of services that it contracts to provide depends on how much the physician group wants to assume in terms of practice and financial risks. The physician group decides how the capitation payments are distributed to each physician in the group. Unlike staff model HMO physicians, group model physicians are somewhat insulated if the HMO fails.
  - Individual Practice Association (IPA) Model HMO: An HMO that contracts directly with physicians in independent practices or contracts with one or more associations of

physicians in independent practice. This form of HMO is organized primarily around solo or single-specialty physician practices. Physicians who belong to an IPA model HMO provide their services to HMO members in their own private offices and see fee-for-service clients as well. IPA primary care physicians are usually paid capitations for members who select them as their primary care physician. Some IPA model HMOs do not use capitation but pay physicians on a negotiated-fee basis. Those who use capitation withhold a certain percentage (withhold amount), which is placed in a "risk pool" or withhold fund. The withhold amount is usually 15% or 20% of the capitation. If, at the end of the year, physician costs or hospital costs are below budgeted amounts, the physician receives the withhold fund. If the physician or hospital costs exceed the budgeted amounts, a portion of, or all of, the withhold fund is used to pay the excess costs. IPA model HMOs are the most difficult to manage fiscally because physicians are in private practice. IPA model HMOs are usually large and have wide market appeal because of the number of hospitals and physicians in the network.

- Network Model HMO: An extension of the group model HMO. This type of HMO contracts with two or more multispecialty physician groups to provide care for their members/enrollees. The physician groups in this organizational form usually do not limit their practice solely to HMO members/enrollees. Like the group model HMO, each multispecialty group is paid on a capitation basis and provides services on a shared-risk arrangement. While a network model HMO may employ solo-practicing physicians, it is predominately organized around several physician group practices.

- Hybrid Model HMO: An HMO that is a combination of at least two other organizational models. A hybrid can be a large staff model HMO that also contracts with an IPA to broaden its geographic appeal or a staff model HMO that also contracts with a few medical groups. Because the HMO is not a "pure model" HMO, it is called a *hybrid*.

- Point-of-Service Model (POS) HMO: The newest form of HMO (also known as an *open-ended HMO*). A POS model HMO allows an HMO member to obtain covered medical services from out-of-plan providers. Typically, an HMO member can receive medical services only from plan-participating providers, and Medical services received from out-of-plan providers are not covered by the HMO unless emergency services are needed. Alternatively, a member of a POS model HMO can elect to use a nonparticipating (nonpar) provider and pay only a portion of the cost instead of 100% of the cost.

- Hold Harmless: A provision in HMO and some PPO provider contracts that stipulates that providers will hold only the HMO (or PPO) solely responsible for payment of covered services rendered to eligible members/enrollees and will not, under any circumstances (including the insolvency of the health plan), charge or attempt to collect payments for services from an HMO (or PPO) member/enrollee except for applicable copayment amounts for covered services. The HMO (or PPO) is the sole guarantor of payment to the provider.

- Incurred-But-Not-Reported (IBNR) Expenses: The estimated expenses incurred by the health plan for which claims for the services rendered have not yet been received for processing.

- Indemnity Insurance: Indemnity insurance is the traditional fee-for-service form of medical insurance that reimburses providers according to the number of services rendered to clients. While many indemnity carriers are switching to managed indemnity plans, they still reimburse providers on a fee-for-service basis. Indemnity insurance principles and fee-for-service reimbursement are still prominent methods of payment in PPOs.

- Lock-In (Lock-In Provision): HMO members are locked into the HMO and HMO-participating providers; they must use HMO-participating providers for all covered services. If they use nonpar providers, they will be financially responsible for the costs. HMOs that participate in Medicare risk programs require Medicare enrollees to sign a lock-in provision so they understand the restrictions and the costs they will have to bear if they use physicians and other providers that are not in the HMO panel. Lock-ins are sometimes used by PPOs, particularly EPOs.

- Managed Indemnity Plan: An indemnity medical plan that has incorporated cost-containment mechanisms to contain service use and costs. Indemnity insurance carriers are now using hospital preadmission certification, concurrent review, second surgical opinions, outpatient procedure services review, and catastrophic case management to help manage service use and costs. In contrast to HMOs and PPOs, they do not have restrictive provider networks, and providers are usually paid on a fee-for-service basis. While managed indemnity plans promote freedom of choice of providers and the continuance of the traditional fee-for-service payment approach, they incorporate many of the cost-containment approaches of managed care plans.
- Member/Enrollee: A person enrolled in an HMO or PPO. Members or enrollees can be subscribers or dependents of subscribers.
- Nonparticipating (Nonpar) Provider: A physician, hospital, or other health service provider that is not on contract with the HMO or PPO to provide covered services to their members/enrollees. Also called *nonpar providers.*
- Open-Enrollment Period: A time during the year when eligible persons are permitted to enroll in the HMO or PPO. Employee groups usually have a 30- to 60-day open-enrollment period on or about the anniversary date of their benefit plan. Some HMOs have year-round open enrollment for certain groups of enrollees (i.e., Medicare and Medicaid).
- Participating Provider: A physician, dentist, hospital, podiatrist, chiropractor. nurse practitioner, clinical nurse specialist, or other health care provider or provider organization that is on contract with the HMO or PPO to provide covered services to HMO or PPO members/enrollees as defined by their applicable health benefit plan.
- Physician-Hospital Organization (PHO): A business arrangement or joint business venture between the hospital and the medical staff. The PHO will contract with a managed care plan on a capitated-risk or other basis for provision of both the hospital and physician services. PHOs can also contract with managed indemnity and other carriers on a risk basis.
- Preadmission Certification/Authorization: A method of screening inpatient admissions before clients are admitted for services. Preadmission review (PAR) is used by HMOs, PPOs, and managed indemnity plans to ensure that the inpatient (hospital or skilled nursing facility) admission meets medical-necessity criteria in terms of severity of illness, service intensity, and the appropriateness of the level of care being proposed. The review is usually conducted by UR nurses and physicians. The purpose of the preadmission certification is to eliminate unnecessary inpatient expenses and to provide the needed services at the most appropriate inpatient facility. When nonemergency inpatient admissions are not certified or authorized in advance, the HMO or PPO member may be responsible for the entire cost of the admission. An HMO member may have to pay the entire bill, and a PPO member may have to pay a higher deductible, higher coinsurance, or both.
- Preferred Provider Organization (PPO): A business arrangement between a group or network of providers and payors in which providers offer health care services to PPO members/enrollees at discounted rates in exchange for increased business volume and quicker payments. PPOs can be sponsored and owned by providers in the community, insurance carriers, business coalitions, employers, and third-party administrators (TPAs). PPO members can use PPO-participating providers or non–PPO-participating providers (nonpar providers). If they choose PPO providers, members have higher service benefit coverage. If they use nonpar providers, members have increased out-of-pocket expenses. PPO hospitals are usually paid on a per-diem or discounted basis—10% to 25% less than reasonable charges. PPO physicians are usually compensated on a fee-for-service schedule that is discounted, usually 10% to 15% below reasonable charges. (Some HMO supporters do not regard PPOs as managed care organizations because some PPOs are not at financial

risk for the services being provided by the organization, and they rely on the traditional fee-for-service forms of reimbursement.)

- Primary Care Physician (PCP): HMO PCPs and some PPO PCPs (if there is a lock-in) are commonly referred to as *gatekeepers*. PCPs assume responsibility for providing directly or arranging for all medical services that an HMO or PPO member/enrollee requires. PCPs provide primary care services in their offices, refer members to specialty physicians, admit members to hospitals, and coordinate other medical services if necessary. PCPs include family practitioners, pediatricians, general practitioners, and internal medicine physicians. Some HMOs also include obstetricians/gynecologists as PCPs. The roles of PCPs vary between health plans. HMO PCPs usually receive a monthly capitation fee and have incentives to provide preventive services and to treat members on an outpatient rather than on an inpatient basis.

- Prospective Payment System (PPS): A payment system that determines the payment amount for a client based on disease criteria before the care is rendered. A PPS gives the provider a financial incentive to use fewer resources in the provision of services, since the provider may retain the difference between what is prepaid and what actual service costs are. DRGs, per diems, and capitation payments are examples of prospective payment systems.

- Reinsurance: To protect the HMO or PPO from catastrophic claims, the health plan turns to an insurance carrier that offers stop-loss reinsurance. A stop-loss reinsurance policy requires the health plan to pay a deductible (i.e., S25,000, $50,000, or $100,000), above which the reinsurer pays a specific claim. The stop-loss amount and the amount the reinsurance carrier pays above it vary. Usually, the reinsurer pays up to $1 million on such a claim. Once this amount is reached, the health plan is liable for the balance.

- Risk Corridor: When capitated providers are at risk, they may accept an agreed-on per-member per-month (pmpm) capitation amount, as long as the actual pmpm cost is within a particular corridor of the agreed-on pmpm payment. The corridor could be at 10% or 15% of the capitation rate. If actual pmpm costs are within

the 10% to 15% corridor, there is no adjustment to the agreed-on pmpm rate.

- Risk Pool (See Withhold).

- Service Area: The geographic area where a health plan ensures the availability and accessibility of covered resources to its members/enrollees. The service area is usually defined by county boundaries or by zip codes.

- Shared Risk: A provider payment arrangement in which the payor, HMO, or PPO shares the financial risk for services that exceed an agreed-on budget amount. If costs exceed the budget amount, the health plan and provider may share the excess costs (loss) at 50%/50%, 25%/75%, or some other agreed-on level. Conversely, if the costs are below the expected budget amount, the payor and provider may share the profit at 50%/50% or at some other agreed-on level. Shared-risk arrangements usually have excess stop-losses for the providers in the event that losses are significant.

- Stop-Loss Provision: A provision in the capitation (risk) contract of a provider (i.e., physician, hospital, or home health agency) that protects the provider from higher-than-expected use and costs as a result of adverse selection and catastrophic illness and injuries. The stop-loss amount could be $1,000, $5,000, or $25,000, depending on the provider. When the stop-loss is reached, the provider is paid on a different payment schedule for the particular case involved.

- Subscriber: A person who enrolls in an HMO or PPO. A subscriber usually is an employee of a company who enrolls himself or herself and all eligible dependents into the HMO or PPO health plan. Medicare beneficiaries and Medicaid recipients are also considered to be subscribers when enrolling in a managed care plan.

- Utilization Management (UM): While UM uses many of the concepts and techniques of utilization review, UM focuses on managing the care of the HMO or PPO member/enrollee rather than managing the use and cost of care delivery. UM incorporates the principles of case management across the entire care continuum. Effective UM programs enable HMO providers to manage the allocation of resources to the benefit of members, providers, and the HMO. UM programs focus on alternative approaches to care, extensive care coordination, continuous monitoring, and aggressive and effective case management by PCPs and professional case managers.

- Utilization Review (UR): A process of examining prospectively, concurrently, and retrospectively the appropriateness of health care services. The purpose of UR is to be certain that the right services are being used at the right time, in the right quantities, at the right location, by the right providers, at the right cost, and at the right quality. How the UR activities are performed varies from one managed care plan to another. UR programs of HMOs typically include the following:
  - Preadmission certification/authorization
  - Concurrent (extended stay) review
  - Discharge planning
  - Second surgical opinions
  - Outpatient procedure reviews
  - Physician specialty reviews
  - Retrospective claims review (hospital)
  - Retrospective emergency care/room reviews
  - Outpatient prescriptions

In addition, HMOs use primary care case management (gatekeepers) and medical case management (catastrophic or large case management).

- Withhold: Withholds are commonly used when there is risk sharing between the health plan and participating providers. It is a common practice in an IPA, for example, to withhold 15% to 20% of a negotiated capitation rate or of an approved provider claim rate. This withhold is placed in a risk pool to pay for unanticipated cost increases or excessive use. When hospital expenses or physician costs exceed the budget, the excess is divided between the health plan and the physicians (providers) participating in the risk-sharing arrangement. If the risk pool has a positive balance, the health plan and the providers split the profits based on an agreed-on formula. If all of the risk pool is needed to pay for excess expenses, the health plan may increase the withhold amount in future budget periods. HMOs and PPOs use withhold funds with PCPs for inpatient services and referral physician care. The risk pool can also be used when capitating a hospital for inpatient care. If there is a surplus in the risk pool, it may be split between the health plan and the hospital.

6 Reimbursement in Home Care

Tina M. Marrelli

Home care reimbursement or payment for services may seem complex to clinicians new to home care. This chapter seeks to provide an overview of home care reimbursement, the multifaceted components of reimbursement or payment, and the nurse's important role in the process. It is important to note at the onset that Medicare is the largest payor of home health care and as such, sets many of the standards for home care services.

HOME CARE NURSE'S ROLE IN REIMBURSEMENT

The professional home care nurse must know and adhere to the rules and regulations that compose the Medicare home care program. The roles that demand a working and correct knowledge of Medicare include the admitting nurse, intake and referral nurses, visit nurse, revisit nurse, case manager, community or hospital liaison, and all other titles. Simply put, all nurses, other clinicians, and administrative, billing, and other team members in home care must have a thorough understanding of Medicare.

HISTORY OF THE MEDICARE PROGRAM

Medicare is the U.S. medical insurance program for the elderly (currently defined as age 65 for qualifying purposes), the disabled, and those with end-stage renal disease (ESRD). The Medicare program provides health insurance for approximately 38 million patients, usually called *Medicare beneficiaries.*

Medicare was signed into law by President Lyndon Johnson in 1965, and the program became operational in 1966. Since the inception of the Medicare program, costs, services, and coverage have expanded significantly. The newspapers frequently report the government's actuarial projections of when the Medicare trust fund will run out of money. These years have varied from 2002 to 2007, but whatever the date, the belief that Medicare funds will be depleted is commonly held, and to date, both Congress and presidents have done little to stem the tide.

A study conducted by the National Coalition on Health Care and the Kellogg Foundation described findings they refer to as the current health care "crisis." Some of the factors related to this crisis follow:

- There are 41 million Americans without health care insurance, and the number is projected to increase to 47 million in 2005.
- By 2007, the United States will spend $1 of every $5 on health care, and health care spending is expected to increase at twice the rate of inflation.

At the same time we read these staggering numbers and projections, it is known that the United States spends more on health care than any other country, yet outcomes such as infant morbidity and mortality are not better than some third-world countries. How can this be? Many consider costly technology and the health care reimbursement system, primarily Medicare, the fuel that has caused spiraling health care costs. Historically cost-based reimbursement, cost reports, and other methods initiated by the government, and maximized in some instances by the health care industry, have also contributed to these costs and problems. Consider also that from a quality perspective, there are no standards for much of the care provided in the United States. One example of the lack of standardized care common in hospitals is the diversity of physician orders related to interventions and medications for patients with similar problems.

Table 6-1 National Medicare Home Health Utilization Statistics			
	1990	1995	Percentage of Change*
Total Medicare beneficiaries	34.2 million	37.6 million	+10%
Beneficiaries who received HHA services	1.9 million	3.48 million	+76%
Total HHA reimbursements	$3.7 billion	$15.4 billion	+316%
HHA percentage of total Medicare program dollars	3.7%	8.7%	+135%
Average HHA reimbursement per patient	$1892	$4438	+135%
Total HHA visits	70 million	250 million	+255%
Average HHA visits per patient	36	72	+100%

From Department of Inspector General, Department of Health and Human Services, July 1997.
HHA, home health agency.
*Percentages may not be exact due to rounding.

Most nurses have worked with physicians who will use only certain catheters or others who prescribe only certain medications, for example. This variation in myriad practice patterns has increased support for standardization of care and care processes. One attempt to standardize care is the practice guidelines of the Agency for Healthcare Research and Quality (AHRQ). These guidelines review the literature, convene a panel of interdisciplinary experts, and determine the best practices for similar conditions. Some of the practice guidelines released to date address incontinence, sickle cell disease, hypertension, congestive heart failure, incontinence, pain, and others. The guidelines are not written only for the clinician; there are also corresponding client education tools to facilitate the goals of care from client and caregiver perspectives. Other tools often used to reduce unnecessary practice variation include clinical paths or pathways, standardized formularies, and case management.

President Clinton's proposed Health Security Act was developed to address three fundamental problems with the U.S. health care system: access, cost, and quality. As the increased payout and projections listed in Table 6-1 show, the focus of the three areas must be cost.

REGULATIONS DESIGNED TO ADDRESS COSTS AND QUALITY ISSUES

The Centers for Medicare and Medicaid (CMS) (formerly the Health Care Financing Administration [HCFA]) published a regulation that significantly changed home care practice and documentation. This is the biggest change since the inception of the home care program from practice and managerial perspectives. Massive reorganizations and educational initiatives are part of any change of this scope and depth. Called the *Outcome and Assessment Information Set (OASIS)*, this comprehensive data set was mandated in February 1997 for all Medicare-certified home care agencies as a part of their comprehensive client assessment. Standard data elements are assessed, collected, and electronically transmitted at defined points in time to the government through the designated state agencies. The data are collected on all adult clients receiving skilled home care services. The only exceptions to date are pediatric, prenatal, and postpartal clients, and clients who receive *only* homemaker services.

With the inception of OASIS, there is now a mechanism for clinicians and organizations to be compared "apples to apples" and for costs and outcomes to be analyzed. OASIS was piloted for years before its implementation and is a part of the Outcome-Based Quality Improvement (OBQI) initiative. Data analysis, outcome and benchmarking, and analysis of evidence-based practice trends are a part of OASIS and its interface with OBQI.

All data from the OASIS tool are incorporated into the organization's own assessment tools, and then varying components are reassessed, collected, and reported at regular times and at the client's discharge from home health services. OASIS is discipline neutral; the data may be collected by any member of the professional team,

Exhibit I   MEDICAL REVIEW   09-94

Department of Health and Human Services Health Care Financing Administration	EXHIBIT I	Form Approved OMB No. 0938-0357

HOME HEALTH CERTIFICATION AND PLAN OF TREATMENT

1. Patient's HI Claim No.	2. SOC Date	3. Certification Period		4. Medical Record No.	5. Provider No.
		From:	To:		

6. Patient's Name and Address	7. Provider's Name and Address

8. Date of Birth:	9. Sex ☐ M ☐ F	10. Medications: Dose/Frequency/Route (N)ew (C)hanged

11. ICD-9-CM	Principal Diagnosis	Date

12. ICD-9-CM	Surgical Procedure	Date

13. ICD-9-CM	Other Pertinent Diagnoses	Date

14. DME and Supplies	15. Safety Measures:

16. Nutritional Req.	17. Allergies:

18. A. Functional Limitations

1 ☐ Amputation	5 ☐ Paralysis	9 ☐ Legally Blind
2 ☐ Bowel/Bladder (Incontinence)	6 ☐ Endurance	A ☐ Dyspnea with Minimal Exertion
3 ☐ Contracture	7 ☐ Ambulation	B ☐ Other (Specify)
4 ☐ Hearing	8 ☐ Speech	

18. B. Activities Permitted

1 ☐ Complete Bedrest	6 ☐ Partial Weight Bearing	A ☐ Wheelchair
2 ☐ Bedrest BRP	7 ☐ Independent At Home	B ☐ Walker
3 ☐ Up as Tolerated	8 ☐ Crutches	C ☐ No Restrictions
4 ☐ Transfer Bed/Chair	9 ☐ Cane	D ☐ Other (Specify)
5 ☐ Exercise Prescribed		

19. Mental Status:

| 1 ☐ Oriented | 3 ☐ Forgetful | 5 ☐ Disoriented | 7 ☐ Agitated |
| 2 ☐ Comatose | 4 ☐ Depressed | 6 ☐ Lethargic | 8 ☐ Other |

20. Prognosis

| 1 ☐ Poor | 2 ☐ Guarded | 3 ☐ Fair | 4 ☐ Good | 5 ☐ Excellent |

21. Orders for Discipline and Treatments (Specify Amount/Frequency/Duration)

22. Goals/Rehabilitation Potential/Discharge Plans

23. Nurse's Signature and Date of Verbal SOC Where Applicable:	25. Date HHA Received Signed POT

24. Physician's Name and Address	26. I certify/recertify that this patient is confined to his/her home and needs intermittent skilled nursing care, physical therapy and/or speech therapy or continues to need occupational therapy. The patient is under my care, and I have authorized the services on this plan of care and will periodically review the plan.
27. Attending Physician's Signature and Date Signed	28. Anyone who misrepresents, falsifies, or conceals essential information required for payment of Federal funds may be subject to fine, imprisonment, or civil penalty under applicable Federal laws.

Form HCFA-485 (C-4) (02-94)   PROVIDER

Fig. 6-1   HCFA Form 485.

such as nurses or therapists, depending on the state and the Medicare rules related to admission and standard of practice.

With the incorporation of OASIS, the bar has been raised related to planning care in a very organized and standardized manner across an organization. It is important to note that OASIS supported Congress' mandate to move home care into its prospective payment system (PPS), which officially began October 1, 2000.

The initial guidelines for home care PPS were published in October 1999. The PPS method of reimbursement for home care services can be analogous to the diagnostic-related group (DRG) method of reimbursement for hospitals, which was enacted as part of the Tax Equity and Fiscal Responsibility Act (TEFRA) of 1982. In the early 1980s, hospital behaviors changed as clinical paths and increased client education emerged as methods for hospitals to stay viable as they moved from cost-based reimbursement to the PPS. In fact, OASIS data play a major role in the home care PPS model. It is imperative that nurses and other clinicians collect accurate and timely OASIS data, because home care reimbursement depends on it. Nurses and other members of the interdisciplinary team must assume professional responsibilities and demonstrate the value of the services provided to payors and consumers of home care services. OASIS may assist in this endeavor.

MEDICARE HOME HEALTH CARE: COVERED SERVICES

Medicare covers home health care to homebound beneficiaries who need skilled care or physical or speech therapy. Medicare does not limit the length of home health coverage, but has a cap of 100 visits under Medicare Part A. Subsequent visits or the 101st visit reverts to payment under Medicare Part B.

To qualify for Medicare home health coverage, the client (Medicare beneficiary) must meet the following four conditions:

1. The physician must have determined that care is medically necessary and that the client will be cared for under a plan of care. This plan of care is usually the *HCFA Form 485*, the "Home Health Certification and Plan of Treatment" form (Fig. 6-1).
2. The care must be intermittent or part-time. Medicare home health does not pay for

full-time care. Covered skilled services include nursing, physical therapy and speech-language pathology or physical or occupational therapy services. Medical–social work services and occupational therapy services can be called in when the three services listed previously are needed to meet the client's needs and are ordered in the client's plan of care.

3. The client must be homebound as defined in the *Medicare Home Health Agency Manual–HCFA Manual 11*. (Visit www. hcfa.gov for the full text regarding homebound clients.)
4. The home health care agency providing services for the client must be a Medicare-certified participating provider. More on the Medicare certification process follows in the next section.

CERTIFICATION: THE FIRST STEP TOWARD REIMBURSEMENT

It is important to remember that Medicare is a federally regulated program. Certain conditions must be met for covered Medicare services to be reimbursed. Because home care is primarily a Medicare Part A benefit, there are Medicare conditions of participation (COPs) that govern home care providers (organizations). The Medicare COPs are conditions or standards that must be met for an organization to care for Medicare clients and receive Medicare reimbursement. The COPs are the core of the Medicare certification process. *Medicare certification* means that the home health agency has met the intent and provisions of the Medicare COPs (for home care) and that the provider organization can bill Medicare for appropriate covered services. The certification becomes the basis for future Medicare reimbursement.

This certification can be seen as the "seal of approval" and may be the first step toward the HHA's receiving other reimbursements (such as from private insurers) or continuing toward accreditation (another level of achievement). At present, the process of certification is going through significant change, with the conditions, standards, and process being revised.

The Medicare certification process typically involves contracts between CMS and the state departments of health. The state departments send survey and certification nurses to the sites of the organizations desiring Medicare certification. For example, the HCFA has a contract with the Ohio Department of Health (ODH) and a new home care organization in Ohio contacts the ODH for their initial Medicare certification. During the certification, visit records are reviewed, home visits are made to clients, and a general overview of the organization and administration of services are thoroughly reviewed by ODH nurses. Standards include assessing that important components of quality are upheld and are demonstrated to the surveyors through objective data gathered during the on-site visit. These data are gathered through client and staff interviews, the record review process, and other methods.

The COPs include standards, which are complex requirements related to particular conditions. (There are only a limited number of COPs, yet the information to explain them, called the *Interpretive Guidelines* in the *State Operations Manual* (SOM), is almost 100 pages!) Here is an example that further explains the Medicare certification process. The first Medicare COP is client rights. This important COP, "notice of rights" includes many components. The first part states, "The HHA must provide the patient with a written notice of the patient's rights in advance of furnishing care to the patient or during the initial evaluation visit before the initiation of treatment." What the surveyor must find to validate compliance with this COP related to client rights is the following: that written notice of the client's rights were given before (in advance of) the furnishing of care to the client during the initial evaluation visit before the initiation of treatment. The surveyors may also interview clients and inquire about the client's rights; ask to see a copy of the written notice of rights that the client signed and was given a copy of; review the client's clinical record, where there may be another copy of the client rights statement signed by the client; and review any documentation by the nurse that these rights were explained to the client before his or her signature and the delivery of care and treatment. This is an example of the relationship between the certification process, the COPs, and the documentation and other supporting information that meets the COPs. It is important to note that certification is not a one-time process, but that surveys occur throughout the tenure of the home health agency for HCFA to determine that the home care agency provides safe and effective care to Medicare beneficiaries.

MEDICARE DOCUMENTATION

Because Medicare is a law, home care nurses and other team members must be aware that their clinical client documentation is the framework for coverage decisions, denials, or payments for appropriate and covered care. The Regional Home Health Intermediaries (RHHI), the specialty payors who contract with the CMS to adjudicate and process all the Medicare home care (and hospice) claims nationally, look to the clinical documentation to support (or not support) covered care. The justification then rests with the visiting clinicians. Justification includes supporting and explaining why the client is homebound every visit, clearly stating the skilled nursing care provided (e.g., injected 100 μg of vitamin B_{12}, changed silicone catheter, provided wound care, taught new ostomy site, and completed observation and assessment). There are 15 nursing duties identified in the Medicare home care program. These follow:

1. Observation and assessment of patient's condition when only the specialized skills of a medical professional can determine a patient's status
2. Management and evaluation of a patient care plan
3. Teaching and training activities
4. Administration of medications
5. Tube feedings
6. Nasopharyngeal and tracheostomy aspiration (suctioning)
7. Catheters
8. Wound care
9. Ostomy care
10. Heat treatment
11. Medical gasses
12. Rehabilitation nursing
13. Venipuncture (not a stand-alone service for qualifying for home care services)
14. Student-nurse visits
15. Psychiatric evaluation, therapy, and teaching

Each of these services has in-depth examples and connotations that must be learned and adhered to for compliance and quality reasons. The specifics of the coverage are discussed in the Medicare *Home Health Agency Manual–Publication 11.* It is important to note that it is not the purpose of this chapter to explain the Medicare home care program, the nuances of nursing coverage, and the required documentation for payment of appropriate care services. Readers should receive a comprehensive orientation to Medicare coverage and documentation by their employing home care organizations.

OTHER SOURCES OF FUNDING IN HOME CARE

Though Medicare is the largest payor of home health services and sets many of the standards, there are other sources of funding in home care. Clients who are not Medicare beneficiaries, such as working baby boomers and children, may have insurance through a health maintenance organization (HMO) or other health insurer models. Medicaid is medical assistance insurance and the payor for clients who have financial difficulty and has been called *state insurance for the poor.* Medicaid, because it is administered by the 50 states, varies widely across the country, with coverage requirements and other rules related to the individual state's Medicaid model. As managed care gains strength in Medicare and Medicaid, more and more clients will need prior authorization for home care visits or services.

The Area Offices on Aging that exist across the country provide support services to the elderly. Again, services may vary widely depending on locale, programs, funding, and client needs.

GRANT OPPORTUNITIES

Grants are one way that many not-for-profit organizations receive funding for special projects. Many of these grants are published through national journals and nursing newsletters. They may serve a certain client population, such as clients with wounds or clients needing spiritual support. One example is the Robert Wood Johnson Grants. Grant writers in home care and hospice care are valued members of the organization because successful grant writing and funding can mean the difference between servicing a special client population and having to end services.

Other often overlooked services include local community agencies, including the United Way, the Cancer Societies (some of which provide direct care and support services), Easter Seals, Crippled Children monies for children, and others as unique as the community.

Regardless of funding, it is important that the professional home care nurse provide a standardized level of care and skillful intervention, not just complete a task. This means assessing and reviewing the client and the plan of care throughout the client's entire course of care. Care coordination and communications with other care team members, including physicians, home health aides, and therapists, are key in quality home care delivery.

SUMMARY

The Medicare home care system is complex and based on federal law and regulation. There are also licensure laws in many states and other applicable laws that impact practice. Home care has undergone massive changes that began with huge budget cuts in the implementation of the Balanced Budget Act of 1997. Congress crafted the act to address spiraling health care costs and limit the growth of home care. Congress and actuaries cannot realistically project the costs of Medicare, given the growth over the past few years.

All clinicians and managers must become aware of these changing rules during their comprehensive orientation and throughout their careers with ongoing education related to Medicare updates and changes. The COPs, the *Home Health Agency Manual–Publication 11,* and other HCFA publications such as the *OASIS Users Manual* should be essential resources of information related to coverage and required documentation. A list of additional readings is provided for the reader at the end of this chapter, some of which incorporate the Medicare coverage and documentation requirements directly into the text.

Other sources of home care funding will continue to be grants, Medicaid, waiver programs, and local community services. As health care dollars become more limited, home care nurses and social workers must work collaboratively to provide linkage for continued services or for referral to other services. This will be the challenge for the future.

As the health care system undergoes significant change, Medicare home care will also change. The competent clinician must keep current with changing regulations and incorporate this knowledge base into daily practice to work effectively with clients and their families. The nurse's role as case manager integrates the most effective use of limited resources as a key component of work. As the nurse works with the physician to create the individualized plan of care, the appropriate use of services and planned interventions related to outcomes will become second nature. Compliance, care planning, and education directed toward self-care will define the effective home care nurse in the future.

ADDITIONAL READINGS

Finkleman A: *Psychiatric home care,* Gaithersburg, Md, 1997, Aspen.

Home Care and Hospice Update is a clinically focused newsletter written for home care and hospice nurses and managers. For a sample issue, call (941) 697-2900 or (800) 993-6397 (NEWS).

Marrelli T: *Handbook of home health orientation,* St Louis, 1997, Mosby.

Marrelli T: *Handbook of home health standards and documentation guidelines for reimbursement,* St Louis, 2001, Mosby.

Marrelli T: *Hospice and palliative care handbook: Quality, compliance, and reimbursement,* St Louis, 1999, Mosby.

Marrelli T: *Mosby's home care and hospice drug handbook,* St Louis, 1999, Mosby.

Marrelli T, Friend L: *Home health aide: Guidelines for care instructor manual,* Boca Grande, Fla, 1997, Marrelli & Associates.

Marrelli T, Hilliard L: *Manual of home health practice: Guidelines for effective clinical operations,* St Louis, 1998, Mosby.

Marrelli T, Krulish L: *Home care therapy: quality, documentation, and reimbursement,* Boca Grande, Fla, 1999, Marrelli & Associates.

Marrelli T, Whittier XX: *Home health aide: Guidelines for care,* Boca Grande, Fla, 1996, Marrelli & Associates.

OASIS user's manual, 1999, *Health Care Financing Administration* www.medicare.gov
www.hcfa.gov
www.hcfa.gov/medlearn/default.htm
www.medicare.gov

PART II

Nursing Competencies in Home Health Care

7 Family Assessment in Home Care

Ann G. Widmer and Ida M. Martinson

Family assessment is the beginning of the nursing process. It is the systematic and careful analysis of the family network in the home environment. Its purpose is to collect information that will aid in developing an effective care plan and providing the support necessary to maintain the highest level of health and quality of life possible for the family and client. Early discharge from acute care is now a reality of home care admission, and assessment requires home care nurses to be highly skilled to meet acute care needs (Thibault, 1997). Family assessment is a systematic evaluative process that leads to decisions about a client's current and potential level of health in a variety of settings.

The family is both the unit of care and the context for the provision of care for an individual. The purpose of this chapter is to present a current overview of the theoretical frameworks and tools necessary to assess and ensure the success of the family and its members in gaining and maintaining health. In the twenty-first century, as in the past, families are significant members of the health care team. They are more responsible than ever in the home care setting for assisting in the care of ill or aging family members.

THE PURPOSES OF ASSESSMENT

The purposes of assessment are to collect data to identify the problem and to assess those aspects of the problem at which intervention will be directed. The essence of family assessment includes identifying physical, intellectual, social, emotional, and spiritual issues that will assist the development and implementation of the care plan. Assessment includes questions about family characteristics and support, health issues, roles, and levels of function. Problems and concerns that surface are examined with the family

with respect to the way they will affect care. Existing family strengths and support networks that can be used are identified. As the assessment progresses, a circle of learning develops. The more the nurse learns about the client and his or her family, the more the family may understand its own situation. Intervention in the form of education and understanding has thus begun, even as the assessment stage is taking place.

NURSING ASSESSMENT ROLES IN HOME CARE SETTINGS

The role of the home care nurse may be more varied and complex than that of the nurse in an institutional setting. As a result of the broadened, more complex level of functioning, the nurse in the home care environment should be prepared to use all available tools to assist in the creative development of the nurse-client relationship. He or she can often begin the assessment phase of the nursing process through the effective assimilation into a client-family–defined and controlled environment. Nurses, social workers, and other health care providers can work together to provide access to resources for the chronically ill or disabled who need extensive environmental support services if they are to remain in their homes (Berkman et al, 1999).

The assessment should provide a broad understanding of a number of areas, which include family health and illness, cultural characteristics, relationships, and behaviors. The nurse must have working definitions of these concepts from which to organize data. Not everything needs to be assessed every time. However, each assessment should provide a fuller understanding of the family, its health and illness situation, and its customs, relationships, and behaviors.

THE FAMILY
Definition of Family

In today's society, families have many forms. They may include, but are no longer restricted to, two adults of the opposite sex in a traditional sexual relationship. A family may now consist of one parent and a child, several brothers and sisters, an unmarried couple of the opposite or same sex, or several people who form an intimate group. It is perhaps better today to define family by purpose rather than by composition. The family creates and maintains a common culture to promote the physical, mental, emotional, and social development of each of its members. It operates within an identity of the group as well as the individual members. Beliefs about health and illness represent an important part of the assessment and differ among families and cultures as these groups interpret what is good for their well-being. Cultural characteristics that relate to health care include beliefs about health and healing, life and death, family roles, communications, diet, and authority. There are also intracultural variations because of generational or economic factors. While knowledge about cultural values and customs is useful in interpreting assessment data, it does not replace actual information obtained from individual family members.

Many of these beliefs and customs enhance and encourage healing and support a healthy lifestyle. The study of cultural characteristics assists the nurse in individualizing care and helps strengthen the nurse-family relationship. Values and attitudes are often shaped by religion and cultural traditions, as are family-based decisions about such things as selection of marriage partners, expression of sexuality, and the cause or purposes of illness or pain. Understanding and valuing a family's beliefs can expedite decision making and provide comfort in times of crisis (Clemen-Stone, 1998). Home health agencies with rich cultures and diverse staffs or agencies that offer continuing diversity training can offer great advantages in recognizing, respecting, and maximizing the strengths of all families (deSavorgnani, 1999).

Characteristics of healthy families include good communication and supportive behaviors; a sense of trust, humor and play; a shared sense of responsibility; and a willingness to seek help from outside the family. Customs and rituals are familial and social patterns of behavior in which members have designated roles or responsibilities. They frequently center on ways of eating, playing, working, observing traditions or religion, and celebrating special occasions or events. Relationships and behaviors are perhaps the most complex of the components. The greater the understanding of the relationships among those in the client-family unit, the more accuracy and sensitivity the nurse will have in understanding by whom and in what way decisions are made, how goals are set and reached, and how development and growth occur. Dellman-Jenkins (2000) noted that contributions from grandchildren and sharing of caregiving responsibilities among family members not only provided more socioemotional aid to older members, but also gave all concerned great satisfaction. Eggebeen and Davey (1998) reached the conclusion from their research that in time of need, children tend to "be there" and that most siblings share in the responsibility of caregiving.

Family Structure

Family structure refers to the characteristics of the family unit and defines the roles, relationships, and positions of family members. Family structure has changed in the Western world during the past few decades. The traditional family composed of husband and wife raising their own biological children is no longer the predominate model. There are married couples without children, and in about one third of the households headed by married couples, one or both of the spouses have been married previously. Single-parent families make up 23% of households with a child under 18 years of age. There are also cohabiting heterosexual and homosexual couples (Hanson, Boyd, 1996). It is important to assess the degree of commitment of family members to the health and well-being of the client. It is an error to assume that certain relationships carry traditional bonds. For example, a spouse may be less involved than close friends, and a daughter-in-law may be closer to a client than his or her own son.

Differentiation refers to the degree to which family members are emotionally separate from each other. It also relates to their ability to distinguish thought from emotion. Highly differentiated people make rational decisions and sustain an identity separate from, yet supportive of, the family. Less differentiated people make decisions that are based on feelings and fuse their identities and opinions with those of family members. Less differentiated people often are more reactive and thus less able to cope with stress (Shepherd, Moriarty, 1996; Goodell, Hanson, 1999). This inability to differentiate should not be confused with the emotional sharing and mutual interdependence that support involvement among family members. Assessing interfamily structure yields benefits in understanding who can be relied on and to what extent internal and external help will be used.

When attempting to understand family structure, it is sometimes helpful to draw a family tree, or genogram, that records family members and their relationships for at least three generations. The process of collecting this information can help the nurse connect with a family in a nonthreatening way and can reveal information about how the family perceives relationships. Family maps are another way to understand family roles and hierarchies. The nurse observes a family interactive situation, then draws a map that details the subsystems, boundaries, and interactive patterns such as alliance, avoidance, or confrontation. Examples of genograms and family maps can be found in Smith and Maurer (2000).

Family Theory in Nursing

Family theory in nursing evolved from many social science theories. The development of family nursing models and theories over the past 40 years has met the challenge of the great diversity in family structure and function. Traditionally, six functions have been performed by families. Families exist to achieve financial stability, to reproduce, to protect, to transfer culture and religion, to educate and socialize, and to confer status in society. In the twenty-first century, these functions have been modified, and new functions have emerged. For example, some married couples have chosen not to have children, and family members are not always dependent on one another to be financially healthy. Functions now include an increased expectation of support in both relationships and health maintenance.

Social Theories of Family

Four major family social theories that have contributed to family nursing theory are (1) struc-tural-functional theory, (2) developmental theory, (3) interactionist theory, and (4) systems theory. A description of each follows.

In structural-functional theory, families are described in terms of how they relate to other major social institutions such as education, government, and the economy. Family members' roles and relationships are measured by how well the family structure performs its functions. Nursing refers to this model in a health care situation when, for example, a single parent is ill and cannot fulfill his or her functions of financial and emotional support. Family assessment includes determining if illness results in a family's inability to perform necessary functions (Friedman, 1998).

Developmental theory addresses the phases and development of family systems over time. Like individuals, families complete tasks and move through phases. In assessment, the family is placed on a continuum of the family life cycle, which provides a basis for forecasting how a family will experience assaults such as illness or death.

Interactionist theory, as it relates to family assessment, views families as communicating and interacting members who judge their own behavior by how they perceive the actions of others toward them. Family norms and role expectations are reinforced and indicate how members act and react. In family assessment, these theories are useful in understanding the clarity and effectiveness of communication and patterns of problem solving (Friedman, 1998).

Systems theory defines a system (the family) that is distinct from the environment in which it exists. The system can be "open" by exchanging resources with the environment or "closed" if it is isolated from its environment. Systems attempt to maintain a steady state through feedback from within and without. Family assessment uses systems theory to determine the effects of illness on the entire family system, the way help is best provided to open and closed systems, and the degree to which family members are able to adapt and change to maintain a steady state.

Roles

Roles within the family structure can be either rigid or flexible according to individual situations. Roles influence almost all behaviors, most notably decision making, dependency or independence, information sharing, and a variety of responsibility-taking or giving behaviors. Traditional roles of husband, wife, parent, or child may have been learned throughout life and deeply ingrained or repudiated.

Family roles change and develop as spouses shift responsibilities for income and support; children are born, grow, and leave home; and goals and activities change at different stages in the family's life. Inner emotional resources are different according to the stage of growth of the family unit. For example, a wife's chronic illness may be responsibly handled until her husband loses his job, and she, by necessity, returns to work. Rather than offering the physical and emotional support necessary when she becomes increasingly ill, the husband may begin to drink. Assessment might show that the anger, guilt, and impotence resulting from his loss of role as husband-provider are central to his drinking. He blames himself for her need to work and increasing illness. Before care can be planned, this perceived guilt and loss of stature must be addressed.

The changing of roles can cause frustration and depression. For example, the wife who must take over the family business or the husband who finds that he is "parent" to both his teenagers and his own mother can be under great stress. The rearrangement of roles by illness, a new baby, or a loss of financial stability may be responsible for any family's inability to organize a healthful environment, comply with a care plan, or even be emotionally supportive of one another.

HOME CARE SETTING

Comprehensive client-family assessment in the home care setting is different from assessment done in the acute care setting. One element of difference is the environment itself. Unlike the hospital, office, or clinic, where the environments are controlled by health care professionals, the home is controlled by the client and family. The nurse does not have the immediate and constant support of rules, policies, and colleagues to aid in planning and compliance. The family, in whose home the nurse is a guest, is often one of several generations, complex relationships, long-term problems, and varying customs. Unlike a health care facility, the home may not be adapted to providing health services. There may be no telephone or hot water, food may be scarce, and in isolated rural settings, the nearest support services may be 30 miles away (Wright, 1997). Other

homes, with wide door openings and safety devices throughout the house, may be more than adequate.

Assessment also differs according to the length of the anticipated client-nurse interaction. In contrast to the short-term relationship of nurse and client in the acute care setting, the relationship with the client and family in the home may last months or even years. The relationship may become extremely personal and intense. For example, a home health care nurse might continue to see a long-term care client even though that nurse is struggling with his or her own illness. While one of the advantages of the home care nurse can be the close relationship that develops over time, appropriate professional boundaries need to be set.

ASSESSMENT MODELS AND INSTRUMENTS
Family Assessment Intervention Model and FS3I

Several assessment models will be presented here, and nurses should select the model or combination of models that best matches their philosophies. The Family Assessment Intervention model reflects a system approach in which the family is the client. Stressors that penetrate its defense systems cause a family to adapt to maintain stability (Hanson, Mischke, 1996). An assessment tool based on this model is the family systems stressor strength inventory (FS3I) (Hanson, Mischke, 1996). This model addresses problem identification and family factors at lines of defense and resistance, family reactions and stability, and restoration of family function. The instrument, FS3I, provides quantitative and qualitative measurement of stressful situations in families and of the families' coping skills. A series of stressors are ranked by family members by their potential to create tension in the family. Members complete the survey independently, the responses are recorded, and a comprehensive synthesis is created by the nurse (Hanson, Mischke, 1996). Data obtained by this instrument can determine the type and amount of intervention necessary to support the families' coping skills.

Friedman Family Assessment Model

Another assessment model, the Friedman family assessment model, is based on elements of several theories, including both developmental and systems theories. The family, defined as an open social system, is a subsystem of society. The Friedman form provides guidelines for family nurses as they interview the family about family structure, functions, socialization, and stress and coping (Friedman, 1998). The family's relationship to other social systems is a focus of this model. An analysis of family responses leads to the identification of problem areas and successful (or unsuccessful) coping strategies (Friedman, 1998).

Calgary Family Assessment Model

The Calgary family assessment model (CFAM) is an integrated, multidimensional framework based on systems theory, cybernetics, communication, and changing theoretical foundations. One strength of this model is the clinical practice emphasis on a method of continuous family assessment. The following concepts from systems theory are most useful:

- A family system is part of a larger suprasystem and is composed of many subsystems.
- The family as a whole is greater than the sum of its parts.
- A change in one family member affects all family members.

A nuclear family living in the suburbs is stressed by multiple conflicts; the entire suprasystem is in disbelief and crisis, and the family members are unable to mobilize their resources. The father is overwhelmed, fearful, and withdrawn. The youngest child shows behavioral problems in school, and the teenage daughter experiments with alcohol. Family members from another part of the country fly in to visit the aging paternal grandmother and express strong negative opinions about her living situation. While this conflict is occurring, the 50-year-old mother is diagnosed with breast cancer.

If the family is to create a balance between change and stability, the family members' behaviors must be understood from a view of circular, rather than linear, causality (Wright, Leahey, 1994). For instance, if the father helps the mother change the dressing from her mastectomy, the mother may express appreciation for this help. In return, the father's fear and anger may subside, and he may be even more willing to continue to help with the dressing changes. As the parents become more communicative, the children may become open to counseling and may be more focused in school.

The cybernetics theory suggests that families possess self-regulating ability through the process of feedback that can simultaneously occur at several different system levels within families. The communication theory offers the concept that all nonverbal communication is meaningful, and that all communication has two major channels for transmission: digital and analogic. Digital communication is the actual content of the message, and analogic communication includes nonverbal communication, such as posture and facial expression. All communications consist of two levels: content and relationship. For example, a mother may say to her daughter, "Come over here, I want to tell you something" (content) or "Get over here, I have something to tell you" (relationship).

The foundation of change theory is that change depends on perception of the problem, on context, and on evolving goals for treatment. It states that understanding alone does not lead to change, does not necessarily occur equally in all family members, and can be related to a myriad of causes. It emphasizes that facilitating change is the nurse's responsibility.

The CFAM consists of three major categories: structural, developmental, and functional. *Structural* refers to family members within a household and their relationships. A genogram is an example of a structural assessment tool. *Developmental* refers to whether the family has young children, school-age children, or teenagers. It might also be used to define an aging family. *Functional* refers to how the family works out issues on a daily basis. Each category has several subcategories, and each nurse decides which subcategories are appropriate to assess with each family at each time (Wright, Leahey, 1994).

By using the CFAM, the nurse can examine who the family is and what the connections are among the members. It helps to identify both internal and external structure. The internal structure has the subcategories of family composition, rank order, subsystem, and boundary. The external structure involves culture, religion, extended family, and social class (Wright, Leahey, 1994).

ASSESSMENT OF SPECIFIC CONCERNS

The family APGAR (adaptability, partnership, growth, affection, and resolve) is a self-administered, five-item questionnaire that offers a quick profile of how the family functions in various areas (McCubbin, Olson, Larson, 1982). It was designed to be a measure of the family's satisfaction with family life. The family inventory of life events and changes examines the quality and quantity of life events or stresses (McCubbin, Patterson, Wilson, 1982). The stresses involved in the caregiver role are complex. The history of the client-caregiver relationship, changes in the caregiver's lifestyle, and the client's willingness to accept help are all important to consider when assessing the strengths and abilities of the family caregiver to provide care and support. Finally, the *burden interview* seen in Box 7-1 can be used to assess the caregiver role (Zarit, Todd, Zarit, 1986).

Risk to the client can sometimes result from caregiving dysfunction. Caregiving risk is determined directly by family environment and resources or, for example, by client-caregiver interaction. Caregiving risk alone can be an appropriate reason for making the choice for institutionalization over home care (McConnochie et al, 1997). Assumptions that there will be agreement among family members and health professionals concerning the ways certain wellness goals are achieved are frequently disproved. Zanetti et al (1999) have reported, for example, contrasts between caregiver and professional observations about functional levels of demented clients. Caregiver depression seems to affect his or her assessment and reporting of performance of activities of daily living (ADLs) in clients with dementia. Even within a disease category such as dementia, there can be variations in caregiver burden. A study by Vetter et al (1999) reports that vascular dementia (VD) clients impose a greater

Box 7-1 The Burden Interview

1. I feel resentful of other relatives who could but who do not do things for my spouse.
2. I feel that my spouse makes requests which I perceive to be over and above what s/he needs.
3. Because of my involvement with my spouse, I don't have enough time for myself.
4. I feel caught between trying to give to my spouse as well as to other family responsibilities, job, etc.
5. I feel embarrassed over my spouse's behavior.
6. I feel guilty about my interactions with my spouse.
7. I feel that I don't do as much for my spouse as I could or should.
8. I feel angry about my interactions with my spouse.
9. I feel that in the past, I haven't done as much for my spouse as I could have or should have.
10. I feel nervous or depressed about my interactions with my spouse.
11. I feel that my spouse currently affects my relationships with other family members and friends in a negative way.
12. I feel resentful about my interactions with my spouse.
13. I am afraid of what the future holds for my spouse.
14. I feel pleased about my interactions with my spouse.
15. It's painful to watch my spouse age.
16. I feel useful in my interactions with my spouse.
17. I feel my spouse is dependent.
18. I feel strained in my interactions with my spouse.
19. I feel that my health has suffered because of my involvement with my spouse.
20. I feel that I am contributing to the well-being of my spouse.
21. I feel that the present situation with my spouse doesn't allow me as much privacy as I'd like.
22. I feel that my social life has suffered because of my involvement with my spouse.
23. I wish that my spouse and I had a better relationship.
24. I feel that my spouse doesn't appreciate what I do for him/her as much as I would like.
25. I feel uncomfortable when I have friends over.
26. I feel that my spouse tries to manipulate me.
27. I feel that my spouse seems to expect me to take care of him/her as if I were the only one s/he could depend on.
28. I feel that I don't have enough money to support my spouse in addition to the rest of our expenses.
29. I feel that I would like to be able to provide more money to support my spouse than I am able to now.

From Zarit SH, Reever KE, Bach-Peterson J: *The Gerontologist* 20(6):649-655, 1980.

burden on relatives than do clients with dementia of the Alzheimer's type (DAT). In severe stages, however, this relationship undergoes a reversal, and caregivers of clients with DAT experience more burden than those of clients with VD. According to the screen for caregiver burden (SCB) (Vitaliano et al, 1991), all six areas of burden measured increased statistically when the client was in late-stage DAT. These areas are (1) activity disturbances, (2) loss of communication, (3) aggression, (4) workload, (5) financial problems, and (6) loss of control. Such increases in caregiver burden are often the result of misconceptions and erroneous information, motives, and roles that individuals have previously played. A holistic approach to the family includes strategies for helping members develop the ability to use resources; grow and develop physically, emotionally, and socially; and adapt to change and variation in lifestyle.

Often, when families are dealing with illness, the nurse needs to help them deal with the following areas: knowledge of the specific illness, adjustment to the changes common with all illness, and adjustment to different stages of illness (Cooley, 1989). A model that addresses the common family reactions to illness according to the stages of illness is the family crisis oriented personal scales (F-COPES). Diagnosis often involves dealing with anxiety and uncertainty. After the illness is identified, the family enters an implementation stage of managing the treatment and daily activities. Other stages of remission and rehabilitation follow. Families may also enter a terminal stage in which the issue of grief must be resolved. The F-COPES measure family responses to these phases (McCubbin, Thompson, 1987).

Other tools can be used to assess more specific family problems. Two that deal with family coping with a child's illness are the chronicity impact and coping instrument:parent questionnaire (CICI:PQ) (Hymovich, 1983) and the Feetham family functioning survey (FFFS) (Feetham, Humenick, 1982).

A short questionnaire called the *geriatric depression scale* measures attitudes, emotional status, and social integration. The questions address depressive symptoms in older persons. For example, the questionnaire asks, "Do you frequently worry about the future?" or "Do you prefer to avoid social gatherings?" (Yesavage et al, 1983). Older persons can read the questions themselves, or the questions can be administered orally by the nurse. Before beginning, the person should be reminded that there are no right or wrong answers and that some answers may seem at times to be both "yes" and "no." Attentive listening without judgmental response by the nurse usually creates the most nonthreatening environment, and the answers may reveal a great deal about the person's emotional status.

Assessment of Emotional Health: Mood and Affect, Hopelessness, and Depression

Illness is often accompanied by loss of privacy, self-esteem, and independence. Anxiety, irritation, powerlessness, and depression, which are by-products of these losses for the client, are sometimes severe enough to require professional attention. There are several assessment tools that are both easy and reliable. It should be noted that separately they do not form the basis for a diagnosis, but are helpful in combination with more extensive counseling.

The geriatric hopelessness scale (GHS) can be used to determine life view and orientation to self and future (Fry, 1984). In these scales, *hopelessness* is defined as negative expectancies toward self, the world, and the future. The GHS can be easily administered orally, which can be a substantial advantage for a client who cannot see or write well.

Questions are presented from both the positive aspect (for example, "I have faith that things will become better for me.") and the negative aspect (for example, "I will always be old and useless."). A "false" response to the former statement and a "true" response to the latter statement both indicate hopelessness.

The scale, which takes approximately 5 minutes to complete and is easily understood by chronically ill, quickly fatigued clients, is highly reliable. Mental health can also be assessed with the CES-D, a 20-item self-report measure of cognitive and affective behaviors and somatic symptoms associated with depression as experienced by clients in the week before the test (Devine, 1985).

Perhaps one of the most difficult assessments for families is that which distinguishes depression from dementia. Frequently there is some combination of depression and dementia in an

Box 7-2 Financial Assessment			
RESOURCES		**MONTHLY EXPENDITURES**	
Yearly income:	_____	Rent/house payments:	_____
Wages:	_____	Medical expenses:	_____
Pension:	_____	Telephone:	_____
Interest income:	_____	Taxes and household incurrence:	_____
Housing subsidy:	_____	Car/transportation:	_____
Stocks:	_____	Food costs:	_____
Dividends:	_____	Drug bills:	_____
Certificates:	_____	Utilities (gas/electric/oil):	_____
Monthly income:	_____	Clothing:	_____
Social Security:	_____	Other monthly recurring expenses:	_____
Rental income:	_____	Unusually nonrecurring expenses	_____
Food stamps:	_____	planned:	
Assets: (other than home/	_____	Total expenditures:	════════
personal property)			
Cash:	_____		
Bonds:	_____		
Savings accounts:	_____		
Total assets:	════════		

individual who has been judged to have either. A number of tools have been developed to measure mental status so that nursing and mental health professionals can coordinate assessment.

The mini-mental state exam (MMSE) is one of the most available and widely used tools for screening cognitive impairment. It comprises 20 items that assess multiple domains of cognitive functioning. It includes tests of language, orientation to time and place, visual-spatial skill, and the ability to sustain attention. The maximum score is 30. Typically, a score of 23 to 24 indicates cognitive impairment such as dementia (Folstein, Folstein, McHugh, 1975). On a cautionary note, a client's failure to respond accurately can be the result of depression.

The assessment of dementia or depression has important implications for treatment, management, and family support. Addington and Fry (1986) note that both groups would respond to treatment with an antidepressant. The true dementia group, however, might have higher susceptibility to these drugs, especially their anticholinergic effect. The most unfortunate (and most common) result of incomplete assessment is that a depressed elderly client is misdiagnosed as demented. Without proper treatment for depression, clients can deteriorate rapidly, compliance is compromised, and recovery is partial or absent. See Chapter 22 for a more thorough discussion of dementia.

Home health care agencies have come to realize the importance of the comprehensive psychosocial component. Without it, the resulting psychosocial care plans would be vague and lack clear goals. While most standard assessments include sections on medications, diet, ADLs, and current health status, the more thorough ones now contain psychosocial components.

Financial Anxiety

The stability and availability of financial resources should be addressed if they are causing undue anxiety in the family. The additional burden of financial worry that is sometimes voiced by families of seriously ill clients can be somewhat decreased if accurate data are available. When the family is able to share financial information, the best use of resources can be made and the search for support, which may be needed immediately or in the future, can be addressed. A few resources are provided in Box 7-2.

Patterns of Sexual Activity

It is not easy for some clients and their partners to initiate dialogue about sexual problems. It is therefore very important that the nurse present a comfortable opportunity to discuss sexual activity. Nurses should take time to explain, paraphrase, and define words. Appropriate questions might include the following:

1. Are you presently sexually active?
2. How does your present sexual activity compare with what you consider to be normal for you?
3. Have any of the physical changes, medications, or anything else created difficulty being intimate or having sexual intercourse? (Examples include pain or difficulty achieving erection, orgasm, or ejaculation.)
4. Do you have any concerns about your present level of sexual functioning?
5. Can you talk about these topics with your partner?

Personal Surroundings

Personal surroundings are important as indicators of social interaction, resources, familial proximity, ego integrity, and activity levels. In addition to the standard safety and functional determinations, considered within broad individual parameters are the following:

1. Are there flowers, pictures, or photographs?
2. Are there mementos of travel, accomplishments, or children?
3. Is there evidence of hobbies or craftwork?
4. Are there clocks, mirrors, or calendars?
5. Are there books, records, or magazines?
6. Is there a pet? A window birdfeeder?
7. Does the client seem proud of or embarrassed by home surroundings?
8. Is trash taken out regularly?
9. Are such things as food and linens clean and properly stored?
10. Are there current mail items and newspapers?

SUPPORT SYSTEMS

Levels of support surround the individual when he or she is ill. They include an inner support system of such attitudes as self-esteem, uniqueness of individuals, world view and resources, space, loss, and needs. An outer or external support system other than the health care team exists, and

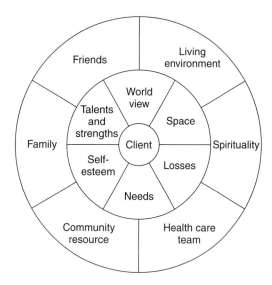

Fig. 7-1 Support systems.

includes, among others, family, friends, living environment, spiritual leader, physician, and community resources (Fig. 7-1). Nurses can support families in several ways. Open and honest communication is important and is done by listening to family concerns and answering questions or assisting the family to get answers. It is important to support the family coping mechanism and foster realistic hope and provide information about options. Family conferences can allow the ventilation of family feelings and help members reach consensus or compromise about client care.

IMPLEMENTING THE ASSESSMENT
Rapport, Trust, and Sensitivity

Before assessment, the nurse establishes rapport with and gains the trust of the client and family. Even in the process of setting the first appointment it is important to be clear and respectful. Arranging a time that allows the most family members to be present is best. This is the necessary beginning of the ongoing mutual respect and cooperation essential to the success of any intervention. The nurse's approach must be genuine. The nurse should show a sincere acceptance of variations such as religion, values, ethnicity, and social behavior. Cultural sensitivity requires the study of traditions and beliefs of other cultures but at the least, the nurse will be aware of his or her own limitations and will strive to become more open and knowledgeable. Clients and families need to be given an opportunity to describe cultural beliefs because there is great variation within, as well as among, cultures.

The nurse should be sensitive to topics that are difficult for the clients and family members to address. Questioning should be sensitive if they are unwilling or unable to answer. Certain areas may be confusing; others may be culturally or emotionally loaded. Responses and problems should be acknowledged and opinions and feelings accepted without judgmental rebuttal. Positive reinforcement can be offered to the client and family to proceed and can elevate feelings of confidence that they are being helpful. Strengths and achievements as well as weaknesses should be identified, and the former should be praised. A therapeutic relationship is built on trust and honesty and exists through good listening skills, caring, and confirmation. Later, this same relationship will form the basis of the rapport necessary to increase cooperation and compliance (Vivian, Wilcox, 2000). Families who share reasonable expectations and make decisions with nurses have a greater commitment to those decisions.

Note-taking is essential, and the client and caregivers should be told that it is important to write things down so that they report symptoms and problems accurately. During the interview, the nurse should not be so absorbed with writing that listening skills diminish. Each entry should be dated so that it does not become confused with future, ongoing entries. When available, data should be entered into the computer-based client record in the system's accepted standardized format and nursing language.

At the conclusion of the assessment, the nurse should summarize the concerns identified so that priorities for action can be jointly established. The client and family members should be given an opportunity to clarify information and express fears and doubts. Open-ended questions often reveal surprising fears and misinformation. The nurse might simply ask, "Is there anything you would like to ask me?"

Important information about environment can be gathered through observation. The sensitive and well-trained observer is able to detect problems that can be reversed or minimized even though they are never verbalized.

Since the family represents the context within which the individual functions, the home gives important clues about that context. The nurse may observe the following:

- Relationship with pets
- Assignment of roles and tasks
- Decor and orderliness
- Preferential seating
- Provision for privacy and interaction
- Quiet or boisterous interaction
- Mutual respect or deference
- Frequency and quality of meals

These are indications of the way this context may or may not support the client's recovery.

That which is observed may add to what is discussed, may alter priorities, or may even contradict what has been stated. Bare cupboards may be a better indication of a client's nutritional intake than a statement that he or she "eats very well." A medicine cabinet full of expired drugs, the smell of stale urine, or cigarette burns in a housecoat all represent situations that are better observed than stated. Signs of an abusive relationship such as physical marks or fearful or servile behaviors by the client should not be overlooked (Wolf, 1999). Perceptions can also be wrong and need verification before action is taken. During observation, it is best to know what situation existed before the illness so that change can be measured. The standards for environment or relationships should be those that were once appropriate for the client, rather than what is suitable to the observer.

SUMMARY

Home care is most often family-centered care, and progress is tied to recognition of the interrelationships of family members, community, and home environment. Psychosocial assessment provides baseline data for comparison as the client's life and health evolve. A good psychosocial assessment, which addresses and plans for cultural and role orientations, financial concerns, communications, decision-making patterns, and inherent strengths and weaknesses in the environment, will positively affect the health of the client and the ability of the family to be supportive caregivers.

Mr. and Mrs. R. have been married 55 years and have lived many of those years in a small coastal town in Oregon. Mr. R., 75 years of age, is very active and mentally alert, works as a real estate agent, and continues to help care for the family farm. Mrs. R., 80 years of age, has never been responsible for housework or cooking. Her primary interests have been playing cards, watching ballgames, attending church services once a week, and playing with her dogs. She is well known for her sense of humor. Trips to Las Vegas and Reno to gamble were a yearly highlight. These roles seemed to be satisfying to Mr. and Mrs. R. Nearly 10 years ago, Mrs. R. began developing cataracts, had unsuccessful eye surgery, and continued gradually to lose her sight. The family helped compensate with aids for the blind, the two most important being enlarged playing cards and an enhanced telephone dial. She continued to make her highly successful gambling trips with someone reading the cards for her! However, 5 years before, she became completely blind and shortly thereafter became confused.

Mrs. R. remains adamantly against institutionalization. Her behavior has become demanding, and she no longer performs personal care tasks. She broke her hip and was hospitalized and has now been brought home, where she is outraged by the presence of home health care staff. Mr. R. has told her they are maids so that she will accept them. Mr. R. is showing signs of fatigue and depression. He constantly worries about how much all of this is costing and about what will happen to Mrs. R. if he gets ill. The children are lobbying to put Mrs. R. in a nursing home.

DISCUSSION

After traditional clinical and environmental factors are assessed, the evaluation tool in Fig. 7-2, which assesses support systems, might be used to advantage. This tool is helpful in recording observations and developing a coordinated psychosocial care plan. Perhaps its greatest advantage is that it encourages communication among client, family, and health care providers and requires the setting of goals and the assessment of responsibilities.

The CFAM would also be useful in measuring expressive functioning. It would include the evaluation of both emotional and verbal communication on the topic of nursing home placement (Wright, Leahey, 1994). The setting of manageable goals is very important. Areas of concern would include the following:

- *The way Mrs. R.'s view of herself and her world contributes to her ability to perform ADLs*
- *The impact of her blindness and other losses on her activities, self-image, and mental alertness*
- *The appropriateness of her environment to maximizing her remaining strengths*
- *Family relationships as they affect her cooperation and health*
- *Family roles as they relate to Mr. R.'s need for understanding and respite*
- *An understanding of financial assets and ways that they can best be used and preserved*

In assigning responsibilities for creating additional support systems, nurses should consider the following:

- *The family relationships with Mrs. R.*
- *Potential support from adult children*
- *Quality and quantity of support from Mr. R. without jeopardizing his mental and physical health*
- *External sources (community/church/friends) to give respite and needed services*
- *Degree and type of support in counseling and team input*

	INNER SUPPORT SYSTEM	
Talents/Strengths	*Losses*	*Needs*
List: Short Term Goal: Responsible Person:	Recent: Short Term Goal: Responsible Person:	List: Short Term Goal: Responsible Person:
Space	*World View*	*Self Esteem*
Control? Identity Cues? Environmental Cues? Short Term Goal: Responsible Person:	Positive: Negative: Continuity of View: Short Term Goal: Responsible Person:	Now: Then: Short Term Goal: Responsible Person:
	OUTER SUPPORT SYSTEM	
Family	*Friends*	*Community Resources*
Local Contact: Short Term Goal: Responsible Person:	Yes/No? Visit Often? Short Term Goal: Responsible Person:	Adequate: Accessible: Short Term Goal: Responsible Person:
Health Care Team	*Spiritual*	*Living Environment*
Recent/ Long standing? Appropriate Discipline: Visitation: Coordinated: Communication: Short Term Goal: Responsible Person:	Important? Organized Group? Is Group Supportive? Short Term Goal: Responsible Person:	Positive? Negative? Behavior Response: Short Term Goal: Responsible Person:
	Care Plan	For:_____
Support System	*Goal*	*Person Responsible*
Inner Support System: Uniqueness: Self-Esteem: Losses: Needs: Space:		
Outer Support System: Family: Friends: Staff: Physician: Spiritual: Environment:		

Fig. 7-2 Assessment and planning tool for psychosocial support. *(Courtesy Doris Weaver, University of Washington.)*

REFERENCES

Addington J, Fry PS: Directions for clinical psychosocial assessment of depression in the elderly. In Brink TL, ed: *Clinical gerontology: A guide to assessment and intervention,* New York, 1986, Haworth Press.

Berkman B et al: Standardized screening of elderly patients' needs for social work assessment, *Health Care and Social Work,* 2(1):9-16, 1999.

Clemen-Stone S, McGuire SL, Eigsti DG: *Comprehensive community health nursing,* St Louis, 1998, Mosby.

Cooley M: A family process model of coping with illness. Paper presented at the meeting of the National Council for Family Relation Theory, New Orleans, Nov 1989.

de Savorgnani AA, Haring RC: Best practice and successes in cultural diversity, *Caring* 18(4):22-27, 1999.

Dellman-Jenkins M, Blankenmeyer M, Pinkard O: Young adult children and grandchildren in primary caregiver roles to older relatives, *Family Relations* 49(2):177-186, 2000.

Devine G, Orme C: CES-D: Center for epidemiologic studies depression scale. In Keyser DJ, Sweetland RC, eds: *Test critiques,* Kansas City, Mo, 1985, Westport.

Eggebeen D, Davey A: Do safety nets work? The role of anticipated help in time of need, *Journal of Marriage and the Family* 60(5):939-950, 1998.

Feetham S, Humenick S: The Feetham family functioning survey. In Humenick S, ed: *Analysis of current assessment strategies in the health care of young children and childbearing families,* New York, 1982, Appleton-Century-Crofts.

Folstein MF, Folstein SE, McHugh PR: "Mini-mental state." A practical method for grading the cognitive state of patients for the clinician, *Journal of Psychiatric Research* 12(3):189-198, 1975.

Friedman M: *Family nursing: Theory and assessment,* ed 4, Norwalk, Conn, 1998, Appleton & Lange.

Fry PS: The development of a geriatric scale of hopelessness: Implications for counseling and intervention, *Journal of Counseling Psychology* 31(2):322-331, 1984.

Goodell T, Hanson S: Nurse-family interaction in adult critical care, *Journal of Family Nursing* 5(1):72-91, 1999.

Hanson S, Boyd S: *Family health care nursing: Theory, practice, and research,* Philadelphia, 1996, FA Davis.

Hanson SMH, Mischke KM: Family health assessment and intervention. In Bormar PJ, Mischke KM, eds: *Nurses and family health promotion: concepts, assessment, and intervention,* Philadelphia, 1996, WB Saunders.

Hymovich D: The Chronicity Impact and Coping Instrument: Parent questionnaire, *Nursing Research* 32(5):275-281, 1983.

McConnochie KM et al: Ensuring high quality alternatives, *Archives of Pediatrics and Adolescent Medicine* 151(4):341, 1997.

McCubbin HI, Thompson AI: *Family assessment inventories,* Madison, 1987, University of Wisconsin-Madison.

McCubbin HI, Olson D, Larson AS: Family crisis oriented personal scales. In Olson D et al, eds: *Family inventories,* St Paul, Minn, 1982, University of Minnesota.

McCubbin HI, Patterson J, Wilson LR: The family inventory of life events and changes. In Olson D et al, eds: *Family inventories,* St Paul, Minn, 1982, University of Minnesota.

McGoldrick M, Gerson R: *Genograms in family assessment,* New York, 1985, WW Norton.

Neuman B: *The Neuman's systems model,* ed 2, Norwalk, Conn, 1989, Appleton & Lange.

Shepherd M, Moriarty H: Family mental health nursing. In Hanson S, Boyd S, eds: *Family health care nursing: Theory, practice, and research,* Philadelphia, 1996, FA Davis.

Smith CM, Mauer FA: *Community Health Nursing,* ed 2, Philadelphia, 2000, WB Saunders.

Thibault L: Home health care management, *Orthopedic Nursing* 16(2):317, 1997.

Vetter PH et al: Vascular dementia versus dementia of Alzheimer's type: Do they have differential effects on caregivers' burden? *Journal of Gerontology* 54B(2):593-598, 1999.

Vitaliano PP et al: The screen for caregiver burden, *The Gerontologist* 31(1):76-83, 1991.

Vivian BG, Wilcox JR: Compliance communication in home health care: A mutually reciprocal process, *Qualitative Health Research* 10(1):103-116, 2000.

Wolf RS: Suspected abuse in an elderly patient, *American Family Physician* 59(5):1319-1320, 1999.

Wright DW: Socially isolated in rural settings without a wide support setting, *Caring* 16(1):26-28, 1997.

Wright L, Leahey M: *Nurses and families: A guide to family assessment and intervention,* Philadelphia, 1994, FA Davis.

Yesavage JA et al: Development and validation of a geriatric depression screening scale, *Journal of Psychiatric Research* 17:37, 1983.

Zanetti O et al: Contrasting results between caregiver's report and direct assessment of activities of daily living in patients affected by mild and very mild dementia: The contribution of the caregiver's personal characteristics, *Journal of the American Geriatrics Society* 42(2):7-12, 1999.

Zarit S, Reever KE, Bach-Peterson J: Relatives of the impaired elderly: Correlates of feelings of burden, *The Gerontologist* 20(6):649-655, 1980.

Zarit S, Todd P, Zarit J: Subjective burden of husbands and wives as caregivers: A longitudinal study, *The Gerontologist* 26(3):260-266, 1986.

8 Skills in Family Teaching

David Arthur

Teaching clients and families how to care for themselves and their loved ones has always been seen as an essential, and in the past, informal part of nursing care. Education has become an integral component of the nursing profession, and its consumers have placed more demands on nurses to be more consumer focused and more accountable in terms of service delivery.

With the information explosion and the advent of consumer rights and empowerment have come demands that the nursing profession be able to provide information in a systematic and therapeutic manner. This is where nursing utilizes the theories and principles of education to strengthen practice. The breadth of education in nursing has widened to incorporate education for clients and their families in both hospital and community situations and in primary, secondary, and tertiary settings. Nursing curricula worldwide are now incorporating family nursing and related education strategies (St John, Rolls, 1996). In addition to the focus on traditional medical and surgical disorders, nurses provide teaching related to human immunodeficiency virus (HIV) and acquired immunodeficiency syndrome (AIDS) awareness; rehabilitation nursing; health-related behaviors and lifestyle-related disorders such as heart disease and diabetes; early intervention in drug and alcohol use; and client-family education for people with mental disorders such as schizophrenia, depression, and dementia. Further, nursing research is endeavoring to identify the therapeutic link between family education and improved clinical outcomes (Brooker, 1990; Reeber, 1992; Youssef, 1987). This chapter narrows the focus of family teaching to home care but encourages readers to consider the depth and breadth of the applications of teaching in nursing. Complementing this chapter are some extra materials to give a more psychosocial dimension to home care and references to stimulate the practitioner to go further afield for information and strategies for use in more complex situations. Family teaching may be done routinely in hospitals, both during the hospital stay and in discharge planning; in clinics; in home care; and wherever else nurses provide care to clients. In actual practice, nurses have long recognized that much of this teaching is done quickly, at whatever time can be found by the nurse, and with a priority that may rank far below other concerns to the client, such as filling out papers for discharge or completing treatments. In some cases, nurses can teach the family strategies for working with a client who is noncompliant or resistive to treatment. This is a more subtle and complicated use of teaching but has applications where disordered cognition, denial, withdrawal, or similar emotions are providing obstruction to the client's welfare.

Family teaching is a complex and essential role for the home care nurse who has become the educational coordinator for the client, family, and health care team. This chapter will discuss general concepts of teaching and learning, theory motivation, learning styles, age-related learning factors, objectives, and teaching strategies that can be used to teach individuals and families in home settings. Family concepts and characteristics that affect home care and family teaching will be described, including family functioning and sociocultural influences. Professional issues on family teaching will be summarized.

GENERAL CONCEPTS OF TEACHING AND LEARNING

Teaching and learning involve both the teacher and the learner as collaborators. If a learner does not participate, nothing happens. The nurse who is trying to teach cannot complete the process alone. The nurse, as the professional provider of educational service, is responsible for taking the lead in adapting teaching techniques to meet the learning needs of the family.

Learning Theory

Hamachek (1995), in a review of major theoretical positions about human behavior, explains how a teacher's beliefs significantly affect his or her teaching practices and relationships with students, whereas Bigge (1976) has noted that theories of learning are based on philosophical beliefs about human nature. For the nurse attempting to apply learning theory to family teaching, it is essential to understand his or her own philosophy about human nature and try to recognize when there are philosophical differences between the teacher and the client.

The most common learning theories based on philosophical beliefs are humanistic theory, behavioristic theory, and cognitive theory. These were developed several decades ago and continue to be used and refined. The writings of Carl Rogers (1969) on becoming a person and Abraham Maslow's concept of self-actualization (1954) based on a hierarchy of human needs are both well-known influences on humanistic learning theory. This theory is generally based on the philosophical view that feelings are as important as knowledge and that the learner intuitively knows what needs to be learned. The role of the teacher is to assist students in developing and finding themselves.

Among the theorists who favor behavioristic learning theory are B.F. Skinner (1953) and Albert Bandura (1969). Behaviorists believe that learning is best achieved by environmental control that shapes new behaviors and offers rewards for changes. The learner changes behavior as a result of stimuli in the learning environment, and the role of the teacher is to reinforce desired behaviors. R.M. Gagne (1984) built on these theories with his ideas on conditions of learning, which need to be identified first by the teacher by looking at the capabilities of the learner, then by the stimulus situation outside the learner. Gagne applied conditions of learning, including intellectual skills, cognitive strategies, verbal information, problem solving, motor skills, and attitudes, to several events relevant to nursing.

The third major learning theory is the cognitive theory, which is based on the belief that all individuals want to learn, and the challenge to the teacher is to provide the right stimuli and assist the learner in self-discovered learning and self-evaluation of learning. Jerome Bruner (1963) and Morris Bigge (1976) have written extensively on this approach (Table 8-1).

The reader is referred to the selected references at the end of the chapter for further information on these theories mentioned. The focus of the chapter is to explore how these theories can assist the home care nurse in teaching families.

Let us look at what happens when there is a philosophical difference between the preferred learning theory of the nurse and the family member. Suppose that the nurse is behavioristic and approaches the teaching and learning process expecting very specific behaviors to change. If working with a family member or group of members who are humanistic in their approach to learning and are more concerned with how they feel emotionally than with what they do be-

Table 8-1	Three Commonly Accepted Learning Theories	
Theory	Theorist	Principles
Humanistic	Carl Rogers Abraham Maslow	Feelings are as important as knowledge, and the learner intuitively knows what he or she needs to know.
Behavioristic	B.F. Skinner Albert Bandura	Learning is best achieved by environmental control that shapes new behaviors and offers rewards for changes.
Cognitive	Jerome Bruner Morris Bigge	All individuals want to learn, and the teaching challenge is to provide the right stimuli and assist the learner in self-discovered learning and self-evaluation.

haviorally, the nurse will need to adjust the teaching process to accommodate and combine these differing philosophies. There are times when a nurse may judge that philosophical issues are seriously hindering progress with a family and may suggest that another nurse work with the family.

There are many possible combinations of philosophical differences between learners and teachers, and the nurse needs to note when questions of congruence of beliefs arise. The learner and the teacher who can accept and incorporate different philosophies will have an advantage of versatility in dealing with respective differences here and in other areas of the nurse-client relationship.

In health education, the predisposing, reinforcing, and enabling causes for educational diagnosis and evaluation (PRECEDE) model for planning programs is basically a combination of the three philosophical variables previously mentioned (Green et al, 1980). In this model, the predisposing factors are those found in humanistic learning theory. The enabling factors are similar to those identified in cognitive learning theory, and the reinforcing factors closely resemble those described in behavioristic learning theory. The use of this model for planning health education is an example of how theory can be used in a practical way.

Motivation

Motivation to learn will be influenced by the family's perceived need for knowledge. Redman (1984) discusses this as a readiness factor in client education. Behaviors that will affect health and family beliefs about health are prime motivators and need to be identified.

Similarly, Miller and Rollnick (1991) see motivation as state of readiness or eagerness to change, which may fluctuate and which may be influenced. In their helpful text on motivational interviewing, they describe strategies to help develop a relationship and to help clients change. Other factors that influence learning may be related to grieving or coming to terms with loss. An understanding of the grief process as described in Chapter 7 is important. People in different stages of coming to terms with their illness may present psychological blocks, which, although quite healthy defense mechanisms, may affect their motivation to learn.

One of the most likely motivators for learning new health-related information and behaviors is the need to cope with a stressful situation that exists in the home. Families who seek home care nursing are experiencing this type of stress and will be highly motivated learners if the stress is not too overwhelming. When a family has accepted the inevitability of change that caring for an ill member requires, the members are usually willing to cooperate in learning activities that will make their adjustment easier. In addition to coping with a new situation, a strong motivator for families is the self-esteem and satisfaction that can be derived from acquiring new skills and increasing knowledge that will positively affect family functioning.

Learning Styles

Learning styles are often closely associated with individual thinking patterns. The most common are based on inductive and deductive reasoning or thinking. People who are basically inductive learn best when confronted with a specific situation, whereas those who are deductive prefer to know general information first and apply this to the specific situation later. Many people fall somewhere between these two approaches, and like those who can function equally with either their right or left hands, some think equally well in either mode.

In helping learners based on their preferred thinking pattern, the nurse would use an actual or simulated situation for an inductive learner; for the deductive learner, the nurse would start with general information and proceed to the specific case. An example of this can be seen in the family who is trying to change the physical activity patterns of a middle-aged member who has recently been discharged from the hospital after a myocardial infarction. If the learning style of the client or primary caregiver is inductive, discussion of specific recent events and the client's exercise patterns would be a more appropriate starting place than a discussion of the general relationship between exercise and cardiovascular function. For those who are primarily deductive, the latter approach would be preferred.

Previous Learning Patterns

A few well-chosen questions can help the nurse and the family to recognize previous successful learning patterns. This also identifies inductive and deductive styles. Motivation for learning can be incorporated into this approach. The nurse might ask, "When you wanted to change the way you were doing something in the past, what was most helpful to you? Did you ever do regular exercise in the past? What made you start? What made you stop?" The answers to these and similar questions give both the nurse and the family some information on appropriate teaching and learning methods.

Age

Developmental theorists have identified factors related to age and learning. Piaget (1952) wrote on learning and cognitive development from infancy to adulthood based on his studies of developmental growth and emotional tasks for different age groups. Erikson's work on developmental growth stages (1963) can help the nurse understand where learner priorities are expected to be based on age-related developmental tasks. These theories can be helpful in working with a family who is caring for a child with a health problem. For example, for a family caring for a school-age child who recently lost a leg in an automobile accident, the teaching plan would take into consideration that this child is at a developmental stage in which cognitively, he leans toward concrete operations. The question, "How will I walk with one leg?" requires a very concrete answer, such as "With the help of this artificial leg we are fitting you for," accompanied by a demonstration of the artificial leg and how it works. The child is not yet ready for abstract details unless he indicates this readiness in his questions. The information that is part of the teaching plan needs to be geared to the learning characteristics of his age group, in addition to other factors that affect him as an individual and family member. For the same child, recognizing that he is working on the industry versus inferiority developmental task as identified by Erikson (1963), the nurse and family can establish goals that will allow the child to be industrious in every possible way, despite the loss of his leg.

Sometimes, learning in adults is complicated by complex variables, including personality and life circumstances. Consequently, responses to health-related problems are diverse. The middle-aged man recently home after a myocardial infarction may be more inclined to change his exercise behavior if he is reminded that he is setting an example for his sons (generativity) than if he is allowed to lose sight of this and become bogged down and self-absorbed in his own health problems. However, another man with the same condition may have great difficulty in modifying his life-style and ignore the advice and teaching. While this may be permanent, in most cases it is a temporary function of coming to terms with a trauma or the loss of previous status. The nurse can recognize this and persist with teaching strategies not only for the client, but also for the family.

To help understand this process of change in adults, it may be useful to consider the process of loss and grief and the model proposed by DiClemente (1991), which describes the stages that people pass through in the course of changing a problem. In this case, the client needs time to work through the stages of contemplation, determination, action, and maintenance. Before actual change takes place, people may go around the process several times. An individual client's readiness to change logically becomes a part of the learning assessment phase described next.

Learning Assessment

Teaching requires assessing the needs of the learners, gathering all that needs to be taught in the particular situation, and mutually setting the educational goals. This is the first phase, and it results in an educational diagnosis and plan. The next steps are to decide how to help this learning process and to choose the appropriate techniques for teaching and learning in the given situation. The nurse can be assisted by physicians, pharmacists, occupational therapists, physical therapists, clergy, social workers, and other professionals. A crucial part of the nurse's role is the coordinating/leading function, and one of the unique characteristics of family teaching is that the client and family members become an integral part of the planning and implementation of the teaching goals.

Before educational intervention, the two most common family situations are (1) the client is the person primarily responsible for implementing his health care behaviors, or (2) the client is unable to take responsibility for his own health care, and another family member has the primary caregiving responsibility. In the first situation, the nurse would put major efforts into teaching the client, as the learner, to handle the responsibility and encourage the family to be supportive without encouraging helplessness on the part of the client. In the second situation, the major effort would be directed toward the family caretaker as the learner while encouraging the client to cooperate in any way possible. Obviously, there are many situations that fall between these two, and the nurse should use professional judgment on the best approach to use at any given time.

Objectives

Objectives serve as guides for implementing and evaluating teaching and are best developed collaboratively by the nurse and the family members involved. Based on the types of learner needs commonly encountered in nursing practice, objectives usually fall into the following categories: cognitive, affective, and psychomotor. In each of these categories, taxonomies or classification systems have been developed describing the complexity of expected behaviors from simple to complex.

Bloom (1956) described a taxonomy for the cognitive domain, or knowledge-based objectives. Krathwohl, Bloom, and Masia (1964) developed a taxonomy for the affective domain, or the objectives that are concerned with values and feelings. Harrow (1972) identified a taxonomy for the psychomotor domain that focused on motor skills. Nurses should become familiar with the terms used in these taxonomies to help in stating behavioral objectives and in strengthening the concept that behaviors can range from simple to complex in any of these categories. The original sources are included in the references at the end of the chapter. The following case study demonstrates how these general concepts can be used to organize a teaching plan in home care.

CASE STUDY

When Mr. K. was discharged from the hospital after surgery for a colostomy, his wife was as concerned and confused as he was. Their two teenaged sons were busy with school, Mrs. K. held a full-time job, and Mr. K. planned to return to his job as soon as possible. The physician at the medical center where the surgery was done, the staff nurses on the unit, and the enterostomal therapist at the hospital had all visited with the K. family members before discharge for instruction on colostomy care and use of equipment that would be needed. The family had also been referred to the local home care agency for follow-up, supervision, and instruction.

APPLYING OBJECTIVES

The general principles and the process of family teaching are basically the same for all families. The challenge for the home care nurse is to adapt them to the needs of each individual family. In this case study, Mr. K. is the primary learner, and other family members will provide support. Mr. K. states he understands how to change his colostomy bag and how to change the appliance that adheres to the skin to hold the bag. He is, however, very worried about the skin irritation around the stoma area. Based on Mr. K.'s statement, and a confirming examination of the skin and perhaps a demonstration by Mr. K. on how he

gives himself colostomy care, the nurse determines the educational needs to be in the following domains:

- *Cognitive: Knowledge about skin care*
- *Psychomotor: Skill to cleanse the skin and attach the appliance*
- *Affective: How he feels about the procedure*

In further assessing the specific needs of this family member, the nurse finds deficits based on the following:

- *Knowledge: He does not understand the importance of cleansing the skin each time he changes the appliance, even if the skin is intact.*
- *Skill: When he does cleanse the skin, he rubs vigorously until the skin is red and irritated from the cleansing.*
- *Emotions: He is having difficulty accepting the amount or time it now takes him to manage what was formerly a simple body function.*

Educational interventions would then include teaching him about skin care and skin integrity, demonstrating the actual procedure for skin cleansing that is appropriate for his skin, and allowing him to discuss his feelings of anger and frustration about his situation. In helping him deal with his feelings, the nurse would probably also refer him to community support services for people with his condition, such as the local Ostomy Club. Following these interventions,

Continued

CASE STUDY—cont'd

within a realistic time period the nurse would work with the client to evaluate the educational outcomes and plan follow-up in accordance with the results.

The nurse would also ask the other family members if they had questions and, in collaboration with Mr. K., explain the difficulties with which he is coping and ways that they might help. Families are usually eager to do what they can to be supportive, and they feel better about themselves as well as the client when concrete suggestions are given. In this case, discussion

about the changes Mr. K. is coping with could help the family to better understand why he takes so much time in the bathroom and why he is sometimes angry and irritable when he has to change his appliance. Understanding this anxiety behavior enables the family to be supportive, rather than angry and blaming. Their quiet support would in turn help Mr. K. to accept his new limitations and feel better about himself and the family. All of these outcomes are intended results of family teaching.

Although it is not the purpose of this chapter to go into great detail on writing behavioral objectives, it is important to understand what makes a sound behavioral objective. It must be valid, observable, and measurable. Box 8-1 presents some examples of terms that can be used when writing objectives in each of the three domains. For the nurse, validity will depend on whether the objective actually addresses the learning problem. For example, in the case study the nurse wants to develop behavioral objectives for Mr. K. After determining, in collaboration with him, that he has learning needs in the three domains, three objectives will be needed. When writing the objectives, the nurse includes the following four characteristics in each one:

1. Who is the learner?
2. What is the anticipated behavior?
3. What are the conditions that will assist in measuring the behavior?
4. How will the behavior be evaluated?

For Mr. K., the following are complete behavioral objectives that address his identified learning needs and include the four parts:

- Cognitive need: Mr. K. will describe to the nurse four of the principles of skin care for his colostomy that they have discussed when she visits in 2 days.
- Psychomotor need: Mr. K. will cleanse his skin in the colostomy area using the techniques that the nurse demonstrated while she observes him during her next visit.
- Affective need: Mr. K. will tell the nurse one area of frustration he is feeling about adjusting to the time demands of his colostomy during each visit for the next 2 weeks.

A word of caution on the limitations of be-

Box 8-1   Examples of Useful *Intended Behaviors* in Objectives

COGNITIVE DOMAIN (KNOWLEDGE)

... *list* three side effects of the medication ...
... *describe* the anatomy of the injection site ...
... *outline* the purpose of daily dressing changes ...
... *state* the three warning signals for indication of side effects of ...
... *explain* the meaning of ...

AFFECTIVE DOMAIN (ATTITUDES)

... *appreciate* the long-term importance of maintaining a low blood glucose level ...
... *accept* that angry feelings are a part of the process ...
... *explore* the feelings of frustration of being regularly hospitalized ...
... *evaluate* the positive and negative features of others' behavior ...
... *believe* in the value of self-care ...

PSYCHOMOTOR DOMAIN (MOTOR SKILLS)

... *insert* the needle into the dermis ...
... *manipulate* the controls on the ...
... *apply* the clean dressing by ...
... *massage* the scar tissue three times each day ...
... *mix* the two solutions together in a glass container ...

---

havioral objectives is in order. They can work well for learning needs that can be corrected by behavioral change. The nurse must be aware that not all needs are in the area of learning and there are times when the behaviors being developed are not sufficient to solve the existing problem. These situations require further assessment, and this is best done in a positive way that does not reflect failure for the client or the nurse but acknowledges that the solution to the problem is only partial and that more time and effort may be required for long-term solutions.

An example of this for Mr. K. would be if, after meeting all of the objectives mentioned, he was still experiencing skin irritation at the site of the stoma. The conclusion would be that he was doing what was needed, but what had been identified as needed was not enough to heal his skin. Further investigation into such things as allergic food reactions and irritation factors from the cleanser or adhesive would be investigated. This can be a very difficult time for the nurse and the client, and it is important that reinforcement for what has been done be given generously while work on solving the problem continues.

The nurse must realize there may be outcomes quite significant to the client's condition that were not mentioned in formulating the objectives. These should be noted in the evaluation, since the objectives are understood to be guides and not chains that limit developments conducive to the growth and healing of the client and to his or her learning experience.

Teaching Strategies

The nurse who is teaching families in a home situation will need a variety of skills and tools. The more varied the available techniques, the more choices there will be available for successful intervention. Some of the common teaching techniques include discussion; demonstration; visual aids, such as handouts, charts, posters, books, and pamphlets; audio cassettes; and audiovisual aids, such as slide presentations or video cassettes. In society today, televisions and radios are common household items, and many learners are more receptive to these methods of gathering information than to reading or listening to an individual. Many home care agencies are developing libraries of materials that will assist the nurse in teaching families. Public libraries may also be community resources for supplying films on needed topics, and agencies and universities with health-related programs work well with community agencies in sharing such teaching aids. The information and technology explosion has seen the widespread use of computers in the home, and many clients and their families have access to the internet. This provides a very valuable source of health care knowledge and has great potential as a teaching strategy in the form of purpose-designed web pages, as well as computer disks loaded with information offering computer-assisted instruction. Some home care agencies now communicate with their clients by e-mail, and this can reinforce teaching as well as communication.

While many clients and their families hunger for information and can freely access it, it may be helpful for the nurse to discuss and interpret some of the internet information, which ranges from highly technical and professional to lay and uninformed. The former may be threatening or confusing and need interpretation; the latter may be misleading and need correcting.

Technology can be a great help to nurses who are teaching, but it is only as effective as the judgment of the nurse who chooses what is appropriate for an individual or family. The information chosen must be judged to determine that it is what the family really needs to know. Its level must match the educational and cultural background of the family so that it is meaningful to them in the context of their lives. As with all teaching interventions, the key factor in this is the nurse's understanding of the characteristics of the family who is learning.

Timing

Another consideration is the art of timing. This is more than learner readiness in the sense discussed previously. It includes an assessment of the other factors impacting the family at the time. For example, it may be very important to teach wound care to a new postoperative client and his family at home. However, if the nurse arrives at the home and finds there has just been a death in the family, one of the children has been hospitalized, or some other family crisis has arisen, it would be appropriate for the nurse to change the dressing with minimal instruction to the family on that day and to spend her time helping the family deal with their major recent concern. Anxiety toward another family concern will interfere with any effort to impart new knowledge about wound care, and the nurse who tries to continue with the teaching agenda will meet with resistance or apathy that can only frustrate all concerned.

Learning Environment

Teaching families in their own homes allows the nurse to use the home environment as a teaching asset. An example is the case of the M. family, in which Danny, age 6, has just been released from the hospital with a diagnosis of diabetes. Although Danny is the client, because of his age and resultant inability to assume total responsibility in managing his disease, the nurse will aim much of the teaching at his parents or other designated caregiver. The nurse can look around the home and note whether fruit or cookies are more available for snacks. The nurse can also observe if kitchen equipment is sufficient to prepare the type of diet needed and if sanitary conditions will allow insulin injections to be prepared without contamination.

Teaching is sometimes mistakenly seen as limited to information sharing. This may be part of a teaching plan, but a comprehensive definition of *teaching,* or *educating,* includes all activities that assist the learner in making behavioral changes. After an assessment of learner needs and an educational diagnosis, the teacher designs the instructional plan and decides what techniques will be best to implement this plan. Evaluation of the teaching plan will then describe the outcome as well as the teaching and learning process. Evaluation findings may also provide direction for revising teaching and implementation strategies.

One application of the use of education in the broader sense is illustrated in recent research, which has shown that education for schizophrenic clients and their families may help reduce rehospitalization rates and improve the quality of life of patients living at home. In some families in which there is a member with schizophrenia, there is a high level of expressed emotion (EE), which is evidenced by a critical, emotional overinvolvement of family members, and it has been shown that this may influence the relapse of the symptoms of schizophrenia (Brooker, 1990; Leff, Kuipers, Berkowitz, 1982). By teaching the patient to recognize and manage stress and by educating the family about new, less critical ways of communicating, the home care nurse may help improve the emotional climate of the family. Of course, the education package for the family will still include information-sharing on medication, diagnosis, and symptom management, but it will have a deeper therapeutic effect with the addition of these theories related to EE.

GENERAL CONCEPTS ON FAMILIES

A family will seek or be referred to home care nursing when they need help in managing their situation. Usually a health-related problem exists. It may be a long-term or chronic problem, or it may be episodic or acute, as when a family member is newly discharged from the hospital after surgery. When a nurse makes an initial visit to the home to assess the situation, a key factor in the assessment is the nature of the family. Who are the members, and how do they function?

Membership in the family can be defined by blood, legal relationship, or function, Although the nurse needs to be aware of blood and legal relationships that exist in families, the basis for care rests more with the caring relationships that exist. For this reason, the concept of family used in this chapter is a unit of interacting persons. This concept allows for the many structures that exist in society today under the general heading of *family,* including nuclear families, single-parent families, groups of communal families, unmarried persons of different sexes living together with or without children, and persons of the same sex living together with or without children.

An important factor in recognizing the various family structures is that the nurse be able to also recognize any bias in his or her own set of beliefs and values about families. Past experience can color attitudes and make nurses more or less sensitive to the families in their care. A nurse who comes from a very traditional background may not think twice about inquiring about a spouse in a family where there are children. A nurse who has been a single parent will probably ask the question carefully (e.g., "Who are the members of your family and where do they work?" versus "What does your husband do for a living?").

A second factor that is important in relation to family structure is the nurse's ability to separate it from family functioning. Nurses should be aware of "solid" families who have severe hidden weaknesses, such as alcoholism and family violence, and "broken" families who have strong abilities to meet the needs of the individual members despite multiple visible problems. If nurses separate structure and function and realize that they are two separate dimensions that may or may not be related, they can avoid confusion in their assessment of the family.

Family functioning is the way in which every family meets the needs of its members as individuals, deals with itself as an entity, and meets its responsibility to the larger community. Some family tasks are specific to health and are necessary when a health problem arises. Freeman and Heinrich (1981) identified the following health-related tasks:

1. Recognizing interruptions of health development, such as illness or a child's failure to thrive
2. Making decisions about seeking health care
3. Dealing effectively with health and non-health crises
4. Providing nursing care to sick, disabled, or dependent members of the family
5. Maintaining a home environment conducive to health maintenance and personal development
6. Maintaining a reciprocal relationship with the community and its institutions

In trying to teach a family skills needed to care for a sick member, the nurse can use these specific tasks to guide health-related teaching plans and to reinforce learning that has occurred in the past. An example of how these tasks can be used to help a client and his family cope with insulin-dependent diabetes in an older adult follows. The numbers in parentheses refer to the health-related tasks listed previously.

Social and Cultural Influences on Teaching and Learning

Families function within the context of the larger community and culture in which they live. The United States is a nation of many cultures and is young when compared to Eastern and European nations. Americans speak of developed and developing countries today and consider the United States among the developed nations because of the many advances in technology and the relative economic advancements. Americans often forget that although the economic and technological advances are great, U.S. history is brief and the culture was developed by people from many

CASE STUDY

Mr. M., age 61, began showing signs of fatigue and had difficulty keeping up with his activities of daily living. He lived with his daughter, who recognized that this was a change in his functional level (#1). She talked with him about what she saw and after much discussion and denial, he agreed to see the family physician (#2). He was subsequently diagnosed as having insulin-dependent diabetes. This situation produced a health-related crisis, since Mr. M. would need to be taught how to give himself insulin, manage his diet and lifestyle, and watch for signs and symptoms of insulin or diabetic reaction (#3). His daughter had a full-time job and was not knowledgeable about the disease.

A family decision was made to have the visiting nurse come to the home to teach the family about managing the new disease condition (#4). While the M. family had maintained a generally healthy home environment, Mr. M.'s chronic illness would call for further adjustments in the home (#5). Arrangements for obtaining, storing, and giving the insulin were needed. Buying low-sugar food products and following a sensible diet were necessary changes. Mr. M. wanted to be sure a phone was always nearby so he could call for help if he had a problem and was alone. The family sought the needed resources to meet this challenge. They also notified friends and neighbors of Mr. M.'s condition to ensure that symptoms of difficulty with the diabetes would be accurately diagnosed and that help would be sought if appropriate. Mr. M. contacted the local support group for diabetics, and this expanded his contacts with others who were managing similar challenges (#6).

other cultures. It continues to develop with an ongoing influx of new Americans from Asia and South America, as well as other countries. In family teaching, nurses must be aware of the cultures from which families have come to adapt the teaching so that it will be acceptable to families within their existing value and belief systems.

One important reason for identifying specific beliefs that govern health practices is to assist the nurse in separating his or her personal health-related beliefs and values from those of the families with whom he or she is working. A second reason is to help the family learn by embracing beliefs and habits that are appropriate to the situation and changing those that are not.

An example of possible misunderstanding between cultural practices of the nurse and the family is seen in the common practice of *coining* used in some Indonesian cultures. When a child is suffering from a cough or other symptoms of illness, a coin is used to rub the skin along the spinal column to stimulate healing. In some children, this produces marks similar to the welts observed from physical blows. The nurse visiting such a child for the first time in the home would understandably be on the alert for child abuse practices. When questioning the parents, she would need to be accepting of their belief in this practice. Her teaching would then be geared toward modifying the pressure used in coining the child to avoid bruising, rather than rejecting the practice as basically wrong.

Language often creates a formidable barrier in trying to teach families from other cultures. Interpreters from community agencies, churches, and health departments can be essential, especially in meeting cognitive and affective learning needs.

Another example of possible misunderstanding can arise when working with Asian families who are influenced by traditional Confucian values. These ideas, which strongly affect families, advocate that relationships between the teacher and learner, the parent and child, and the professional and client are based on authority, and the subordinate (e.g., the learner, the child, the client) should respectfully listen to and comply with instructions. This contradicts many of the Western ideas of education, assessment, and communication, which advocate equality in the relationship to help with the process. Donnelly (1992) suggests that attempting to introduce equality into a relationship for a client deeply entrenched in such values may be problematic. To combat this problem, nurses working with families holding such values should identify, as part of the family assessment process, the opinion leader in the family to find out to whom the identified client is more likely to listen. Very often a senior, respected family member may have more potential to influence change than the home nurse. Teaching strategies may need to be targeted more broadly.

The nurse who is working with an interpreter can better enhance the nurse-client-family relationship if he or she has at least an overall understanding of the family's ethnic background to improve her knowledge of their cultural values relative to health and illness. By using nonverbal communication skills such as maintaining frequent eye contact with the family during the interview and positioning herself nearby in relaxed posture, the nurse can lessen the impact of language barriers. The nurse should know that some of the full context of teaching and the determination of the degree of learning can be lost with the use of interpreters.

USE OF EDUCATIONAL PROCESS IN FAMILY TEACHING

Educational process, like nursing process, is based on problem solving and is circular in nature. It differs from nursing process in its focus, which is on those problems solvable by behavioral changes that can be accomplished through educational intervention. An economic problem that can only be solved by obtaining more funds requires a noneducational solution: funding. This problem may heavily impact health and the ability of the family to meet its health needs, but it is an economic rather than an educational need. Similarly, a medical need such as diagnosing a disease process is not amenable to educational intervention. Learning how to manage money to pay for medical treatments or how to care for the family member who requires medical treatment is an educational need and is thus appropriate for educational intervention.

Assessment

Assessing the family is usually best done in the home environment. It is worth the advance planning required to find a mutually convenient time for an interview that will allow a thorough initial assessment. In addition to serving as a basis for assessment and planning, the initial interview allows the family and the nurse to become acquainted and forms a basis of trust for the teaching and learning process and other nursing interventions. The development of a good rapport followed by a systematic gathering of data about lifestyle (Miller, Rollick, 1991) will help establish the client and family's readiness for change, help identify the unique social-cultural values within the family's, and help identify which family members hold the strongest opinions.

Assessing the educational needs of the family requires information from family members and health professionals. In some hospitals and home care agencies, there are liaison nurses whose primary function is to gather the information needed for this assessment and make appropriate referrals. This person is a valuable source of information to home care nurses. In the absence of an identified liaison nurse, the staff nurses perform these tasks.

Family-focused educational assessment includes identifying the structural and functional patterns of the family, as well as the learning characteristics of the individual members involved. Learning deficits may vary among family members, and during the assessment phase, the nurse can validate differences.

Educational Diagnosis

Nurses are familiar with nursing diagnoses. An educational diagnosis also calls for a critical decision and a professional judgment of learning deficits that impact health and can be modified through appropriate teaching interventions. An educational diagnosis is based on assessment. It identifies specific weaknesses in knowledge, skill, and motivation in relation to managing existing health problems. It serves as the basis for planning mutually acceptable goals and objectives that will assist the family.

Planning

The planning stage of the process results in developing learning objectives mutually acceptable to the family and the nurse. Appropriate strategies based on the needs of each family are also developed at this stage. Learner-focused objectives become the basis for evaluation. Thus it is worth the time and energy required to develop realistic and measurable objectives, keeping in mind both short- and long-term goals.

Implementation

As the nurse and family implement strategies for learning, it is important for all concerned to be aware of what is happening. Some families feel more comfortable when they have a written record of progress as their objectives are being implemented. The nurse can provide this with simple written statements that describe the sequence of behaviors and consequent outcomes. It is handy for both the nurse and the family to have a copy of this.

Evaluation

Evaluation is the final and crucial step in the education process and includes evaluation of both the outcome and the process used to arrive at the outcome. The outcome evaluation is based on whether or not the client and family have met the learning objectives developed in the planning stage. If these objectives were well defined based on the assessment and resultant educational diagnosis, outcome evaluation is simplified.

Evaluation of the educational process looks at how well the strategies for implementing the process worked. When focusing on families, the nurse must evaluate learning for the individual members and for the family as a whole as defined in the plan. Ruzicki has discussed many additional issues on the evaluation of patient education that also impact family teaching (Smith, 1987).

Documentation of learning outcomes in the family record is an expected activity in evaluating professional nursing. Accurate documentation assists administrators who must make cost-effective decisions on use of agency resources and the value of staff time spent in family teaching. Documenting effective teaching techniques and existing learning resources can also assist other staff who teach families.

ISSUES IN FAMILY TEACHING

Some of the sobering realities that confront the nurse trying to teach the family in home care situations are those affecting resources of both the family and the home care agency. Family resources may be so strained that education seems relatively unimportant. In this situation, the nurse will need to remove the barriers to learning by helping the family find solutions to other problems and by increasing their knowledge of resources. The nurse can help the family see how learning new coping strategies will ultimately help in the solution of the existing problems.

A common limitation of resources in the agency is justification of time and expertise spent on the teaching role of the nurse when the agency is accountable to third-party payors who minimize the importance of this aspect of nursing care. An important strategy to use here is educating the policy makers for third-party payors about the value of individual and family teaching. Since an important consideration for insurers is cost effectiveness, it is crucial that nurses document what they have done in family teaching and what outcomes have resulted from their intervention, because specific and accurate documentation of client learning may be tied to reimbursement. Chapter 6 describes the issues related to reimbursement in home health care nursing. Education of clients and families is part of comprehensive health care services.

Other issues that contribute to the gap between the real and the ideal in home care nursing practice are the beliefs that all nurses are prepared to teach during their basic nursing programs and that it is a licensure and certification requirement for professional nurses to perform client and family teaching. However, few basic nursing programs require formal education courses. Client teaching is taught as part of every clinical course, but it is usually based on the nursing role in a specific clinical area rather than a separate process that can be generalized to any setting. Faculty evaluation of the nursing students' teaching process is often minimal when nursing faculty have to make difficult choices, such as whether to supervise students in their group who are doing technical procedures or those who are doing client teaching. For all these reasons, the nurse practicing in home care may need to seek further education on how to teach families. Home care agencies are often faced with the challenge of providing this education to their staff.

SUMMARY

This chapter has described some of the general concepts of teaching and learning used to educate individuals and families in the home care setting. The education process, like the nursing process, includes the steps of assessing, planning, implementing, and evaluating. The primary learner in the family must be identified and his or her learning needs assessed. After this assessment, a mutually acceptable plan to meet the identified educational needs is developed by the nurse/teacher and client/learner. Appropriate teaching strategies are used to implement the plan, and it is mutually evaluated, with the evaluation serving as a basis for further decisions.

General concepts about families that affect teaching and learning include the structure and function of the family, family development and health tasks, and sociocultural influences.

Professional issues that impact family teaching in home care must be identified. Barriers and facilitators to teaching are found in the family, in the nurse, and in the home care agencies.

REFERENCES

Bandura A: *Principles of behavior modification,* New York, 1969, Holt, Rinehart & Winston.

Bigge ML: *Learning theories for teachers,* ed 3, New York, 1976, Harper & Row.

Bloom BS, ed: *Taxonomy of educational objectives: The classification of educational goals,* Handbook I: Cognitive domain, New York, 1956, David McKay.

Brooker C: Expressed emotion and psychosocial intervention: a review, *International Journal of Nursing Studies* 27(3):267-276, 1990.

Bruner JS: *The process of education,* New York, 1963, Random House.

DiClemente CC: Motivational interviewing at the stages of change. In Miller WR, Rollnick S, eds: *Motivational interviewing: Preparing people to change,* New York, 1991, The Guilford Press.

Donnelly PJL: The impact of culture on psychotherapy: Korean clients' expectations of psychotherapy, *Journal of the New York State Nurses Association* 23(2):12-15, 1992.

Erikson EH: *Childhood and society,* New York, 1963, WW Norton.

Freeman RB, Heinrich J: *Community health nursing practice,* ed 2, Philadelphia, 1981, Saunders.

Gagne R: *The conditions of learning,* ed 4, New York, 1984, Holt, Rinehart & Winston.

Green LW et al: *Health education planning: a diagnostic approach,* Palo Alto, Calif, 1980, Mayfield.

Hamachek D: *Psychology in teaching, learning, & growth,* ed 5, Boston, 1995, Allyn & Bacon.

Harrow AJ: *A taxonomy of the psychomotor domain: a guide for developing behavioral objectives,* New York, 1972, David McKay.

Krathwohl DR, Bloom BS, Masia BB: Taxonomy of educational objectives, the classification of educational goals, *Handbook II: Affective domain,* New York, 1964, David McKay.

Leff J, Kuipers L, Berkowitz R: A controlled trial of social intervention in the families of schizophrenic patients, *British Journal of Psychiatry* 141:121-134, 1982.

Maslow A: *Motivation and personality,* New York, 1954, Harper & Row.

Miller WR, Rollnick S: *Motivational interviewing: Preparing people to change,* New York, 1991, The Guilford Press.

Piaget J: *The origins of intelligence in children,* New York, 1952, Interactional Universities Press.

Redman BK: *The process of patient education,* ed 5, St Louis, 1984, Mosby.

Reeber BJ: Evaluating the effects of a family education intervention, *Rehabilitation Nursing* 17(6):332-336, 1992.

Rogers C: *Freedom to learn,* Columbus, Ohio, 1969, Charles E Merrill.

Skinner BF: Science and human behavior, New York, 1953, Macmillan.

Smith CE: *Patient education: Nurses in partnership with other health professionals,* Orlando, 1987, Grune & Stratton.

St John W, Rolls C: Teaching family nursing: Strategies and experiences, *Journal of Advanced Nursing* 23(1):91-96, 1996.

Youssef FA: Discharge planning for psychiatric patients: The effects of a family patient teaching program, *Journal of Advanced Nursing* 12(5):611-616, 1987.

ADDITIONAL READINGS

Bartlett E: Behavioral diagnosis: a practical approach to patient education, *Patient Counseling and Health Education* 4(1):29-35, 1982.

Becker MH, Maimam L: Strategies for enhancing patient compliance, *Journal of Community Health* 6(2):113-132, 1980.

Bille D, ed: *Practical approaches to patient teaching,* Boston, 1981, Little, Brown.

Cross P: *Adults as learners,* San Francisco, 1981, Jossey-Bass.

Dolphin P, Holtzclaw B: *Theories of adult learning: Continuing education in nursing: strategies for lifelong learning,* Reston, Va, 1983, Reston Publishing.

Duval E: *Family development,* ed 4, Philadelphia, 1971, JB Lippincott.

Knowles MS: *The modern practice of adult education: From pedagogy to andragogy,* Chicago, 1980, Cambridge Books.

Mager RF: *Preparing instructional objectives,* ed 2, Palo Alto, Calif, 1975, Fearon.

Squyres W: *Patient education: An inquiry into the state of the art,* New York, 1980, Springer.

9 Use of the Omaha System

Karen S. Martin and Kathryn H. Bowles

The art and science of diagnostic reasoning are increasingly important to health care providers. The term *diagnostic reasoning* has a long history when it is used similarly or even synonymously with the scientific method and the problem-solving process. A milestone occurred when Florence Nightingale used sophisticated and powerful methods to collect, analyze, and display data from Scutari in the 1850s. Another milestone occurred when the importance of using discrete categories for medical diagnoses was described in nineteenth century literature.

Nearly a century passed before nurses focused on diagnostic reasoning again. The concepts of client problems, nursing diagnoses, and nursing process appeared in the nursing literature during the 1950s. Werley and her colleagues worked to identify a classification framework or minimum data set useful for the entire profession during the 1970s; their efforts produced the Nursing Minimum Data Set a decade later (Marek, 1997; Werley, Grier, 1981; Werley, Lang, 1988). Development of the Omaha System and North American Nursing Diagnosis Association (NANDA) began early in the 1970s, resulting in the first systematic vocabularies. During the 1980s and 1990s, additional vocabularies were developed. To date, the American Nurses Association has recognized 11 languages for consideration by nurses: the Omaha System, NANDA, Home Health Care Classification, Nursing Interventions Classification, Nursing Outcomes Classification, Patient Care Data Set, Perioperative Nursing Data Set, SNOMED®RT, Nursing Minimum Data Set, Alternative Link, and International Classification for Nursing Practice (Lang, 1995; American Nurses Association, 1999, 2001). In less than 50 years, nursing practice, education, and research have made remarkable progress with the development, use, and acceptance of diagnostic reasoning, standardized vocabularies, and automated documentation systems.

HOME HEALTH CARE PRACTICE

Traditionally, nursing care has been the primary service of home health care agencies. Most employees and many agency administrators have been nurses. However, physical therapists, occupational therapists, speech pathologists, registered dietitians, social workers, home health aides, physicians, and volunteers are important members of the multidisciplinary team. Often, the team leader is a nurse.

Characteristics of home care nurse-client contacts are different than nurse-client contacts in most institutional settings. The home care nurse enters the home of the client as a guest. Because home care nurses are usually alone when they conduct home visits, they practice independently, use the equipment they bring with them, and adapt to the client's physical environment. To quickly and accurately collect enough client data needed for the diagnostic process, the nurse must function as a partner or collaborator with the client. Widmer further describe concepts related to the client and the assessment phase of the nursing process in Chapter 7. Many other chapters in this book address effective home care nursing interventions. Two such examples, communication and coordination, are especially important in home care because the nurse is a member of a multidisciplinary team and often functions as the coordinator of care. The nurse must communicate data quickly and accurately to other team members, including the client's physician. In addition, the nurse identifies other community resources that the client needs and coordinates the steps of that process.

Clients, families, agency administrators, accreditors, payors, politicians, and the public are some of the competing forces that are changing home care nursing practice. Decreased reimbursement, increased productivity requirements for nurses, and shorter hospital stays for clients are trends that encourage nurses to focus on the primary reason for referral, physiological concerns, and the individual's needs rather than the family's needs. Such trends are the result of demands initiated by managed care companies and prospective payment plans to limit home care services, by payors to decrease more expensive types of services such as hospitalization and emergency department care, and by politicians to decrease national health care expenditures. At the same time, clients, families, payors, politicians, and the public are demanding seamless health care services and quantitative data about the outcomes of the services provided by home health care agencies. In addition, the philosophy of rapidly expanding programs such as hospice and home infusion therapy emphasizes a holistic, family-centered approach to care and the power of the client in determining and achieving the desired outcomes (Martin, 2000).

Thoughtful, experienced home care nurses and agency administrators recognize the necessity of addressing competing forces to provide effective care. Principles of group dynamics and group effectiveness help explain the impact of the individual on the family and the family on the individual, as well as health habits and client actions. Lewin's field theory includes concepts of group cohesiveness and group locomotion; the relationships among conformity, cohesiveness, and communication are always dynamic, never static (Deutsch, Krauss, 1965; Hollander, 1971). Family members serve as positive or driving forces as they collaborate with home care staff members and provide physical care, comfort, and advice to the client. It is important that home care nurses accurately identify and respect individual and family values and goals, thus avoiding confusion and conflict. Addressing the unique factors that motivate individuals and families increases the probability that client outcomes will be positive, permanent, and economical (Stanhope, Lancaster, 2000).

OVERVIEW OF THE OMAHA SYSTEM

Home care nurses use a variety of methods to communicate assessment, intervention, and evaluation data to other nurses, members of the multidisciplinary team, physicians, and the community. A standardized vocabulary, such as the Omaha System, provides a communication tool to integrate clinical practice, the nursing process and diagnostic reasoning, and an automated or paper-pen client record. The remainder of this chapter will describe the components of the Omaha System and how those components can be used by home care nurses.

The Omaha System is an example of a research-based, standardized vocabulary. It offers a holistic framework to assess and diagnose client or family care needs, track nursing interventions, and evaluate client progress. The Omaha System was inductively developed and refined during three research projects by the Visiting Nurse Association (VNA) of Omaha, funded by the Division of Nursing, U.S. Department of Health and Human Services between 1975 and 1986. Further research funded by the National Institute of Nursing Research, National Institutes of Health, between 1989 and 1993 addressed reliability, validity, and usability of the Omaha System. Practicing nurses at the VNA and seven diverse sites throughout the country participated in the four research projects. Further details about the initial Omaha System development and research are found in electronic and other publications (Martin, Scheet, 1992a; Martin, 1999; Martin, Norris, Leak, 1999). As others built on the Omaha System research foundation, the diversity of subjects, settings, and designs has expanded.*

The Omaha System follows the principles of taxonomy. It consists of terms and codes arranged from general to specific and allows for expansion by including space for additional terms. Terms are intended to be familiar, clear, concise, and useful to nurses, members of other disciplines, and even to the general public. The Omaha System consists of the Problem Classification

---

*Bowles, 1999, 2000a, 2000b; Coenen, Marek, Lundeen, 1996; Doran et al, 1997; Elfrink, 1999; Hays, 1992; Marek, 1996; Marek et al, 1998; McGourthy, 1999; Naylor, Bowles, Brooten, 2000; Nightingale Tracker Field Test Nurse Team, 1999; Sampson, Doran, 1998; Zielstorff et al, 1998.

Box 9-1   Problem Classification Scheme

DOMAIN I. ENVIRONMENTAL

Material resources and physical surroundings both internal and external to the client, home, neighborhood, and broader community.

01. Income
02. Sanitation
03. Residence
04. Neighborhood/workplace safety
05. Other

DOMAIN II. PSYCHOSOCIAL

Patterns of behavior, communication, relationships, and development.

06. Communication with community resources
07. Social contact
08. Role change
09. Interpersonal relationship
10. Spirituality
11. Grief
12. Emotional stability
13. Human sexuality
14. Caretaking/parenting
15. Neglected child/adult
16. Abused child/adult
17. Growth and development
18. Other

DOMAIN III. PHYSIOLOGICAL

Functional status of processes that maintain life.

19. Hearing
20. Vision

DOMAIN III. PHYSIOLOGICAL—cont'd

21. Speech and language
22. Dentition
23. Cognition
24. Pain
25. Consciousness
26. Integument
27. Neuro-musculo-skeletal function
28. Respiration
29. Circulation
30. Digestion-hydration
31. Bowel function
32. Genito-urinary function
33. Antepartum/postpartum
34. Other

DOMAIN IV. HEALTH RELATED BEHAVIORS

Activities that maintain or promote wellness, promote recovery, or maximize rehabilitation

35. Nutrition
36. Sleep and rest patterns
37. Physical activity
38. Personal hygiene
39. Substance use
40. Family planning
41. Healthcare supervision
42. Prescribed medication regime
43. Technical procedure
44. Other

From Martin KS, Scheet NJ: *The Omaha System: Applications for community health nursing,* Philadelphia, 1992, WB Saunders.

Scheme, the Problem Rating Scale for Outcomes, and the Intervention Scheme.

Problem Classification Scheme

The Problem Classification Scheme is an orderly, nonexhaustive, mutually exclusive, client-focused taxonomy of domains, problems, and signs and symptoms. The four domains represent the broad areas of nursing practice; the domains and the problems are listed in Box 9-1. Client problems are the 40 nursing diagnoses that represent matters of difficulty and concern that historically, presently, or potentially have an adverse effect on any aspect of the client's well-being. Each of the problems may be referenced as health promotion, potential, or deficit/impairment/actual, as well as individual or family problems. Actual problems are accompanied by a descriptive cluster of signs and symptoms. Box 9-2 illustrates three problems and their respective problem-specific signs and symptoms. In conjunction with practice and documentation, the Problem Classification Scheme is used by the home care nurse and other clinicians to formulate a list of client problems to address during the episode of care.

Problem Rating Scale for Outcomes

The Problem Rating Scale for Outcomes is a framework for measuring a client's problem-specific knowledge, behavior, and status. It is a guide for practice and a method for evaluating

---

Box 9-2   Examples of Problems and Their Signs and Symptoms

08 ROLE CHANGE

Health promotion
Potential impairment
Impairment
01. involuntary reversal of traditional male/
    female roles
02. involuntary reversal of dependent/
    independent roles
03. assumes new role
04. loses previous role
05. other

26 INTEGUMENT

Health promotion
Potential impairment
Impairment
01. lesion
02. rash
03. excessively dry
04. excessively oily

26 INTEGUMENT—cont'd

05. inflammation
06. pruritus
07. drainage
08. ecchymosis
09. hypertrophy of nails
10. other

36 SLEEP AND REST PATTERNS

Health promotion
Potential impairment
Impairment
01. sleep/rest pattern disrupts family
02. frequently wakes during the night
03. somnambulism
04. insomnia
05. nightmares
06. insufficient sleep for age/physical condition
07. other

From Martin KS, Scheet NJ: *The Omaha System: Applications for community health nursing,* Philadelphia, 1992, WB Saunders.

Table 9-1   Problem Rating Scale for Outcomes

Concept	1	2	3	4	5
Knowledge: Ability of the client to remember and interpret information	No knowledge	Minimal knowledge	Basic knowledge	Adequate knowledge	Superior knowledge
Behavior: Observable responses, actions, or activities of the client fitting the occasion or purpose	Never appropriate	Rarely appropriate	Inconsistently appropriate	Usually appropriate	Consistently appropriate
Status: Condition of the client in relation to objective and subjective defining characteristics	Extreme signs/ symptoms	Severe signs/ symptoms	Moderate signs/ symptoms	Minimal signs/ symptoms	No signs/ symptoms

From Martin KS, Scheet NJ: *The Omaha System: Applications for community health nursing,* Philadelphia, 1992, WB Saunders.

---

and documenting client progress. The scale is depicted in Table 9-1. Each Likert-type ordinal subscale has five categories or degrees for response. When selecting one category and establishing the initial ratings for client problems, the user creates an independent data baseline, capturing the condition and circumstances of the client at a given point. The clinician uses the admission baseline to compare and contrast the client's condition and circumstances with the ratings completed at

Box 9-3   Intervention Scheme

I. HEALTH TEACHING, GUIDANCE, AND COUNSELING

Activities that give information, anticipate client problems, encourage client action and responsibility for self-care and coping, and assist with decision-making and problem-solving; overlapping concepts that occur on a continuum with the variation due to the client's self-direction capabilities.

II. TREATMENTS AND PROCEDURES

Technical activities directed toward preventing signs/symptoms, identifying risk factors and early signs/symptoms, and decreasing or alleviating signs/symptoms.

III. CASE MANAGEMENT

Activities of coordination, advocacy, and referral that involve facilitating service delivery on behalf of the client, communicating with health and human service providers, promoting assertive client communication, and guiding the client toward the use of appropriate community resources.

IV. SURVEILLANCE

Activities of detection, measurement, critical analysis, and monitoring to indicate client status in relation to a given condition or phenomenon.

TARGETS

01. anatomy and physiology
02. behavior modification
03. bladder care
04. bonding
05. bowel care
06. bronchial hygiene
07. cardiac care
08. caretaking/parenting skills
09. cast care
10. communication
11. coping skills
12. day-care/respite
13. discipline
14. dressing change/wound care
15. durable medical equipment
16. education
17. employment

TARGETS—cont'd

18. environment
19. exercises
20. family planning
21. feeding procedures
22. finances
23. food
24. gait training
25. growth/development
26. homemaking
27. housing
28. interaction
29. lab findings
30. legal system
31. medical/dental care
32. medication action/side effects
33. medication administration
34. medication set-up
35. mobility/transfers
36. nursing care, supplementary
37. nutrition
38. nutritionist
39. ostomy care
40. other community resource
41. personal care
42. positioning
43. rehabilitation
44. relaxation/breathing techniques
45. rest/sleep
46. safety
47. screening
48. sickness/injury care
49. signs/symptoms—mental/emotional
50. signs/symptoms—physical
51. skin care
52. social work/counseling
53. specimen collection
54. spiritual care
55. stimulation/nurturance
56. stress management
57. substance use
58. supplies
59. support group
60. support system
61. transportation
62. wellness
63. other

From Martin KS, Scheet NJ: *The Omaha System: Applications for community health nursing,* Philadelphia, 1992, WB Saunders.

later intervals and at client dismissal. The comparison or change in ratings throughout the period of service provides a method to track the client's progress in relation to interventions and the effectiveness of the care plan.

Intervention Scheme

The Intervention Scheme is a taxonomy of nursing actions or activities designed to help users identify and document plans and interventions. The scheme offers a research-based effort to link the effectiveness of interventions with diagnoses. The first level of the Intervention Scheme is composed of four comprehensive categories; the second level is an alphabetical listing of 62 targets. The categories and targets are listed in Box 9-3. Targets are defined as objects of nursing activities that serve to further describe problem-specific intervention categories. The third level of the Intervention Scheme is designed for client-specific information. Users generate pertinent, concise words or phrases as they develop plans or document care for specific clients. Although

not part of the research project, VNA of Omaha staff organized the care plan ideas they used frequently into care planning guides. These guides provide suggestions for clinicians, enabling them to develop their own care plans more quickly and effectively (Martin, Scheet, 1992b).

APPLICATION OF THE OMAHA SYSTEM

Application of the Omaha System is illustrated in the following paragraphs and in Table 9-2. The case study describes the home care admission visit for Mr. Decker, a typical client referred for home care and nursing services after hospitalization. Table 9-2 illustrates a summary of the admission assessment findings, outcome ratings, and interventions for the priority problems only. It is not intended to illustrate complete documentation of the nursing encounter. The interventions were limited to those the home care nurse was able to realistically accomplish during one visit, although many other interventions were planned for future visits. The actual clinical

Table 9-2 Case Example Using the Omaha System

Domain	Client Data	Problems, Signs, and Symptoms	Ratings	Interventions
Environmental	No significant findings			
Psychosocial	Had to leave his home and move in with daughter until capable of self care. Feels he is a burden. Daughter says he is "frustrated that he can't do much."	08 Role change 02 involuntary reversal of dependent/ independent roles	K = 3 B = 3 S = 3	
Physiological	Temperature 99.6° F; blood pressure 170/94 mm Hg; pulse 110 bpm, regular.	29 Circulation 08 abnormal blood pressure reading	K = 3 B = 4 S = 2	I 07, 48, 50 III 31 IV 50

	Sternal incision red, edematous, tender. Remains open at distal edge 1 inch long and ¼ inch wide with a small amount of serous drainage, no odor.	26 Integument
		  05 inflammation
		  07 drainage
		  10 other—incision not approximated
			K = 4
			B = 4
			S = 3
				I 48, 50
				IV 14, 50

	Takes pain medication only at night. Avoids deep breaths and sits in a chair all day because it hurts too badly to move.	24 Pain
		  01 expresses discomfort/pain
		  05 facial grimaces
			K = 2
			B = 3
			S = 3
				I 32, 42
				IV 32, 50

Continued

Table 9-2	Case Example Using the Omaha System—cont'd			
Domain	Client Data	Problems, Signs, and Symptoms	Ratings	Interventions
Health-Related Behaviors	Sleeping poorly. Cannot turn over without waking up. Restless, sleeps only 4 hours at night. Naps all afternoon, then has difficulty falling asleep at night. Feels tired and sleepy all day.	36 Sleep and rest patterns 02 Frequently wakes during night 03 Somnambulism 06 Insufficient sleep/ rest for age/ physical condition	K = 4 B = 3 S = 2	I 32, 42 IV 33, 45
	Admits to drinking 2 to 3 cocktails per night. His daughter does not want him to have them.	39 Substance use Potential problem	K = 3 B = 3 S = 5	I 57 IV 50, 57

record would be more detailed and comprehensive to provide an easy-to-follow audit trail for the primary nurse, other nurses, members of other disciplines, auditors, and accreditors.

BENEFITS OF THE OMAHA SYSTEM

Using the Omaha System to assess, plan, evaluate, and document care offers many benefits for clinical practice, education, and research. For clinical practice, the four domains of the Problem Classification Scheme provide a comprehensive framework for assessing clients' needs in a systematic, standardized manner. The Omaha System ensures that all domains of client need are considered when integrated with other data sets such as the Outcomes and Assessment Information Set (OASIS); OASIS must be completed for Medicare reimbursement in conjunction with the prospective payment system (Crisler, Campbell, Shaughnessy, 1997). The Omaha System offers an integrated framework that is compatible with practice when the Problem Rating Scale for Outcomes and the Intervention Scheme are also used and linked to client problems, unlike when other assessment tools are used alone. The result is a comprehensive picture about the needs of home care clients that is linked to the home care nurse's actions and the outcomes of care. Many agencies are implementing automated client record and management information systems to avoid time-consuming, costly content analysis of

free-form handwritten clinicians' notes and to capture, analyze, and disseminate outcomes of care, costs, and other essential information rapidly and accurately. From the perspective of clinicians, administrators, quality improvement staff, and information management, such data are essential for agency survival.

When the Omaha System is used in educational settings, it offers a comprehensive assessment framework to identify clients' needs and an audit trail to track students' activities with particular clients. Developments in technology and communication, such as the Nightingale Tracker, provide access to students' care plans and real-time evaluation of their diagnostic reasoning (Elfrink, 1999; Nightingale Tracker Field Test Nurse Team, 1999). In addition, some colleges of nursing have integrated the Omaha System into their courses or based their curricula on its concepts (Merrill et al, 1998).

Researchers benefit from the standardized, comprehensive data generated through the use of the Omaha System. The relatively small number of data and discrete categories that compose the three schemes of the Omaha System make data collection more reliable and efficient. Aggregate client data can be used to make health policy decisions and to evaluate quality and cost issues in relation to the needs of the clients, the types of nursing interventions conducted, and the outcomes of care.

CASE STUDY

Mr. Decker was hospitalized for an aortic valve re-placement. During his 5-day hospital stay, he developed a fever of 101° F and required vancomycin (Vancocin) for probable infection of his surgical incision. He is 71 years of age, was widowed 3 years ago, lives alone, and has a supportive daughter who lives nearby. He admits to two or three alcoholic drinks each day. His medical history includes hypertension and arthritis.

At discharge, Mr. Decker was referred to the Visiting Nurse Association and discharged to his daughter's home until he became stronger. His sternal incision was considered unstable. He received discharge instructions for enalapril (Vasotec), 20 mg once a day; warfarin (Coumadin), 5 mg once a day; docusate (Surfak), 240 mg once a day; erythromycin, 250 mg every 6 hours; and flurbiprofen (Ansaid), 200 mg twice a day. He was told not to lift more than 10 pounds, to take his temperature daily, and to call his physician if his temperature was higher than 100° F. Mr. Decker's home care nursing orders included (1) cardiopulmonary assessment, (2) cardiac teaching, (3) medication teaching, (4) incision assessment, (5) wound care and temperature monitoring, and (6) blood specimen collection to monitor anticoagulant therapy.

The home care nurse used an assessment form organized according to the Problem Classification Scheme. The form helped the nurse identify Mr. Decker's signs and symptoms, diagnose his problems, and indicate whether the appropriate modifiers for those problems were health promotion, potential or actual and individual or family. Using this problem list, the nurse formulated a prioritized plan of care.

The home care nurse noted that Mr. Decker had six problems within three of the four domains of the Problem Classification Scheme. Mr. Decker was accustomed to living alone and being independent and active. He expressed concern that he was a burden to his daughter and, according to his daughter, became "frustrated that he can't do much." The nurse noted that the problem, #08 Role change, was a family problem. Realizing that not all problems can be addressed on the first visit, the nurse planned to help Mr. Decker and his daughter cope with these temporary changes at future visits.

Mr. Decker's recovery from aortic valve surgery was complicated by continued hypertension with a blood pressure of 170/94 mm Hg and an increased heart rate of 110 bpm. He continued to have a low-grade fever of 99.6° F with a very tender, red, and edematous sternal incision. The presence of these signs

and symptoms confirmed the actual problems, #29 Circulation and #26 Integument, and prompted the nurse to provide interventions as seen in Table 9-2.

The tender incision also affected Mr. Decker's sleep. He reported awakening frequently from discomfort each time he tried to change position, napping all afternoon, and being unable to sleep at night. Because of these data, the home care nurse noted #36 Sleep and rest patterns on his care plan as an actual problem. Mr. Decker told the nurse that pain inhibited his movement and deep breathing but that he took his pain medication "only at night." This information and the objective pain scale data collected by the home care nurse indicated that pain management was an issue. The nurse recorded #24 Pain as an actual problem.

Finally, the nurse documented #39 Substance use as a potential problem. Mr. Decker usually had two or three cocktails per day. His daughter voiced concern that this behavior was inappropriate for his condition, especially in "her house." The nurse planned to further monitor Mr. Decker's behavior for signs of an actual problem and to make him aware of the damaging effects of excessive alcohol consumption.

Once problems were identified and the assessment completed, the Omaha System facilitated further application of the nursing process, specifically the evaluation and intervention steps. Thus the home care nurse used the three Likert-type 0-5 subscales of the Problem Rating Scale for Outcomes to identify, evaluate, and document Mr. Decker's knowledge, behavior, and status data in relation to each priority problem. When the scale is used during admission, at regularly scheduled intervals, and at discharge, the nurse has another evaluation tool to monitor Mr. Decker's progress or decline.

As shown in Table 9-2, the home care nurse rated knowledge, behavior, and status for priority problems, including #24 Pain. The knowledge rating was 2 (minimal knowledge), based on data that Mr. Decker took his medication at night even though the pain was severely limiting his activity during the day. This indicated minimal knowledge about pain management and the importance of deep breathing and moving after surgery. His behavior was rated 3 (inconsistently appropriate) because, although he took pain medication for his discomfort, he took it only at night. The status was rated 3 (moderate signs and symptoms) based on a score of 5 when the nurse used a pain scale of 0 to 10 during the visit.

When the initial ratings were completed, the nurse referred to the four intervention categories of

Continued

CASE STUDY—cont'd

the Intervention Scheme: Health teaching, counseling, and guidance; Treatments and procedures; Case management; and Surveillance. In addition, the nurse reviewed the 63 targets, the terms at the next level of the Intervention Scheme. Use of the Intervention Scheme is illustrated in Table 9-2 and described later.

For the problem, #29 Circulation, the nurse taught Mr. Decker how to take his temperature and pulse and reviewed the signs and symptoms that warrant calling the nurse or physician. Health teaching, guidance, and counseling is the intervention category and #07 cardiac care and #48 sickness/injury care are

the intervention targets that appear on Table 9-2 to document this nursing intervention. The nurse also took Mr. Decker's vital signs and listened to his heart and lungs. These interventions were documented using the category, Surveillance, and the target, #50 signs/symptoms-physical. The nurse chose the category, Case management, and the target, #31 medical/dental care, to document a telephone call to Mr. Decker's physician regarding his elevated blood pressure, pulse rate, and other findings. Further teaching was planned related to target #32 medication/side effects and target #44 relaxation/breathing techniques, but could not be accomplished on the first visit.

SUMMARY

The Omaha System has existed for nearly 30 years. The diversity of settings using the Omaha System and their national and international locations are expanding rapidly. Many of these settings are implementing automated versions, although some continue to use paper-pen versions (Martin, 1999). Research and testing of the Omaha System has also expanded to care settings beyond those that are community focused.*

REFERENCES

American Nurses Association: ANA recognizes languages for nursing management and patient assessment, *Am Nurse* 31(5):11, 1999.

American Nurses Association: Recognized languages for nursing, *Nursing World* (on-line) 2001, http://www.nursingworld.org/nidsec/class1st.htm

Bowles KH: Application of the Omaha System in acute care. *Research in Nursing and Health* 23(2):93-105, 2000a.

Bowles KH: The Omaha System: Bridging hospital and home care, *On-line Journal of Nursing Informatics* (On-line), 3:7-11, 1999, http://cac.psu.edu/~dxm12/ojni.html.

Bowles KH: Patient problems and nurse interventions during acute care and discharge planning, *Journal of Cardiovascular Nursing* 14(3):29-41, 2000b.

Coenen A, Marek KD, Lundeen SP: Using nursing diagnoses to explain utilization in a community nursing center, *Research in Nursing and Health* 19(5):441-445, 1996.

Crisler KS, Campbell BM, Shaughnessy PK: *OASIS basics: Beginning to use the outcome and assessment information set,* Denver, 1997, University of Colorado Center for Health Services and Policy Research.

Deutsch M, Krauss R: *Theories in social psychology,* New York, 1965, Basic Books.

Doran K et al: Clinical pathway across tertiary and community care after an interventional cardiology procedure, *Journal of Cardiovascular Nursing* 11(2):1-14, 1997.

Elfrink V: The Omaha System: Bridging nursing education and information technology. On-line Journal of Nursing Informatics (On-line), 3:15-19, 1999, http://cac.psu.edu/~dxm12/ojni.html.

Hays B: Nursing care requirements and resource consumption in home health care, *Nursing Research* 41(3):138-143, 1992.

Hollander E: *Principles and methods of social psychology,* ed 2, New York, 1971, Oxford University Press.

Lang NM, ed: *Nursing data systems: The emerging framework,* Washington, DC, 1995, American Nurses Publishing.

Marek KD: Nursing diagnoses and home care nursing utilization, *Public Health Nursing* 13(3):195-200, 1996.

Marek KD: Measuring the effectiveness of nursing care, *Outcomes Management for Nursing Practice* 1(1):8-13, 1997.

Marek KD et al: Implementation of a clinical information system in nurse-managed care, *Canadian Journal of Nursing Research* 30(1):37-44, 1998.

---

*Bowles, 2000a, 2000b; Coenen, Marek, Lundeen, 1996; Doran et al, 1997; Elfrink, 1999; Hays, 1992; Marek et al, 1998; Naylor, Bowles, Brooten, 2000; Sampson, Doran, 1998; Zielstorff et al, 1998.

Martin KS: Home health care, outcomes management, and the Land of Oz, *Outcomes Management for Nursing Practice* 4(1):7-12, 2000.

Martin KS: The Omaha System: Past, present, and future. On-line Journal of Nursing Informatics [On-line], 3:1-6, 1999. Available: http://cac.psu.edu/~dxm12/ojni.html

Martin KS, Norris J, Leak GK: Psychometric analysis of the Problem Rating Scale for Outcomes, *Outcomes Management for Nursing Practice* 3(1):20-25, 1999.

Martin KS, Scheet NJ: *The Omaha System: Applications for community health nursing,* Philadelphia, 1992a, WB Saunders.

Martin KS, Scheet NJ: *The Omaha System: A pocket guide for community health nursing,* Philadelphia, 1992b, WB Saunders.

McGourthy RJ: Omaha and OASIS: A comparative study of outcomes in patients with chronic obstructive pulmonary disease, *Home Care Provider* 4(1):21-25, 1999.

Merrill AS et al: Curriculum restructuring using the practice-based Omaha System, *Journal of Nursing Education* 23(3):41-44, 1998.

Naylor MD, Bowles KH, Brooten D: Patient problems and advanced practice nurse interventions during transitional care, *Public Health Nursing* 17(2):94-102, 2000.

Nightingale Tracker Field Test Nurse Team: Designing an information technology application for use in community-focused nursing education, *Computers in Nursing* 17(2):73-81, 1999.

Sampson BK, Doran KA: Health needs of coronary artery bypass graft surgery patients at discharge, *Dimensions of Critical Care Nursing* 17(3):158-164, 1998.

Stanhope M, Lancaster J, eds: *Community and public health nursing,* ed 5, St Louis, 2000, Mosby.

Werley HH, Grier MR, eds: *Nursing information systems,* New York, 1981, Springer.

Werley HH, Lang NM, eds: *Identification of the Nursing Minimum Data Set,* New York, 1988, Springer.

Zielstorff RD et al: Mapping nursing diagnosis nomenclatures for coordinated care, *Image—The Journal of Nursing Scholarship* 30(4):369-373, 1998.

10 Symptom Control and Medication Management

Jo Ann Wegmann

Client care for advanced, chronic conditions, as well as terminal care, has progressively moved away from the acute care hospital into extended care settings and the home. This has resulted in the transfer of professional nursing care delivery to settings that demand creativity and flexibility to provide comfort and safety to those in need. While addressing a client's physical needs, caregivers must also remain aware of quality-of-life issues for all involved in the care setting. Bland (1997) states that quality of life reflects psychosocial, emotional, and physical outcomes of health care and involves controlling physical symptoms while preserving a functioning psychosocial environment as much as possible. This chapter explores successful therapies for symptom management in the home. It is assumed that much of the nursing care described here will be provided by advanced practice nurses, and references are made to such roles.

It is important to briefly identify changes in care delivery that professional nurses face in the current health care environment. Murray (1998) performed a qualitative study to determine stressors of nurses leaving acute care settings and moving into home settings. Adaptations required to minimize role stress were also identified. This researcher found that nurses moving into the home setting felt they dealt with limited access to peer support and equipment, experienced a sense of isolation because of decreased opportunities for professional interaction, relinquished traditional responsibilities to their client's family members or other caregivers, and experienced an increased need for documentation for reimbursement of services. These stressors assume

immense importance in areas of symptom management, requiring advanced practice medication administration and advanced technology to meet the demands of the rapidly changing physical status of clients.

Adaptations that were identified by Murray's subjects (1998) include adjusting to performing nursing care on the client's turf and making decisions without the presence of other health care team members. Nurses moving into home care of chronically ill clients had to learn to manage their time effectively and independently, without the support of the oncoming shift. Clinical competence had to be accomplished in a variety of areas different from the acute setting. Also, these nurses had to become accountable for practice that was more independent and often more creative than their previous experience or education indicated. These adaptations will be further explored and defined in the various treatment approaches described in this chapter.

Symptom management for the chronically or terminally ill client at home involves far more than treatment of physical manifestations and maintaining quality of life. Hogan (1997) reports that advocating on behalf of clients and those they hold dear becomes a significant part of symptom management. She further states that ensuring optimal symptom control is a tangible measurement of such advocacy that must be nurtured, guarded, and continually strengthened. To this end, symptom-control measures in the home are explored. Etiologies of the problems presented are not described; rather, symptom-management approaches are discussed.

PHYSIOLOGICAL PROBLEMS

Quality-of-life issues and symptom management are of extreme importance and fall within the

The contributions of Jane Cady, RN, MS, are gratefully acknowledged.

realm of practice of the professional nurse within the home setting. Depending on factors such as diagnosis, client age, and progression or disease, many physiological challenges may be present. Some of these are specifically addressed elsewhere in this book. For purposes of this chapter, the following areas are discussed: pain, nausea and vomiting, fatigue, and mucositis and stomatitis.

Pain

The treatment and prevention of pain associated with chronic illness and terminal disease remain challenges, even in the new millennium. In the last decade, efforts have been directed at defining pain, understanding and accepting the client's declaration of pain, establishing guidelines for pain control, and promoting adequate pain relief through self- and caregiver-management techniques. Pain-control techniques include pharmaceutical interventions, potentially invasive methods, and noninvasive client-controlled methods. Many nurse scholars have offered important contributions to these pain-control approaches, and the reader is directed to explore the works of McCaffrey and Beebe (1989), Ferrell, McGuire, and Donovan (1993), Grant (1997), and McGuire (1997). Of importance here is the concept that pain is multidimensional, may be unnecessarily incapacitating to the client, and can be effectively managed by the nurse in the home setting.

Although the nurse in the home may act in isolation (Murray, 1998), the recognition and effective treatment of pain should entail a multidisciplinary effort. Depending on the underlying disease process and type of pain, treatment approaches may consist of chemotherapy, radiotherapy, surgery, anesthetic techniques, behavioral or cognitive methods, Oriental medicine approaches, and medications, among others (McGuire, 1993). Even in the presence of a nurse practitioner with prescriptive capabilities, multidisciplinary approaches to pain management demand the participation of a team of professionals that includes the nurse, pharmacist, physician, therapist, family members, and client.

Assessment of pain often falls into the nurse's domain, and there are a variety of tools to assist in this function. Several of the most frequently used for ease and rapidity in obtaining client data are described here.

The McGill pain questionnaire (short form) has been effectively used by nurses for several years. This tool measures physiological, sensory, and affective interpretations of pain and is used for clients with acute, postoperative, and musculoskeletal pain. It is a brief, simple questionnaire that the client completes, using a Likert scale for responses. It is well tested and easily administered within the home (McGuire, 1992; Melzak, 1987).

The brief pain inventory (BPI) is another multidimensional instrument for measuring pain and offering suggestions for appropriate intervention (McGuire, 1997). It successfully measures cancer, arthritic, and chronic orthopedic pain. Clients rate their pain on this instrument on a scale of 0 to 10, with 0 indicating no pain and 10 indicating pain as bad as can be imagined. Although these responses may be viewed as subjective, an ongoing record of the client's responses can provide an effective mapping of his or her perception of pain and the effectiveness of the interventions.

The last pain scale described here is the *visual analogue scale* (VAS). Use of this scale (typically a representation of a facial expression) to be either completed by the client or to be selected by the client as representative of his or her pain, has become common by nurses seeking to quickly and effectively determine status of pain. Another use of the VAS for pain measurement consists of a 10-cm horizontal line with verbal anchors at each end. The verbal anchors reflect no pain (left side) and pain as bad as it could possibly be (right side) (McGuire, 1997). The client then indicates where on the scale his or her pain falls, again offering an ongoing pain assessment over time.

These analogues have been used to measure different phenomena such as fatigue and nausea, as well as pain (Maxwell, 1978). The effectiveness of the VAS is that it is easy to use, has been validated with extensive use, and can be adapted to different age, disease, and ethnic and language groups. The challenge of using self-report pain measurement is to identify the most effective interventions for pain management.

The use of nonininvasive, self-controlled methods is described abundantly in the literature and includes music therapy, biofeedback, self-hypnosis, relaxation therapy, and imaging, among others. For example, we have seen an increase in the use of acupuncture in recent years, complete with documentation indicating success.

Pharmacological methods of pain control remain significant among approaches to this universal problem and remain suspect for problems of overuse and addiction. Current pharmacological treatments are discussed in the next section.

Nausea and Vomiting

Perhaps two symptoms most dreaded by clients are nausea and vomiting. These physiological problems are often the result of chemotherapy and other treatment regimens. Nausea and vomiting directly affect quality of life and, if left untreated, can impair potential curative therapeutic regimens (Grant, 1997). Effective treatment of nausea and vomiting has been demonstrated to positively impact physical, psychological, social, and spiritual well-being. Furthermore, therapeutic advances in the last 2 decades clearly identify the nurse as an individual instrumental in the measurement of nausea and vomiting and as an effective resource in the treatment of nausea and vomiting (Fessele, 1996).

Many interventions, both pharmacological and nonpharmacological, have been investigated for the management of nausea and vomiting. Several are explored here. From the pharmacological standpoint, one of the truly remarkable advances for this problem has been the development and use of the serotonin antagonists as antiemetics (Morrow, Hickock, Rosenthal, 1995). These drugs, also known as 5-HT3-receptor antagonists, include ondansetron (Zofran) and granisetron (Kytril), both of which can be administered orally or intravenously. These drugs are recognized as being very effective in the prevention and treatment of chemotherapy-induced nausea and vomiting. Cunningham (1997) states that 5-HT3-receptor antagonists are particularly effective in combating nausea and vomiting induced by cisplatin (Platinol) and doxorubicin (Adriamycin). Although these drugs are expensive, they are easy to administer in the home every 12 hours either orally or intravenously and offer a significant solution to controlling nausea and vomiting.

Another important group of medications for control of nausea and vomiting are the phenothiazines. These drugs include prochlorperazine (Compazine) and thiethylperazine (Torecan), which can be administered orally, intramuscularly, or rectally. Side effects may include ex-

trapyramidal symptoms of drowsiness, irritation, dry mouth, and anxiety. Other drugs commonly used for nausea and vomiting include benzamides (e.g., metoclopramide [Reglan]), cannabinoids, steroids, and benzodiazepines (e.g., lorazepam [Ativan]) (Goodman, 1997).

As with pain management, nonpharmacological management of nausea and vomiting has received much attention. Again, many of these methods can be implemented by the nurse within the home, and effects of intervention can be measured by tested instruments. King (1997) describes behavioral interventions as self-hypnosis, progressive muscle relaxation, biofeedback, guided imagery, and systematic desensitization. Other interventions include acupuncture or acupressure and music therapy. Nonpharmacological approaches can be of particular benefit when used with prescribed antiemetic therapies.

Fatigue

As with the symptom of pain, fatigue is also difficult to describe precisely. Fatigue is defined as complex, multicausal, and multidimensional in nature. Causes can be physiological (e.g., anemia), psychological (e.g., depression), or pharmacological (e.g., beta blockers) (Piper, 1997). The etiology of fatigue is discussed elsewhere; of interest to the home care nurse are the accurate assessment of, interventions for, and evaluation of fatigue.

Clark and Lacasse (1998) note that the assessment of fatigue is similar to the assessment of pain. Both are subjective phenomena and are often best identified by the patient. Assessment tools should be easily understood and quickly completed. As with pain, fatigue lends itself to self-reporting on visual analogue scales, using a horizontal line scale with verbal anchors at each end. The client can indicate his or her current level of fatigue on the line, thus producing an ongoing record of fatigue throughout his or her care.

Another widely tested and used fatigue scale measures four dimensions of subjective fatigue. Through these dimensions, the nurse can determine the timing of the client's fatigue in terms of onset, pattern, and duration. Emotional manifestations of fatigue can be better understood. Signs and symptoms of fatigue and their intensities can be determined, and severity of the fatigue experience can be evaluated (Winningham et al, 1994). By reviewing exacerbating factors of fatigue, the nurse may add depth to the assessment and better guide interventions (Clark, Lacasse, 1998).

Through their research, Winningham et al (1994) have identified three categories of interventions as education, exercise, and attention-restoring activities. Education includes preparing patients for anticipated fatigue, such as with cancer treatment, anemia, and dyspnea. Through education, the client and family members may better choose the most appropriate interventions for fatigue. For example, a balance of activity and rest may prove more helpful for chronic fatigue. Attention-restoring activities are valuable when the presentation of new information is not appropriate. These are activities within the natural environment in a safe and nonthreatening manner. The client's home is an ideal setting for such activities.

Physiological interventions for fatigue include oxygenating the blood and maintaining proper nutrition. Anemia is a side effect of many disease treatments or is a sequela of the disease itself. Epoetin alfa is a new medication used for individuals with anemia that directly affects hemoglobin levels, leading to decreased fatigue and decreased need for transfusions (Glaspy et al, 1997). This is a remarkable intervention available for use at home. It is important for the home care nurse to identify clients at risk for anemia to monitor their response to epoetin alfa and to teach clients and family members the administration of epoetin alfa. This is discussed further in the section on medication administration.

Clark and Lacasse (1998) offer sound strategies for conserving a client's energy in the home, workplace, and outside activities. These include doing as many activities or tasks as possible sitting down. Activities, such as shopping, should be planned for less busy times. Workplaces should be arranged to provide easy access for frequently used items. These authors suggest performing leisure activities with a companion and balancing activities with rest. Finally, the authors note that when working with the client experiencing fatigue, nurses have opportunities to develop research-based guidelines for practice and to improve the quality of life for him or her. Further family teaching and home care guidelines are presented in Table 10-1.

Mucositis and Stomatitis

Mucositis is an inflammatory reaction that can occur to any of the mucous membranes within the body. Mucositis is generally recognized as a side effect of disease treatment, particularly the cancers treated by chemotherapy and radiation therapy, and involves a number of sequelae. The specific foci of this section are assessment and treatment of this common painful and potentially dangerous condition.

Mucositis can develop from cell tissue sloughing in the genitourinary tract, leading to vaginitis. Mucositis also affects the gastrointestinal (GI) tract, with mucus and blood in the stools. Oral mucositis or stomatitis, also in the GI tract, commonly presents early in the course of chemotherapy and can cause profound problems for the client.

Problems resulting from mucositis involve local tissue reaction with pain, burning, itching, bleeding, development of sores, and potential for infection. Genitourinary mucositis is treated appropriately with topical medications such as miconazole (Monistat). GI mucositis is treated with nutrition and hydration supplements, local anesthetic cream to the anal area, and treatment of anal or rectal bleeding.

Within the home, it is possible to thoroughly assess the oral cavity for signs of impending stomatitis. Hyland (1997) describes historical approaches to oral assessment, noting that the oral cavity is often categorized into specific areas scored according to the severity of stomatitis. Scales range from no evidence of tissue disruption to severe tissue disruption. Such approaches rely on direct visualization of the oral cavity and depend on the nurse's ability to objectively quantify findings. The nurse must also be able to distinguish between actual stomatitis and its complications, edema, and infection.

It is suggested for home assessment purposes that a simple rating scale developed by the World Health Organization (1977) be used. This five-point scale is as follows:

Grade 0   No change
Grade 1   Soreness, erythema
Grade 2   Erythema, ulcers; patient can eat solids
Grade 3   Ulcers; patient requires liquid diet only
Grade 4   Alimentation not possible

Assessment data may be recorded, offering an ongoing measure of this physiological

Table 10-1   Family Teaching and Home Care Guidelines

Potential Problem	Care Guidelines
Physical injury caused by unsteady gait	Obtain equipment (wheelchair, bedside commode, walker, three-prong cane, guard rail for bathroom, stool for shower).
	Take up throw rugs to prevent tripping.
	Wear nonskid shoes when out of bed.
	Eliminate the need to ambulate up and down steps.
	Obtain assistance with physical care through home health aide and visiting nursing service.
Decreased mobility caused by physical disability	Obtain hospital bed if necessary to change position and assist with care needs.
	Perform range-of-motion exercises four times daily.
	Provide a physical therapy consult.
	Provide an occupational therapy consult.
	Change position in bed every 4 hours.
Skin breakdown caused by immobility and chronic steroid use	Bathe every 2-3 days using a nondeodorant soap.
	Apply aloe-based or Eucerin cream daily, especially to pressure points.
	Massage pressure points daily to simulate blood flow.
	Change position every 4 hours.
	Keep the perineum dry.
Oral fungal infections	Perform oral hygiene three times daily.
	Inspect the oral cavity for white plaque buildup.
	Use nystatin (Mycostatin) mouth wash.
High blood sugar caused by steroid use	Medical Management: Sliding scale insulin administration may be used.
	Test blood glucose level as directed:
	Record Tes-Tape values as instructed.
	Fingerstick glucose monitoring may be initiated.
	Report appropriate levels to doctor or nurse:
	Tes-Tape urine values over 200 should be reported.
	Phone number: _____
	Report unusual symptoms to your doctor such as:
	Increased thirst
	Dry mouth
	Flushed skin
	Polyuria
	Nausea and vomiting
Stomach irritation and possible ulcer formation caused by chronic steroid use	Eat small meals frequently.
	Use Riopan or Maalox to minimize stomach upset.
	Avoid caffeine.
	Eat foods that are soft, easy to eat, and easy to digest.
	Use a soft feeding tube to maintain nutrition, if necessary.

Modified from Wegman JA: Central nervous system cancers. In Groenwald S et al, eds: *Cancer nursing principles and practice*, ed 3, Philadelphia, 1993, JB Lippincott.

Table 10-1	Family Teaching and Home Care Guidelines—cont'd
Potential Problem	Care Guidelines
Fatigue, dizziness, muscle weakness, and joint pain caused by immobility	Conserve energy for activities individual enjoys. Be out of bed as much as possible. Walk out of doors daily as tolerated. Use nonsteroidal antiinflammatory agent as needed for joint pain. Vary activities to combat fatigue. Avoid sleeping during the day if possible. Use removable splinting for weakened muscles, as necessary. Slide items rather than lifting and carrying.
Difficulty with dressing and personal hygiene caused by decreased mobility and/or perception	Assess basic functional abilities to identity effective assistance devices. Provide garments that are easy to put on, with large fasteners in easily accessible areas. Use nonskid shoes with Velcro closings. Assess need for raised toilet seat, shower stool, tilted mirrors, and large faucets. Lower closet rods. Store frequently used items within easy reach, in consistent places.
Memory impairment, perceptual deficits, and cognitive processing impairments	Establish habitual use of safety devices and routines. Provide compensatory cognitive devices: Labels Written instructions Reminders Memory logs Minimize environmental stimuli, which may contribute to decreased sleep.
Urinary incontinence caused by confusion, loss of muscle control	Note patterns of incontinence. Establish habit retraining, based on time intervals. Assess need for mechanical methods of urine collection. Maintain positive attitude and recognize incontinence as a symptom, not a disease.
Impending death related to anticipated cardio-pulmonary failure and advanced disease	Perform family assessment of: Diminishing level of consciousness Decreased oral fluid intake Oliguria Labored, irregular breathing Bubbling in throat and chest Progressive cyanotic mottling in lower extremities Encourage participation in home hospice program. Determine unfinished business. Encourage worship and prayer that are consistent with family beliefs.

complication, which can add to the strong client database established regarding the client's pain, nausea, and fatigue. Ongoing assessment for stomatitis should also include the client's ability to eat, drink, talk, and swallow and the degree of associated pain (Hyland, 1997).

With any type of mucositis, pain relief and good hygiene remain paramount. Gentle bathing or rinsing of the area is recommended, and various nurse researchers have experimented with different solutions, temperatures of solutions, and combinations of solutions for this purpose. The reader is referred to the case study at the end of this chapter to see how one client is successfully avoiding and managing her stomatitis. Dodd et al (1996) experimented with several solutions for the treatment of stomatitis. These authors concluded that sterile water is as effective as chlorhexidine in preventing therapy-induced stomatitis. This study also suggests that a protocol of twice daily self-assessment and mouth care is effective in reducing both the incidence and the severity of stomatitis. Such measures involve client and family education and planning for this simple approach to a serious problem.

MEDICATION ADMINISTRATION

Recent pharmacological and technological advances have promoted home-based administration of medication regimens once performed only in hospitals. Administration of therapeutic agents for symptom control is discussed here. Specific disease treatments are discussed elsewhere in this text. Various routes of administration are presented with examples of medications applicable to the specific route. Components of client and family teaching in the home are discussed.

Reymann (1993) identifies routes of administration for chemotherapeutic agents. She presents modes of administration that still remain outside the domain of home use. For use within the home, the following modes are explored: topical, oral, intramuscular (IM), subcutaneous (SQ), and intravenous (IV).

Topical medications are used for the treatment and prevention of various skin conditions. Over-the-counter lotions and creams are used to prevent or improve dryness and to prevent skin breakdown, pruritus, and rashes. Topical medications are also used to treat mucositis or stomatitis and include sprays containing diphenhydramine (Benadryl) and occasionally antibiotics.

Topical medications are also used to treat musculoskeletal and neuropathic pain. Ketamine ointment is an example of an N-methyl-D-aspartate (NMDA) blocker that is applied topically. This medication works at receptors found throughout the central and peripheral nervous systems and interrupts afferent pain from peripheral nerves. Recently available commercially, it can be obtained with prescription from the pharmacy at Loma Linda University, Loma Linda, California (Crowley, 1998).

Topical medication administration requires client education regarding safe handling and storing; use of appropriate equipment, such as gloves; hygiene regarding handling; and correct method of application. Observation for expected, as well as untoward, results is included in education. Other topics include dressings if necessary and things to avoid, such as fabrics and direct sunlight (Reymann, 1993).

Oral administration of medications remains the route of easiest delivery. Drugs commonly given orally include analgesics, nutrition supplements, and antibiotics. A significant oral medication used in the home is extended-release morphine, known as oxycodone (MS Contin or OxyContin). These medications are taken two to four times per day and are used for cancer pain, as well as for other chronic, nonterminal pain. They are triplicate-form medications requiring careful monitoring by the prescriber. One problem that has been encountered with the use of extended-release oral morphine is the lack of availability of these drugs in significantly large quantities by pharmacies. This problem can be avoided with careful planning and communication between the prescriber and the provider (Puryear, 1998). Client education regarding oral medications includes issues of storage and handling, safety with other medications, and conditions of administration, such as with food. Such effects, including possible nausea, vomiting, and changes in bowel habits, must be explained. The importance of maintaining an accurate medication schedule must also be emphasized.

IM and SQ administration of medications are techniques that can be taught to both client and caregivers within the home. These medications include hormones (e.g., insulin), antibiotics, analgesics, and several drugs used to offset factors of disease treatment, such as anemia. Two are discussed here.

Epoetin alfa (Epogen) is derived from recombinant human erythropoietin. This substance is produced in the kidney and is used in the presence of chronic renal failure to stimulate red blood cell production (Glaspy et al, 1997). It is administered subcutaneously or intravenously usually three times per week. Use of this drug enhances hemoglobin production, alleviating symptoms of anemia. This drug is used successfully in the home, administered by the client or family member for hospice and other home care clients (Puryear, 1998).

Neupogen is a human granulocyte-stimulating factor produced by recombinant DNA technology. It is used to prevent infection by increasing the number of white blood cells and to decrease neutropenia caused by immunosuppression. It is administered subcutaneously or intravenously, and may be given immediately after chemotherapy to maintain levels of white blood cells. This drug is also used successfully in the home, administered by the client or family member (Puryear, 1998).

Continuous or long-term IV access has facilitated IV medication administration but adds other concerns and challenges. These involve selection of the most appropriate device, usage, maintenance, procedures, and complication management (Reymann, 1993). Devices include five broad categories of catheters, as shown in Box 10-1.

These devices are inserted surgically in an outpatient setting, usually under general anesthesia. With proper care, they may be left in place indefinitely. The exception to this is the subclavian line, which is usually inserted when there is an immediate need for a central line, generally at the bedside. This discussion therefore focuses on long-term catheters, the most common of which are PICC lines, Hickman and Groshong catheters, and Port-a-Cath devices (Puryear, 1998).

Family members are taught correct technique for care of the insertion site, as well as care of the actual catheter. Insertion site care requires sterile technique until granulation tissue has formed, at which time care includes gentle bathing and dressing placement. The catheters may be multilumen and may be used for drawing blood and administering medication (Reymann, 1993).

Many medications, hyperalimentation solutions, and some blood products can be given through a long-term venous access device in the home setting. The reader is referred to the chapters on specific diseases for further information. Of importance here is the incidence of fungal infections in immunosuppressed clients and the treatment with IV lipid-based amphotericin B. Through clinical trials, this medication has been developed into amphotericin B colloidal dispersion (ABCD) and has been used in the home to treat fungal infections (Rust, Jameson, 1998). Dosage is specific, and the client is at risk for toxicities. This requires that home administration be performed by the professional nurse.

Medication Management of Severe or Chronic Pain

Individualized treatment plans for severe pain through pharmacological approaches represent a significant component of home care. This section addresses three specific medication regimens for pain control. These include the use of nonsteroidal antiinflammatory agents (NSAIDs), opioids, and antidepressants. Guidance in the use of analgesics is offered by the World Health Organization (WHO) (1996), which advocates the use of a three-step analgesic ladder (Figure 10-1). According to this guideline, clients are treated with analgesics appropriate to the severity of their pain.

NSAIDs include acetaminophen, aspirin, naproxen, and indomethacin, among others. These oral medications are most often used for clients with mild to moderate pain. They may also

---

Box 10-1   Categories of Long-Term Vascular Access Devices

Nontunneled central venous catheter (e.g., subclavian line)
Peripherally inserted central catheter (PICC line)
Tunneled central venous catheter (e.g., Hickman, Groshong)
Implantable port (e.g., Port-a-Cath)
Peripheral port (e.g., PAS-Port)

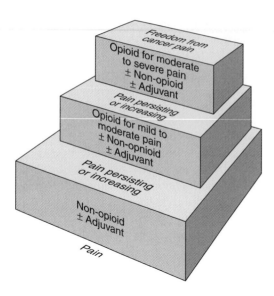

Fig. 10-1 Analgesic ladder outlining the use of nonopioid analgesics, opioid analgesics, and analgesic adjuvants for severe pain. *(From World Health Organization:* Cancer pain relief and palliative care, *ed 2, Geneva, 1996, The Organization.)*

be used for an addictive effect in conjunction with opioids. The administration of NSAIDs is monitored for effect, generally after 1 week of use. Effective dosage is determined by client response (Cunningham, Thorpe, Ruger, 1998).

Side effects of NSAIDs must be monitored. They include GI upset, platelet dysfunction, headache, and depression. These medications are available in over-the-counter products, with stronger doses available by prescription.

Opioids are narcotic medications that relieve pain by binding to opiate receptor sites in the brain and spinal canal. Opioids include, but are not limited to, morphine, methadone, hydromorphone, codeine, and hydrocodone. Opioids are administered orally, rectally, intravenously, subcutaneously, and intramuscularly. Weaker opioids, such as codeine and hydrocodone, may be given in conjunction with NSAIDs. This requires monitoring for renal and hepatic toxicities (Cunningham, Thorpe, Ruger, 1998). Opioids are available through triplicate prescription only.

Nursing's role in the home administration of opioids includes significant client and family teaching. Fears or hesitations regarding use of these drugs need to be explored, with adequate and realistic information conveyed. Nurses should watch for signs of opioid overdose, such as lethargy, respiratory depression, and inadequate oxygenation. Use of opioids in the home requires availability of opioid antagonists, such as naloxone, with clear directions for antagonist use and access to a physician or nurse.

Antidepressants represent another classification of medications that are used for analgesia. Tricyclic antidepressants inhibit the neuronal reuptake of serotonin and norepinephrine, thereby inhibiting pain (Cunningham, Thorpe, Ruger, 1998). They may also be used for potentiation of opioids. These medications include amitriptyline (Elavil), nortriptyline (Pamelor), and desipramine (Norpramin), among others. They are administered orally, usually at night to avoid the sedative effect of the drug. Potential side effects include dry mouth, drowsiness, dizziness, and blurred vision. These medications are available through prescription.

Along with pharmacological management, there are many other methods for pain treatment. These include, but are not limited to, relaxation, biofeedback, guided imagery, and hypnosis. Physical modalities used in pain treatment include, but are not limited to, use of heat and cold, massage, electrotherapy, and transcutaneous electrical nerve stimulation (TENS) (Thorpe et al, 1998). These authors note that nonpharmacological pain interventions require coordinated, multidisciplinary efforts, including thorough client assessment and knowledge of the underlying pathophysiology of the client's pain.

The ability to administer many medications in the home has greatly impacted the delivery of nursing care. Involvement of client and family caregivers, through education and participation, cannot be overemphasized. The role of the home care nurse is paramount in symptom management, largely through effective administration of medications. In particular, the nurse practitioner with prescriptive abilities can have a profound effect on the success of home care.

The actual experiences of living with a life-threatening illness, receiving treatments as an outpatient, and coping with numerous problems are worth investigating. The situations in which nurses provide home care require flexibility, creativity, and the support of the client's loved ones. For these reasons, a case study of an individual who is confronting the problems described in this chapter is presented.

CASE STUDY

Jane Doe and her housemate are both registered nurses, an important factor in the problem-solving occurring in this particular case. Jane is a 50-year-old woman. She was diagnosed with breast cancer 2 years ago. She underwent a mastectomy, began a course of tamoxifen (Nolvadex), and initially did well after surgery. An occasional complicating factor has been her long history of insulin-dependent diabetes mellitus.

Two years after her initial diagnosis, over a 2-month period, she developed progressive skeletal pain. Nothing was identified by x-ray examination and the pain was treated with ibuprofen (Motrin), methocarbamol (Robaxin), and acetaminophen with hydrocodone (Vicodin). Because her pain continued, her physician ordered a CEA, which was elevated to 115 (normal <5 µg/dl). She was referred to an oncologist, and tests were performed to seek bone metastases.

A bone scan revealed involvement in a number of areas but did not reveal depth of bone involvement. A

chest x-ray examination revealed significant pleural effusion. The treatment plan was to discontinue (D/C) tamoxifen (Nolvodex), discontinue Vicodin, and begin megestrol (Megace) and morphine (MS Contin) and begin chemotherapy every 3 weeks for the next year. Initial chemotherapy included cyclophosphamide (Cytoxan), doxorubicin (Adriamycin), and fluorouracil (5-FU). Current chemotherapy is paclitaxel (Taxol) and doxorubicin (Adriamycin).

As Jane Doe continues outpatient chemotherapy and home care, the problems and solutions listed in Table 10-2 have occurred.

At the time of this writing, Jane Doe was 4 months into chemotherapy and doing well. She provided invaluable information to assist others in their home care and treatment journeys. Her advice includes staying on top of side effects and problems and being proactive and not reactive. Also, she was pain free without the use of any pain medications.

Table 10-2   Resolving Problems Caused by Chemotherapy

Problem	Solution
Pain	Initial treatment with MS Contin every 12 hours has good results.
Unavailability of MS Contin, fentanyl (Duragesic) patches, and oxycodone (Percocet) in local pharmacies	This is a problem that should not have to occur. The solution involved searching for, and changing to, a small pharmacy that was willing to work with Jane and her housemate and recognize the importance of making needed medications available in a more convenient way. It is suggested that a nurse practitioner work with pharmacies to avoid this problem.
Sudden pruritus, rash, and wheezing from MS Contin	MS Contin should be D/C and use of Duragesic patches 150 mg and Percocet started.
Confusion	The strength of Duragesic patch is gradually decreased while the effect of pain relief is maintained. Jane Doe is currently pain free with no pain medications required.
Periods of severe sickness during the first 6 weeks of treatment	Jane should plan for friends and family to be within the home. A baby monitor can be used within the home to alert others to the need for assistance.
Venous access	A Port-a-Cath should be placed.
Nausea and vomiting related to reactions to pain medications	Frequent popsicles and small servings of food should be offered. Music should be played during chemotherapy. Ondansetron (Zofran) should be administered up to 2 days after chemotherapy then PRN as necessary.

Continued

Table 10-2	Resolving Problems Caused by Chemotherapy—cont'd
Problem	Solution
Decreased appetite	Her appetite initially decreased and then gradually returned. Eating small, frequent amounts of food she liked or craved was helpful. Also, she began to take Megace, which is an appetite stimulant as well as an anticancer medication.
Anxiety, possible panic attacks, diagnosed by the physician after the development of shortness of breath	Alprazolam (Xanax) was prescribed, with good results, especially with use the day before chemotherapy. Also, she noted the shortness of breath was minimized as soon as Cytoxan was discontinued.
Leukopenia (white blood cell count decreased to 600 μl)	Neupogen SQ every day for 7-10 days and antibiotics should be administered. Jane should avoid crowds and use mask when in crowds.
Vaginitis from antibiotics taken for leukopenia, 10 days, then 7 days, then 2 days after chemotherapy, lasting 10 days	Monistat should be started with the first onset of symptoms (itching, burning).
Stomatitis	Bland, easy-to-eat foods, such as cottage cheese, cucumber slices, popsicles, and creamsicles, should be offered. Oral swish solution should be used four times every day: 1 L water, 1 tsp salt, 1 tsp baking soda. Ice should be eaten during chemotherapy administration. Other helpful swish and spit solutions: 3 Tbs calcium carbonate (Maalox) with 1 Tbs diphenhydramine (Benadryl) Ulcer Ease Also use of Chloraseptic throat spray and Orabase B (oral analgesic)
Elevated blood glucose level from dexamethasone (Decadron), premedication for paclitaxel (Taxol)	Insulin should be increased for 5 days after chemotherapy.
Vaginal spotting with initiation of chemotherapy, continuing to the present	This problem was not incapacitating and was treated with ferrous sulfate and the use of tampons or pads.
Constipation	Colace should be administered every day, and fluid intake should be increased.
Fatigue	She notes that this is still her biggest problem but improves the week after chemotherapy. Therefore they plan for and adjust activities accordingly. She notes that compared to other side effects, this "ain't so bad."
Disruption in plans for long-distance travel	She should plan with her oncologist, monitor blood counts, and wear a mask while on the airplane.
Difficulty maintaining hope and positive attitude	Prayer and the support of loved ones and friends, including the sharing of laughs and tears, can help. She should participate in church. They perform an activity of centering prayer twice per day. Also, Jane keeps in touch with a group of family and friends through journaling and sharing her experiences through e-mail.

SUMMARY

More and more individuals are managing chronic health problems, often with complicated treatments, while remaining at home. Remarkable advances in technology and therapies make this possible. Home care nursing practice continues to evolve to meet increasing client care needs effectively and compassionately. Without such nursing care, the management and resolution of symptoms and problems described in this chapter would not be possible in the home.

Therapeutic nursing interventions provide measurable data to assess client response to treatments. An outcome of nursing interventions that may not be so easily quantifiable is the placebo effect. Kwekkeboom (1997) notes that placebo effects occur in up to 90% of nursing interventions. This author states that once placebo effects occur, nurses may then use the effects to enhance response to treatment.

The impact of professional nursing care within the home is profound, promoting symptom relief and improved quality of life. Challenges for home care nursing are great and will continue to grow. Through ongoing practice and client outcome evaluation, these challenges will be successfully met.

REFERENCES

Bland KI: Quality-of-life management for cancer patients, *CA—A Cancer Journal for Clinicians* 47(4):194-197, 1997.

Clark PM, Lacasse C: Cancer-related fatigue: Clinical practice issues, *Clinical Journal of Oncology Nursing* 2(2):45-53, 1998.

Crowley KL: Personal communication, April 15, 1998.

Cunningham RS: 5-HT3-receptor antagonists: A review of pharmacology and clinical efficacy, *Oncology Nursing Forum* 23(suppl)(7):33-41, 1997.

Cunningham ML, Thorpe DM, Ruger TF: Pharmacologic approaches to cancer pain management, *Strategies for Pain Management* 1(2):1-32, 1998.

Dodd JJ et al: Randomized clinical trial of chlorhexidine versus placebo for the prevention of oral mucositis in patients receiving chemotherapy, *Oncology Nursing Forum* 23(6):921-927, 1996.

Ferrell BR, McGuire DB, Donovan MI: Knowledge and beliefs regarding pain in a sample of nursing faculty, *Journal of Professional Nursing* 9(2):79-88, 1993.

Fessele KS: Managing the multiple causes of nausea and vomiting in the patient with cancer, *Oncology Nursing Forum* 23(9):1409-1417, 1996.

Glaspy J et al: Impact of therapy with epoetin alfa on clinical outcomes in patients with nonmyeloid malignancies during cancer chemotherapy in community oncology practice, *Journal of Clinical Oncology* 15(3):1218-1234, 1997.

Goodman M: Risk factors and antiemetic management of chemotherapy-induced nausea and vomiting, *Oncology Nursing Forum* 24(suppl)(7):20-32, 1997.

Grant M: Introduction: Nausea and vomiting, quality of life, and the oncology nurse, *Oncology Nursing Forum* 24(suppl)(7):5-8, 1997.

Hogan CM: Cancer nursing: The art of symptom management, *Oncology Nursing Forum* 24(8):1335-1340, 1997.

Hyland SA: Assessing the oral cavity. In Frank-Stromborg M, Olsen S, eds: *Instruments for clinical health-care research,* ed 2, Boston, 1997, Jones & Bartlett.

King C: Nonpharmacologic management of chemotherapy-induced nausea and vomiting, *Oncology Nursing Forum* 24(suppl)(7):41-48, 1997.

Kwekkeboom KL: The placebo effect in symptom management, *Oncology Nursing Forum* 24(8):1393-1408, 1997.

Maxwell C: Sensitivity and accuracy of the visual analogue scale: A psycho-physical classroom experiment, *British Journal of Clinical Pharmacology* 6(1):15-24, 1978.

McCaffrey M, Beebe A: *Pain: Clinical manual for nursing practice,* St Louis, 1989, Mosby.

McGuire DB: Comprehensive and multidimensional assessment and measurement of pain, *Journal of Pain and Symptom Management* 7(5):312-319, 1992.

McGuire DB: Pain. In Groenwald SL et al, eds: *Cancer nursing principles and practice,* ed 3, Boston, 1993, Jones & Bartlett.

McGuire DB: Measuring pain. In Frank-Stromborg M, Olsen SJ, eds: *Instruments for clinical health care research,* ed 2, Boston, 1997, Jones & Bartlett.

Melzak R: The short form McGill pain questionnaire, *Pain* 30:191-197, 1987.

Morrow GR, Hickock JT, Rosenthal SN: Progress in reducing nausea and emesis, *Cancer* 76(3):343-357, 1995.

Murray TA: From outside the walls: A qualitative study of nurses who recently changed from hospital-based practice to home health nursing, *Journal of Continuing Education in Nursing* 29(2):55-60, 1998.

Piper BF: Measuring fatigue. In Frank-Stromborg M, Olsen SJ, eds: *Instruments for clinical health care research,* ed 2, Boston, 1997, Jones & Bartlett.

Puryear J: Personal communication, April 14, 1998.

Reymann PE: Chemotherapy: Principles of administration. In Groenwald S et al, eds: *Cancer nursing principles and practice,* ed 3, Philadelphia, 1993, JB Lippincott.

Rust DM, Jameson G: The novel lipid delivery system of amphotericin B: Drug profile and relevance to clinical practice, *Oncology Nursing Forum* 25(1):35-48, 1998.

Thorpe DM et al: Nonpharmacologic approaches to cancer pain management, *Strategies for Pain Management* 1(3):1-18, 1998.

Wegmann JA: Central nervous system cancers. In Groenwald S et al, eds: *Cancer nursing principles and practice,* ed 3, Philadelphia, 1993, JB Lippincott.

Winningham ML et al: Fatigue and the cancer experience: The state of knowledge, *Oncology Nursing Forum* 21(1):23-36, 1994.

World Health Organization: *WHO handbook for reporting results of cancer treatment,* Geneva, 1977, The Organization.

World Health Organization: *Cancer pain relief and palliative care,* Geneva, 1996, The Organization.

11 Rehabilitation in the Home

Leslie Jean Neal, Raija Kuisma, Janet Sit, and David W.K. Man

Rehabilitation nursing as a specialty practice in the home setting is a fairly new concept. Although most home care nurses use principles of rehabilitation nursing to guide their practice, they do so unwittingly unless they have a background or certification in rehabilitation nursing (Neal, 1999). The goals of home care nursing and rehabilitation nursing are very similar, and many of the same theoretical constructs are used to underpin both areas of nursing practice. Rehabilitation nurses practicing in the home setting have used the inherent creativity of the rehabilitation professional to implement their roles in various ways within the home care setting.

The health care environment has changed over the years, and the trend has been toward early discharge of ill and disabled clients to the home setting. Changes in the delivery of health care and the increased acuity of clients cared for in the home support the increasing need for health care professionals whose primary goal is to promote client independence and self-care.

This chapter will discuss the principles of rehabilitation nursing and their congruence with the goals of home care nursing. In addition, several ways in which the rehabilitation nursing role has been implemented within home health care will be described.

GOALS OF REHABILITATION NURSING

According to the *Standards and scope of rehabilitation nursing practice* (Association of Rehabilitation Nurses, 1995), rehabilitation nursing is "the diagnosis and treatment of human responses of individuals and groups to actual or potential health problems relative to altered functional ability and lifestyle." The primary goal is "to assist the individual who has a disability and/or chronic illness in restoring, maintaining, and promoting his or her maximal health. This includes preventing chronic illness and disability." According to Hoeman (2001), rehabilitation nurses do the following as they work with their clients and their families:

- Set goals for maximal levels of interdependent functioning and activities of daily living
- Promote self-care and prevent complications or further disability
- Reinforce positive coping behaviors
- Ensure access to home care with continuity of services and care
- Advocate for clients' optimal quality of life
- Improve outcome for clients
- Contribute to reforms in the character, structure, and delivery of health care in the United States

Assisting the client in achieving maximal health and independence also necessitates teaching clients to "adapt" to their altered lifestyle. Often the concept of *functional substitution* is used to accomplish this. Functional substitution is a method by which the client is taught to perform or accomplish a task in a way that is different from how it would be accomplished under normal conditions. Sometimes adaptive or assistive aids are used, such as with eating or ambulating. At other times, functional substitution is as basic as learning to write with the left hand instead of the right hand. In any case, adaptations of some type must be made during the rehabilitation process. In the case of rehabilitation in the home, the client adapts to the home setting what he or she may have learned in the institutional or outpatient setting. In addition, the rehabilitation nurse is expected to assess for and prevent potential risk factors and complications. Typical client problems such as decreased endurance and strength and poor balance and mobility will invariably increase the risk of accidents in the home.

Given the definition of *rehabilitation nursing* and the goal of the rehabilitation nurse, it is clear that rehabilitation nursing can be practiced with almost any client population. For example, the client who has a wound that is extensive enough to limit independent function or to alter his or her lifestyle might be considered to have a disability (Neal, 1995b). Consequently, although any nurse experienced with wound care could conceivably care for this client, it is the rehabilitation nurse or the nurse who uses rehabilitation nursing principles who will assist the client in regaining optimal health and independence. This nurse will view the wound as a disability and will focus on what the client is able to do while encouraging and teaching methods of functional substitution to the client.

Similarly, the rehabilitation nurse's approach to a client with acquired immunodeficiency syndrome (AIDS) would be one of optimizing the client's functional ability (Neal, 1997b). As AIDS manifests itself in various ways depending on how long the client has had the disease and how his or her body has responded to it, the client may have different levels of function from one phase of the illness to the next. Both physical and psychosocial changes in function and lifestyle are addressed with the primary goals being maintenance and maximization of self-care and independence.

Diagnoses or Conditions Cared for by the Rehabilitation Nurse

Although almost any client, regardless of diagnosis, can potentially benefit from rehabilitation nursing, the diagnoses or conditions most commonly associated with rehabilitation nursing include, but are not limited to, the following:

- Neurologic conditions, such as traumatic brain injury and spinal cord injury, multiple sclerosis, stroke, and Parkinson's disease
- Musculoskeletal conditions, such as total hip and total knee replacement, arthritis, amputations, and fractures
- Geriatric complaints, such as incontinence and limited mobility and sensory-perceptual ability
- Pediatric complaints, such as limited mobility and sensory-perceptual ability

- Various cardiac conditions, such as recovery from coronary artery bypass graft surgery or myocardial infarction
- Chronic obstructive pulmonary disease
- Pain
- Wounds
- Sexual dysfunction
- Communication, cognitive, and behavioral disorders

Self-care and independence are the fundamental goals of rehabilitation for all clients, regardless of the health care setting. Several theories provide the conceptual framework to support these fundamental principles. Some of these theories are discussed here.

Theoretical Frameworks (Box 11-1)

Orem's (1995) theory of self-care agency is the theoretical construct that is perhaps the most familiar to rehabilitation nurses. Orem describes

---

Box 11-1   Major Concepts of Nurse Theorists

OREM

The nurse provides care that is *supportive-educative, partly compensatory,* or *wholly compensatory.*

ROY

The nurse's role is to facilitate the *adaptation* of the client to an altered lifestyle resulting from illness or disability.

HENDERSON

The nurse is a *substitute, helper,* or *partner* for or with the client.

NEAL

The nurse must *adapt and make adaptations* to provide quality care in the home.

ALBRECHT

There are many interrelated factors linked by *structure, process,* and *outcome* that modify the care of the home care client.

RICE

The nurse, the client, and the family caregiver work as a *unit toward a sense of independence.*

the role of the nurse with clients in the context of the extent of the client's self-care deficit. Clients who require maximal care, such as a bed-bound comatose client, would receive wholly compensatory care from the nurse. That is, the nurse would provide for all of the needs of the client because the client cannot meet his or her own self-care needs. It is important to add, however, that a conscious bedbound client would be assisted and encouraged to participate in self-care to whatever extent possible, such as brushing the hair or shaving.

Clients, according to Orem (1995), who are capable of meeting some of their self-care needs or requisites would require only partly compensatory nursing care. In this case, the nurse assists only when the client cannot perform self-care requisites alone. Finally, nurses caring for clients who are able to perform independent self-care but need instruction, emotional support, or encouragement practice in a supportive-educative role. The requisites described by Orem are the following (Pratt, 1996; Thomason, 1998):

- Maintenance of sufficient intake of air, water, and food
- Provision of care associated with eliminative processes and excrements
- Maintenance of balance between activity and rest
- Maintenance of balance between solitude and social interaction
- Prevention of hazards to life, functioning, and well-being
- Promotion of normalcy

Henderson (1978) considers health and independence to be equivalent states. The nurse can be a substitute for the client when the client is unable to perform independently, such as during serious illness. The nurse becomes a helper for the client as the client convalesces and then works with the client in a partnership during the development and implementation of the health care plan. The nurse alters the client's environment as necessary to foster independence and promote health and works with the client toward a goal of full independence or a peaceful death. Henderson's philosophy is applicable not only to rehabilitation nursing, which strives to treat the client as the director of the plan of care and to assist the client in attaining maximal independence, but also to the home setting because it considers the

environment as a vital element of the client's ability to become and remain independent.

Roy (Roy, Andrews, 1999) views the nurse's role as facilitating the adaptation of the client to the alteration in lifestyle that has resulted from the illness or disability. Roy contends that the client, the recipient of care, interacts with a changing environment and must make adaptations to respond to and cope with the demands made by that changing environment. "At any point [along the continuum of health and illness] he will have a variety of stimuli acting on him to which he must respond" (Roy, Andrews, 1999). Roy explains that a client can raise his or her adaptation response. By repeating an action, such as placing his or her hand in hot water, the ability to adapt, in this case to the hot water, is increased. The nurse's role, Roy goes on, is to encourage adaptation by the client so that the client is free to respond to other stimuli that might enter the environment. The subsequent energy saved is available for healing. The modes of adaptation, or the ways in which a client adapts, can be physiological or psychological (self-concept, role function, and interdependence) (Pollock et al, 1994).

Another theory (Neal, 1998) that is not yet well known but is based on recent research with home care nurses describes the importance of the adaptations the nurse must make to care for clients in their homes. The Neal theory of home health nursing practice contends that on entering the field of home care nursing, nurses proceed through the following three-step process toward the attainment of autonomy of practice:

- Stage One: Dependence. The nurse is overwhelmed with learning the clinical and logistical components of home health care. This stage lasts approximately 6 months to 1 year.
- Stage Two: Moderate Dependence. The nurse is comfortable with some of the clinical and logistical aspects of home care and is able to answer some questions about home care practice from nurses new to home care. This stage lasts approximately 1 year.
- Stage Three: Autonomy. The nurse is confident and competent in all areas of home care practice. If the nurse encounters an unfamiliar situation, he or she is temporarily moderately dependent in that the nurse must

locate the information to prepare to care for the client. However, the nurse knows where and how to obtain the information. The nurse's autonomy is also temporarily restricted when the physician will not approve an order, when a payor refuses to allow a visit or supplies, when the client or caregivers are nonadherent, or when office procedures present a barrier to effective communication and smooth job performance by the nurse. This stage is attained after approximately 2 years practicing in home care and is maintained throughout the remainder of the nurse's practice.

The research, using grounded theory methodology to study 30 home care nurses (this study has since been followed with another qualitative survey that validated the original research and refined the specific qualities of the home care nurse), concluded that the core category or key concept of home care nursing practice is *adaptation*. Home care nurses must be adaptable and make adaptations to function effectively and successfully in home care (Neal, 1998). Because home care nursing practice occurs within the home environment and each home environment is different, as are the client's resources, both tangible and intangible, the nurse is constantly adapting to meet the needs of the client.

GOAL OF HOME HEALTH CARE NURSING PRACTICE

The goal of home health care nursing parallels that of rehabilitation nursing. According to *A statement on the scope of home health nursing practice* (American Nurses Association, 1992), the goal of home health care is to "initiate, manage, and evaluate the resources needed to promote the client's optimal level of well-being. Nursing activities necessary to achieve this goal may warrant preventive, maintenance, and restorative emphases to avoid potential deficits from developing."

Theoretical Frameworks

The home care setting is ideal for practice that is based on nursing theory because of the unique conditions that it presents (Clarke, Cody, 1994). The home setting is a unique care setting because of the potential influences of the client's environment on the care provided (Mundinger, 1983).

Theories that support the practice of home care nursing also include the works of Orem and Henderson. In addition to Neal, two other theorists have recently published conceptual frameworks specific to home care nursing practice.

Albrecht (1990) views home health care as dynamic and complex. She devised a model based on a review of the literature and on her own professional and teaching experiences related to home care. The model developed by Albrecht was based on 18 concepts that she deemed important to home care nursing and their interrelationships. The model links the concepts based on their elements of structure, process, or outcome.

The concepts listed by Albrecht (1990) are accessibility, accountability, availability, client classification, comprehensiveness, continuity, coordination, cost effectiveness, client/consumer, demand, efficiency, intervention, nurse, productivity, provider, quality of care, satisfaction, and the use of home care. Albrecht identifies the client, family, provider agency, professional nurse, and health team as being impacted by or modified by the following factors: type of care, coordination of care, interventions toward satisfaction with care, quality of care, cost effectiveness, health status, self-care capability, and the use of home care.

The Rice model of dynamic self-determination (Rice, 1994, 1996) is a client-focused model for home care nursing practice. It supports a nursing goal of successful management of care by the client on discharge from home health care. The nurse's role is to facilitate the client's independence at home through education, advocacy, and case management. "Dynamic self-determination allows patients to bridge the gap between need and goal attainment" (Rice, 1994). Health care is considered, in the model, to be related to intrapersonal harmony or a state in which frustration and unmet needs do not exist. Clients are part of a health care unit that includes the caregiver and the environment. The relationship between this unit and the nurse proceeds through the phases of dependence, interdependence, and independence. Rice described the caregiver as an "extension of the patient and the patient's needs" and stated that "as with the patient, the caregiver will require respect, support, nurturing, and other elements of 'caring' for goal attainment to occur"(1996).

IMPLEMENTING THE REHABILITATION NURSING ROLE IN THE HOME HEALTH CARE SETTING

Rehabilitation in any setting inherently includes comprehensive therapies or services. Rehabilitation is accomplished not by one discipline but within the context of a team approach. Throughout the rehabilitation process, the client is considered most significant, having unique and complex physical, psychological, and spiritual attributes contributing to his or her identity (McCourt, 1993). Alterations in any of these areas affect the function of the total being. Therefore, similar to institution-based rehabilitation, home rehabilitation is not the exclusive domain of any professional discipline but requires a collaborative team effort to help the client reach his or her maximal potential. The team is typically interdisciplinary in that activities are performed by different team members to reach a mutually agreed-on goal; problem solving and responsibility are shared equally or transdisciplinarily, in which the boundaries of team-member roles are blurred so that the functions of each team member can overlap the functions of the others.

The composition of a rehabilitation team varies according to the needs of the client. The core team typically includes the physician, rehabilitation nurse, physical therapist (PT), occupational therapist (OT), social worker, and, most important, the client and his or her family or significant others. Other specialists such as the home health aide, speech therapist, clinical psychologist, psychiatrist, rehabilitation and vocational counselors, and dietitian, as well as experts in prosthetics and orthotics, may also be involved in the rehabilitation team.

Core Functions of the Rehabilitation Team

McCourt (1993) identified the core functions of the home rehabilitation team as follows:
1. Assessment of the client's needs and functional ability
2. Development and documentation of an interdisciplinary treatment plan based on mutually agreed-on goals
3. Implementation of the treatment plan in an interdisciplinary team approach

4. Evaluation of the treatment plan. This includes continuous monitoring of intervention outcomes to the extent to which goals are achieved by the client. All disciplines in the rehabilitation team are involved in the evaluation and review of the client's progress.

Case Manager

In home health care, the nurse is typically the case manager for the client, regardless of the other disciplines involved in the case. The nurse often makes the referrals to other disciplines and then coordinates the team to ensure optimal collaboration. It is the responsibility of the case manager to ensure that the client's chart reflects that there are physician orders to cover all of the care provided, that the payor is aware and supportive of the care delivered to the client, and that all appropriate community resources (both formal and informal) have been garnered for the client.

Documentation of services and of orders to provide service is key to reimbursement. Clients who receive skilled home care services are expected to meet specific criteria, such as being homebound or able to leave the home only with great difficulty. The case manager, each clinician who documents service, and the staff assigned to perform utilization review must take responsibility for justifying service through documentation for Medicare, Medicaid, and other third-party payors.

TEAM MEMBERS
Rehabilitation Nurse

The rehabilitation nurse is a nurse first. That is, the rehabilitation nurse is skilled in performing the rudiments of nursing care, such as a thorough physical and psychosocial assessment, wound care, medication instruction, and various clinical procedures. As a nurse, he or she advocates for the client and protects the rights and interests of the client while the client is under his or her care.

The rehabilitation nurse strives to promote the client's optimal functioning and independence. To do so, he or she collaborates with inpatient and home-based rehabilitation team members through ongoing communication and monitoring. He or she mobilizes appropriate, available, and accessible resources and also coordinates all of the care provided to ensure the continuity and cost effectiveness of each service.

While providing hands-on nursing care, the rehabilitation nurse promotes client and caregiver participation. The nurse does "with" the client, not "for" or "to" the client (Preston, 1990). This is a significant difference from the care provided by nurses without a rehabilitation perspective. The nurse teaches the client self-care, and when the client is incapable of learning, the nurse teaches the caregiver to perform the care while the nurse supervises the client's activities. Teaching is a key role of both rehabilitation and home care nurses. However, the guiding purpose of teaching should be to make the client independent of health care professionals. Consequently, instruction must begin from the first contact with the client and not be delayed until discharge is imminent. For example, as the nurse performs wound care, he or she teaches the client or caregiver to perform wound care.

Frequently, rehabilitation nurses must invest a lot of time teaching caregivers to permit clients to do what they can for themselves. The process by which the client performs self-care is often slow, and caregivers become anxious and impatient. Rehabilitation nurses reinforce the principle that self-care is very therapeutic to the client, both physically and psychologically.

Rehabilitation nurses, along with the other members of the interdisciplinary or transdisciplinary team, assess the client, caregiver, and environment for the suitability of care delivery in the home and for the potential for independent care. The client is assessed using the usual methods of nursing assessment, with particular attention paid to the performance of activities of daily living (ADLs) and instrumental activities of daily living (IADLs). Most home care clients have significant impairments in both of these areas; otherwise they would not likely meet the homebound criterion to receive skilled home care services.

The assessment of the caregiver includes assessing his or her ability to assist the client with self-care and correctly use any equipment that may be needed. Assessment also covers the caregiver's ability to obtain respite and emotional support. Caregiving imposes stress and strain that may ultimately lead to caregiver illness. The caregiver or the family is as much a recipient of the home care practice of the nurse as is the client.

Role of Physical Therapist

The PT has specialized knowledge and skills based on his or her orientation to human structure and function and expertise in the assessment and treatment of musculoskeletal, neurological, respiratory, and cardiovascular impairment and disabilities that are related to movement and function. The roles of the PT in the home include assessment, education, and treatment. The outcomes of physical therapy are best measured by gains in the client's functional capacity and quality of life.

Some examples in which the PT works in the home setting include the initial or follow-up assessment of the client in his or her own environment to help the client adapt after discharge from a hospital or other institution. Preventing venous and respiratory complications in immobile clients and assisting clients in attaining maximal mobility are primary goals of the PT. Prevention of falls in elderly people by early detection and elimination of hazards at home is one of the most valuable physical therapy services in the home. Relatives and caregivers or other professionals concerned with the client are instructed regarding the physical therapy program for the client to support, assist, and encourage the client to comply with the program.

Role of Occupational Therapist

OTs typically work with clients to achieve maximal upper body function. They use assistive and adaptive devices to help the client perform self-care and ADLs. In addition, they instruct clients and caregivers regarding the performance of IADLs and the importance of rest and energy conservation. OTs help clients make therapeutic adaptations. *Therapeutic adaptation* refers to the design or restructuring of the physical environment to assist in self-care, work, and leisure. The following categories of adaptation are frequently used in occupational therapy:

1. Orthotics: provision of dynamic or static splints and slings to relieve pain, maintain joint integrity, improve function, and decrease deformity
2. Assistive or adaptive equipment: the provision of special devices to assist in performance such as the mobile arm support, dressing equipment, feeding and communication equipment, and equipment for personal hygiene

3. Environmental modification in the home: increased lighting, contrasting colors of rooms, neatness of the room, and stability of furniture and grab bars

ENVIRONMENTAL AND FUNCTIONAL ASSESSMENT

Both the tangible and intangible aspects of the client's environment and the way the client functions within the environment should be assessed by the team. The purpose of this assessment is to assess the degree of safety, accessibility, function, and comfort in the home; to identify the need for adaptive equipment; to promote independence in ADLs; and to have more in-depth and reliable evaluation of existing family and social support.

Tangible Environment

Each member of the interdisciplinary team, frequently the first discipline to admit the client to home care, conducts a thorough home safety assessment. Information obtained is fundamental to planning for the removal or modification of environmental hazards and for the promotion of self-care.

Each member of the team has the responsibility for conducting a thorough assessment of the client's ability to function within the environment. Included in the admission assessment is the type of dwelling; number of steps; availability of an elevator if the dwelling is a multistory building; availability of a caregiver during the day, evening, and night; and availability of telephone service and the use of any equipment or assistive devices in the home before the illness or disability. Moreover, access to transportation, community facilities, and a social system is also evaluated. The physical environment may be cluttered and dirty regardless of the client's financial status and may make care delivery a challenge for team members. In addition, the client may have a pet that needs care, and the client cannot be receptive to health care instruction until he or she knows the pet's needs are being met.

Intangible Environment

The dynamics of the family or support network directly influence the client's care. For example, there may be a family member who has not been in contact with the client for years and yet may be the only source of financial support during the client's illness. Informal support networks, such as neighbors and religious organization members, frequently fill in gaps left by the lack of family participation or support.

Both tangible and intangible aspects of the environment influence care planning and implementation. These are most accurately assessed by the rehabilitation professional because his or her training provides cues to barriers to mobility and self-care.

Many of these areas are assessed when the nurse or therapist uses the Outcomes Assessment Information Set (OASIS), now required by the Centers for Medicare and Medicaid Services (CMS) on every admission to home care. The OASIS is a 75-question tool (not including demographic questions) intended to assess the client's need for skilled care in the home and to measure the outcomes of home health care. Home health care agencies are responsible for targeting specific areas on the OASIS for quality improvement and assurance. In addition, the OASIS is used to influence reimbursement under the prospective payment system that began in home care in the fall of 2000. It is important that the information gleaned from the OASIS be used to formulate a comprehensive plan of care that includes the entire team, particularly the client and caregivers. Team members are expected to respond to the OASIS questions with consistency so that the data help paint a picture of the condition of the client.

SPECIALTY REHABILITATION NURSING CLIENTS
Geriatric Clients

The goals of rehabilitation for geriatric clients in the home setting include the control of the underlying disease process to maintain function and minimize impairment, functional substitution balanced by rest, the prevention of secondary disabilities, and the preservation of the client's dignity and self-image (Girard, 1997; Pratt, 1996). Rehabilitation nurses working with homebound geriatric clients must consider the impact of comorbidities, as well as a high incidence of cognitive deficits, the likelihood of polypharmacy, and the frequent absence of social support networks while working toward maximal self-care and independence (Pratt, 1996). Sensory-perceptual changes and physical changes resulting from the normal aging process can also be sequelae to disease processes and must be carefully assessed to determine etiology and to plan care appropriately.

Pediatric Clients

Children cared for by rehabilitation home care nurses typically have chronic illnesses or either congenital or acquired disabilities (Brothers, 1998). More children are receiving care in the home than before (Dittbrenner, 1994; Brothers, 1998). However, social conditions for children have changed related to an increase in step-families and blended families, the likelihood of both parents working outside the home, and the lack of health insurance for many children (Mc-Clinton, 1997). Rehabilitation nurses provide both acute and nonacute care for these clients in the home setting.

Clients with Wounds

The rehabilitation home care nurse can orchestrate interventions that may be required from other health care professionals in addition to providing nursing interventions that will have an impact on the wound's healing process. The rehabilitation home care nurse has the ability to look at the sum of the parts and map out interventions that include more than just wound dressings (Griffitt, 1998). A wound that renders a client homebound and thus qualified to receive skilled nursing care in the home is a wound that is likely to interfere with the client's everyday activities and function. The rehabilitation nurse views the wound as a disability (Neal, 1995b) and treats the wound within the context of a holistic view of treating the entire person. The goal is to assist the client in performing self-care functions, including learning how to care for the wound and how to prevent further disability while managing ambulation and other ADLs.

Clients with Cardiac or Pulmonary Conditions

Rehabilitation nurses in the home setting also treat cardiac and pulmonary conditions as disabling. That is, the client's ability to breathe and to perform ADLs and IADLs is impaired. Formal cardiac and pulmonary rehabilitation programs instituted in conjunction with the client's physi-

cian and PT may be coordinated and directed by the rehabilitation nurse. Also, informal programs such as reinforcing (along with other members of the team) the importance of diet, exercise, smoking cessation, medication compliance, and regular medical examinations are typical. Nurses use creative methods to devise charts and incentives to instruct and encourage clients to participate in these programs. Energy-conservation techniques and graded exercise programs are common reasons for consulting rehabilitation home care nurses.

Clients with AIDS

AIDS is a syndrome of chronic illnesses that eventually causes disability related to its systemic effects. Rehabilitation home care nurses are expert at caring for clients with chronic illness or disabilities, and although AIDS is not a chronic illness typically associated with rehabilitation nursing, it is a syndrome that promises to benefit from rehabilitation nursing expertise. Nutrition, pain management, exercise, infection control, and medication compliance are areas nurses commonly target when caring for clients with AIDS. However, issues such as fatigue, sexual function, bowel and bladder incontinence, and neurologic changes are especially suited to the interventions of the rehabilitation nurse. To maximize self-care and independence at home, nurses must dispel the fear caregivers express about having clients participate in household activities. These fears are usually related to infection-control issues and to concerns about the client's energy level (Neal, 1998).

EVALUATION OF REHABILITATION OUTCOME

Periodic evaluation of the plan of care and rehabilitation outcome using an interdisciplinary approach is one of the important aspects of rehabilitation. Evaluation of rehabilitation outcomes is dynamic, ranging from functional aspects to psychological and social aspects. Daus (1996) emphasizes that for clients who suffer from chronic illnesses or permanent disabilities, outcome information is typically not about improving function but about maintaining function and providing an adequate quality of life and satisfaction with services. For example, a client with stroke or multiple sclerosis may not achieve outcomes that reflect his or her ability to show continuous improvement in independence in ADLs, but the outcomes may have more to do with the individual's sense of well-being; physical, emotional, and social adjustment toward the illness or disability; comfort with people around him or her; and ability to reintegrate into the community.

Therefore, apart from the physical aspect of recovery, such as functional capacity and independence in ADLs, the outcome criteria have to be sensitive to reflect realistically what could be expected to occur in psychosocial aspects of recovery. In evaluating rehabilitation outcomes in home care, it is important to consider the rate of emergency room use and rehospitalization, the use of outpatient clinic services, and the costs of providing rehabilitation at home versus longer lengths of stay in hospitals, skilled nursing facilities, nursing homes, and rehabilitation centers.

When evaluating the client's health status after rehabilitation services in the home, the incidence and types of complications, overall general health status, quality of life (as measured by the client), vocational status, and the ability to participate in leisure activities and reintegrate into the community must be considered in addition to functional ability, level of self-care, and independence. In addition, the client's and caregiver's satisfaction with the care provided must be taken into account when evaluating the outcome of services rendered.

ADDITIONAL REHABILITATION NURSING ROLES IN HOME HEALTH CARE
Certification

Nurses can obtain certification in rehabilitation nursing at either the basic or advanced practice levels. The Association of Rehabilitation Nurses offers certification to those who have practiced rehabilitation nursing in any of a variety of settings, including home care, and who have passed a certification examination.

In addition, certification in case management is useful to the rehabilitation nurse practicing in home care. Rehabilitation nurses practice in a case-management role in many different settings. However, rehabilitation nurses seem particularly suited to case managing clients in home care because they consider the primary care planning goal to be maximal self-care and independence. This is also the ultimate goal of home health care. The American Nurses Association (ANA) offers a certificate in nursing case management. In addition, the ANA sponsors a home care nurse certificate. This certificate requires experience in home care and a passing score on a standardized examination.

Advanced Practice Rehabilitation Nurse

Rehabilitation clinical nurse specialists (CNSs) and adult or family nurse practitioners play important roles in home care. "The APN in rehabilitation, who is a master's prepared nurse with specialty expertise in rehabilitation nursing, educates clients, families, and interdisciplinary staff and performs the roles of clinician, consultant, liaison, and researcher" (McCourt, 1993; Daus, 1996).

> Within the home care setting, the CNS has almost unlimited potential for practicing CNS roles and for possibly gaining a larger degree of autonomy than is usually enjoyed in the institutional setting. CNSs in home care, however, face the challenge of obtaining recognition for their potential contributions and must be willing and able to design and develop their own role (Neal, 1997a).

"The APN [advanced practice rehabilitation nurse] in rehabilitation already possesses most of the qualities required of the APN of the 21st century: knowledge about and experience in interdisciplinary collaboration, client self-care, client-directed healthcare, and health promotion strategies" (Daus, 1996). Home care practice offers almost limitless opportunities for flexibility, creativity, and ultimately expansion of the advanced practice roles. As rehabilitation principles are clearly congruent with the principles of home care practice (Neal, 1999), advanced practice rehabilitation nursing appears a perfect fit within community practice. It is up to rehabilitation APNs to explore possibilities for insinuating and expanding their roles within home care and to publish and disseminate information and research regarding the effects of their roles on positive outcomes in home care.

Alternative Rehabilitation Teams (Box 11-2)

"The rehabilitation nursing team can make a significant impact on the quality of patient care provided in the home setting" (Neal, 1995a). This concept has been implemented in home care in a variety of creative ways.

One approach (Neal, 1995a) consists of a team of certified rehabilitation nurses who each manage their own caseload but share consultation for clients throughout the home care agency. The team meets regularly to share current information that ensures evidence-based practice and to discuss difficult cases. In addition, members of the team share their expertise via inservices to other staff in the agency. This approach encourages agency staff and administration to learn about and acknowledge the value of rehabilitation nurses, because consultation opportunities and inservices clearly differentiate rehabilitation nursing practice from generalist nursing practice.

Another approach to the rehabilitation nursing team is a multilevel approach (Neal, 1995c, 1998). This approach includes the following levels of care: "acute rehabilitation, subacute rehabilitation, skilled nursing facility (SNF) rehabilitation, and rehabilitation nurse case-managed care" (Neal, 1995c, 1998). The program is monitored by an interdisciplinary team and case managed by a rehabilitation home care nurse. This program includes "intensive interdisciplinary rehabilitation" (Neal, 1995c, 1998) in the home.

Another approach involves training all of the home care nurses within an agency to practice as rehabilitation nurses. This method is consistent with the congruence of rehabilitation and home care theoretical constructs. A formal and lengthy mandatory training program is undertaken to train nurses with the intent of the following (Schuster, 1998):

- Providing appropriate care to clients because of increasing acuity and shorter inpatient lengths of stay
- Responding to shortages of specialty therapists in home health care
- Correcting inappropriate referrals to therapy
- Ensuring compliance with agency standards for timely interventions
- Coping with capitation imposed by managed care

Each of these approaches has been used successfully. These approaches do not preclude attempts to devise other methods and alternative teams.

Choosing an effective approach depends on many factors, such as the size and composition of the agency and the rehabilitation nursing staff, the location (urban or rural) of the agency, the skills of the rehabilitation professionals, and the receptivity of the administration and the therapists to an alternative team approach. It is important to design a thorough plan to present to administrators with the assumption that compromises will inevitably be made by everyone involved before beginning to implement an alternative team approach. In addition, rehabilitation nurses must make clear to agency therapists that the chosen method is not intended to threaten the practice or professionalism of the therapy staff. Whenever possible, therapy staff should be included in planning and implementing the al-

---

Box 11-2 Alternative Rehabilitation Teams

APPROACH 1

Rehabilitation nurses form a specialty group of nurses who manage their own caseloads and meet regularly to share information and educate agency staff.

APPROACH 2

Four levels of care are monitored by an interdisciplinary team and case managed by a nurse.

APPROACH 3

All home care nurses within an agency are trained to function as rehabilitation nurses.

Mrs. A., a 60-year-old non–insulin-dependent diabetic housewife, was discharged from the hospital with a left below-the-knee amputation. Mrs. A's diabetes had been controlled with an oral hypoglycemic agent for several years. She lived with her 66-year-old retired husband in an apartment accessible from the outside by six steps. Sue, Mrs. A.'s daughter, was married and lived in the same neighborhood.

A few weeks before, she accidentally injured her left big toe while cutting her toenails with a knife. Initially, because the wound was slightly swollen, she applied some herbs to it. The swelling subsided 2 days later. The following week, the big toe turned black, and the whole leg was very swollen with a large amount of foul-smelling, greenish discharge coming from the wound. Mrs. A. experienced tremendous pain and was very worried about the condition. Her husband eventually took her to the physician.

After consultation with her physician, Mrs. A. was admitted to the hospital and underwent a below-the-knee amputation. She recovered well from her operation and her rehabilitation started in the hospital. Mrs. A. received care of the stump wound with a pressure dressing to prevent edema. Shortly after surgery, she was fitted with a temporary prosthesis and began working on mobility with the PT. The PT used parallel bars, crutches, and walkers to help her learn to walk.

PROBLEM LIST

On admission of Mrs. A. to home care, the rehabilitation nurse notes the following:

- *Knowledge deficit related to diabetes management*
- *Knowledge deficit related to diet*
- *Nonadherence with medications*
- *Lower extremity wound*
- *Poor access to living quarters and within living quarters, including safety and environmental hazards*
- *Alteration in body image*
- *Alteration in mobility*
- *Alteration in self-care*

PLAN

The rehabilitation home care nurse formulates the following plan to care for Mrs. A.:

- *Confer with the payor to determine the allowable number of nurse visits and the disciplines from which the nurses will visit.*

- *Establish mutually agreed-on and realistic short- and long-term goals with Mrs. A. and her family*
- *Obtain physician orders for the following referrals:*
  1. *Home health aide to temporarily assist with personal care*
  2. *PT to assist with prosthesis fitting, gait training, balance training, mobility, strengthening exercises, and evaluation for adaptive and assistive devices within the home*
  3. *Medical-social worker to assist Mrs. A. and her husband to explore alternative living arrangements, evaluate financial assets to meet food and medication needs, and locate the appropriate community resources to assist them after discharge from home care*
  4. *Dietitian to instruct Mrs. A. and her family in the proper diabetic diet*
- *Obtain orders for and perform wound care and teach Mrs. A. and her family to perform wound care*
- *Instruct Mrs. A. and her family in medications, their precautions, and the need for adherence*
- *Instruct Mrs. A. and her family in diabetes management*
- *Instruct Mrs. A. and her family regarding the reduction of safety hazards in the home*
- *Create an environment for open discussion about the alteration in body image and allow Mrs. A. and her husband to ventilate their feelings*
- *Open a discussion and provide instruction about sexual activity after the amputation*
- *Update the physician weekly and confer as needed for orders*
- *Convene weekly case conferences, preferably in Mrs. A.'s home, to include Mrs. A., her husband, and her daughter, as well as the rest of the team*
- *Order supplies and equipment as needed*
- *Monitor compliance with payor allowances*
- *Evaluate outcomes of care with the team, Mrs. A., and her family*
- *Discharge the client when goals have been met and skilled needs are no longer present*

ternative approach so that the method will truly reflect a rehabilitation team approach.

SUMMARY

The primary goal of both rehabilitation and home care nursing is to help the client achieve maximal independence and self-care. The nurse who uses rehabilitation principles to guide nursing practice in the home setting collaborates with the client and caregiver and the rest of the interdisciplinary team. Rehabilitation professionals work with the client to accomplish realistic, mutually established goals. Changes in health care will increasingly require the competencies and knowledge of the rehabilitation home care nurse and the inherent creativity and ingenious role diversification for which rehabilitation nurses are noted.

REFERENCES

Albrecht MN: The Albrecht model for home health care: Implications for research, practice and education, *Public Health Nursing* 7(2):118-126, 1990.

American Nurses Association: *A statement on the scope of home health nursing practice,* Kansas City, 1992, The Association.

Association of Rehabilitation Nurses: *Standards and scope of rehabilitation nursing practice,* Glenview, Ill, 1995, The Association.

Brothers F: The rehabilitation home health nurse and pediatric clients. In Neal LJ, ed: *Rehabilitation nursing in the home health setting,* Glenview, Ill, 1998, Association of Rehabilitation Nurses.

Clarke PN, Cody WK: Nursing theory-based practice in the home and community: The crux of professional nursing education, *Advanced Nursing Science* 17(2):41-53, 1994.

Daus C: Bringing geriatric rehabilitation into the home, *The Interdisciplinary Journal of Rehabilitation* 9(1):53-59, 1996.

Dittbrenner H: Opportunity and responsibility, *Caring* 13(12):1, 1994.

Girard N: Gerontological nursing in acute care settings. In Matteson MA, McConnell E, Linton A, eds: *Gerontological nursing,* ed 2, Philadelphia, 1997, WB Saunders.

Griffitt R: The rehabilitation home health nurse and clients with wounds. In Neal LJ, ed: *Rehabilitation nursing in the home health setting,* Glenview, Ill, 1998, Association of Rehabilitation Nurses.

Henderson V: The concept of nursing, *Journal of Advances in Nursing* 3(2):113-130, 1978.

Hoeman SP: *Rehabilitation nursing: Process and application,* ed 3, St Louis, 2000, Mosby.

McClinton D: Editor's note, *Continuing Care* 16(1):4, 1997.

McCourt A, ed: *The specialty practice of rehabilitation nursing: A core curriculum,* ed 3, Skokie, Ill, 1993, Association of Rehabilitation Nurses.

Mundinger MO: *Home care controversy,* Rockville, Md, 1983, Aspen.

Neal LJ: The rehabilitation clinical nurse specialist in the home health care setting, *Clinical Nurse Specialist* 9(6):293-298, 1995a.

Neal LJ: The rehabilitation nurse in the home setting: Treating the chronic wound as a disability, *Rehabilitation Nursing* 20(5):261-264, 1995b.

Neal LJ: The rehabilitation nursing team in the home health setting, *Rehabilitation Nursing* 20(1):32-36, 1995c.

Neal LJ: Characteristics of the advanced practice nurse in rehabilitation. In Johnson KMM, ed: *Advanced practice nursing in rehabilitation,* Glenview, Ill, 1997a, Association of Rehabilitation Nurses.

Neal LJ: The rehabilitation nurse in the home care setting: Care of the client with HIV/AIDS, *Rehabilitation Nursing* 22(5):239-242, 1997b.

Neal LJ: The Neal model of home health nursing practice. In Neal LJ, ed: *Rehabilitation nursing in the home health setting,* Glenview, Ill, 1998, Association of Rehabilitation Nurses.

Neal LJ: Research supporting the congruence between rehabilitation principles and home health nursing practice, *Rehabilitation Nursing* 24(3):115-121, 1999.

Orem DE: *Nursing: Concepts of practice,* ed 5, St Louis, 1995, Mosby.

Pollock SE et al: Contributions to nursing science: Synthesis of findings from adaptation model research, *Scholarly Inquiry for Nursing Practice: An International Journal* 8(4):361-372, 1994.

Pratt JR: Home health care: A dynamic complex field requiring dynamic, competent managers, *Home Health Management & Practice* 8(2):6-14, 1996.

Preston KM: A team approach to rehabilitation, *Home Healthcare Nurse* 8(1):17-23, 1990.

Rice R: Procedures in home care conceptual framework for nursing practice in the home: The Rice model of dynamic self-determination, *Home Healthcare Nurse* 12(2):51-53, 1994.

Rice R: *Home health nursing practice: Concepts and application,* St Louis, 1996, Mosby.

Roy C, Andrews HA: *The Roy adaptation model,* ed 2, New Jersey, 1999, Prentice Hall.

Schuster L: The rehabilitation nursing team in home health care: Approach 1. In Neal LJ, ed: *Rehabilitation nursing in the home health setting,* Glenview, Ill, 1998, Association of Rehabilitation Nurses.

Thomason SS: Rehabilitation nursing. In Neal LJ, ed: *Rehabilitation nursing in the home health setting,* Glenview, Ill, 1998, Association of Rehabilitation Nurses.

12 Nutritional Aspects of Home Health Care

Juliann G. Sebastian and Maria G. Boosalis

As more health care is provided in the home, it has become increasingly important for nurses to have a thorough understanding of nutritional issues in home care. Nutritional status is an important outcome of home care nursing, and it influences other health outcomes. For example, a client's perception of quality of life may be influenced by nutritional status and ability to enjoy his or her food (Grindel, Whitmer, Barsevik, 1996). A client's ability to feed himself or herself is one of the basic activities of daily living and, as such, is reflected in the Outcome and Assessment Information Set (OASIS) (Shaughnessy et al, 1994) for Medicare beneficiaries. Social and cultural life is heavily linked to food and sharing meals. Clients' and families' nutritional status, preferences, and economic constraints must be clearly understood to work most effectively with them in designing therapeutic adaptations to nutritional patterns. The purpose of this chapter is to examine the nutritional issues that commonly arise in the home and to provide home care nurses with current information on nutritional assessment, intervention, and outcomes measurement. A case study is woven throughout the chapter illustrating the major points.

With client acuity higher than ever and increasing pressure placed on home care agencies to reduce the length of service, helping clients and families learn how to manage nutritional challenges effectively has become a major concern. Not only are home care nurses caring for extremely ill clients, they are often caring for clients who have developed iatrogenic malnutrition. Early studies demonstrated that a majority of clients discharged from hospitals are malnourished and that this represents a decline from preadmission nutritional status (Konstantinides, 1986). While many of the factors contributing to iatrogenic malnutrition may decrease once the individual returns home, some may not. Two examples are the drug-drug and drug-food interactions that may be experienced by clients taking multiple medications in the home and by those who may be self-medicating with complementary and vitamin-based therapies (Rimmer, 1998).

Home care nurses also work with clients for whom therapeutic diets have been prescribed. Chronically ill clients often require nutritional interventions to treat their health problems effectively. Examples include the dietary modifications in carbohydrates, fat, and sodium frequently prescribed for people with diabetes, cardiovascular disease, and hypertension, respectively. Those with certain chronic illnesses, such as cancer, diabetes, and cardiovascular problems, may experience difficulty metabolizing certain nutrients (Konstantinides, 1986). Clients with short-term problems (such as those recovering from surgery and those with infections) require optimal nutritional intake to facilitate healing. The hypermetabolic state of many of these clients further compounds their needs. Clients whose usual mode of eating has been altered as a result of disease or surgery require both intensive psychological support and assistance in modifying eating habits. In addition to the primary client, the nurse must consider the family and caregivers in planning nutritional interventions. Incorporating the dietary intervention into the lifestyle of the family can pose its own challenges. Consider the case of Mrs. Bell. This case is fictional, but it highlights common nutritional issues in home care.

CASE STUDY

Mrs. Bell is a 78-year-old widow recently diagnosed with protein-calorie malnutrition. She had been following the same low-fat, "heart healthy" diet as her husband, George, while he was alive. Since George's death 3 months ago, Mrs. Bell has remained on the low-fat food plan. This plan includes avoiding all sources of saturated fat and consuming no more than 15 grams of fat from other sources daily. Mrs. Bell was recently seen in the outpatient geriatrics clinic at the local medical center and referred to the geriatric home follow-up team for assessment and dietary teaching. Sharon Collier, BSN, RN, is the nurse assigned to work with Mrs. Bell.

Questions

- How should Sharon begin the nutritional assessment of Mrs. Bell? Which questions should Sharon ask initially? What physical observations would you recommend that Sharon make?
- Why might Sharon be concerned about the fact that Mrs. Bell has remained on the low-fat diet that had originally been prescribed for her husband?

THEORY-BASED APPROACHES TO NUTRITIONAL CARE

Because clients, families, and caregivers ultimately bear the responsibility for nutritional care in the home, nurses should use a theory base to guide care aimed at providing clients, families, and caregivers with the skills and knowledge necessary to assume self-care. Three theoretical bases will guide the discussion in this chapter, although individual nurses might select differing approaches based on other theoretical frameworks. Orem's self-care theory (1995) is a nursing theory base consistent with promoting individual and family self-care. Both self-efficacy theory (Bandura, 1977) and the health belief model (Becker, 1974) provide useful guidance for organizing health education to help clients develop self-care skills.

Orem argues that three types of self-care are necessary for promoting health and preventing illness. Therapeutic self-care is specifically aimed at providing interventions designed to correct a health problem. Nurses often provide therapeutic care for clients but focus on helping clients gradually meet as many of their own care requirements as possible.

To do this, nurses must work with clients, families, and caregivers to do a thorough assessment of their readiness to learn the care. Such an assessment should be guided by a search to understand what the client believes about the severity of the problem, his or her own susceptibility to the problem, and his or her own ability to do something about the problem. The health belief model emphasizes the importance of clients' prior beliefs about their own susceptibility and their perceptions of the seriousness of the problems as key to changing behaviors (Becker, 1974). According to the health belief model, the benefits of adopting new self-care behaviors and the barriers to the adoption of those behaviors help predict the likelihood of taking action. Use of the health belief model also directs the nurse in understanding the cultural aspects of dietary practices and in working with clients and families in designing culturally appropriate nutritional care.

Self-efficacy theory emphasizes the importance of clients' confidence in their abilities as key to learning new skills and changing behavior (Bandura, 1977). This theory would suggest that the nurse serve as role model for new skills. The nurse should help clients learn skills through a planned sequence of small steps. Clients learning to change dressings around intravenous sites for parenteral feedings might learn how to don and remove sterile gloves before learning anything about cleaning around the line insertion site. According to self-efficacy theory, as individuals experience success with small components of a new skill, they increase their readiness to learn more complex components of that same skill. Assessment, diagnosis, planning, intervention, evaluation, and revisions should all be based on a theoretical framework. Self-care theory, the health belief model, and self-efficacy theory serve as the basis for the nutritional care described in the remainder of the chapter.

INTERDISCIPLINARY ASPECTS OF NUTRITIONAL CARE

In addition to their partnership with clients and families, home care nurses collaborate with other health professionals to provide nutritional care.

Registered dietitians, physicians, pharmacists, and social workers all contribute to development of comprehensive nutritional care plans. Gunning, Saffel-Shriner, and Shane-McWhorter (1998) reported on an interdisciplinary nutritional evaluation and intervention program for elders at high risk for nutritional problems. In this program, nurses evaluate older adults in their homes using a nutritional risk assessment instrument. Registered dietitians complete in-home dietary assessments, and pharmacists evaluate the potential for drug-food interactions among the participants. Targeted interventions for people at high risk of nutritional problems should include nutritional care plans and plans for minimizing the potential for drug-nutrient interactions (Gunning, Saffel-Shriner, Shane-McWhorter, 1998).

Registered dietitians (RDs) are key players on any interdisciplinary health care team and can interact with the home care nurse on three levels. First, the registered dietitian can develop nutritional screening or nutritional assessment tools. Such tools can assist in the recognition or identification of signs of malnutrition (including undernutrition and overnutrition) in home care clients. Second, once malnutrition is suspected or identified in a client, the registered dietitian can consult with the nursing staff about which nutritional interventions might be most beneficial. Finally, the registered dietitian can perform the required nutritional intervention in the most complicated situations.

NUTRITIONAL ASSESSMENT

A nutritional assessment contains four components: anthropometric, biochemical, clinical, and dietary data (Boosalis, Stiles, 1995a). For home care clients, it is important to add a fifth component: environmental assessment (Sanville, 1994). While information regarding the client's environment is routinely collected during the clinical and dietary assessments, making it a separate category emphasizes its importance. The environmental assessment makes it possible to incorporate information related to the client's social and home environment, as well as physical and financial resources. Only after examining data gathered from each of these components can the nurse make an appropriate nutritional evaluation and subsequent nutritional recommendations.

Anthropometric Assessment

Routine anthropometric measurements include height, weight, weight history (including amount or percentage of weight loss or gain, if any), and body mass index (BMI). Recording a weight by itself provides little useful clinical information unless the nurse has also obtained and recorded a measured height. For example, a client who weighs 160 pounds and is 5 feet tall is too heavy for his or her height. On the other hand, if he or she is 6 feet 2 inches tall, the client may be undernourished at 160 pounds. Home care nurses should always measure the client's height. If the client is unable to stand or is kyphotic, a knee height can be obtained using a specially designed caliper (Ross Products Division, Abbott Laboratories, Columbus, OH), and a standing height may be calculated using the following formula (Chumlea, Roche, Steinbaugh, 1989):

$$\text{Stature} = 1.83 \times \text{Knee height} - [0.24 \times \text{age}] + 84.88$$

A weight history is important to obtain for several reasons. Serial weight data help evaluate trends or patterns in weight loss or weight gain. For example, infant growth patterns can be determined only through repeated measurements of length and weight. Generally, any unintentional weight loss or gain requires further investigation. Finally, helping clients identify their own weight patterns provides them with information necessary for self-care. Home care nurses should keep a standard height and weight chart among the materials they carry with them on home visits. Such charts may be easily obtained from life insurance companies.

BMI is calculated by dividing the individual's weight in kilograms by his or her height in meters squared (BMI = kg/m^2). This value gives a relative measure of weight to height and is associated with morbidity and mortality (Bray, 1995). Generally, less than 22 kg/m^2 implies a person is underweight, and greater than 27 kg/m^2 implies a person is overweight. There is a greater association of morbidity and mortality when the BMI falls below 19 or 20 kg/m^2 or is above 30 and especially above 40 kg/m^2 or when the client weighs more than 100% over his or her ideal weight (the latter is referred to as *morbid obesity*) (Barkauskus et al, 1998). Ideally the BMI, depending on age, falls between 20 and 25 kg/m^2 for adults un-

der 35 years of age and 22 and 27 kg/m² for elders (Gallagher-Allred, 1993; NHLBI, 1998).
While a BMI between 27 and 30 kg/m² does not
increase a client's morbidity and mortality as
much as a BMI over 30 kg/m², it is predictive
when present with other comorbidities such as
diabetes, hypertension, or cardiovascular disease.
For example, even a 10% weight loss in a client
with diabetes may improve glucose or glycemic
control. Regarding interpretation, very muscular
clients may have a BMI in the 25 to 27 or 28
range but would not be considered overweight or
obese.

A trained health professional may use other
types of anthropometric measurements, such as
skinfold thicknesses and circumferences. For example, a commonly used measure is the waist-
to-hip ratio (WHR), which to date is the most
practical surrogate measure available for obtaining a client's relative amount of abdominal or
visceral fat (St Jeor, Silverstein, Shane, 1996). Although controversial, a WHR greater than 0.8 for
women and 1.0 for men has been used, along
with body fat of more than 30% for women and
25% for men, and an elevated BMI (as described
earlier), to define obesity and acknowledge an increased health risk as a result of body fat distribution (National Task Force on Prevention and
Treatment of Obesity, 1993).

Home care nurses may also measure the mid-
arm muscle circumference (MAMC) (Barkauskus et al, 1998). Since tape measures are lightweight and inexpensive, they are easily included
in the nurse's supplies. Serial measurements of
MAMC provide an indication of patterns in
weight gain or loss.

Another indicator of undernutrition or overnutrition is the triceps skinfold (TSF) measurement, which is calculated using specially designed calipers. For many home care clients such
as Mrs. Bell, major nutritional problems result in
weight loss and protein catabolism. Repeated
measurements of the TSF thickness over a period
of time can demonstrate fairly objective changes
in status. However, the use of standardized
norms is of limited usefulness in evaluating isolated sets of data for elderly clients who have an
increased proportion of fat to muscle. For example, in determining triceps skinfold thickness, the
nurse should pinch a fold of skin at the midpoint
between the acromion and olecranon processes,

measuring the distance between the parallel sides
with a pair of calibrated calipers.

Biochemical Assessment

The biochemical component of nutritional assessment includes laboratory tests to determine
macronutrient (protein, carbohydrate, lipid) and
micronutrient (vitamin and mineral) status, as
well as organ function. A detailed explanation of
each of these categories follows.

When macronutrient levels are evaluated,
protein status generally is assessed by measuring
the circulating levels of various visceral proteins,
in particular albumin or thyroxine-binding prealbumin (or transthyretin). Thyroxine-binding
prealbumin has a shorter half-life (2 days) than
albumin (18 to 21 days) and can indicate short-
term changes in protein status. A low serum albumin level (below 3.4 g/dl) is an indication of
undernutrition and is associated with problems
in wound healing and immune function
(Barkauskus et al, 1998).

While circulating levels of transferrin or
retinol-binding protein may also be used to assess protein malnutrition, they afford no advantages over thyroxine-binding prealbumin and
therefore are not routinely used on a clinical basis. In addition, circulating levels of transferrin
are influenced by iron status. For example, iron
deficiency will elevate circulating levels of transferrin, and therefore iron status must be known
to interpret the significance of serum transferrin
levels.

With respect to carbohydrate status, a fasting
blood glucose level is used to screen for glucose

CASE STUDY

When Sharon visited Mrs. Bell, she found that Mrs. Bell was 5 feet 5 inches tall and weighed 97 pounds. Mrs. Bell reported having lost 10 pounds since her husband died. She told Sharon that she had lost interest in eating since George's death and that preparing meals was no longer enjoyable.

Questions
• What was Mrs. Bell's BMI?
• Would you consider her weight loss to be significant? Why or why not?
• What would you do at this point?

intolerance and diabetes. Once an individual has been diagnosed with diabetes, glycosylated alpha-1 hemoglobin levels are used to screen for long-term glucose control.

Lipid status is usually first assessed by using the serum concentration of total cholesterol as a screening measure. If the total cholesterol level is elevated, further investigation may be warranted through determination of circulating levels of LDL and HDL cholesterol. In addition, measurement of serum triglyceride levels may also be warranted. In an elder, a serum cholesterol level of 160 mg/dl or below is used as a possible indicator of protein-calorie malnutrition (Gallagher-Allred, 1993). Evaluation of the hepatic and renal systems is necessary for determination of nutrient load and intake of a client, and in particular, protein and solute loads.

If a deficiency of a particular vitamin or mineral is suspected, then appropriate blood or urine tests should be conducted (Table 12-1). One common finding in the elderly population is depressed zinc status, which is usually identified by a decrease in the circulating level of zinc (Boosalis, Stuart, McClain, 1995). Another common finding is that of a nutritional anemia, which may be caused by a deficiency or compromise in iron, folic acid, or vitamin B_{12} status.

Generally, an iron deficiency anemia is microcytic, whereas a deficiency of either folic acid or vitamin B_{12} results in a macrocytic or megaloblastic anemia. Anemia of chronic disease is ac-

Table 12-1   Tests Used to Evaluate Levels of Selected Nutrients

Nutrient	Blood	Urine*	Others
Protein	Protein (P)	Total nitrogen	
	Albumin (P)	Urea	
	Albumin (S)	Creatinine	Creatinine-height index
	Transferrin (S)	Hydroxyproline	
	RBP (S)		
	Amino acids (P)		Nitrogen balance
	Lymphocyte counts		
	Hemoglobin		
Iron	Hematocrit		Complete blood count (CBC);
	Transferrin (S)		size and color of cells
	Iron (S)		
Vitamin A	Vitamin A (P)		
	Carotene (P)		
Vitamin C	Vitamin C (S)	Vitamin C	Vitamin C load test
	Vitamin C (WBC)		
Thiamine	Transketolase (E)	Thiamine	
Riboflavin	Glutathione reductase (E)	Riboflavin	
Niacin		N-methyl nicotinamide	
Vitamin B_6	GOT (E)	Xanthurenic acid	Tryptophan load test
	GPT (E)	Pyridoxine	
Folic acid	Folic acid (S)	FIGLU (formiminoglutamic acid)	CBC; size and color of cells
Vitamin B_{12}	Vitamin B_{12} (S)	Iodine	
Iodine			

From Kamath S: Nutritional assessment. In Malasanos L et al: *Health assessment,* ed 3, St Louis, 1986, Mosby.
P, Plasma; *S,* serum; *RBP,* retinol binding protein; *WBC,* white blood cell; *E,* erythrocyte; *GOT,* glutamine-oxaloacetic transaminase; *GPT,* glutamic-pyruvic transaminase.
*Urine values are often considered per unit weight of creatinine excreted.

Ed: This is the asterisk for this font.

tually a different type of anemia that, while not exactly nutritional in nature, can resemble an iron deficiency. Although the etiology of each differs, each may present as a microcytic anemia. However, the provision of iron in the anemia of chronic disease will not correct the anemia and may in fact exacerbate an infection because of the decrease in the circulating level of transferrin. If the concentration of the transport protein of iron (in this case, transferrin) is low and iron is given, the level of "free" or unbound iron circulating in the blood may increase and could serve as a growth factor (nutrient) for bacteria, resulting in an infection. In iron-deficiency anemia the level of transferrin or the total iron capacity of the blood is increased.

If a macrocytic or megaloblastic anemia is suspected, it is critical to determine if it is due to a folic acid or vitamin B_{12} deficiency. If the anemia is due to a deficiency of vitamin B_{12} but the client is treated with folic acid, the anemia will correct, but the neurological manifestations of a vitamin B_{12} deficiency will continue unnoticed and will result in an irreversible peripheral neuropathy. Generally, determining the etiology of this type of anemia requires that the concentration of serum levels of both nutrients be measured.

A word of caution is warranted when interpreting certain biochemical tests in the presence of an acute-phase or systemic inflammatory response. An acute-phase response is a series of systemic metabolic and physiological processes that occur as the host responds to acute trauma, microbial or viral invasion, or the presence of chronic disease or inflammatory processes (Baumann, Gauldie, 1994; Gordon, 1985; Kushner, 1982; Steel, Whitehead, 1994). As part of this response, circulating levels of albumin, thyroxine-binding prealbumin, transferrin, iron, and zinc decrease, whereas circulating levels of copper generally increase.* Recent evidence suggests that circulating levels of certain antioxidants also decrease during an acute-phase response (Boosalis et al, 1996; Louw et al, 1992). Therefore, if an acute-phase or systemic inflammatory response is suspected or confirmed by an increase in the circulating levels of C-reactive protein (Dina-

rello, 1984; Stuart, Lewis, 1988), then interpretation of the aforementioned tests may be altered.

Clinical Assessment

The clinical component of the nutritional assessment includes a complete history and physical examination that targets signs of malnutrition or nutritional compromise. This component includes, but is not limited to, checking oral health (e.g., dentition and swallowing), gastrointestinal function (e.g., absorption, elimination, and liver and pancreatic function), skin changes (e.g., rash and turgor), and musculoskeletal system status for signs of wasting or weakness, loss of mobility, arthritis, and any compromise in functional status. Functional status is important because it may affect the client's ability to obtain and prepare food (Boosalis, Stiles, 1995b). As part of the clinical assessment, the individual's mental status and ability, level of physical activity, overall perception of well-being and energy, and current medications should be assessed.

The purpose of the assessment, as well as the actual and potential health problems, should guide the nurse in determining the depth and breadth of the assessment. The nurse should ask the client about food preferences; intolerances; availability of food; financial, cultural, and religious influences on food choices; impact of dietary choices on other family members; and food preparation and storage routines. History

---

*Boosalis et al, 1986, 1987, 1988, 1989; Stahl, 1987; Wilmore, 1974.

CASE STUDY

Sharon checked the results of Mrs. Bell's most recent labwork. She found that Mrs. Bell's serum cholesterol was 154 mg/dl, and her thyroxine-binding prealbumin level was 18. Her hemoglobin level was 10 gm/dl, and her hematocrit level was 32.

Questions
- How do these values compare with norms for Mrs. Bell's age?
- What are the clinical implications? Based on these findings, on what aspects of clinical and environmental assessment would you recommend that Sharon focus at this point?

taking should include symptomatology related to nutritional and metabolic patterns and problems anywhere in the alimentary canal that could affect food intake, absorption, use, and elimination. Questions about recurrent infections will yield information about potential immunocompetency. The nurse should ask about symptoms such as dental problems, including dentures, loose teeth, and pain; dysphagia; indigestion; abdominal pain; vomiting; hematemesis; constipation; diarrhea; melena; and frequent or persistent upper respiratory infections.

Information should be obtained about the client's appetite and willingness to eat. Children dependent on long-term home parenteral nutrition may lose the desire to eat and drink (Vargas et al, 1987). Elderly clients who live alone sometimes lose interest in food resulting in part from eating alone.

Home care clients may require special emphasis on socioeconomic areas such as financial concerns related to nutritional support, coping ability when nutritional support methods are used, and the effects of therapeutic diets or nutritional support methods on family members. The ability of clients and families to understand the purpose of therapeutic diets and the appropriate methods for their implementation is critical to therapeutic effectiveness. While the specific data to be gathered will vary with the age of the client, the client's health problems, and the type of nutritional therapy being used, certain commonalities do exist for most clients. Fig. 12-1 is a sample history form that can serve as the basis for most nutritional evaluations.

Physical examination data may be gathered in several ways. First, the anthropometric and biochemical measurements related to nutritional status have already been discussed. The nurse should begin the clinical appraisal with an evaluation of the client's overall appearance, including skin color (e.g., pale or sallow), emaciation, or obesity. This should be followed by inspection and palpation of the client's skin to identify dryness, decreased turgor and elasticity, and lesions, including reddened areas suggestive of impending skin breakdown, frank ulcerations, rashes, and dermatitis. The appendages of the skin (hair and nails) also should be inspected for dryness, brittleness, and decreased luster. Oral mucosa should be evaluated for signs of dryness, which suggest dehydration.

Other organs that undergo changes with nutritional imbalances should be included in the clinical appraisal. Examination of the eyes will yield useful data, since problems such as xerophthalmia (corneal opacities) and corneal injection (Kamath, 1986) are possible results of vitamin deficiencies. Xanthelasma, particularly near the inner canthus of the eye, suggests hypercholesterolemia, especially in young adults. Enlargement of the thyroid may result from iodine deficiency; therefore palpation of the thyroid should be included in the clinical appraisal. The abdomen should be inspected for abnormalities of contour (such as protuberance suggestive of alcoholic cirrhosis), auscultated for the presence of normal bowel sounds, percussed to identify fluid or unusual amounts of flatus, and palpated to identify areas of tenderness. The lungs should be auscultated for adventitious sounds suggestive of edema, and the feet and ankles should be palpated for peripheral edema.

Dietary Assessment

The dietary component of the nutritional assessment consists of an evaluation of the client's routine or typical food intake. Numerous methods, such as interview, recording, and direct observation, are available for obtaining this information. The nurse may obtain a 24-hour dietary recall from the client, or the caregiver may report or record the client's dietary intake. This dietary intake must then be analyzed to determine if it is adequate or if it needs to be modified to meet the client's dietary needs. In addition to determination and analysis of food intake, dietary assessment also includes the identification of any drug-nutrient interactions or incompatibilities, use or misuse of any dietary supplements, level of physical activity, and identification of any food allergy or intolerance (if this specific information was not obtained in the clinical component of the nutritional assessment).

The analysis of dietary intake can involve the exact determination of all of the major nutrients, or the nurse may compare the client's dietary intake to daily recommendations on the Food Guide Pyramid. The Food Guide Pyramid recommends 6 to 11 servings of breads/cereals/

Client name: _____   Family/caregiver: _____

Age: _____   _____

Gender: _____   _____

Primary medical diagnosis: _____

Primary nursing diagnosis: _____

Other health problems or comorbidities: _____

_____

_____

_____

_____

Weight: _____

Weight history: _____

Frame (small, medium, large): _____

Allergies (food or drug): _____

Medications: Describe dosage schedule for medications (including whether taken with meals or on an empty
stomach).

_____

_____

_____

_____

_____

_____

Food preferences: _____

_____

_____

_____

Food intolerances or restrictions: _____

_____

_____

Therapeutic diet or nutritional support prescription: _____

_____

_____

_____

_____

Cultural patterns related to dietary practices: _____

_____

_____

_____

Fig. 12-1   Nutritional history guidelines for home care clients.   *Continued*

Client and caregiver understanding of the therapeutic diet or nutritional support plan:

_____

_____

What do the client and family/caregiver find to be the easiest and most difficult parts of the therapeutic diet or nutritional support plan?

_____

_____

What, if anything, would the client or family/caregiver like to change about the therapeutic diet or nutritional support plan?

_____

_____

Client and family/caregiver learning needs related to the therapeutic diet or nutritional support plan:

_____

_____

_____

Availability of food:
  Who does the shopping? _____
  Where: _____
  Transportation for shopping: _____
  Any seasonal limitations related to food availability: _____

Financial resources:
  Source of reimbursement for nutritional therapy: _____
  Aspects of the diet or nutritional therapy for which the client does not have adequate financial resources:

_____

_____

Home environment:
  Electricity, gas? _____
  Running water? _____
  Functioning stove, oven? _____
  Refrigeration? _____
  Hygiene? _____

Fig. 12-1, cont'd   For legend see p. 147.

grains per day a minimum of 5 servings of vegetables and fruits per day; 2 to 4 servings of dairy products; and 2 to 3 servings from the meat/poultry/fish/eggs/dry beans group (USDA, 1992).

Environmental Assessment

Finally, the nurse must assess the client's or the caregiver's ability to provide nutritional care and the adequacy of the environment to support such care. This assessment should be initiated before discharge from the hospital or in the physician's office or clinic before hospitalization, especially if the client will receive a formal nutritional support intervention in the home. Registered dietitians are key members of the interdisciplinary home nutrition support team and can contribute

---

CASE STUDY

Mrs. Bell's 24-hour dietary recall showed that she had consumed the following food and beverages:
    Breakfast:
    2 cups decaffeinated coffee with sugar substitute
    1 slice of white toast with strawberry jelly
    Lunch:
    American cheese sandwich with lettuce and
        fat-free mayonnaise
    1 small dish of applesauce
    Dinner:
    1 bowl of bran cereal with banana slices
        and skim milk
    ½ dish of canned peaches
    1 dish of fat-free chocolate yogurt
    Evening snack:
    3 fat-free fig cookies and 8 ounces of skim milk
    During the assessment, Sharon learned that among her other medications, Mrs. Bell takes a thiazide diuretic for mild hypertension.

Questions

- How does Mrs. Bell's intake for the previous 24 hours compare with the recommendations on the Food Guide Pyramid?
- What dietary recommendation would you make to help Mrs. Bell compensate for the loss of potassium from the thiazide diuretic she is taking?
- If you were Sharon, would you recommend any other dietary changes to Mrs. Bell? If so, what would they be, and why would you make these recommendations?

---

important assessment and planning information (American Dietetic Association, 1994). Home health care agencies might find it useful to develop their own brief nutritional assessment forms to send to the agencies from which they receive referrals and request that these be implemented before discharge.

Fig. 12-2 gives an example of what such a form might entail and is a modification of Fig. 12-1, the assessment form recommended for use by the home care nurse. This makes it possible to integrate the hospital- or home-based nutritional evaluations to promote seamless care delivery. These assessments should represent an interdisciplinary effort among nursing, medicine, dietary, pharmacy, and social work. Early assessment facilitates appropriate teaching plans and timely arrangements for equipment delivery or physical modifications to the home (e.g., ordering a pump for the client receiving parenteral nutritional support). The hospital-based assessment serves to identify physical needs, potential problems, and specific educational and psychological needs of the client and family. The nutritional assessment by the home care nurse should be initiated within 24 hours after hospital discharge to verify referral data and identify special modifications of the care plan that may be necessary for that client.

Data that are important in determining how best to support the family or caregiver include first identifying who in the household is willing and able to handle food preparation for the client on a therapeutic diet. Is the caregiver able to learn a complex set of menu choices, or will the nurse need to assist with menu development? Is the social environment supportive of the client's diet, or will household members tend to sabotage the client's efforts? The lack of necessary foodstuffs and the presence of favored items not on the client's diet exemplify intentional or unintentional sabotage. Is the physical environment adequate for the client's nutritional needs? For example, is refrigeration available? Does the home contain adequate storage for the client's supplies (Sanville, 1994)? Is the level of hygiene suitable for the client receiving parenteral nutrition? Can the family afford the special diet? One method of assessing these issues is to note the types of foods in the refrigerator and on the cupboard shelves, as well as the general level of hygiene. Finally,

Client name: _____

Age: _____

Gender: _____

Reason for the referral:

_____

_____

_____

Primary medical diagnosis: _____

_____

Primary nursing diagnosis: _____

_____

Height: _____

Weight: _____

Weight history: _____

Frame (small, medium, large): _____

Allergies (food or drug): _____

Medications: _____

_____

_____

_____

_____

Family or caregiver: _____

_____

Home environment:

   Electricity, gas? _____

   Running water? _____

   Functioning stove, oven? _____

   Refrigeration? _____

Nutritional support (therapeutic oral diet, parenteral or enteral support): _____

_____

_____

_____

Other health problems:

_____

_____

_____

Fig. 12-2   Hospital-based nutritional referral form.

what effect might nutritional support of the client have on the family dynamics over a period of time? Does the family possess the coping skills to make the major lifestyle changes nutritional support often requires without resorting to destructive patterns, such as neglect or abuse? If no caregiver is available, the nurse should work with the client to determine other ways to support the client, such as arranging for home-delivered meals.

In addition to the client's immediate home environment, the home care nurse should be thoroughly familiar with nutritional support services available in the client's community. It is equally important to be knowledgeable about the referral procedures to facilitate seamless service delivery to the client. Examples of community-based nutritional support services are Meals on Wheels; the Women, Infants, and Children programs available through health departments; senior citizen congregate meals; and government surplus food commodity programs. Local drug-

stores supply special formulas for infants and enteral nutrition. It is helpful if the nurse has a well-developed network of colleagues in community-based agencies to whom he or she can turn for help or assistance in troubleshooting for clients.

In summary, while the bases for nutritional assessment remain the same in the home as in the hospital, the focus differs because of the shift to a heavier emphasis on client self-care and health promotion. Obtaining such simple measurements as fluid intake and output and monitoring quantity and quality of food eaten are dependent on the understanding and participation of the client and caregiver. Home care nurses must determine the client and family's levels of understanding, perceptions of the severity of and personal vulnerability to nutrition-related problems, levels of confidence in providing nutritional self-care, and technical aspects of providing nutritional care. Evaluating the availability, accessibility, and acceptability of community resources dealing with nutrition is a high priority for nutritional assessment of the home care client.

Assessment Issues Across the Lifespan

Infancy, childhood, and adolescence Increasing numbers of children are being referred to home care agencies, and more of these children are receiving home nutritional support than in the past (American Dietetic Association, 1994; Howard et al, 1995). These children might be quite healthy and seen in relation to health promotion (e.g., visits to parents and newborns by lactation nurses). Conversely, the children may be quite ill, as for example, children with cancer, Crohn's disease, or acquired immunodeficiency syndrome (AIDS). The rapidly changing metabolic needs of children at various ages result in a wide variety of nutritional issues.

In addition to assessing nutritional requirements as they are affected by the child's health status and age, the home care nurse should evaluate the meaning of diet for the family and the cultural and emotional aspects of therapeutic dietary regimens for the child and family. Feeding children is often closely associated with emotional feelings of nurturance and parenting. Thorough evaluation of patterns of control, hostility, and passivity and an evaluation of the social

---

CASE STUDY

When Sharon assessed Mrs. Bell's home, she noted no fresh food in the refrigerator other than the remains of a head of lettuce. Instead, she found many high-carbohydrate, prepackaged foods such as jelly, bagels, and English muffins. Two sherbet containers and a quart of yogurt were in the freezer, and several boxes of fat-free cereals were in the cupboard. She observed pretzels and fat-free chips, along with a can of water-packed tuna and bread in the cupboard. The sink was filled with dirty dishes, and she noted roaches around the baseboards. When she asked about family, Mrs. Bell said her daughter lived in the next county and visited every couple of weeks. "I don't want to be a burden, so I try not to call her much," Mrs. Bell shared. "I have always done for myself, and I don't intend to change now," she stated firmly.

Questions

- What preliminary nursing diagnoses would you make at this point?
- In which areas would you want to provide nutritional counseling for Mrs. Bell?
- Which community resources might be helpful to Mrs. Bell?

pressures experienced by the child and family in relation to dietary fads are important. Simple sugars offered as rewards for good behavior and food withheld for misbehavior may compromise the nutritional well-being of healthy children and contribute to the physical and emotional problems of children already in poor health. When conducting nutritional assessments in the home, nurses may find that parents are more relaxed and better able to articulate their concerns regarding their child's eating patterns than in the hospital.

Examples of common, minor health problems that may contribute to nutritional imbalances are nausea, vomiting, diarrhea, iron-deficiency anemia, being overweight or underweight, pica, and recurrent abdominal pain (Bowden, Dickey, Greenberg, 1998). Major health problems affecting nutritional status that may be seen in children at home include a variety of congenital malformations such as cleft lip or palate, pyloric stenosis, short bowel syndrome, juvenile rheumatoid arthritis, leukemia, diabetes, eating disorders, obesity, Crohn's disease, ulcerative colitis, and duodenal ulcers. Adolescent pregnancy and pregnancy-related disorders such as hyperemesis gravidarum require thorough nutritional assessment. Treatment modalities may necessitate special emphasis on nutritional assessment. For example, children in full body casts have such limited mobility that eating may be difficult, and they may lose weight as a result.

Children with long-term illnesses require special considerations in relation to their nutritional status (Bowden, Dickey, Greenberg, 1998). These considerations may be categorized as those relating to the physiological effects of the illness itself and those based on the psychosocial responses of the family to having a child with a long-term illness. Because of the pathological condition itself, the child may be smaller than the average child of the same age, thus having lower caloric and nutritional needs. The child may have physical handicaps, such as weakened musculature of the trunk (making it difficult to sit up) or of the mouth and facial muscles (resulting in difficulty in biting and chewing). Fatigue can also be a problem for the weakened child.

Families may respond to sick children with overindulgence, permissiveness, or a tendency to provide nutrient-deficient treats. If the diet is monotonous, it will be difficult for the child to follow and particularly difficult for the family to integrate into the normal meal structure. Behavior patterns that develop concomitantly with the sick may negatively influence nutritional status. For example, if the child watches long hours of television and accompanies this with snacks, he or she may associate food with television viewing, thus potentiating obesity. Parents may find it difficult to resist acquiescing if the child repeatedly asks to be served nonnutritious foods that have been heavily advertised on television. The nurse should also assess the effect of the special diet on siblings. Parental emphasis on the needs of one child may create difficulties in the behavior of the other children in the family. Assessment of physical limitations and patterns of family interaction deserve special attention for the family and child coping with long-term illness.

The nurse should be aware of the tendency of adolescents to diet stringently or to consume high-calorie, high-fat foods. Adolescents most likely to be seen by home care nurses are those who are pregnant, who have just delivered a high-risk infant, or who have children with health problems. Also, some adolescents with gastrointestinal problems that require parenteral nutrition may receive home care. Nutritional imbalances are of concern in the healthy adolescent because adolescents are still building bone and muscle mass and have high needs for adequate calcium and protein. Preconceptual nutritional status is important in adolescent females, particularly because folate deficiencies may lead to problems in the developing fetus. Nutritional imbalances are also of concern in the adolescent faced with child rearing. The teratogenic effects of poor nutritional status on the developing fetus of a pregnant adolescent can be immense and can have long-term physical, social, and economic consequences.

For adolescents preparing to receive parenteral nutrition at home, the cultural and emotional connotations of food and dietary practices, as well as the ability of teenagers to cope with peer pressures, must be carefully evaluated. Teenagers may find it difficult to follow dietary restrictions when at parties with their friends or eating at restaurants. Careful assessment may reveal this and could lead to a plan to save some of the day's allotment of oral fluids for this type of occasion. Bender and Faubion (1985) reported a case of an adolescent girl who so valued slimness that she skipped parenteral nutrition sessions to reduce her caloric intake. Careful evaluation of such factors prior to implementation can promote individualization of plans and prevent problems. The nurse also should assess adolescents for signs and symptoms of depression and screen for suicide risk. Paradoxically, those with short-term problems have been found to have more difficulty adjusting to parenteral nutrition than those with long-term problems, who often view nutritional supplementation as a relief (Bender et al, 1985).

Adulthood Young and middle-aged adults seen in the home are often those recovering from acute short-term problems, such as surgery, trauma, or infection. For these clients, it is important to assess the match between caloric need and intake, as well as protein status. For some clients with the hypermetabolic demands of surgery or infection, caloric needs may be as much as 65% higher than the caloric demands of the basal metabolic rate (Busby, Seiffert, 1986). Food diaries followed by calorie counts may be required. Adults recovering from acute problems may have difficulty adjusting to nutritional therapy, owing in part to their poor physiological status and the possibility of being in the denial phase of adaptation to their illnesses. Using the health belief model, it may be necessary for the home care nurse to evaluate the client's and family's perceptions of the client's susceptibility to nutritional problems and the importance of the nutritional therapy. Self-efficacy theory suggests that the nurse assess not only the clients' and family's understanding of how to implement the therapy, but also their confidence in their abilities to do so. Complicating the client's pathophysiological status and psychological phase of adaptation is the possibility that he or she may have simply been too sick in the hospital to understand the instructions provided for the new diet or nutritional support method. Cost-containment pressures have led to admission of only the sickest individuals to hospitals and early discharges before recovery has been completed and before resumption of a regular diet. The high acuity of most hospitalized clients influences their readiness and ability to learn therapeutic self-care. It is not unusual to see clients who save their hospital menus for continuous repetition at home because they either did not understand the dietary instructions or because they have forgotten them.

Adults with chronic illness such as hypertension, atherosclerotic cardiovascular disease, and Crohn's disease may need to make much more substantial, long-term alterations in lifestyle to maintain nutritional status. It is probably as important to assess the social effects of the nutritional support modality for these patients as it is to assess the adequacy of the nutritional support itself in meeting caloric and nutrient needs. For patients on ambulatory hyperalimentation, for example, it is necessary to identify any problems the client may have integrating this therapy into his or her lifestyle. Examples of these questions are listed in Box 12-1.

Box 12-1 History-taking with Adults Receiving Parenteral Nutrition

- Does the client have coping mechanisms sufficient to adapt to parenteral nutrition?
- Is he or she depressed about this form of treatment?
- How is the family responding to this modality?
- How do the client and family view parenteral nutrition in relation to the sick role?
- Do they view this as a confining methodology and confirmation of the client's role as an invalid?
- Do they, on the other hand, see this as a way of freeing the client to function more normally? What effects does it have on employment, hobbies, and sports?
- Is the client fearful of participating in previously favored activities, or does the client feel liberated?
- What effect does the ambulatory parenteral nutrition have on the client's body image?
- Does he or she feel embarrassed or restricted by the catheter, vest, or equipment?
- What is the impact on his or her sexual relationships with significant others?
- Are appropriate facilities available in the workplace for changing bags and initiating or discontinuing infusions?
- Does the mesh vest fit comfortably and snugly?
- Does the client's job pose any potential hazards, such as equipment that might rupture the bags, entangle the lines, or damage the catheter insertion site?
- Does the client understand the concept of sterility and the technique involved?

Certain questions are appropriate if the client is on a cycle necessitating parenteral nutrition during all or part of the work day. Examples of these questions also are listed in Box 12-1. These include evaluation of availability of appropriate facilities and adaptive equipment to enable the client to manage the therapy during the workday. Other important areas are related to the client's body image and home life, including sexuality. Thorough evaluation of relational patterns and discussion of potential problems with the client and his or her significant other are priorities. Financial resources are a critical issue to evaluate. Although payors may reimburse the cost of home nutritional support, some clients may still have no coverage or inadequate coverage. In addition, the hidden costs of therapy may not be covered (Bender, Faubion, 1985). Examples of hidden costs include transportation to and from office visits, long-distance phone calls for clients living in rural areas, and home modifications. Also, payors may cover only particular types of supplies, whereas some clients may function at a higher level with more costly or more convenient supplies (such as premixed solutions).

Using the anthropometric, biochemical, clinical, dietary, and environmental (A, B, C, D, E) framework for nutritional assessment makes it possible to customize the nutritional assessment for adult clients with specific chronic diseases. For example, diabetics and their families should be thoroughly evaluated for the degree to which they are able to follow their diets, with consideration given not only to an understanding of the basic mechanics of the diet plan, but also to their ability to plan menus that are flexible, palatable, and economical and that fit the family's lifestyle. To what extent has the family felt the need to radically modify aspects of their usual habits (such as eating out) to comply with the diet? The Food Guide Pyramid should be used as the basis for evaluating modifications of all therapeutic and regular diets.

Conversely, have clients found the diet so cumbersome that they have simply abandoned it as the only acceptable coping mechanism? Do they have reasonable choices available to them for unusual days, such as sick days, holidays, and social events, such as weddings? The nurse should assess all diabetic patients for their knowledge of diet and their adherence to the diet, rather than make the assumption that long-term diabetics already have sufficient knowledge. For those who have not forgotten their dietary regimens but have simply gotten into habits of inappropriate modifications, such a refresher may restore waning motivation.

Patients with cardiovascular diseases, including hypertension and atherosclerosis, should receive similar reevaluations and dietary updates. These patients may experience dietary problems related to their medication regimens that should be assessed. Loss of appetite, decreased taste sensation, and drug-nutrient interactions should be assessed in particular. Drug-nutrient interactions can occur in the following five ways (Moore, 1997): (1) drugs can affect appetite, (2) drug absorption may be influenced by foods, (3) drugs may modify taste sensitivity, (4) drug action may be affected by foods, and (5) drugs may affect nutrient absorption, metabolism, and excretion. For example, digitalis preparations may decrease appetite, cause diarrhea, and result in nutrient malabsorption (Moore, 1997). Certain hypocholesterolemics reduce fat absorption and absorption of fat-soluble vitamins, as well as vitamin B_{12}. Some potassium supplements can also interfere with vitamin B_{12} absorption. Potassium deficits can affect the action of digitalis and antiarrhythmic drugs (Moore, 1997).

Older Adults   The problems older adults have in maintaining good nutritional status are multidimensional and relate to the potential presence of one or more chronic illnesses, use of multiple medications, slowed gastrointestinal functioning, diminished taste sensation, decreased appetite, loneliness, economic problems, and transportation and mobility problems (with the resulting difficulties in shopping and cooking). In one study of frail older adults living in the community (Ritchie et al, 1997), a large proportion of older adults were found with BMIs under 24 or with serum albumin concentrations less than 3.5 g/dl. Nutritional risk was strongly correlated with dental problems. Another study found that nutritional risks were related to hospitalization (Mowe, Bohmer, 1996), suggesting that home care nurses might help prevent hospitalization by promoting adequate nutritional status among frail older adults. Although the Older Americans Act included provisions for nutritional support for older people, it is still quite common for the home care nurse to encounter elderly people living on a diet of prepared foods, such as peanut butter, ice cream, day-old bakery products dipped in tea, and even canned icing. These problems may be related to lack of mobility to nutrition centers, social isolation, or discomfort with seeking help.

It is inappropriate to extrapolate norms developed for children and young adults to older adults. The elderly have very different metabolic processes than younger adults and are extremely heterogeneous. This heterogeneity provides the basis for some of the assessment data the home care nurse should obtain, including information about usual diet, presence of chronic illnesses, dietary restrictions, and drug use (including prescription drugs, over-the-counter medications, and vitamins).

Moehrlin, Wolanin, and Burnside (1981) have identified several common nutritional problems in the elderly that should be evaluated. These include frank malnutrition and fluid imbalances (overload and dehydration), anemia, dental problems, vitamin and mineral imbalances (in particular, toxicities and osteoporosis), and alcoholism. In addition to problems with intake of food and fluids, many elderly have difficulty procuring, choosing, and preparing foods. Reading and interpreting nutrition information on package labels may be difficult for some. Elderly people who order groceries over the phone or internet may not be aware of the full variety of food products available. Some may have difficulty opening cans or packages, whereas others find it difficult to read or follow recipe instructions. Elderly clients, such as Mrs. Bell in the case presented in this chapter, who follow low-fat, "heart healthy" diets to the extreme are at risk for serious protein-calorie malnutrition.

The elderly are at risk for a wide variety of nutritional problems, and it is difficult to obtain accurate and meaningful databases on elderly clients. Many of these clients are too proud to give accurate historical data about their potentially poor nutritional intakes, or their memories may not be accurate. A proud elder might explain his or her edentulous state by saying, "I lost my teeth," or "My teeth don't fit." The difficulty experienced by many elderly in remembering recent events, such as dietary intake, may further compound the problems in establishing a sub-

jective database in relation to food and fluid intake. Not only are historical data difficult to establish, but physical examination data are also difficult to evaluate accurately. For example, it is often hard to determine if the elderly client has poor skin turgor or just decreased elasticity resulting from the aging process. With some clients, it is hard to determine if they have multiple ecchymotic areas because of tissue fragility related to poor nutritional status or if they are victims of abuse. Also, interpretation of laboratory findings in the elderly is difficult, since most norms are based on young, healthy adults.

Recognizing the problems with both biochemical and anthropometric evaluations of elderly in the community (i.e., logistic, economic, and special equipment needs), Wolinsky and colleagues (1986) developed a 16-item nutritional risk index for use with this population. The factors they determined to be associated with high nutritional risk in the elderly included use of dentures, concomitant presence of illness or use of medications, digestive discomfort, and limitation of the senses of taste and smell. More recently, the Nutritional Screening Initiative extended this work and developed the "DETERMINE" nutrition checklist (Gallagher-Allred, 1993). This simple screening tool helps older adults think about the major risk factors for poor nutritional health and stimulates them to consider getting assistance if they possess multiple risk factors. The tool (Fig. 12-3) contains 10 yes/no questions that ask about illness, eating habits, oral pain, financial problems, social contact, polypharmacy, weight loss and gain, functional status, and age. Home care nurses could provide feedback this to their clients before discharge from home services to better prepare clients for ongoing self-monitoring.

Other health problems experienced by the elderly that affect nutritional status include cancer and chronic obstructive lung disease. The gastrointestinal problems associated with cancer chemotherapy and radiation are well known and have particularly devastating effects on the elderly, whose reserves for coping with these stressors are limited. In addition, the diminished liver metabolic capacity and decreased renal efficiency impair the ability of the elderly client to cope with cytotoxic drugs. Individuals with chronic lung disease may experience anorexia as a result of their

The Warning Signs of poor nutritional health are often overlooked. Use this checklist to find out if you or someone you know is at nutritional risk.

DETERMINE YOUR NUTRITIONAL HEALTH

Read the statements below. Circle the number in the yes column for those that apply to you or someone you know. For each yes answer, score the number in the box. Total your nutritional score.

	YES
I have an illness or condition that made me change the kind and/or amount of food I eat.	2
I eat fewer than 2 meals per day.	3
I eat few fruits or vegetables, or milk products.	2
I have 3 or more drinks of beer, liquor or wine almost every day.	2
I have tooth or mouth problems that make it hard for me to eat.	2
I don't always have enough money to buy the food I need.	4
I eat alone most of the time.	1
I take 3 or more different prescribed or over-the-counter drugs a day.	1
Without wanting to, I have lost or gained 10 pounds in the last 6 months.	2
I am not always physically able to shop, cook and/or feed myself.	2
TOTAL	

Total Your Nutritional Score. If it's —

0-2 **Good!** Recheck your nutritional score in 6 months.

3-5 **You are at moderate nutritional risk.** See what can be done to improve your eating habits and lifestyle. Your office on aging, senior nutrition program, senior citizens center or health department can help. Recheck your nutritional score in 3 months.

6 or more **You are at high nutritional risk.** Bring in this checklist the next time you see your doctor, dietitian or other qualified health or social service professional. Talk with them about any problems you may have. Ask for help to improve your nutritional health.

These materials developed and distributed by the Nutrition Screening Initiative, a project of:

 AMERICAN ACADEMY OF FAMILY PHYSICIANS

 THE AMERICAN DIETETIC ASSOCIATION

 NATIONAL COUNCIL ON THE AGING

Remember that warning signs suggest risk, but do not represent diagnosis of any condition. Turn the page to learn more about the Warning Signs of poor nutritional health.

Fig. 12-3 The warning signs of poor nutritional health. Reprinted with permission by the Nutrition Screening Initiative, a project of the American Academy of Family Physicians, the American Dietetic Association and the National Council on the Aging, Inc., and funded in part by a grant from Ross Products Division, Abbott Laboratories Inc.

**The Nutrition Checklist is based on the Warning Signs described below.
Use the word DETERMINE to remind you of the Warning Signs.**

Disease

Any disease, illness or chronic condition which causes you to change the way you eat, or makes it hard for you to eat, puts your nutritional health at risk. Four out of five adults have chronic diseases that are affected by diet. Confusion or memory loss that keeps getting worse is estimated to affect one out of five or more of older adults. This can make it hard to remember what, when or if you've eaten. Feeling sad or depressed, which happens to about one in eight older adults, can cause big changes in appetite, digestion, energy level, weight and well-being.

Eating poorly

Eating too little and eating too much both lead to poor health. Eating the same foods day after day or not eating fruit, vegetables, and milk products daily will also cause poor nutritional health. One in five adults skip meals daily. Only 13% of adults eat the minimum amount of fruit and vegetables needed. One in four older adults drink too much alcohol. Many health problems become worse if you drink more than one or two alcoholic beverages per day.

Tooth loss/mouth pain

A healthy mouth, teeth and gums are needed to eat. Missing, loose or rotten teeth or dentures which don't fit well or cause mouth sores make it hard to eat.

Economic hardship

As many as 40% of older Americans have incomes of less than $6,000 per year. Having less—or choosing to spend less—than $25-30 per week for food makes it very hard to get the foods you need to stay healthy.

Reduced social contact

One-third of all older people live alone. Being with people daily has a positive effect on morale, well-being and eating.

Multiple medicines

Many older Americans must take medicines for health problems. Almost half of older Americans take multiple medicines daily. Growing old may change the way we respond to drugs. The more medicines you take, the greater the chance for side effects such as increased or decreased appetite, change in taste, constipation, weakness, drowsiness, diarrhea, nausea, and others. Vitamins or minerals when taken in large doses act like drugs and can cause harm. Alert your doctor to everything you take.

Involuntary weight loss/gain

Losing or gaining a lot of weight when you are not trying to do so is an important warning sign that must not be ignored. Being overweight or underweight also increases your chance of poor health.

Needs assistance in self care

Although most older people are able to eat, one of every five have trouble walking, shopping, buying and cooking food, especially as they get older.

Elder years above age 80

Most older people lead full and productive lives. But as age increases, risk of frailty and health problems increase. Checking your nutritional health regularly makes good sense.

The Nutrition Screening Initiative, 2626 Pennsylvania Avenue, NW, Suite 301, Washington, DC 20037
The Nutrition Screening Initiative is funded in part by a grant from Ross Laboratories, a division of Abbott Laboratories.

A5944/MARCH 1992

Fig. 12-3, cont'd   For legend see opposite page.

CASE STUDY

"Honey, I don't want you to worry about me. I am doing just fine," Mrs. Bell assured Sharon. She went on to say that she did not eat apples, carrots, or any meats that were at all difficult to chew because her dentures did not fit well. In completing the health history, Sharon learned that Mrs. Bell had been treated for breast cancer 7 years earlier, with no apparent recurrence. Mrs. Bell's physician had told her that she had a "touch of sugar," although she was not being treated for diabetes. She was taking a diuretic for hypertension and a daily multivitamin, as well as an antacid for calcium supplementation and "some extra vitamins that my neighbor gets for me from the health food store."

Questions

- Based on what Mrs. Bell has indicated about her diet, current health problems and medications, and nutritional supplementation, what other information would you want to obtain from her and why?
- What are some potential problems that result from high levels of intake of certain vitamins?

chronic hypoxia, as well as fatigue when eating. Problems with appetite, fatigue, dyspnea, glossitis, stomatitis, pharyngitis, digestion, and elimination experienced by clients with cancer or chronic lung disease should be thoroughly evaluated.

High-Risk Populations

Populations at high risk for nutrition-related problems include people with multiple comorbidities (particularly diabetes, cardiovascular disease, and immunodeficiencies) predisposing them to debilitation; the very young and very old; those with hypermetabolic needs (e.g., clients recovering from surgery, those with overwhelming infections and burns, and pregnant women); clients more than 20% above or below their ideal weights; those requiring artificial nutritional support, such as parenteral or enteral nutrition; and those with socioeconomic risk factors. Some types of socioeconomic risk factors are poverty and social isolation. Any client referred to home care with one or more risk factors should receive further evaluation of his or her nutritional status before discharge from hospital or nursing home. In this way, nutri-

tional care plans can be developed in a timely fashion, with no gaps in service to the client. If this is not possible, the home care nurse should consider screening clients for nutritional risk and conducting more detailed assessments of those determined to be at high risk for nutrition-related health problems (Gunning, Saffel-Shriner, Shane-McWhorter, 1998; Lyman, Marquart, 1997). Nurse case managers in the home health care agency may be called on to work with client groups that the agency has found to be the highest volume and most problem prone.

NURSING DIAGNOSES RELATED TO NUTRITIONAL NEEDS

The diagnostic phase is crucial in planning home care services appropriately. Because nutritional modifications influence a key aspect of clients' lifestyles, it is imperative that the nurse, along with the family and the rest of the health care team involved in the client's care, identify the strengths and positive factors on which the client and family can draw and the potential problems they are facing. For example, clients who have always enjoyed cooking and trying new recipes may find that it is not too difficult to adapt to a modified diet if they are helped to find appropriate recipes and sources of new ingredients. Other clients and families with a low tolerance for stress and frustration may need more frequent visits from the home care nurse when implementing home enteral or parenteral feedings for assistance in troubleshooting areas such as clogged gavage tubes or assessment of deep-line insertion sites.

The North American Nursing Diagnosis Association (NANDA) has developed a list of approved diagnoses, many of which are related to nutritional-metabolic problems. A number of the diagnoses found in this functional pattern (Gordon, 1993) reflect problems of home care clients. These are listed in Box 12-2. Several diagnoses, such as "effective breastfeeding," reflect the nurse's assessment of client strengths. In addition to nursing diagnoses focused on the client, the nurse must determine the strengths and needs of the family to plan the services best suited to that family's needs. The OMAHA system (Martin, Sheets, 1992) and Saba's home health system (Stanhope, Lancaster, 1996) also contain nursing diagnostic labels related to nutritional care of clients in the home.

NUTRITIONAL-METABOLIC PATTERN

Altered nutrition: High risk for more than body requirements or High risk for obesity
Altered nutrition: More than body requirements or Exogenous obesity
Altered nutrition: Less than body requirements or Nutritional deficit
Ineffective breastfeeding
Effective breastfeeding
Interrupted breastfeeding
Ineffective infant feeding pattern
High risk for aspiration
Impaired swallowing or Uncompensated swallowing impairment
Altered oral mucous membrane
High risk for fluid volume deficit
Fluid volume deficit
Fluid volume excess

From Gordon M: *Manual of nursing diagnosis*, St Louis, 1993-1994, Mosby.

NUTRITIONAL PLANNING WITH CLIENTS AND FAMILIES

With increasing emphasis on limiting length of service for home care clients, nurses should work closely with clients, families, and caregivers to plan care that will maximize the client's and caregiver's abilities to manage the nutritional interventions after discharge from home care. It is important to work in partnership with families to predict the length of home care service (number of visits per week, length of visits, and number of total visits), as well as the nature of service (e.g., teaching, coaching, changing dressings, monitoring tube or line placement). Nurses need strong skills in client and family education, including skills in assessing readiness to learn and planning incremental learning consistent with families' abilities and needs.

Clients who have been referred to a home health care agency and have received their first visit from the nurse should participate in planning the types of interventions most appropriate and acceptable to them. This planning should focus on the means of ensuring adequate nutritional intake, as well as on the identification of

support persons and services available to help. Planning should include health promotion and primary, secondary, and tertiary preventive interventions. This is a more comprehensive approach than simply emphasizing nutritional therapy or nutritional support in isolation. For example, clients such as Mrs. Bell, who are undernourished and at risk for complications related to currently existing comorbidities (hypertension in this case), should be helped to learn dietary modifications to correct the undernutrition and to prevent further deterioration of health (both tertiary preventive measures).

It may be necessary for the client and family to make some choices about interventions. During the planning phase, the nurse should help them identify alternatives and recognize consequences and determine with them which sets of alternatives and consequences are most acceptable in terms of the various costs: financial, emotional, physical, and social. The costs of services should be compared with the benefits of the services.

It may be prudent to assist clients and families preparing to implement enteral or parenteral nutritional support at home to discuss with their insurer which services and goods will be covered and whether any special circumstances must be considered. For example, does the therapy need to be considered a permanent feeding modality? Is reimbursement limited to specific vendors or types of products? In this way, the nurse, physician, and social worker can work with the client and family to individualize and optimize the necessary treatment and look for creative sources of reimbursement if necessary. This can spare the client and family unpleasant and perhaps debilitating financial surprises later and reduce the stress of worrying about financial responsibilities related to treatment.

In addition to determining the impact of finances on the choices of modalities and services, other priority-setting factors should be discussed with the family. They will no doubt be facing some lifestyle changes. It is often difficult for clients under such circumstances to clearly delineate values, priorities, capabilities, and potential problems. The nurse should assist the family with discussing such areas as past practices in relation to meals and dietary preferences and ways that these will be altered by the new routines. He or she should help the family articulate how they feel about the new routines and freely verbalize any negative reactions. For example, a mother faced with repeated gavage feedings for her infant may have very strong but difficult-to-articulate feelings about not being able to feed the baby in a more traditional fashion, such as nursing or bottle feeding. It is important to have determined the impact the client's illness and treatment may have already had on the family. In this way, interventions can be planned that will draw on the family's strengths and avert potential problems.

Other common examples of major changes in lifestyle are related to the care of clients who live alone. Clients in these circumstances may move in with family or friends, or these support persons might move in with the client. One additional pattern is that the support person will spend long periods staying with the client during the day. The impact of these new routines on eating habits must be taken into account when planning nutritional services.

Once the priorities and the constraints have been determined, the nurse and family should work together to quantify the extent of nursing services required. While the needs of the client and family will dictate the preferred frequency of visits, the policies of the reimbursement source will no doubt have an impact on the frequency of visits. These issues should be discussed early with the client and family (preferably on the first visit) and will help set the stage for termination of services.

Home care nurses have long been experts at the identification and use of community resources for their clients, and this is no less important in the area of nutritional services. Referrals to community agencies should be discussed with family members to obtain their agreement and to explain the proposed benefits of such a referral. The nurse should also explain what would be expected of the family, such as when and where to go to obtain the services and the financial obligations associated with the referral (Sebastian, 1996). Families are just as interested in knowing that services will be offered without charge as they are in knowing what the particular costs will be. Some examples of widely available community services include the Women, Infant, and Children's (WIC) nutritional support program; Meals on Wheels or other home-delivered meals;

food stamps, school meals, and government surplus commodities; food banks and soup kitchens; local charities; homemakers' programs (which can offer help with cooking and light housework); and support groups. Resources may be found in a number of ways, such as by looking in the community services section of the telephone book or a social service directory, contacting a social worker or hospital discharge planner, or working through a local community service coordinating agency. Nurse case managers can help with resource identification and coordination.

NURSING INTERVENTIONS FOR NUTRITIONAL PROBLEMS

Nutritional interventions are among the six classes of interventions included within the domain of basic physiological support in the Nursing Interventions Classification (McCloskey, Bulechek, 1996). Some interventions are specific to the type of nutritional therapy used, whereas others are more general interventions that are tailored to meet the client's nutritional needs, such as client and family teaching. These interventions are listed in Table 12-2.

Client and Family Teaching

Client and family teaching related to nutritional interventions in the home is particularly significant considering how difficult it is for acutely ill clients to learn self-care while they are hospitalized. The current emphasis on reducing costs in home care by empowering clients to manage their own care as quickly as possible makes it even more important that home care nurses develop systematic plans for client nutritional education. Effective self-care requires that clients and family or other caregivers and support persons learn how to (1) manage therapeutic diets and regular, health-promoting diets; (2) monitor the effectiveness of the diet; (3) procure and prepare food; (4) monitor for side effects or adverse effects (e.g., in the case of enteral or parenteral support), as well as for food-drug interactions; (5) manage adverse effects (e.g., diarrhea); and (6) provide direct care (e.g., cleaning a peripheral or central venous access site or administering a tube feeding). Nurses should work with the interdisciplinary health team to adapt diet therapy and teaching plans in a manner consistent with the cultural preferences of clients and families.

Table 12-2	Nutritional Interventions in the Nursing Interventions Classification

NIC Domain: *Physiologic support, basic*
NIC Domain Class: *Nutrition support*
NIC Interventions

NIC Intervention Code	Intervention Name
1020	Diet staging
1030	Eating disorders management
1050	Feeding
1056	Enteral tube feeding
1080	Gastrointestinal intubation
1100	Nutrition management
1120	Nutrition therapy
5246	Nutritional counseling
1160	Nutritional monitoring
1803	Self-care assistance: Feeding
1860	Swallowing therapy
5614	Teaching prescribed diet
1200	Total parenteral nutrition (TPN) administration
1874	Tube care: Gastrointestinal
1240	Weight gain assistance
1260	Weight management
1280	Weight reduction assistance

From McCloskey JC, Bulechek GM: *Nursing Interventions Classification (NIC): Iowa Intervention Project,* ed 2, St Louis, 1996, Mosby.

The nurse should be aware of the importance of teaching, even with clients who have been following a particular diet for a long time. A wide variety of materials are available to assist in teaching dietary regimens to home care clients; however, the nurse must be cautious not to select materials inappropriate for the client's reading or comprehension level. It is useful to provide printed material for clients, but these should be supplemented with verbal instructions, demonstrations, and return demonstrations as necessary. In addition, it is necessary to determine if clients can see, can read (and at what level), and can read in English before providing printed materials. Teaching materials should be available in Spanish in areas with large Hispanic populations, or in other languages as appropriate for the pop-

ulation mix. Such materials also should be available in pictorial form for clients with low literacy levels. Videotaped client education, computerized information on CD-ROMs, and information on the World Wide Web are other examples of teaching venues that can be used with clients with different levels of readiness and resources (such as access to computers). Telehealth technology makes it possible to deliver some teaching over interactive video, which has advantages for areas with large rural populations. Client and caregiver teaching should be documented on a checklist to facilitate monitoring the client's progress (Sanville, 1994).

The amount of time necessary for the client to learn his or her care depends on the individual client. Some clients or families may learn how to administer tube feedings in only one or two sessions. Structured teaching programs by interdisciplinary teams that begin before insertion of the feeding tube and continue after discharge to the home have shown good results (Hull et al, 1993). Supplementation of home-based follow-up and instruction with telephone counseling provides clients and families with reassurance and the opportunity to ask questions in a timely manner (Hull et al, 1993).

Learning how to manage parenteral therapy can be time consuming and overwhelming for some clients and families. After evaluating the client and caregiver's readiness to learn, the nurse should organize the teaching into manageable segments with a logical flow. According to self-efficacy theory (Bandura, 1977), people are more likely to feel confident about new procedures if they have the opportunity to experience sequential small successes. Furthermore, the nurse should allow the client and caregiver time to practice each new skill and ask questions as necessary. Self-efficacy theory also emphasizes the importance of feedback, so the nurse should allow adequate time for this.

Specific Approaches to Therapeutic Nutritional Interventions

Approaches to nutritional therapy for home care clients may be divided into three categories: supplementation of the content of the diet, modification of the content of the diet, and administration of feedings in a nontraditional manner (commonly referred to as *nutritional support). Dietary supplementation* refers to any type of therapeutic additions to the client's diet, from vitamin supplementation for children and pregnant women to hydration therapy for the elderly. *Dietary modification* refers to therapeutic alterations made in the client's diet, as a low-sodium or low-fat diet would illustrate. *Nutritional support* has come to refer to either enteral or parenteral routes of feeding the client and may be administered on a supplemental basis, an intermittent basis (e.g., for clients experiencing periodic remissions and exacerbations with Crohn's disease), or a long-term basis.

In addition to these particular approaches to nutritional care, the nurse may use teaching, referral, or psychosocial support as the primary intervention modality. For example, with some elderly clients on therapeutic diets, the major focus of the nurse's efforts may be on reinforcing appropriate food choices and on facilitating referrals to sources of nutritional assistance. Simply encouraging some clients to try some of the community services for which they are eligible is key to helping them balance their desires for independence with their nutritional needs.

EVALUATION AND OUTCOME ASSESSMENT

Evaluation and follow-up of the client's nutritional needs at home focus on monitoring the effectiveness of the plan, making revisions as appropriate, and determining an appropriate discharge date. Monitoring activities are simply a modification of the assessment process in which the emphasis is on making quantitative and qualitative judgments with the client and family on changes in the client's condition. Both improvements and deterioration in status should be noted. Subjective data comprise a large part of the information used in this process; objective data, including physical assessment parameters and laboratory analysis, are also involved. The frequency of collection of specific types of data is often jointly determined among the physician, nurse, and client. Requirements of third-party payors also are critical considerations. The effects of the client's illness and treatment on family functioning are also important but may be difficult to document because so many agencies view the patient as the primary client.

Outcome measures and indicators will relate to the specific goals developed for that client. Generally they will include factors such as sufficient intake of carbohydrates, proteins, fats, fluids, vitamins, and minerals. Indicators such as body weight within normal limits, good skin turgor and elasticity, total lymphocyte count, and normal levels of albumin, serum glucose, and the rapid-turnover proteins are also commonly used. Survival is one broad indicator of success (Detsky, 1995), especially with long-term parenteral nutrition, since it is the most invasive support method in use. Improvement in functional status, including return to school, work, or other usual activities of daily living, is a key outcome indicator. Resumption of oral nutrition is an appropriate outcome criterion for clients receiving home parenteral or enteral nutrition for whom oral nutrition can reasonably be expected. Quality of life is a critical outcome of nutritional support as is cost effectiveness (Detsky, 1995). Recommendations for evaluating clients' responses to nutritional support are found in Table 12-3 (Moore, 1997). The Medicare Outcomes Assessment Instrument,

---

CASE STUDY

Sharon explained the importance of adequate protein, fat, and calories in the diet to Mrs. Bell and reinforced the information with a colorful chart depicting appropriate food choices. Mrs. Bell indicated that she would be willing to attend adult day care 3 days a week for a trial period. "I really don't know if I want to go over there and be with all those old people, dear," she commented. "Besides, I have my things to do here at the house, and I just don't know if I have time." However, she agreed to try it out for 2 months and to eat the lunches served at the center.

Sharon contacted the nurse manager at the adult day care center and discussed Mrs. Bell's dietary needs. She followed up with a written referral form that included a dietary prescription that had been developed in collaboration with the home care agency's dietitian and Mrs. Bell's physician.

Questions

- Do you agree with Sharon's decision to recommend an adult day care center for Mrs. Bell? Explain why or why not.
- How would you choose between making that type of referral as opposed to a program such as Meals on Wheels?

Table 12-3 Assessing Response to Nutritional Support

Parameter	Frequency of Measurement*	Purpose/Comments
ANTHROPOMETRIC MEASUREMENTS		
Weight	Daily	Indicator of efficacy, client should have steady gain; use usual or IBW for guide to desirable weight; a gain of >0.1-0.2 kg (0.25-0.5 lb.) a day
Skinfolds, mid-arm circumference		Indicator of efficacy
Length or height (pediatrics only)		Indicator of efficacy; see pediatric growth charts for expected growth pattern
PHYSICAL ASSESSMENT		
State of hydration	Daily	*Overhydration:* check for edema of dependent body parts, shortness of breath, rales in lungs, fluid intake consistently greater than output *Dehydration:* look for poor skin turgor, dry mucous membranes, complaints of thirst, output greater than intake (measure stool volumes if liquid), greater than 10% difference between blood pressure when lying and standing
Gastrointestinal motility (tube-fed individuals)—i.e., presence of bowel sounds, signs of abdominal distention, passage of flatus or stool, nausea or vomiting, gastric residual volumes (RV) obtained from feeding tubes	Every 2-4 hr. during initiation of feedings; every 8 hr. when stable	Indicators of GI motility and feeding tolerance; RV over 200 ml during nasogastric feeding or 100 ml during gastrostomy feeding may indicate delayed gastric emptying and should be reported to a physician†
HEMATOLOGIC AND BIOCHEMICAL MEASUREMENTS		
Serum glucose and electrolytes	Daily until stable, then 2-3/wk	Indicates whether intake is adequate or excessive
BUN	1-2/wk	*Increased:* inadequate fluid intake, renal impairment, or excessive protein intake *Decreased:* inadequate protein intake is possible
Serum Ca, P, Mg	1-2/wk	Measure of adequacy of intake
Complete blood count	1/wk	Indicator of adequacy of Fe, protein, folic acid, and vitamin B_{12}
Serum triglycerides (during TPN)	After each increase in lipid dosage; 2-3/wk when stable	Elevated levels indicate inadequate lipid clearance and possibly a need for reduction in lipid dosage.
Serum albumin, transferrin, or prealbumin	1/wk	Indicator of efficacy in maintaining or improving protein nutriture

From Moore MC: *Pocket guide to nutritional care,* ed 3, St Louis, 1997, Mosby.

IBW, ideal body weight; *BUN,* blood urea nitrogen; *Ca,* calcium; *P,* phosphorus; *Mg,* magnesium; *Fe,* iron.

*These are suggested frequencies only. Individual patients may need more or less frequent assessment.

†Check residual volumes with a large (60 ml) syringe to avoid collapsing the feeding tube; return RV to the patient and then irrigate the tube thoroughly with water. Measuring RV increases the risk of clogging small-bore feeding tubes, and these tubes collapse easily, making it questionable whether RV is measured accurately. Therefore some clinicians do not advocate measuring RV in patients with small-bore tubes. Even with large RV, feedings can usually continue with careful monitoring of physical findings and abdominal radiographs.

"Mrs. Bell, this is wonderful! You have gained 10 pounds over the last 2 months. Your most recent labwork shows that your hemoglobin is up to 13 and you are eating a very well-balanced diet. I know what hard work this has been for you, and I want to tell you how pleased I am with the progress you have made." Sharon patted Mrs. Bell's hand and smiled at the older woman.

"Well, dear, if you had not encouraged me to eat differently, I would have continued following George's diet. I thought if his doctor said it was good enough for George, then it was good enough for me. I must say that I do feel better. Now I have the energy to take care of my roses the way I used to." Mrs. Bell looked outside her living room window at the roses blooming in her front yard and smiled.

OASIS, provides a means for collecting certain key outcomes data related to home care, including nutritional indices (Shaughnessy et al, 1994).

Finally, in addition to evaluating the outcomes of care, nurses should evaluate the processes of nutritional care and whether those processes seem to be directly related to the desired outcomes. One instrument available for monitoring the processes of home care nursing is the Schmele Instrument to Measure the Process of Nursing Practice in Home Health (Schmele, Allen, 1990; Schmele, Foss, 1989). This 60-item instrument has been used to evaluate the processes of nutritional care by home care nurses (Davis, 1996), with promising results.

ENTERAL AND PARENTERAL NUTRITIONAL SUPPORT
Selection of Candidates

The use of home nutritional support therapies has grown dramatically since the late 1980s and is one of the most expensive therapies in use in home care (Howard et al, 1995). Clinical practice patterns have changed from using these modalities primarily for long-term therapy toward greater use as a short-term therapy (Howard et al, 1995). Roughly one third of clients receiving home parenteral nutrition also receive "at least one other infusion therapy" (Sanville, 1994), such as fluid replacement, intravenous antibiotics, or chemotherapy. Numerous physical indices have been published as criteria for the selection of candidates for enteral or parenteral nutritional support. Although the very young and very old were less likely to receive home enteral or parenteral therapy in the past, more recently, clients of all ages are increasingly being treated with these modalities (Howard et al, 1995). In addition to the physical indices, others have suggested environmental characteristics and socioeconomic considerations in accepting clients for home parenteral nutrition (Bender, Faubion, 1985; Blackburn, Baptista, 1984; Decker, 1984). Sanville (1994) says that one of the most critical concerns is the "willingness of the client and/or caregiver to participate in the care."

The clients for whom oral nutrition is not a possibility are candidates for enteral or parenteral nutrition. Most experts agree that those who have intact gastrointestinal function should receive enteral nutrition, whereas those whose gastrointestinal tracts are not functioning normally should receive parenteral nutrition. Other advantages of enteral feeding include lower cost than parenteral nutrition, lower complication rates, and ease of administration (Shike, 1996). Some examples of conditions necessitating enteral support include pharyngeal or esophageal strictures, neurological disorders resulting in dysphagia, psychotic disorders (resulting in anorexia or refusal to eat), coma, and in children, problems including prematurity, cystic fibrosis, and gastroesophageal reflux (Kleinman, 1998).

The choice of access devices depends on the extent to which the gastrointestinal tract is functioning, the expected duration of therapy, the degree to which the client can participate in self-care, and the extent to which the home environment can support therapy (Loan et al, 1997). Clients receiving short-term therapy (less than a few weeks) may have either a nasoduodenal or a nasojejunal feeding tube in place. Nasojejunal feeding tubes have the advantage of delivering formula past the duodenum, which decreases pancreatic stimulation for clients with pancreatic cancer (Loan et al, 1997). Both types of tubes have small bores and clog easily, making them poor choices for long-term therapy in the home.

Enteral access devices better suited to long-term home therapy are gastrostomy tubes (either surgically implanted or percutaneous endoscopic gastrostomy tubes [PEG] tubes), percutaneous endoscopic gastrostomy/jejunostomy (PEG/J) tubes, or surgical jejunostomy tubes (Loan et al, 1997). Gastrostomy tubes are not recommended for clients with delayed gastric emptying, gastric ulceration or bleeding, previous gastrectomy, ascites, peritonitis, morbid obesity, gastric tumor, or gastric outlet obstruction (Loan et al, 1997).

Generally clients who cannot sufficiently digest, absorb, or move nutrients through the digestive tract are considered candidates for either full or partial parenteral nutritional support. This includes clients with cancer, Crohn's disease, AIDS, gastrointestinal motility disorders, ischemic bowel infarctions, chronic bowel obstructions, inflammatory bowel disorder, radiation enteritis, short bowel syndrome, and congenital bowel defects (Davis, 1996; Howard et al, 1995). Blackburn and Baptista (1984) noted that candidates most likely to benefit from home parenteral nutrition are those with sufficient motivation, learning abilities, and the physical characteristics (such as good eye-hand coordination) necessary to participate in this treatment. Of course, some clients are unable to provide self-care because of extreme infirmity or age and are therefore cared for by someone else in the home.

Enteral Nutritional Support Interventions

In providing enteral support, the physician, nurse, and dietitian should work together to determine the most effective access device and feeding site based on the client's physiological needs, prognosis and anticipated length of therapy, home environment, and ability to provide self-care. The choice of formula depends on the client's physiological and therapeutic needs, the nature of the access device chosen (Loan et al, 1997), and financial considerations.

Feedings may be prescribed as continuous, intermittent, or bolus, depending on the physiological capabilities and needs of the client, as well as on the various needs and capabilities of the caregivers. For example, people with Crohn's disease have been successfully treated with cyclic home enteral nutrition (e.g., administration of enteral nutrition throughout the night and supplementation with "low residue and low fat foods" during the day) (Matsueda et al, 1995).

Specific instructions on placing the tube, checking the position of the tube, and maintaining tube patency may be found in any current nursing skills manual and will not be repeated here (Metheny, Eisenberg, McSweeney, 1998). Research now indicates that checking gastric pH is a more reliable method of confirming gastric tube placement than the auscultatory method often used, although x-ray confirmation is the most definitive approach (Metheny et al, 1998). Families or caregivers are often taught to check the position of the tube before initiating feeding, to aspirate gastric contents to determine if the feedings are being sufficiently digested, and to elevate the head of the bed to prevent aspiration by the client. Generally, a consistent gastric residual of 100 ml or more over a 2-hour period is considered an indication that the feeding is not being sufficiently digested and should be withheld. Repeated episodes of large amounts of residual should be reported to the physician. Families should be taught to report frequency of diarrhea, as well as to cope with the incontinent family member with diarrhea to prevent skin breakdown.

The home care client often must be taught to irrigate the tube periodically to ensure patency. Generally it is best to flush the tube with approximately 30 to 50 ml of warm water (Loan et al, 1997) after each feeding. This must be taken into account when calculating the appropriate dilution of the formula and the 24-hour total fluid intake. Certain medications tend to clog feeding tubes; these include hydrochlorothiazide, ibuprofen, psyllium, and theophylline (Theodur) sprinkles (Loan et al, 1997). "Feeding tubes should be flushed with 30 to 50 ml water before and after medication administration" (Loan et al, 1997). It is best to check with a pharmacist before dissolving medications, since this is not appropriate in every case. Furthermore, the nurse should avoid mixing medications, since some combinations will precipitate interactions. Home care nurses should ensure that those drugs that should be administered into the stomach are not administered directly into the small bowel. If the client's access site is not compatible with the medication, either the access site or the medication should be changed (Loan et al, 1997). "Hypertonic liquid medications should be diluted with 60 to 90 ml of water before administration because they are irritating to the gastrointestinal tract" (Loan et al, 1997). Examples of these drugs include furosemide, digoxin, and potassium chloride (Loan et al, 1997).

Families need to know the appropriate storage method for the tube feeding formulas, since they are highly perishable once opened. Some families keep the unopened cans in a warm room over a radiator; this can result in spoilage even when the cans are unopened. Also, caregivers or clients who mix their own formulas will need assistance to learn how to do this in a manner unlikely to result in spoilage and to do it accurately to prevent the development of nutritional imbalances.

One study found that bacterial contamination of enteral formula was more common in the home than in the hospital (Patchell et al, 1994). The researchers found that formulas to which the caregiver added other ingredients were particularly likely to be contaminated. They also speculated that the practice of topping off formulas after 4 hours to prevent formula from hanging very long at one time may have been responsible for contamination. In a later study (Patchell et al, 1998), researchers found that hanging enough formula for 24 hours (rather than 4) and using a strict protocol for the conditions under which the formula and hanging bag were assembled led to a reduction in contamination rates from 62% to 6% in the home. It may be most helpful for the home care nurse to visit at times when caregivers are preparing and administering formulas to evaluate their techniques and provide feedback as appropriate.

For infants receiving routine gavage feedings, the concomitant use of nonnutritive sucking devices has long been recognized as a useful developmental adjunct (Bowden, Dickey, Greenberg, 1998; Schwartz et al, 1987). Infants meet developmental and nutritional needs through the more traditional feeding modalities of nursing and bottle feeding by virtue of their sucking activity. When this is bypassed by the use of the gavage tube, the addition of a pacifier to satisfy the baby's sucking needs assists with that developmental task. Parents may need assistance in understanding the rationale for this, although they may intuitively recognize the need for sucking.

Parenteral Nutritional Support Interventions

Nursing interventions related to home parenteral nutrition (HPN) focus on monitoring the therapeutic efficacy of nutritional support, teaching clients and caregivers how to administer the infusate and how to prevent complications, ensuring client safety, and promoting client and family adaptation and quality of life. Clients should be given a toll-free telephone number they can call for support and assistance (Sanville, 1994). They must learn how to use aseptic technique when performing functions related to parenteral nutrition, how to properly care for their venous access site, and how to handle their solutions (which may include adding vitamins or minerals to the formulas). They must also learn how to handle problems with the infusion pump. In addition to mastering these skills, they must cope not only with their initial anxiety at confronting this complex technology on which they are dependent, but also with the emotional ramifications of not eating and perhaps the social isolation of being left out at mealtimes.

The choice of formulas for HPN is usually determined through evaluation of the client's total calorie, protein, and fat requirements. Total kilocalorie requirements are calculated using the Harris-Benedict equation, and total protein requirements are "based on the patient's level of stress and any nitrogen losses occurring from nasogastric suction, diarrhea, or ostomy output. Fat emulsions are used to prevent essential fatty acid deficiency and as a caloric source" (Sanville, 1994). Home parenteral nutrition formulas also contain electrolytes, fluid, vitamins, trace minerals, and dextrose (Sanville, 1994). The nurse should consult with a pharmacist if the client is scheduled to add iron to their formulas, since iron is incompatible with lipids. Some clients will need to add insulin to their formulas, and others may require an H_2 antagonist or heparin (Sanville, 1994; Veerabagu et al, 1995). Individuals who will receive replacement parenteral supplementation as a result of "large ostomy outputs, diarrhea or nasogastric suctioning," should receive this formula as a separate infusion (Sanville, 1994).

Understanding the principles involved in the strict application of aseptic technique may be difficult for some clients because of the abstract nature of this concept. However, it is absolutely critical that the nurse spend sufficient time teaching the application of this concept to the client through handwashing techniques, maintenance of a clean area for preparation of the infusate, and catheter care. Catheter sepsis is the most frequently noted complication (Bender, Faubion, 1985; Sanville, 1994; Steiger et al, 1985), with infection related to the solution a common problem (Busby, Seiffert, 1986). One study found that patients receiving total parenteral nutrition and intralipid therapy in the home were more likely to develop bloodstream infections if needleless infusion devices were used than if protected needle systems were used (Danzig et al, 1995). The researchers suggest that paying greater attention to aseptic technique and determining the most appropriate standard for frequency of changing the injection caps are needed to ensure patient safety.

Numerous improvements have been made and continue to be made in venous access devices. Hickman catheters have enjoyed wide popularity because of their wide lumens, the ease with which blood specimens may be obtained, and their elasticity. Implantable central venous access discs offer convenience for clients because of the decreased frequency with which they must be flushed with heparin and the diminished potential for infection. Peripherally inserted central catheters (PICC lines) combine the advantages of both peripheral and central catheters. They are usually less expensive to insert than central lines. Also, they are better suited to home care than central venous catheters because they still permit infusion of very hypertonic solute concentrations while removing the risk of pneumothorax (Moore, 1997).

Basic principles involved in care of the catheter insertion site include the use of aseptic technique, frequent dressing changes (approximately one to three times a week), and careful inspection of the site for any signs of infection (Munro-Black, 1984). Every agency should have its own individualized protocols printed in a procedure manual. These may reflect the recommendations of the vendor most frequently used by that agency's clients, as well as the clinical experiences of the physicians and nurses involved. The clients may have been taught slight variations in the procedure by the hospital staff. Generally, it will reduce client anxiety if the nurse will assess the procedure the client has learned and reinforce that technique, rather than teach a new one. Another approach is for agencies to adopt a common standard of care. Home care agencies often use videotapes to supplement and reinforce client teaching related to parenteral nutrition.

Although most clients will have received continuous feedings while in the hospital, they will generally be switched at home to a schedule of cycling in which a large volume of solution will be infused over a 10- to 12-hour period (generally at night) to permit as normal a schedule during the waking hours as possible. This may be troublesome for some clients because they will need to void several times throughout the night because of the large amount of fluid infusing. The pump may have an automatic tapering feature that will begin and end the infusion at a lower rate. If the pump does not have this feature, clients and caregivers will need to learn to manage the tapering schedules themselves (Sanville, 1994). For clients who cannot tolerate the large amounts of infusate over the 10- to 12-hour period, ambulatory vests are available that can be worn under the client's clothing.

Special problems of parenteral nutrition with infants and children include maintaining safety of the lines and preventing clogging of the tubing. Parents should be taught to tape all connections securely to prevent them from being dislodged. In addition to the difficulty of disciplining a child with a visible health problem, the nature of the catheter itself can precipitate further problems. Increased intrathoracic pressure from crying can result in blood backing up into the permanent right atrial catheter, which then necessitates additional heparin flushes to maintain the patency of the catheter. This can cause some problems in disciplining the child, especially an older child who may learn to use this to his or her advantage (Bender, Faubion, 1985).

Catheter-related sepsis is a problem for children as it is for adults (Bowden, Dickey, Greenberg, 1998). In a retrospective chart review of 102 pediatric clients, Vargas and colleagues (1987) found that catheter infection had occurred in 42% of the clients. The authors noted that of the nine client deaths attributed to catheter-related sepsis, three could have been prevented if the parents had recognized fever as a sign of possible infection and had brought the child in for prompt treatment. Home care nurses must emphasize this point with parents of children receiving parenteral nutrition.

School-age children should be able to return to any age-appropriate activities, although certain activities should be cleared with the physician.

Bender and Faubion (1985) point out the importance of educating a child's teacher about the parenteral nutrition to increase the teacher's comfort with regard to the child. The child's classmates will no doubt be aware that the child is "different" in some way, and the teacher who feels comfortable about the normalcy of the child can serve as a buffer in these situations. The school nurse may be a valuable resource in promoting the child's adaptation, and the home care nurse can enhance service integration by coordinating the child's care with that individual.

On the first visit to the client at home, the nurse should determine that the correct solutions are available; the venous access is patent; the pump is operating correctly; all the necessary supplies are available (including the prescribed solution for flushing the tubing); a 24-hour telephone number (e.g., a toll-free number) is available if the client has questions (Sanville, 1994); and the client has established a reasonable schedule of cycling infusions that will not interfere with the usual activities of school, work, or other activities. Subsequent visits should focus on the client's physical status, the use of correct techniques, the functioning of the equipment, and the family dynamics.

Outcome Indicators of Nutritional Support for Children

Home enteral nutrition has been found to be an effective strategy for improving or maintaining nutritional status for children with many clinical conditions (Papadopoulou et al, 1995). Appropriate outcome indicators include serial anthropometric measurements (height, weight, mid-arm circumference, and skinfold thickness) (Papadopoulou et al, 1995). Children requiring repeated placement of gavage tubes and those receiving parenteral nutrition need continual assessment of cardiopulmonary status (to evaluate for aspiration pneumonia and fluid overload) and condition of the nasopharyngeal areas and the access site and laboratory evaluation of fluid and electrolyte status.

In addition, children receiving parenteral nutrition should have neck and arm circumferences monitored because it is possible for them to develop nontender deep vein thrombosis, which may be apparent only by edema (Bender, Faubion, 1985). The condition of the catheter site must be monitored because sepsis is such a com-

mon complication.* Bender and Faubion (1985) noted that it is particularly important to monitor the child's weight when the child is in the transition phase from parenteral to enteral nutrition, since this is a time when weight loss may easily develop. Children who have had long-term parenteral nutrition may need help in learning how to choose "a nutritious diet or control ostomy outputs" (Bender, Faubion, 1985).

Outcome Indicators of Nutritional Support for Adults

Howard et al (1995) reviewed statistics from Medicare Part B and the North American Home Parenteral and Enteral Patient Registry from 1985 to 1992 to determine the impact of both forms of nutritional support on four outcomes: (1) mortality, (2) resumption of oral nutrition, (3) functional status and work-related rehabilitation, and (4) complications. They concluded that for clients who died or had poor rehabilitative outcomes, the client's primary diagnosis exerted more of an influence on the outcome than did the therapy itself. While the very old tended to have poorer outcomes than those who were younger, the outcomes of older adults were still good. Certain clinical parameters should be regularly evaluated by home care nurses working with clients receiving one of these forms of nutritional support.

Enteral Support   Long-term enteral support can be a successful strategy for maintaining nutritional status in clients unable to swallow. Hull et al (1993) report good outcomes for 49 dysphagic patients receiving PEG feedings for an average of 175 days. They measured outcomes in terms of complications in the following three areas: (1) infectious (gastrostomy site infection), (2) mechanical problems (clogged PEG tubes, or tubes or hubs requiring replacement), and (3) gastrointestinal intolerance (nausea and vomiting, diarrhea, and constipation).

In addition to these categories, metabolic status should be monitored (Howard, 1993). Serum electrolyte levels should be evaluated on a regular basis for clients receiving enteral feedings to ensure that they have not developed hyponatremia or hypernatremia, hypokalemia, excess carbon dioxide levels, or hyperglycemia. These compli-

---

*Bender, Faubion, 1985; Dudrick et al, 1984; Kathan, 1985; Pollack et al, 1981; Robb et al, 1983; Steiger, Srp, 1983.

cations of tube feedings are related to factors such as fluid overload, dehydration, diuretic or large-dose insulin therapy, and intake of excessive calories (particularly carbohydrate calories) (Konstantinides, Shronts, 1983). Clients who have just begun enteral therapy will require more frequent assessment of serum electrolyte levels (e.g., weekly) than will those who have been using this treatment modality for longer periods of time (e.g., once every 2 months).

Careful assessment at each visit of any signs of complications or negative emotional reactions is necessary. Auscultating the client's lungs, checking the amount of gastric residual, assessing the condition of the client's nares or the skin around the ostomy site, assessing the client's output (including diarrhea or constipation), and palpating the skin to determine the presence of diaphoresis or edema are important aspects of the evaluation process, as is noting the presence of palpitations (possible indications of the dumping syndrome) (Konstantinides, Shronts, 1983). Table 12-4 lists

Table 12-4   Management of Feeding Tube Complications

Complication	Possible Cause	Suggested Intervention
Pulmonary aspiration*	Feeding tube in esophagus or respiratory tract	Confirm proper placement of tube before administering any feeding; check placement at least every 6-8 hr during continuous feedings.
	Regurgitation of formula	Consider giving feedings into small bowel rather than stomach; keep head elevated 30 degrees during feedings; stop feedings temporarily during treatments such as chest physiotherapy; tint formula with food coloring to make it easier to detect formula in the respiratory tract.
Diarrhea	Antibiotic therapy	Antidiarrheal medications may be ordered if the possibility of infection with *Clostridium difficile* has been ruled out; lactobacillus-containing medications or yogurt are sometimes used in an effort to establish benign gut flora.
	Hypertonic formula or medications (e.g., KCl or medications containing sorbitol)	Deliver formula continuously, decrease volume; dilute enteral medications well; evaluate sorbitol content of medications.
	Malnutrition/ hypoalbuminemia	Dilute formula or deliver slowly initially; use continuous rather than bolus feedings.
	Bacterial contamination	Use scrupulously clean formula preparation and administration techniques; hang formula no longer than 4-8 hr; refrigerate home-prepared, reconstituted, or opened cans of formula until ready to use, and use all such products within 24 hr.
	Predisposing illness (e.g., short bowel syndrome, inflammatory bowel disease, AIDS)	Consider use of elemental formula; use continuous feedings.
	Lactose intolerance	Use a lactose-free formula.
	Fecal impaction	Perform digital examination to rule out fecal impaction with seepage of liquid stool around the obstruction.
	Intestinal mucosal atrophy	Consider use of formula containing fiber or addition of pectin to formula.

From Moore MC: *Pocket guide to nutritional care*, ed 3, St Louis, 1997, Mosby.
*Signs and symptoms of pulmonary aspiration include tachypnea, dyspnea, hypoxia, and infiltrate on chest radiographs.
†Fluids such as cranberry juice or Coca-Cola are sometimes used as irrigants in the mistaken belief that they are better than water at preventing tube occlusion. Research has shown cranberry juice to be inferior to, and Coca-Cola no better than, water.

Continued

Table 12-4	Management of Feeding Tube Complications—cont'd	
Complication	Possible Cause	Suggested Intervention
Constipation	Lack of fiber	Fiber-containing formula may be helpful, unless contraindicated; stool softeners may be ordered.
Tube occlusion	Administration of medications via tube	Avoid crushing tablets and administer medications in elixir or suspension form whenever possible; irrigate feeding tube with water before and after giving medications; never mix medications with enteral formulas, since this may cause clumping of formula.
	Sedimentation of formula	Irrigate tube with water† (Metheny et al, 1988) every 4-8 hr during continuous feedings and after every intermittent feeding; one study (Metheny et al, 1988) found less clogging of polyurethane than silicone rubber tubes; irrigate tubes well if gastric residuals are measured, since gastric juices left in the tube may cause precipitation of formula in the tube; instilling pancreatic enzyme into the tube may clear some occlusions.
Delayed gastric emptying	Serious illness, diabetic gastroparesis, prematurity, surgery, high fat content of formula	Consult with physician regarding whether feedings can be administered into the small bowel, feeding volume can be temporarily reduced, a lower fat formula can be used, or cisapride or metoclopramide can be administered to stimulate gastric emptying.

From Moore MC: *Pocket guide to nutritional care,* ed 3, St Louis, 1997, Mosby.
*Signs and symptoms of pulmonary aspiration include tachypnea, dyspnea, hypoxia, and infiltrate on chest radiographs.
†Fluids such as cranberry juice or Coca-Cola are sometimes used as irrigants in the mistaken belief that they are better than water at preventing tube occlusion. Research has shown cranberry juice to be inferior to, and Coca-Cola no better than, water.

strategies for managing complications of tube feedings (Moore, 1997).

In addition, the nurse should monitor for the sociopsychological effects of the treatment on the family and client. In some unfortunate situations, the stress of the treatment may result in active or passive abuse of the client. For example, the vulnerable client may be left by himself or herself while a tube feeding is being administered by gravity drip, thus risking aspiration. Another example of neglect would be permitting the tube feeding to sit in the feeding bag for so long that it spoils and then administering it.

Parenteral Support   The most common complications of parenteral nutritional support are bacteriologic, mechanical or technical, and metabolic (Rodgers, 1984). The most frequently reported complication is bacteriologic (e.g., sepsis). The source may be the catheter itself or the infusate. Mechanical or technical complications may arise from a malfunctioning pump, kinked tubing, and rarely, displacement of the catheter.

Air embolus is an additional potential hazard, although this is less likely to occur with the use of a micropore filter. Central venous thrombosis is a serious mechanical problem that is a particular risk for clients on long-term home parenteral nutritional support (Veerabagu et al, 1995). This complication is especially problematic because subclinical presentations are more common than clinical presentations of the problem (Veerabagu et al, 1995). Clinical signs of central venous thrombosis include the following (Veerabagu et al, 1995): "1) pain and swelling of the head and neck region or the extremity near the central venous catheter with or without fever; and 2) difficulty or pain on infusing parenteral nutrition." Minidose warfarin has been found to be effective in preventing most thrombotic events while reducing the hemorrhagic complications associated with long-term therapeutic doses of warfarin. For clients who do develop thromboses, switching them to therapeutic warfarin dosages is appropriate (Veerabagu et al, 1995).

Table 12-5	TPN Complications	
Complication	Signs/Symptoms	Intervention
Catheter-related sepsis	Fever, chills, glucose intolerance, positive blood culture	Maintain an intact dressing, change if contaminated by vomitus, sputum, etc.; use aseptic technique whenever handling catheter, IV tubing, and TPN solutions; hang a single bottle of TPN no longer than 24 hr., lipid emulsion no longer than 12 hr.; use an in-line 0.22 μm filter with TPN to remove bacteria.
Air embolism	Dyspnea, cyanosis, tachycardia, hypotension, possibly death	Use Luer-Lok system or secure all connections well; Groshong catheter, which has valve at tip, may reduce risk of air embolism; use an in-line 0.22 μm air-eliminating filter; have patient perform Valsalva's maneuver during tubing changes; if air embolism is suspected, place patient in left lateral decubitus position and administer oxygen; immediately notify physician, who will attempt to aspirate air from the heart.
Central venous thrombosis	Unilateral edema of neck, shoulder, and arm; development of collateral circulation on chest; pain in the insertion site	Follow measures to prevent sepsis; repeated or traumatic catheterizations are most likely to result in thrombosis.
Catheter occlusion or semiocclusion	No flow or sluggish flow through the catheter	Flush catheter with heparinized saline if infusion is stopped temporarily; if catheter appears to be occluded, attempt to aspirate the clot; if ineffective, physician may order thrombolytic agent such as streptokinase or urokinase instilled in the catheter.
Hypoglycemia	Diaphoresis, shakiness, confusion, loss of consciousness	Do not discontinue TPN abruptly, taper rate over several hours; use pump to regulate infusion so that it remains ±10% of ordered rate; if hypoglycemia is suspected, administer oral carbohydrate; if oral intake is contraindicated, physician may order a bolus of IV dextrose.
Hyperglycemia	Thirst, headache, lethargy, increased urination	Monitor blood glucose at least daily until stable; TPN is usually initiated at a slow rate or with a low dextrose concentration and increased over 2-3 days to avoid hyperglycemia; the patient may require insulin added to the TPN if the problem is severe.

From Moore MC: *Pocket guide to nutritional care,* ed 3, St Louis, 1997, Mosby.

Metabolic complications are routinely evaluated during outpatient visits, although the home care nurse must assess for the early development of such problems as well. These problems are more likely to occur after prolonged therapy, although the change in activity for the client recently discharged from the hospital may precipitate problems also. Types of metabolic complications that may occur include fluid or electrolyte imbalances; imbalances of vitamins, trace elements, or fats; weight loss or excessive weight gain; and erratic metabolization of prescription drugs (Grant et al, 1985; Rodgers, 1984). Table 12-5 lists potential complications of HPN and suggested interventions (Moore, 1997).

Overall, evaluation of the client's intake and output, as well as serial measurements of weights, body circumferences, and periodic laboratory tests, provides the most useful data in monitoring the effectiveness of parenteral nutrition. Clients may return for outpatient visits to their physicians as often as biweekly or as infrequently as every 3 months, depending on their clinical stability. Typical evaluative parameters include weights, oral intakes, urine and stool outputs, vital signs, chemistry, and serum enzyme levels (Blackburn, Baptista, 1984; Grant et al, 1985). The home care nurse should be familiar with the results of laboratory testing and any changes in formula, flow rate, or assessment parameters requested by the physician. In addition, a thorough medication history should be obtained to screen for potential drug-nutrient interactions. Carefully recorded flow sheets, which the client brings to follow-up visits with the physician, help minimize confusion and maximize evaluation of the client's progress.

Psychological indices are important to evaluate as well. Often, this is the most disabling aspect for the client. Body image changes with resulting reactive depression, sexual difficulties, delirium, dependency, and sleep disturbances are among the problems for HPN clients that have been noted (Bender, Faubion, 1985; Blackburn, Baptista, 1984; Gulledge, 1985; Rodgers, 1984). One study, which was based on patients' perceptions of psychosocial interferences attributed to parenteral nutritional therapy, found that the majority of the respondents did not report interference with any routine daily activity other than sleep (Robb et al, 1983). The authors concluded that the majority of the patients in that particular program did have a reasonable quality of life and that the supportive atmosphere in the program might be conducive to this kind of adjustment. They noted that "support from family and friends, the HPN team, and other HPN patients is very important" and reported tangible methods of promoting such support. For example, newsletters to which the patients contributed and nightly parenteral nutrition cycles (thus permitting a more normal daily schedule) were part of the program. Johnston (1981) reported that the use of newsletters as a form of support was helpful to clients and families when geographical distances made support groups impractical. Gulledge (1985) has cautioned, however, against assuming that all negative emotional states were reactions to the therapy and has suggested that physical causes for the behavioral manifestations should be considered as well. For example, etiological factors for anxiety states in these clients may include infections, anemia, and fluid or electrolyte imbalances.

Clinical pathways provide a useful tool for monitoring client responses to home parenteral nutritional support. The value of this approach is that it facilitates care coordination and monitors therapeutic efficacy by interdisciplinary teams. Clients can be provided with copies of pathways modified for appropriate readability levels that they can use to promote self-care, and monitoring can be more standardized, promoting cost-effective care. One home care agency has developed disease-specific clinical pathways for enteral support, parenteral support, and transition from parenteral to enteral nutritional support (Ireton-Jones, Orr, Hennessy, 1997). Excerpts from these pathways are shown in Figures 12-4 to 12-6. An evaluation of the use of these pathways over a 1-year period shows an average 22% variance from the pathways. This is close to the recommended 20% average variance level for clinical pathways and suggests that further development of pathways for home nutritional support is warranted (Ireton-Jones, Orr, Hennessy, 1997).

NUTRITIONAL POLICY ISSUES

Numerous issues surround access to home nutritional care, quality and appropriateness of care, and cost of care. Access issues result from reimbursement requirements. Although Medicare, Medicaid, and most third-party payors provide coverage for nutritional support services such as enteral or parenteral nutrition, they may not pay for lengthy services or for the more expensive supplies from which some clients benefit, such as pumps for tube feedings or premixed formulas. Home parenteral nutrition is covered by Medicare Part B as a prosthetic device, although clients must meet the "test of permanency." This requires that the therapy "replace a permanently inoperative internal body organ or its function . . . for a duration of at least 90 days" (Sanville, 1994).

Home Enteral Monitoring

Dates							
Parameters	**Baseline**	**Day 3**	**Week 2**	**Week 3**	**Week 4**	**Week 6**	**Week 8**
Laboratory Studies	Chemical Profile, Mg, CBC, PT				Chemical Profile, Mg, Zn		
CNN Clinical Assessment							
1) Physical & Nutrition Assessment -Pt/therapy compliance	√	√ Phone Contact	√		√		
2) Quality of Life -SF-36	√				√		√
3) Karnofsky Functional Scale	√				√		√
Communications Quarterly Summary							

Dates							
Parameters	**Week 12**	**Month 4**	**Month 5**	**Month 6**	**Month 9**	**Month 12**	**Month 18**
Laboratory Studies	Chemical Profile, Mg, Fe			Chemical Profile, Mg, Fe		Chemical Profile, Mg, CBC, Fe	Chemical Profile, Fe
CNN Clinical Assessment							
1) Physical & Nutrition Assessment -Pt/therapy compliance	√			√		√	√
2) Quality of Life -SF-36				√		√ then every 6 months	
3) Karnofsky Functional Scale				√		√ then every 6 months	
Communications Quarterly Summary	√			√	√	√	

Fig. 12-4   Home enteral monitoring portion of a sample human immunodeficiency virus clinical pathway for home nutrition support for adults. Courtesy Coram Healthcare Corp, Denver.

Home TPN Monitoring

Dates							
Parameters	**Baseline**	**Week 1**	**Week 2**	**Week 3**	**Week 4**	**Week 6**	**Week 8**
*Laboratory Studies**	Chemical Profile, Mg, CBC, PT	Chemical Profile, Mg, CBC, Trig	Chemical Profile, Mg,		Chemical Profile, Mg, CBC	Chemical Profile, Mg	Chemical Profile, Mg, CBC
CNN Clinical Assessment							
1) Physical & Nutrition Assessment -Pt/therapy compliance	√	2-4	0-1	0-1	0-1	√	2/month- 2nd month
2) Quality of Life -SF-36	√				√		√
3) Karnofsky Functional Scale	√				√		√
Communications Quarterly Summary							

Dates							
Parameters	**Week 12**	**Month 4**	**Month 5**	**Month 6**	**Month 9**	**Month 12**	**Month 18**
*Laboratory Studies**	Chemical Profile, Mg, CBC, Fe	Chemical Profile, Mg	Chemical Profile, Mg	Chemical Profile, Mg, CBC, Trig	Chemical Profile, Mg, CBC, PT, Fe	Chemical Profile, Mg, CBC, Fe	Chemical Profile, Fe, CBC (then every 6 months)
CNN Clinical Assessment							
1) Physical & Nutrition Assessment -Pt/therapy compliance	1/month- 3rd month			√ then every 6 months		√	√
2) Quality of Life -SF-36				√		√	√ then every 6 months
3) Karnofsky Functional Scale				√		√	√ then every 6 months
Communications Quarterly Summary	√			√	√	√	

*Protime will be checked when: PT >14.5; Elevated LFT; Patient receiving antibiotics; Patient on anticoagulant.

Fig. 12-5　Home total parenteral nutrition (TPN) monitoring portion of a sample immunodeficiency virus clinical pathway for home nutrition support for adults. Courtesy Coram Healthcare Corp, Denver.

Preauthorization may be required by some managed care and indemnity insurers. Some clients simply may fall between the cracks of coverage. Others have found that, although they may qualify for financial assistance, they may not return to employment without risking loss of their disability coverage with subsequent financial difficulties (Robb et al, 1983).

Quality and appropriateness of care are also related to reimbursement requirements. Allowing sufficient time for the client and family to learn the care involved in nutritional support before discharge from a hospital is an additional problem area. While as long as 2 weeks have been recommended for clients who will be instituting parenteral nutrition, this is costly and, in many cases, impractical from the perspective of reimbursement. Length of service is a particular concern with the initiation of prospective payment for home care. Home health care agencies must

Transition from TPN to Enteral Therapy							
Dates							
Parameters	**Week 1**	**Week 2**	**Week 3**	**Week 4**	**Week 5**	**Week 6**	**Week 8**
TPN Prescription	Progressively decrease days on TPN every 1-2 weeks				Discontinue TPN		
Laboratory Studies	Lytes, Mg, Phos, BUN/Creat	Lytes, Mg, Phos, BUN/Creat	Lytes, Mg, Phos, BUN/Creat	Lytes, Mg, Phos, BUN/Creat		Lytes, Mg, Phos, BUN/Creat	Lytes, Mg, Phos, BUN/Creat
CNN Clinical Assessment							
1) Physical & Nutrition Assessment -Pt/therapy compliance	√	√	√	√			√
2) Quality of Life -SF-36	√			√			√
3) Karnofsky Functional Scale	√			√			√

Fig. 12-6 Transition from total parenteral nutrition (TPN) to enteral therapy portion of a sample human immunodeficiency virus clinical pathway for home nutrition support for adults. Courtesy Coram Healthcare Corp, Denver.

develop strategies that will enable client teaching to be done in an effective and efficient manner. Home care nurses could work with nurses working in ambulatory clinics to develop teaching and preparatory programs on an outpatient basis for nonemergency cases before the initiation of parenteral nutrition in the hospital.

Selection of appropriate nutritional therapy for terminally ill clients with short-term prognoses is an ethical issue and one that is related to quality and appropriateness of care. Home enteral and parenteral nutrition require significant self-care or caregiver involvement and may detract from quality of life for some terminally ill clients in the final stages of illness (Howard, 1993). Cancer patients with metastatic disease and those who are terminally ill may show little benefit from this therapy (Shike, 1996). Shike (1996) reported that studies to date show no clear benefit from home parenteral nutrition either for cancer patients receiving chemotherapy or for cancer patients after surgery (although some studies have shown benefits from administering home parenteral nutrition preoperatively). Terminally ill clients receiving substantial doses of pain medication may not be sufficiently alert to safely manage self-care (Howard, 1993). Howard (1993) noted that the Medicare prosthetic device benefit does not cover simple intra-

venous hydration and electrolyte therapy, so some clients who might otherwise opt for this less intensive form of treatment may instead choose parenteral nutrition. Client autonomy, justice, beneficence, and maleficence are ethical issues related to decisions about using increasingly invasive and technologically intense forms of nutritional therapy in the home and choosing the optimal point along the illness trajectory for using one of these therapies.

Another issue of concern is determination of the legitimate client. Most agencies are organized to deal with individual clients and to receive reimbursement for individual clients, but inevitably, the needs and abilities of the family as a whole influence the client, particularly in the area of nutrition. How can agencies reconcile the resultant problems without denying care to clients?

The use of an interdisciplinary team in the provision of nutritional care in the home is often advocated, but many home health care agencies do not have registered dietitians on their staffs. The American Dietetic Association (1994) urges the addition of a registered dietitian to the staffs of home health care agencies, noting that these professionals are cost-effective from both the agency's and the client's perspectives. One agency has reported the development of screening protocol designed to help nurses identify clients at the highest nutritional risk and consult with the registered dietitian for the development of nutritional plans of care for them (Rebovich, 1981). Also, the dietitians provided in-service education to the nurses in areas such as nutritional assessment. Community-based nurses have long worked with informal networks of multidisciplinary sharing, but more formal linkages such as this may be more effective.

Finally, expansion of nutrition services to vulnerable members of the population is an area of need. The nutrition education mandated by the Older Americans Act amendments of 1984 with the accompanying meal programs is helpful for many elderly, but much more needs to be done. Many elderly individuals do not have sufficient transportation to the services that are available and may not qualify for the meals they need at home. The numbers of soup kitchens available have increased, but hunger continues to be a problem for many younger people as well, compromising the health of women of childbearing years, their children, and the chronically ill.

Some home health care agencies have begun discussing the feasibility of moving into the area of health promotion, and others have initiated adult day care programs. Issues that need to be addressed include the match of these activities with the mission and goals of the agency, overlaps with other local services, and the most cost-effective ways of accomplishing goals related to health promotion. Not the least problematic area is that of reimbursement. Third-party payors are reluctant to fund nutrition education for those on therapeutic diets and can be expected to be most resistant to funding either illness prevention or wellness-oriented education (although some are offering incentives to subscribers who take positive steps in these directions). Private payment for this type of service is certainly feasible, and appropriate marketing may result in heightened public interest.

Nutrition in home care is an area in need of research to determine the most cost-effective and least stressful assessment modalities, nutritional interventions with the least potential for disrupting family dynamics, and coping strategies for those with modified intakes. Because the focus of home care may be either rehabilitative or maintenance (as is the case with some federally funded programs), identifying the most effective and

efficient ways of returning the client to optimal nutritional status requires different strategies for the acutely and the chronically ill. The potential effects of nutritional interventions in the home on family dynamics are unknown and have been recognized as an area where research is needed (Moore, Guenter, Bender, 1986). Also, because so many home care clients are at the age extremes, it is important to identify the best ways to intervene in the client's nutritional status and maintain normal developmental progress. For example, the infant's need for sucking or the adolescent's need to solidify a sense of identity must be nurtured. In addition, it is not known what the minimum daily requirements are for the healthy elderly or what the physical or laboratory norms are for this group (Schneider et al, 1986).

SUMMARY

Nutrition in home care is a key aspect of comprehensive care with the increased acuity level of home care clients, as well as the technological advances that have stimulated more activity in this direction. Nurses must plan their services in an organized fashion, with a view toward planning for future nutritional needs based on demographic and sociopolitical trends. Home health care agencies are ideal centers for research to assist in determining the best approaches to meet these clinical challenges.

REFERENCES

American Dietetic Association: Position of the American Dietetic Association: Nutrition monitoring of the home parenteral and enteral patient, *Journal of the American Dietetic Association* 94(6):664-666, 1994.

Bandura A: Self-efficacy: Toward a unifying theory of behavioral change, *Psychological Review* 84(2):191-215, 1977.

Barkauskus VH et al: *Health & Physical Assessment*, ed 2, St Louis, 1998, Mosby.

Baumann H, Gauldie J: The acute phase response, *Immunology Today* 15(2):74-80, 1994.

Becker MH: *The health belief model and personal health behavior*, Thorofare, NJ, 1974, CB Slack.

Bender JH, Faubion WC: Parenteral nutrition for the pediatric patient, *Home Healthcare Nurse* 3(6):32-39, 1985.

Blackburn GL, Baptista RJ: Home TPN: State of the art, *American Journal of Intravenous Therapy and Clinical Nutrition* 11(2):20-32, 1984.

Boosalis MG et al: Serum copper and ceruloplasmin levels and urinary copper excretion in thermal injury, *American Journal of Clinical Nutrition* 44(6):899-906, 1986.

Boosalis MG et al: Serum and urinary silver levels in thermal injury patients, *Surgery* 101(1):40-43, 1987.

Boosalis MG et al: Serum zinc response in thermal injury, *Journal of the American College of Nutrition,* 7(1):69-76, 1988.

Boosalis MG et al: Relationship of visceral proteins to nutritional status in chronic and acute stress, *Critical Care Medicine* 17(8):741-747, 1989.

Boosalis MG et al: Acute phase response and plasma carotenoid concentrations in older women: Finding from the Nun Study, *Nutrition* 12(7-8):475-478, 1996.

Boosalis MG, Stiles NJ: Nutritional assessment in the elderly: Biochemical analyses, *Clinical Laboratory Science* 8(1):31-33, 1995a.

Boosalis MG, Stiles NJ: Nutritional needs of the elderly, *Surgical Care of the Elderly: Oral and Maxillofacial Surgery Clinics of North America,* 1995b.

Boosalis MG, Stuart MA, McClain CJ: Zinc metabolism in the elderly. In Morley, Glick, Rubenstein, eds: *Geriatric nutrition,* ed 2, New York, 1995, Raven Press.

Bowden VR, Dickey SB, Greenberg CS: *Children and their families: The continuum of care,* Philadelphia, 1998, WB Saunders.

Bray GA: Measurement of body composition: An improving art, *Obesity Research* 3(3):291-293, 1995.

Busby HC, Seiffert W: Management modalities: Gastrointestinal system. In Hudak CM, Gallo BM, Lohr T, eds: *Critical care nursing: A holistic approach,* ed 4, Philadelphia, 1986, JB Lippincott.

Chumlea WC, Roche AF, Steinbaugh ML: Anthropometric approaches to the nutritional assessment of the elderly. In Munro HN, Danford DE, eds: *Nutrition, aging and the elderly,* New York, 1989, Plenum.

Danzig LE et al: Bloodstream infections associated with a needleless intravenous infusion system in patients receiving home infusion therapy, *Journal of the American Medical Association* 273(23):1862-1864, 1995.

Davis JH: Total parenteral nutrition (TPN) at home: Prototype high-tech home care nursing, *Gastroenterology Nursing* 19(6):207-209, 1996.

Decker K: Home parenteral nutrition: Evaluating community services, *Nutritional Support Services* 4(4):14-16, 1984.

Detsky AS: Evaluating a mature technology: Long-term parenteral nutrition, *Gastroenterology* 108(4):1302-1304, 1995.

Dinarello CA: Interleukin-1, *Review of Infectious Diseases* 6(1):51-95, 1984.

Dudrick SJ et al: 100 patient years of ambulatory home total parenteral nutrition, *Annals of Surgery* 199(6):770-781, 1984.

Gallagher-Allred CR: *Implementing nutrition screening and intervention strategies,* Washington, DC, 1993, The Nutrition Screening Initiative.

Gordon AH: *Acute phase response to injury and infection: The roles of interleukin one and other mediators,* Amsterdam, 1985, Elsevier.

Gordon M: *Manual of nursing diagnosis, 1993-94,* St Louis, 1993, Mosby.

Grant JP et al: A home total parenteral nutrition monitoring system, *Nutritional Support Services* 5(3):16-18, 1985.

Grindel CG, Whitmer K, Barsevick A: Quality of life and nutritional support in patients with cancer, *Cancer Practice* 4(2):81-87, 1996.

Gulledge AD: Common psychiatric concerns in home parenteral nutrition, *Cleveland Clinic Quarterly* 52(3):329-332, 1985.

Gunning K, Saffel-Shriner S, Shane-McWhorter L: Medication use and nutritional status in elderly patients receiving home care, *The Consultant Pharmacist* 13(8):897-910, 1998.

Howard L: Home parenteral and enteral nutrition in cancer patients, *CANCER* (suppl) 72(11):3531-3541, 1993.

Howard L et al: Current use and clinical outcome of home parenteral and enteral nutrition therapies in the United States, *Gastroenterology* 109(2):355-365, 1995.

Hull MA et al: Audit of outcome of long-term enteral nutrition by percutaneous endoscopic gastrostomy, *The Lancet* 341(8849):869-872, 1993.

Ireton-Jones C, Orr M, Hennessy K: Clinical pathways in home nutrition support, *Journal of the American Dietetic Association* 97(9):1003-1007, 1997.

Johnston JE: Home parenteral nutrition: The "costs" of patient and family participation, *Social Work in Health Care* 7(2):49-66, 1981.

Kamath S: Nutritional assessment. In Malasanos L et al, eds: *Health Assessment,* ed 3, St Louis, 1986, Mosby.

Kleineman RE, ed: *Pediatric Nutrition Handbook,* Elk Grove Village, Ill, 1998, American Academy of Pediatrics.

Koithan M: Home total parenteral nutrition complications, *Journal of the National IV Therapy Association* 8(3):231-237, 1985.

Konstantinides NN: Malnutrition. In Kneisl CR, Ames SW, eds: *Adult health nursing: A biopsychosocial approach,* Menlo Park, Calif, 1986, Addison-Wesley.

Konstantinides NN, Shronts E: Tube feeding: Managing the basics, *American Journal of Nursing* 83(9):1312-1320, 1983.

Kushner I: The phenomenon of the acute phase response, *Annals of the New York Academy of Science* 389:39-48, 1982.

Loan T et al: Enteral feeding in the home environment, *Home Healthcare Nurse* 15(8):531-536, 1997.

Louw JA et al: Blood vitamin concentrations during the acute-phase response, *Critical Care Medicine* 20(7):934-941, 1992.

Lyman B, Marquardt P: Nutrition screening tool: Development and utilization for home care patients, *Home Healthcare Nurse* 15(12):835-841, 1997.

Martin KS, Sheets NJ: *The OMAHA System: Applications for community health nursing,* Philadelphia, 1992, WB Saunders.

Matsuedea K et al: Therapeutic efficacy of cyclic home elemental enteral alimentation in Crohn's disease: Japanese cooperative Crohn's disease study, *Gastroenterology* 30(suppl 8):91-94, 1995.

McCloskey JC, Bulechek GM: *Nursing Interventions Classification (NIC): Iowa Intervention Project,* ed 2, St Louis, 1996, Mosby.

Metheny N, Eisenberg P, McSweeney M: Effect of feeding tube properties and three irrigants on clogging rates, *Nursing Research* 37(3):165-169, 1988.

Metheny N et al: Testing feeding tube placement: Auscultation vs. pH method, *American Journal of Nursing* 98(5):37-42, 1998.

Moehrlen BA, Wolanin MO, Burnside IM: Nutrition and the elderly. In Burnside IM, ed: *Nursing and the aged,* ed 2, New York, 1981, McGraw-Hill.

Moore MC: *Pocket guide to nutritional care,* ed 3, St Louis, 1997, Mosby.

Moore MC, Guenter PA, Bender JH: Nutrition-related nursing research, *Image: Journal of nursing scholarship* 18(1):18-21, 1986.

Mowe M, Bohmer T: Nutrition problems among home-living elderly people may lead to disease and hospitalization, *Nutrition Reviews* 54(1):S22-S24, 1996.

Munro-Black J: The ABC's of total parenteral nutrition, *Nursing* 14(2):50-56, 1984.

National Task Force on Prevention and Treatment of Obesity, US Department of Health and Human Services, National Institutes of Health. *Understanding adult obesity,* Pub No 94-3680, Washington, DC, 1993, US Government Printing Office.

National Heart, Lung and Blood Institute: NHLBI Obesity Task Force clinical guidelines on the identification, evaluation, and treatment of overweight and obesity in adults: The evidence report, *Obesity Research* 6(suppl 2):51s-209s, 1998.

Orem DC: *Nursing concepts of practice,* ed 5, St Louis, 1995, Mosby.

Papadopoulou A et al: The nutritional response to home enteral nutrition in childhood, *Acta Pediatrica* 84(5):528-531, 1995.

Patchell CJ et al: Bacterial contamination of enteral feeds, *Archives of Disability in Children* 70(4):327-330, 1994.

Patchell CJ et al: Reducing bacterial contamination of enteral feeds, *Archives of Disability in Children* 78(2):166-168, 1998.

Pollack PF et al: 100 patient years experience with the Broviac Silastic catheter for central venous nutrition, *Journal of Parenteral and Enteral Nutrition* 5(1):32-36, 1981.

Rebovich EJ: Innovative home care programs: One alternative for nutrition services, *Home Health Review* 4(2):19-24, 1981.

Rimmer LM: What every home healthcare nurse should know about complementary therapy, *Home Healthcare Nurse* 16(11):760-764, 1998.

Ritchie CS et al: Nutritional status of urban homebound older adults, *American Journal of Clinical Nutrition* 66(4):815-818, 1997.

Robb RA et al: Subjective assessment of patient outcomes of home parenteral nutrition, *American Journal of Hospital Pharmacy* 40(10):1646-1650, 1983.

Rodgers BL: Home parenteral nutrition: Principles and management, *Nurse Practitioner* 8(30):46-52, 1984.

Sanville MH: Initiating parenteral nutrition therapy in the home, *Journal of Intravenous Nursing* 17(3):119-126, 1994.

Schmele JA, Allen MF: A comparison of four nursing process measures of quality in home health, *Journal of Nursing Quality Assurance* 4(4):26-35, 1990.

Schmele JA, Foss SJ: A process method for clinical practice evaluation in the home health setting, *Journal of Nursing Quality Assurance* 3(3):54-63, 1989.

Schneider EL et al: Recommended dietary allowances and the health of the elderly, *New England Journal of Medicine* 314(3):157-160, 1986.

Schwartz R et al: A meta-analysis of critical outcome variables in nonnutritive sucking in preterm infants, *Nursing Research* 36(5):292-295, 1987.

Sebastian JG: Vulnerability and vulnerable populations. In Stanhope M, Lancaster J, eds: *Community health nursing,* St Louis, 1996, Mosby.

Shaughnessy PW et al: Measuring and assuring the quality of home healthcare, *Health Care Financing Review* 16(1):35-65, 1994.

Shike M: Nutrition therapy for the cancer patient, *Hematology/Oncology Clinics of North America* 10(1):221-234, 1996.

Stahl WM: Acute phase protein response to tissue injury, *Critical Care Medicine* 15(6):545-550, 1987.

Stanhope M, Lancaster J: *Community health nursing*, St Louis, 1996, Mosby.

Steel DM, Whitehead AS: The major acute phase reactants: C-reactive protein, serum amyloid P component and serum amyloid A protein, *Immunology Today* 15(2):81-88, 1994.

Steiger E, Srp F: Morbidity and mortality related to home parenteral nutrition in patients with gut failure, *American Journal of Surgery* 145(1):102-105, 1983.

Steiger E et al: Total parenteral nutrition and fluid/electrolyte therapy in the home: Nine years experience, *Cleveland Clinic Quarterly* 52(3):317-327, 1985.

St Jeor ST, Silverstein LJ, Shane SR: Obesity. In Krummel DA, Kris-Etherton PM, eds: *Nutrition in women's health*, Gaithersburg, Md, 1996, Aspen.

Stuart J, Lewis SM: Monitoring the acute phase response, *British Medical Journal* 297(6657):1143-1144, 1988.

Turner NC: Nutritional support at home: Parenteral and enteral hyperalimentation, *Caring* 38(11):21-27, 1984.

US Department of Agriculture, Human Nutrition Information Service: *The Food Guide Pyramid. Home and Garden Bulletin Number 252,* Washington, DC, 1992, Government Printing Office.

Vargas JH, Ament ME, Berquist WE: Long-term home parenteral nutrition in pediatrics: Ten years of experience in 102 patients, *Journal of Pediatric Gastroenterologic Nutrition* 6(1):24-32, 1987.

Veerabagu MP et al: Warfarin and reduced central venous thrombosis in home total parenteral nutrition patients, *Nutrition* 11(2):142-144, 1995.

Wieczorek RR, Natapoff JN: *A conceptual approach to the nursing of children: Health care from birth through adolescence,* Philadelphia, 1981, JB Lippincott.

Wilmore DW: Nutrition and metabolism following thermal injury, *Clinics in Plastic Surgery* 1(4):603-619, 1974.

Wolinsky FD et al: Further assessment of the reliability and validity of a nutritional risk index: Analysis of a three-wave panel study of elderly adults, *Health Services Research* 20(6):977-990, 1986.

13 Complementary Therapies

Donna M. Guyot and Gretchen M. Oliver

OVERVIEW OF COMPLEMENTARY APPROACHES

Harold was feeling hassled. A seasoned home care nurse, Harold was finding it difficult to keep up with organizational changes in his agency, the new forms that had just been introduced, and all the new drugs that he was encountering as he cared for his clients. How was he supposed to be able to answer the many clients that were now asking him about specific herbs for their symptoms or whether or not treatments he had never heard of would help? Harold found himself wondering why so many clients were either using or inquiring about different ways of dealing with their illnesses and symptoms. Harold also wondered just what he, as a home care nurse, should do about it. It would be a fairly safe assumption that Harold is not unlike many other home care nurses whose patients are using herbs and other healing modalities.

Harold is encountering something that is happening throughout the United States as more and more individuals are turning to what can be called *complementary approaches* to health and healing. Contrast Harold's experience with the experience of Sarah, another home care nurse. After over 10 years of hospital nursing, Sarah recently became a home care nurse. An enthusiastic supporter of complementary approaches to health and healing, Sarah has been studying energy healing, imagery, relaxation therapies, the use of herbs, and other healing modalities. Sarah turned to complementary approaches after experiencing some health issues of her own. Using a blend of allopathic and complementary approaches, Sarah finds herself enjoying good health and renewed commitment to her nursing practice. However, because of how quickly clients are discharged from hospitals, Sarah wanted the

opportunity to serve clients in their homes over longer periods of time. Sarah felt she would have more opportunities to incorporate complementary modalities that are within the scope of nursing practice in a home care setting.

After a review of some definitions and a discussion of the most recent information on the prevalence of this phenomenon, some of the major principles and systems of complementary approaches will be highlighted. The remainder of the chapter will then focus on the implications for home health care nursing practice, including complementary modalities within the scope of nursing practice and case histories that demonstrate these principles in practice.

Definitions, Prevalence, and Trends

Even the name, *alternative therapies,* describes how rapidly this area of health care is changing. A landmark study published in 1993 (Eisenberg et al) defined *alternative medical therapies* as "interventions neither taught widely in medical schools nor generally available in U.S. hospitals." Because what is taught in medical schools and what is offered in hospitals is subject to change, what was considered alternative therapy yesterday may be mainstream today. Nurses should question the use of the word *medical* between the words *alternative* and *therapies.* Most of the therapies considered alternative have several significant differences from what is commonly understood to be medicine. A further problem with the use of the word *alternative* is that it indicates an either/or situation. A more favored term today is *complementary.* This term indicates that one approach may be used to complement or add to another approach. The term *complementary* is also relative because it must be understood what is being complemented. In the industrialized nations, biomedicine or allopathy is the dominant health care focus, and approaches to health and healing that are not part of the allopathic focus can be added to facilitate an increased state of well-being in a client. Thus the client would be engaging in complementary therapies. For example, the client who uses inhalers for asthma and also uses acupuncture for asthma is using one approach (acupuncture) to complement the other (Western medicine or allopathy).

In more recent years, the term *integrated health care* has gained favor. This refers to a system, yet to be created, that combines allopathic and complementary approaches in one care delivery system. Many clinicians and researchers believe an integrated health care system would provide the best care for patients. Inadequate research and unresolved issues regarding reimbursement are some of the barriers to providing integrated health care today.

A recent study (Eisenberg et al, 1998) indicates that 42.17% of the U.S. population is using alternative therapies. There was an 8.37% increase in alternative therapy use from 1990 to 1997. According to the researchers, this increase represents a greater proportion of individuals using alternative therapies, rather than an increase in the number of visits per patient to alternative therapy providers. Overall, more women than men use alternative therapies, and currently there is a greater use of alternative therapies by younger and middle-aged individuals than by older individuals. Individuals are also paying enormous sums of money out-of-pocket for alternative therapies because most of these therapies are not yet covered by third-party payors. More than $21 billion was spent on alternative therapies in the United States in 1997.

Although one of three individuals seeing a physician uses some form of alternative therapy, more than 61% of those using alternative therapies do not tell their physicians that they are also using alternative therapies. Individuals used alternative therapies to treat existing illness (42% of the sample, mostly treating chronic illness), and 58% of the sample used alternative therapies to promote health and prevent illness (Eisenberg et al, 1998).

One national survey (Astin, 1998) found that use of complementary approaches to health was not predicted by age, race, income, or education. Contrary to popular belief, this survey also found that individuals were not using complementary approaches because they were dissatisfied with allopathic care. Rather, perceived benefit of the complementary approach and congruency with personal values and beliefs were the most significant reasons individuals gave for using complementary approaches. Most individuals used both alternative and conventional treatments. According to this researcher, "results . . . lend support to the notion that for many individuals, the use of alternative health care is part of a broader orientation and set of cultural beliefs."

More and more medical schools now offer courses on complementary alternative medicine, also known as *CAM*. To date, the number of nursing schools offering curricula on complementary healing is unknown. Another indicator of how important alternative or complementary therapies have become is the creation of the Office of Complementary and Alternative Medicine (OCAM), part of the National Institutes of Health. Founded in 1992 with a budget of $2 million, the OCAM budget in 1999 was $50 million. Currently 10 research centers across the United States are funded, research is moving from emphasis on the exploratory phases to evidence-producing studies, and the OCAM has been renamed the National Center for Complementary and Alternative Medicine (NCCAM) (Marwick, 1998). The mission of NCCAM includes conducting research and serving as a clearinghouse of information about complementary approaches to health and healing.

Harold, the hassled home care nurse, would likely be relieved to know there is a central clearinghouse of information related to complementary approaches to health and healing. Harold would, no doubt, also benefit from a continuing education approach to catch up on the latest information in this field. Of great importance to this dedicated home care nurse will be learning more about how complementary approaches to health and healing relate to his nursing practice. Harold will have much to offer Sarah in terms of orientation to home care nursing, and Sarah will have much to offer the home care team in terms of complementary approaches to health and healing.

PRINCIPLES AND APPROACHES

The phrase *complementary approaches to health and healing* does not simply refer to a variety of healing modalities. *Complementary healing* refers to a set of principles that describe what can be thought of as a world view or perspective. This is a dynamic perspective, and although there are implications for all aspects of living, the focus of this discussion is limited to health and healing. It should be emphasized that healing is not simply achieving the absence of disease. Exactly how *healing* is defined is very important and is relative to who is defining it. Specifically, a provider of complementary healing techniques would want to know how the client, as opposed to patient, defines *healing*. Often the complementary healing provider conceives of healing as restoring balance to the forces within the individual and his or her environment to restore optimal health and well-being.

In this dynamic, complementary perspective, the body is seen as a dynamic energy field within the energy field of the environment, however *environment* may be defined. Symptoms, disease, and disability are seen as processes that are to be understood, not merely eradicated. There is a search for patterns or possible signals of imbalance within the individual and environment fields. Although the individual is not responsible for the disease, the individual must be responsive to it. Emphasis is placed on human values, the professional as a caring partner, minimal intervention and an intervention as natural as possible, client autonomy, the body-mind-spirit perspective, a holistic approach to the whole of the client's life, and the achievement of maximal well-being. There is also significant emphasis on the body's innate healing potential. Most often, the various modalities used in complementary healing work from the principle of stimulating or restoring this innate healing potential. In this model, the healing comes from within the client or patient and is merely facilitated by the practitioner (Ferguson, 1987; Micozzi, 1996).

Does this paradigm shift also require a shift in perspective where research is concerned? On one hand, proponents of complementary approaches to health and healing seem to be advocating that rigorous research is necessary, but how that research is done and the assumptions held about research in biomedicine or allopathy are in question. On the other hand, opponents of complementary approaches to health often complain that adequate rigorous research on complemen-

tary modalities is lacking, and since empirical data to support these modalities are lacking, the modalities should not be used. Although debate of the various ways of "knowing" is beyond the scope of this chapter, it must be pointed out that a significant amount of modern medicine is without empirical data to support the practices that are now standard (Box 13-1).

The scientific paradigm of biomedicine holds that for an observer to "know" something, the dictates of objectivism, reductionism, positivism, and determinism must be present. In other words, the observer must be separate from what is observed, what is "known" must be able to be reduced to its smallest parts and then reconstructed, the phenomena of study must be physically measurable, and predictions must be able to be made from scientific law and the set of initial conditions.

If a clinical phenomenon is observed, such as reduced symptoms of asthma after acupuncture treatment with no additional variable, should acupuncture not be used and not be covered by insurance because there is no explanation for how acupuncture works? Or should the set of assumptions inherent in our scientific paradigm be adjusted instead?

It is already known in physics that the observer is not separate from what is observed. It is known that the synergism inherent in biology and ecology cannot be reduced to its smallest components and then rebuilt. It is also known that not all phenomena are measurable. For example, how is consciousness measured? (Dossey, 1995; Micozzi, 1996).

Box 13-1	History of Medicine
2000 BCE	Here, eat this root.
1000 CE	That root is heathen. Here, say this prayer.
1850 CE	That prayer is superstition. Here, drink this potion.
1940 CE	That potion is snake oil. Here, swallow this pill.
1985 CE	That pill is ineffective. Here, take this antibiotic.
2000 CE	That antibiotic doesn't work anymore. Here, eat this root.

Source: Unknown.

What is at question here is not whether complementary approaches to health and healing should be thoroughly researched and tested, but rather how that research and testing should be done. Additional questions follow: who is going to pay for research and testing, since it is unlikely to reap as great a financial reward as pharmaceuticals? If by clinical observation it is known that something works without causing harm, how much more evidence is needed? Given the trends previously discussed, it appears that the majority of the U.S. population and an increasing number of health care providers are not waiting for more answers before using complementary approaches to health and healing.

Table 13-1 lists important features of several approaches commonly used in complementary healing. These approaches, clustered according to how they are categorized by the NCCAM, are further described.

Table 13-1	Complementary Healing at a Glance		
Approach	NCCAM Category	Underlying Principles	Treatment Modalities
Chinese Medicine	Alternative Medical Systems	Yin and Yang forces are balanced.	Diet, exercise, acupuncture, herbal medicine, acupressure, and moxibustion
Homeopathy	Alternative Medical Systems	Law of Similars can cure disease.	Homeopathic preparations known as *remedies*
Ayurveda	Alternative Medical Systems	Forces of Vata, Pitta, Kelpha are balanced.	Diet, exercise, meditation, and medications
Naturopathic	Alternative Medical Systems	Body's natural healing ability is stimulated.	Diet, exercise, hydrotherapy, massage, herbs, relaxation therapy, and vitamin and mineral treatment
Indigenous healing	Alternative Medical Systems	Various: balance and harmony of spirit, including with community	Herbal treatments, ceremonial healing, prayer, ritual, and laying on of hands
Chiropractic	Manipulative and Body-based Methods	Alignment of spine restores health.	Manual adjustment of spine and body
Massage and bodywork	Manipulative and Body-based Methods	Manipulation of body tissue restores health.	Massage, Rolfing, osteopathy, reflexology, Alexander Technique, Feldenkrais, Trager Method, others
Energy healing	Manipulative and Body-based Methods (Biofield Therapy) and Mind/Body Interventions (Prayer and Mental Health)	Balance and flow of energy in the individual energy field contributes to health.	Healing touch, therapeutic touch, Reiki, Shen therapy, and biofield therapy
Herbalism	Biologically based Treatments	Plant and plant products contain what is needed for healing.	Treatment through herbal preparations
Aromatherapy	Biologically-based Treatments	Essential oils promote health and stimulate body's innate healing potential.	Ingestion, topical application, and inhalation of essential oils

Continued

Table 13-1	Complementary Healing at a Glance—cont'd		
Approach	NCCAM Category	Underlying Principles	Treatment Modalities
Spiritual healing	Mind/Body Interventions	Healing through spiritual intervention	Prayer, laying on of hands, and ritual and ceremonial healing
Imagery	Mind/Body Interventions	Positive images trigger the body's healing response and connect mind/body, conscious, and unconscious to improve well-being.	Imagery used with trained professional
Relaxation therapy	Mind/Body Interventions	Relaxation triggers healing response and increases well-being.	Guided, progressive, autogenic, meditation, biofeedback, others
Bach Flower Remedies	Not classified by NCCAM	Plant essences bring balance to consciousness, creating greater health.	Bach Flower Remedies

Alternative Systems of Medical Practice

Chinese Medicine The Taoist philosophers developed the principles of health and disease in China over 5000 years ago. The first recorded text of Chinese medicine is the 2000-year-old Yellow Emperor's Classic of Internal Medicine, which sets forth a system based on the concept of health as harmony and balance within the individual and between the individual and the universe. The body reflects the same dynamics and is subject to the same governing laws as the universe at large. Balance of the forces of Yin and Yang must be achieved and maintained for optimal health. Diet, exercise, and harmonious thought and feelings are necessary to achieve this balance. Diet principles include balancing Yin and Yang, and exercise is often a form of T'ai Chi or Qigong. Treatment of disharmony, or dis-ease, is often multifaceted, with a client receiving herbal prescriptions that chemically balance the body and acupuncture or acupressure to redirect the flow of energy within the body toward balance (Eliopoulos, 1999; Ergil, 1996).

Homeopathy The physician-chemist Samuel Hahnemann (1753-1843) developed the system of homeopathy. Hahnemann was interested in developing treatments that were less violent and harmful than some of the treatments of the day, such as bloodletting and the use of mercury. Hahnemann felt that the symptoms produced by the body in the presence of disease are evidence of the body's own ability to heal itself, and these symptoms should be encouraged rather than suppressed. Hahnemann developed what is called the *Law of Similars,* which states that like can be cured by like. In other words, substances that produce the symptoms of a disease in a healthy person will, in very dilute concentrations, cure the disease in a stricken individual. Homeopathic preparations are highly diluted substances meant to stimulate the body's innate healing response by causing mild symptoms of a given disease or condition. Combining the correct remedy with the individual's innate healing potential results in healing of the individual. Homeopathy is a holistic system that includes the mental and emotional states of the client and the client's physical condition.

There are now several well-conducted, peer-reviewed studies documenting that homeopathic remedies offer benefit beyond placebo in some conditions. Based on research and clinical observation, the remedies are not harmful. However, the fact that infinitesimally small, and sometimes unmeasurable, doses achieve greater effect than larger doses does not fit the allopathic model and has been an obstacle to the acceptance of homeopathy in the United States. This is less the case in Europe (Jacobs, Moskowitz, 1996; Skinner, 1996).

Ayurveda   The Ayurvedic principles come from India and are over 5000 years old. Like Chinese medicine, Ayurveda emphasizes the balance and harmony of the individual as the basis of health. In the system of Ayurveda, the body has a unique balance of three primary universal forces, or doshas. These are the energy of Vata (air), Pitta (fire), and Kelpha (physical substance). Imbalances in these three energies are thought to originate in the consciousness of the individual. When Vata, Pitta, and Kelpha are in balance within the individual, health is maintained. Keeping the forces in balance requires knowledge of the unique blend of these energies in an individual's body. The Ayurvedic physician has the responsibility of interpreting the individual's need for maintenance of balance by diet, movement, meditation, and treatments (NCCAM, 2000; Zysk, 1996).

Naturopathic   Founded at the beginning of the twentieth century, naturopathy emphasizes the natural ability of the body to restore health. Naturopathic medicine incorporates holistic and preventive perspectives. The mental and emotional states of the client are important in this type of practice, since the natural healing powers of the body may be hindered by emotions and ideas that create stress and imbalance. Depending on the client's condition, diet, vitamin and mineral therapy, herbs, hydrotherapy, massage therapy, acupressure, and relaxation therapy are prescribed as part of the naturopathic practice. Today, naturopathic medicine combines natural healing methods with modern allopathic diagnostic methods (National Center for Complementary and Alternative Medicine, 2000; Pizzorno, 1996).

Indigenous healing   Indigenous peoples around the globe practice healing traditions specific to their own culture. However, there are similarities among the many indigenous healing traditions. Spirituality is emphasized in these healing traditions. There is a belief in a transcendent power, and the healer, often known as a *shaman,* is someone who is trained to alter his or her own consciousness to obtain information from the spirit world to assist an individual or community. The healer may perform any variety of healing ceremonies, may use herbs, may use a variety of techniques such as energy healing or extractions, and may counsel the individual or the community regarding necessary changes in lifestyle to promote and maintain health. Ritual and ceremony serve a variety of functions for the indigenous peoples, including marking major life transitions.

An important common theme among indigenous cultures is that all life is connected and related. Trees, plants, animals, the earth, water, and the air, as a few examples, are felt to have spirit and to be vitally interconnected. This circle of life includes humans, or "two leggeds," but humans are not the center of the circle. We are merely a part of the circle. Life and death are part of the circle also. Some of the implications are that individuals are seen in relation to the social and ecological environment and that the community has an important role in healing work. In fact, illness in an individual may be a result of imbalance in the community. Today there is a growing interest in Native American medicine by American Indians and other people of the United States (Cohen, 1998; Krippner, 1995).

Manual Healing

Chiropractic   Daniel David Palmer (1845-1913) originated the system of chiropractic from a healing practice in Davenport, Iowa. Palmer was looking for a way to heal without the use of drugs, which he considered harmful. While treating a patient in his practice for sudden onset deafness that occurred during heavy exercise, Palmer pushed a misaligned vertebrae on the patient's spine into alignment, and the patient's hearing was restored. Thus Palmer began to experiment with the principle that disease was caused by misalignment of the spinal vertebrae and pressure on the spinal nerves. Health could be returned by restoring proper alignment of the spine. Adjustments are most often done with the hands of the practitioner pushing the spine into alignment. However, some newer systems of chiropractic, such as Network Chiropractic, use energy healing techniques to create the adjustments in the spine.

Today, chiropractic science continues to focus on the relationship between structural changes and their effects on the nervous system. Chiropractic treatment can be useful in the areas of orthopedics, neurology, and sports medicine (NCCAM, 2000; Redwood, 1996).

Massage therapy and bodywork   Massage is an ancient form of therapy in which the soft tissues of the body are manipulated by the hand of the therapist. Massage therapies can affect superficial or deep tissue, depending on the type of massage used by the therapist. Bodywork includes techniques that may teach movement, posture, and balance, as well as manipulate soft tissue. Massage therapy and bodywork have been found to be useful in stress reduction, chronic edema, reduction of anxiety and depression, and recovery from soft tissue trauma. Specific techniques include Swedish massage, Rolfing, Hellerwork, Shiatsu, Feldenkrais, Alexander Technique, and Trager work (Eliopoulos, 1999).

Energy healing   Energy healing is based on the belief in a universal healing energy that can be directed by a trained healer, usually through the hands, to improve a patient's condition. As with many other holistic approaches, balance and harmonious flow of universal energy are equated with health and wellness. This universal energy is known by different names throughout the world. Some of those names are *prana* in India, *chi* in the traditions of Chinese medicine, and *mana* in the Hawaiian indigenous healing system. Two energy healing methods that have gained recognition in nursing are Healing Touch and Therapeutic Touch. Reiki is a Tibetan and Japanese technique that is also a form of energy healing. The theoretical basis for energy healing ranges from ancient Indian texts to the laying on of hands in the Christian traditions to quantum physics. Most nurses cite the work of nurse theorist Martha Rogers as a theoretical basis for energy healing. Since 1995, "energy field disturbance" has been listed as a nursing diagnosis (NANDA, 1995-1996).

Energy healing is classified by NCCAM as a type of manual healing known as *biofield therapy*. However, energy healing is often equated with laying on of hands, which is classified by NCCAM as prayer and mental healing under the category of mind/body control. The presence of spirituality seems to be the key factor in differentiating energy healing, which is a mind/body control approach, from energy healing, which is a manual

therapy. In actual practice, the division between the two categories blurs and individual practitioners may draw from both approaches (NCCAM, 2000; Slater, 1995).

Herbal Medicine

Herbalism   Herbalism, prevalent in ancient cultures around the globe, promotes the study and use of plants and plant products for the cure of disease and enhancement of health. An important component of many systems of healing, herbalism is a holistic practice that takes into account the body, mind, and spirit of each individual and their relationship to their environment. Herbalism embodies the concept that the whole plant or part of the plant, not just the active ingredient, is important in making the healing process more natural, effective, and gentle.

There is a growing interest in and demand for the inclusion of herbalism in health care in the United States, where currently herbs are marketed as food supplements. Some of the barriers to further integration of herbalism include the fact that, unlike European regulations, the United States does not follow the World Health Organization's guidelines, which recognize historical use as a valid method of determining effectiveness and safety. The focus in the U.S. herbal research on a specific active component, rather than on the whole herb as one active component, as is done in Germany, significantly increases the cost of research in the United States (Meserole, 1996; NCCAM, 2000).

Aromatherapy   A French chemist, René-Maurice Gattefossé, is credited with the discovery of aromatherapy. Aromatherapy uses the essential oils, the oils forming the odoriferous parts of plants, for therapeutic purposes. The extracts from many different trees, roots, and flowers can be used. The oils can be used as inhalation therapy, mixed with carrier oils and massaged into the skin, or prepared to be taken internally (orally, vaginally, or rectally).

Aromatherapy has been used since ancient times, and it has been used around the globe. While it has been established by research that some essential oils have an antimicrobial effect and that others can alter brain wave states, research into the use of aromatherapy is incomplete. Aromatherapy is incorporated as part of nursing practice in England, and a good deal of research is being conducted there (Buckle, 1997; Stevensen, 1996).

Mind and Body Control

Spiritual healing   Spiritual healing is a concept found in almost every culture today. Spiritual healing, sometimes referred to as *faith healing,* is healing that takes place by or through spiritual intervention. Spiritual healing may be understood as the intervention of a higher power in answer to prayer, the intervention of ancestor spirits on behalf of the client, the exorcism of harmful spirits, or the actions of spirit guides working through a healer. Founded by Mary Baker Eddy, Christian Science is one of the largest Christian faiths that practice spiritual healing. Medicare has reimbursed practitioners of Christian Science healing for these treatments.

Spiritual healing may or may not involve organized religion. *Religion* can be described as a particular belief system, whereas *spirituality* refers to a search for and understanding of purpose, as well as relationship with, a transcendent power. Individuals may reach for spiritual healing through their personal concepts of god(s) and their relationship in the universe, or through more formal doctrines and ceremonies. A significant body of research has demonstrated benefit of religious commitment, and a well-conducted study documented benefit of intercessory prayer in coronary care unit clients (Eliopoulos, 1999).

Imagery   Imagery is a technique that seeks to influence the mind-body connection by creating images in the mind, that trigger a specific healing response in the body. Imagery is used to facilitate healing of emotional and physical issues. Often one or more senses are involved in the imagery process. In some types of imagery, the images come from the client and can provide greater understanding of disease conditions, achieve relaxation, promote circulation, and link the mind and body of a client to bring about healing. The field of psychoneuroimmunology offers increasing understanding of these mind-body linkages. Relaxation is often used to facilitate the imagery process in the client.

Although use of imagery may require practice by the client, it has been shown to be useful and effective in the healing process. Studies document benefit in cancer, perioperative states, and many other situations. Before using imagery with clients, practitioners should be trained and certified. There are a variety of types of imagery practice, including creative visualization, guided imagery, interactive imagery, and integrative imagery (Eliopoulos, 1999; Miller, 1998; Schaub, Dossey, 2000).

Relaxation therapies   Relaxation therapies use various techniques to achieve a state of deep relaxation through stimulation of the relaxation response. This state of relaxation is characterized by reduced sympathetic nervous system arousal. Deep relaxation has been shown to help with conditions such as chronic pain, insomnia, and hypertension, and there is documented increase in overall well-being. Some of the various types of relaxation therapies include progressive muscle relaxation, autogenic training, meditation, biofeedback, self-hypnosis, and a variety of breathing techniques (Anselmo, Kolkmeir, 2000; Eliopoulos, 1999).

Therapies Not Classified by NCCAM

Bach Flower Remedies   The Bach flower remedies are the work of Dr. Edward Bach (1886-1936), an English physician. Bach believed that the cause of disease was within the personality and character of the client and the healing of disease could be achieved through treatment of the disharmonious and excessive aspects in the client's consciousness. Bach researched the wild flowers and plants in his native English countryside and devised a system of healing using the distilled essences of wild plants and trees. He published his work in 1933 in a volume entitled *The Twelve Healers and Other Remedies.* The Bach Flower Remedies are taken orally in a solution usually preserved with brandy. Only a few drops are taken at a time, and they are held on the tongue until absorbed. Unlike homeopathy, Bach's Remedies do not use the Law of Similars. The Bach Remedies are like the tinctures used in homeopathic medicine in that the amount of plant substance contained within the remedies is very dilute, as it is with homeopathic remedies. Both homeopathic medicine and the Bach Remedies are best understood as the absorption of the vibrational essence of a plant or substance to stimulate changes. The Bach Remedies work to stimulate changes in the personality, emotions, and character patterns of the client.

There is an increasing variety of essences being developed and marketed through health food stores, direct mail, and the internet. Most represent the imprinting of an essential component of a source, such as flowers or crystals, on a base fluid, such as water (Bach, 1952; Weeks, Bullen, 1964).

NURSING PRACTICE AND COMPLEMENTARY APPROACHES

Nursing can be described as the art and science of healing. Nursing has always been concerned with healing rather than curing disease. In ancient times, there was less differentiation between nursing and medicine. From tribal cultures in which a shaman or "wise" village woman (who would later be called a *witch*) tended the sick and injured to midwifery throughout the ages; from the first hospitals that were temples of pagan gods to the religious orders, guilds, and charities of today; from the battlefields of the Crimea and the U.S. Civil War to the apprenticeship models of diploma nursing programs and to today's "science of caring," people have tended their sick with the intent to improve physical and mental well-being and comfort (Brooke, 1997; Donahue, 1985). The reader is certain to notice the commonalities between nursing as the art and science of healing and the principles of complementary approaches to health and healing.

Nightingale's early definitions of *nursing* also reflect some of the previously discussed principles of complementary approaches. Nightingale described nursing as helping people to live and the role of the nurse as putting "the patient in the best condition for nature to act upon him" (Skeet, 1980). As additional evidence of nursing's healing heritage, in the 1960s, Virginia Henderson discussed the role of the nurse in terms of helping move an individual toward health or the recovery of health (Henderson, 1991). With the movement of nursing into higher levels of academia, nursing theory assumed a greater importance, and even early nurse theorists of the twentieth century described nursing as a holistic art and science involved with healing.

Nursing Theory and Complementary Approaches

One of the earliest holistic nurse theorists of the twentieth century was Myra Levine. According to Levine, the goal of nursing is to identify the specific pattern of adaptation of a client and design a plan that would conserve that client's energy, as well as structural, personal, and social integrity. She saw humans as holistic beings in an environment (Chinn, Kramer, 1991).

Moving beyond Levine's description of a holistic human in an environment, the visionary academic, Martha Rogers, described humans as evolutionary beings and stated that humans and nature (environment) are not separate. Ahead of her time, Rogers saw science as humanistic rather than mechanistic and combined principles from branches of science as diverse as anthropology and quantum physics in her theory of nursing. For Rogers, a human being was more than the sum of its parts. She conceived of humans and the environment as two energy fields that are in continuous, creative, noncausal change and interaction. Humans were described as energy fields that were dynamic and without end. Patterns, which continually change, characterize energy fields. Human and environmental energy fields, being in continuous interaction, are always transforming into increasingly diverse and complex patterns. Humans and environments exist on a nonlinear dimension without spatial or temporal bounds. According to Rogers, nursing's goal is to contribute to the achievement of an individual's or a group's greatest possible well-being (Rogers, 1970; Sarter, 1988).

Building on the work of her predecessors, Margaret Newman described health as the expansion of consciousness. Rejecting the dualism inherent in a polarized view of health and disease, and like Rogers, calling on several branches of science, Newman instead saw disease as a meaningful aspect of health and a reflection of the whole. Disease is seen as an integrating factor and is important in the evolution of the individual. Speaking of nursing as a partnership with a client, Newman stressed the importance of the professional's awareness of "being" rather than "doing," as in the fixing of things. The nurse must first observe, learn, and take in what the client is reflecting to ascertain the pattern of the whole, which is what Newman saw to be the focus of nursing. The whole of an individual, according to Newman, is a pattern. The parts of this pattern cannot stand alone; rather, the relationship between the parts is also of great importance. Nursing's task, then, is to help individuals recognize the innate and inherent power within to move to higher levels of consciousness (Newman, 1994).

Holistic Nursing Practice Today

The paradigm shift toward complementary approaches to health and healing is well reflected by the holistic nursing movement. Reclaiming nursing's healing heritage, the holistic nursing movement emphasizes healing the whole person. Using nursing theory, such as that of Rogers and Newman, and theory from other branches of science and using clinical expertise and intuition, nurses partner with their clients to help them move toward greater well-being, whatever that may mean for each individual client.

The American Holistic Nurses Association (AHNA) is the professional organization representing and working for nursing and holistic nurses in particular. Founded in 1981, the organization today offers professional development, networking, curricula, research, scholarships, and a professional journal devoted to holistic nursing, as well as links with other nursing organizations. There is now a national holistic nursing examination, leading to certification by the American Nurses Credentialing Center. The association has also developed standards that define and describe the scope of holistic nursing practice. A major tenet of the AHNA, which is reflected in the standards of holistic nursing, is that the nurse must be committed to self-care. This self-care includes personal and professional development (Dossey, Guzzetta, 2000).

There has been an increase in the number of holistically oriented programs at all levels of nursing education. Some institutions offer optional courses with an emphasis on complementary modalities. A number of complementary modalities are clearly within the scope of nursing practice and are increasingly the focus of nursing research. Common examples include imagery, relaxation therapies, massage therapy, and energy healing.

Perhaps the best known example of a complementary modality within the scope of nursing practice is energy healing. Introduced by Dolores Kreiger into academic nursing in the 1970s, Therapeutic Touch is the best-researched type of energy healing. Healing Touch, which is a combination of energy healing techniques and perspectives, began as a specific program of study in 1989 and has had over 50,000 students (Hutchison, 1999). Currently, a significant amount of research is being conducted on Healing Touch, and

both Therapeutic Touch and Healing Touch are written into nursing policy and procedure in many institutions throughout the United States.

Imagery, another modality well within the scope of nursing practice, is also the subject of increasing study. Some institutions have designed programs that incorporate imagery into perioperative nursing, creating a unique niche for nurses. Other modalities, such as aromatherapy, are pioneering activities for nurses. Although seemingly well incorporated into nursing practice in the United Kingdom and certainly a healing practice that has been used around the globe for centuries, it is yet to be specifically determined whether or not aromatherapy is within the realm of nursing practice according to most of the various state practice acts in the United States. It should be noted that aromatherapy has been approved in some states.

Knowing that certain modalities are within the scope of nursing practice is not the same as knowing the modalities. All these complementary approaches require additional training, education, and experience. In addition, the nurse is well advised to review the state practice act and institutional policy and procedure for the state and institution in which he or she works. A benefit of a professional organization such as the AHNA is that the organization can link an individual nurse with local professional holistic nursing colleagues who can offer much guidance and support in locating quality continuing education programs and promoting the incorporation of complementary modalities in health care institutions. Although some effort is required in the beginning, new roles for nurses are being created as interest in complementary approaches to health and healing increases throughout the country.

COMPLEMENTARY APPROACHES TO HEALING IN HOME CARE NURSING

Our complementary healing–savvy nurse, Sarah, is correct that there are some very attractive features of home care when it comes to incorporating complementary approaches in nursing practice. Despite the increasing complexity of home care clients and despite the many challenges home care nurses face in today's health care system, many aspects of home care are very conducive to using complementary modalities. At home, clients are likely to feel freer to disclose the use of complementary modalities or to add complementary modalities to their existing plan of care.

Home Setting and Complementary Therapy

The home provides a unique setting for the introduction and practice of complementary therapy. In a hospital or clinical setting, clients are removed from their natural environments. They exist in environments created, organized, and sustained for and by professional health care workers. The schedule, activities, food, medicine, and even the time and amount of interaction with family are governed for the client by the institutional setting. Observation and interaction with a client or family in these controlled environments may not reveal key physical, emotional, mental, and spiritual factors that impact the client in their surroundings at home.

In the home setting, the nurse sees the client in the environment in which he or she naturally relates and functions. The nurse is able to observe and interact with the client in the setting that he or she creates and, for the most part, controls. Nurses are better able to understand whether or not the plans they generate for greater health and wellness of their clients will be integrated into their clients' lives. In the home care setting, nurses observe and interact with clients in their holistic totalities. Complementary therapies, which may be applied to nursing diagnoses, may be most realistic and practical in the home setting.

In addition to the client, the home care nurse observes and interacts with the client's family. Today this family might be the traditional mother, father, wife, husband, and/or children, or it might be the client's partner and friends. Whatever its exact make-up, the family is a vital part of the care plan for any home care client. Part of the role of the home care nurse is to empower the family members to participate in the care of the client to the extent that they are able and willing to do so. Therefore the home care nurse must understand the family dynamic and the cultural context in which the client's illness and treatment will take place. Complementary therapies that are acceptable both culturally and personally to the client and the client's family can enhance the ability of the family to participate in the care of the client.

Assessment

Assessment of the home care client must begin with a thorough history and a complete physical assessment. To be useful in determining the appropriateness of complementary approaches for a client or to determine whether or not a client is using complementary approaches, the assessment must include additional information. Important areas of such an assessment include the client's cultural beliefs, spiritual or religious practice, and attitudes and feelings about his or her diagnosis, treatment, and conceptualization of health and healing. In addition, the home care nurse considering application of complementary therapy should obtain information about the client's past and present attitudes toward complementary therapy. If the client has used a complementary therapy in the past and wishes to continue treatment with that therapy, the nurse must evaluate the therapy for possible conflicts with the current medical treatment. Some herbal preparations, for example, may enhance or inhibit the effectiveness of medications that may be part of the treatment plan. It is important to include the client's evaluation of the effectiveness of any complementary therapy previously used and whether or not the client intends to continue using these therapies.

Resource considerations are an important aspect of the assessment. At present, most complementary approaches requiring a licensed provider, such as acupuncture or chiropractic care, are typically paid for by the client, rather than a third party. The home care nurse may need to assess availability of financial resources, insurance status, preferred provider lists, and local resources and referral networks.

Another important aspect of the assessment in relation to complementary approaches to healing is how the nurse approaches the subject. A nonjudgmental attitude in the beginning may go a long way toward eliciting honest responses from the client. It is often helpful to understand why clients desire to explore complementary approaches. Although the home care nurse may not be responsible for determining what a medical evaluation should consist of, he or she is well advised to explore whether or not the client has undergone adequate evaluation of symptoms. Complementary modalities should not delay or prevent needed allopathic treatment. Instead, the home care nurse may be in a position to support an integrated approach.

Serving as a resource regarding the use, safety, and efficacy of complementary modalities can be compared to providing information about medication use, safety, and efficacy. Just as the home care nurse provides information about community resources for transportation, durable medical equipment, and care providers, the nurse may be the client's best link to a network of licensed and professional providers of complementary modalities (Box 13-2). Although the

---

Box 13-2   Resources

American Holistic Nurses Association
    P.O. Box 2130
    Flagstaff, AZ 86003-2130
    1-800-278-AHNA
    www.ahna.org
The AHNA web site provides a multitude of links to relevant topics and web sites.
The National Center for Complementary and Alternative Medicine
    NCCAM Clearinghouse
    P.O. Box 8218
    Silver Springs, MD 20907-8218
    1-888-644-62226
    http://nccam.nih.gov

---

home care nurse is certain to discuss with the client questions to ask of the physician, the nurse should also discuss with the client questions to ask of the provider of complementary modalities. It is also important to review with the client the outcome of any interventions or modalities. Assisting the client with a symptom diary will be very helpful both before and after the implementation of complementary interventions (Eisenberg, 1997; Hughes, 1997).

An assessment tool with a holistic perspective and suitability for use in home care is available (Potter, Guzzetta, 2000), and a validated tool for assessing the human energy field is also available (Wright, 1991). While it may be advantageous to use an assessment tool developed for holistic nursing, most home care assessment tools provide a good foundation to which the previously mentioned areas of focus can be added.

The following case studies profile two home care clients. Their diagnoses, home environments, and major complaints are typical of clients found in home care settings today. The case studies demonstrate how the home care nurse, either experienced in complementary approaches to health and healing or a novice in the field, might assess and develop a plan of care that includes complementary therapies for his or her clients.

CASE STUDIES

GARY

Gary, a 47-year-old gay man who has been HIV positive since 1989, suffers with cytomegalovirus (CMV) retinitis and disseminated CMV, wasting syndrome, and severe peripheral neuropathy. As a result of significant visual impairment, Gary has been referred for ongoing intravenous care. He lives with his partner Peter, who is also HIV positive but in better health. Gary's major complaints are weakness, exhaustion, pain in both feet caused by neuropathy, and occasional nausea and vomiting. Sleeping has become a problem because of neuropathic pain, although once he falls asleep, Gary generally sleeps through the night. Peter has become increasingly focused on Gary's weight, insisting on daily weighing and large meals. Gary finds it difficult to cope with Peter's focus on the need for Gary to eat more and to gain weight.

Gary's medical regimen includes both oral and intravenous medications.

On her first visit to their home, Sarah notes that Gary's partner Peter is very interested and concerned with Gary's care. She concludes from this observation that Peter might be able and willing to learn simple complementary therapies that might be helpful to Gary. After obtaining Gary's history and completing her baseline physical examination, Sarah expands this basic information to include what she needs to know to assess the appropriateness of complementary approaches in Gary's plan of care. She learns that Gary has tried acupuncture for his neuropathic pain and that he found it helpful. Gary also indicated that he would like to continue receiving acupuncture. It will, however, be necessary to coordinate home treatment, since Gary can no longer make it up the steep

Continued

flight of stairs to the office of the acupuncturist. Being aware of possible herb-medication interactions and that the acupuncturist often prescribes herbs, Sarah instructs Gary to inform the acupuncturist of all medications being used. She also discusses with Gary the importance of informing his physician that he will continue acupuncture. Knowing that some physicians are strongly opposed to the incorporation of complementary approaches, Sarah discusses with Gary what he knows of his physician's opinions on this matter. Gary explains that his doctor actually recommended acupuncture because the standard medications used for neuropathy were not adequately controlling Gary's pain and because he had side effects with higher doses. Had the physician not been receptive to complementary approaches, Sarah would support Gary by advocating for his choices as a health care consumer and would review methods of discussing this with his physician. Sarah asks if Peter would like to learn some simple acupressure techniques that might help diminish Gary's nausea. Peter is receptive and enthusiastic, and Sarah hopes this will also help to alleviate the tension between Peter and Gary that seems to result from Peter's frustrated attempts to encourage Gary to eat more food.

Sarah then begins her evaluation of Gary's complaint of difficulty falling asleep. Her questions include an examination of both Gary's diet and his evening routine. She finds that Gary is fond of watching movies at night and usually enjoys several sodas during the evening. Sarah reminds Gary and Peter that movies can be a stimulant, exciting the nervous system and thoughts, and might be a contributing factor to Gary's sleep difficulty. In addition, she notes that there is caffeine in the soda Gary drinks and suggests an alternative that contains no caffeine. She asks Gary if he would be interested in trying a technique that is likely to assist him with falling asleep. She describes a simple imagery exercise that Gary could either do by himself, with Peter, or by using a personalized cassette recording. Peter indicates that he would like to offer this type of assistance to Gary, and they both ask Sarah to teach them more about imagery to promote sleep. Sarah records in her plan that this will be a focus of the next visit.

During her assessment of Gary's diet, Sarah observes a pattern of large meals taken three times daily. She listens to Peter's frustration as he describes Gary's resistance to his efforts. Sarah suggests that Gary try eating smaller, more frequent meals and avoid consuming large amounts of food and soda late in the evening because this could contribute to difficulties falling asleep. Finally, Sarah asks Gary if he might be interested in energy healing. She explains energy healing and how it works. Gary and Peter are less enthusiastic but are willing to consider trying energy healing if they could get more information. Sarah promises to bring information about Healing Touch on her next visit.

With this assessment, Sarah is able to develop a plan of care that includes active participation of Gary's partner, addresses the major complaints of the client, and includes safe and acceptable complementary therapies. Most of the conversation between Sarah, Gary, and Peter takes place during Gary's routine intravenous care. This allows Sarah to complete a thorough assessment, including complementary approaches, without adding significant time to the visit.

ALISON

Alison, a 51-year-old woman, recently underwent mastectomy and radiation for cancer of the right breast. Currently she is receiving chemotherapy, necessitating home care nursing for care of her venous access. She is of American Indian ancestry and lives with her husband and two children. Both her children are in college and are available to help with her care on a part-time basis. She states she is hopeful about her prognosis, as is her family, but she is frightened at the possibility of a recurrence, and she lies awake at night afraid she will die and not live long enough to see the grandchildren she hopes to have. Her major problems are weakness and tenderness at the surgical site, swelling of her right hand and forearm, and anxiety and depression.

During the examination, Harold notes significant lymphedema of Alison's right hand and arm. The swelling has made it difficult for Alison to meet some of her daily care needs. Having just learned about new approaches to lymphedema, Harold discusses the possibility of therapeutic massage and Alison readily agrees. Because of the particular insurance coverage and the provider network available to Alison, a referral can easily be made and Harold does so.

As Harold completes his physical assessment, Alison begins to talk about the fact that she is having difficulty sleeping. Sometimes Alison feels so scared and anxious that she begins breathing fast, becomes dizzy, and starts to panic. Other times Alison is tearful and depressed. She is resistant to mental health evaluation and states she absolutely does not want to take more medications. Besides, her doctor told her this was often part of dealing with a cancer diagnosis. Harold wonders if Alison has maintained any cultural ties with her American Indian heritage, and he asks Alison about it. Alison becomes tearful and tells Harold that she has not had much contact with her cultural and spiritual traditions since childhood but that she has very fond memories of gatherings and ceremonies that her great-grandmother conducted. Harold suggests that Alison might consider seeking support from her cultural traditions. As Harold leaves, Alison resolves to contact her mother and ask for support from their tribal elders. While Harold will be referring Alison to others to address her needs, Harold has identified physical, emotional, and spiritual issues that need to be included in Alison's plan of care.

Planning, Intervention, and Evaluation

As with most aspects of home care nursing, planning the client's care must take into account the uniqueness of the individual client and the environment in which the client exists. Based on the assessment, individualized plans are formulated for each identified problem. Although incorporating complementary approaches to healing creates a wider range of available options, planning is essentially the same standard process. The client's role as co-planner is emphasized in complementary approaches to healing.

The nurse may carry out complementary interventions, since several complementary modalities are well within the scope of nursing practice. In some situations, an agency policy and procedure may be required. The plan of care may include the need for the nurse to refer the client to qualified practitioners, with the nurse then serving as a case manager coordinating the care. Complementary interventions will need to be prioritized and are very often introduced in phases. This prevents a client from feeling overwhelmed and confused. As every home care nurse knows, too much information or stimulation at one time leads to decreased effectiveness of teaching.

Evaluation is a dynamic and ongoing process. Probably the most significant factor to consider is that once a client has been referred to a complementary practitioner, the home care nurse's role is not complete. Ongoing evaluation is the responsibility of the nurse whether or not the nurse is actively involved in implementing the intervention described in the plan. Open lines of communication between complementary and conventional providers of care are necessary to ensure optimal client outcome. The case studies of Gary and Alison will illustrate how Sarah and Harold put these principles into action.

CASE STUDIES

GARY

Sarah returns to the office with the completed assessment of Gary from her visit this morning. Using the standard care planning form, Sarah designs a plan reflecting Gary's need for teaching and support in his intravenous therapy. Taking care to respect Gary's needs and wishes, she makes certain that her plan includes interventions to meet his need for pain control, nutritional support, and disturbances in sleep patterns. Sarah incorporates the complementary therapies that were of interest to Gary. Remembering his interest in acupuncture and his intention to continue treatment at home, Sarah adds this information to the plan. She documents her patient's positive past results with this complementary approach and notes her case-management role as coordinator of continuing treatment at home. She is careful to include the follow-up with Gary, which must be done to evaluate the effectiveness of acupuncture as a complementary approach to his pain. Finally, Sarah reminds herself to be sure to inform Gary's physician of his decision to continue acupuncture as part of his treatment plan.

Sarah then turns to the teaching portion of her plan of care for Gary. There is a need for teaching in many areas. During the assessment visit, Sarah began the instruction to assist Gary and Peter with the nutritional problems Gary has been having. She documents her teaching concerning Gary's diet—eating smaller, more frequent meals and avoiding caffeine late in the evening—and notes within her plan the follow-up evaluation that she must do. Acupressure was discussed during her assessment of Gary's nausea, and in the care plan, she includes her intention to instruct both Gary and Peter in the use of two forearm points that have been documented to relieve nausea. In discussing sleep disturbances, both Gary and Peter expressed interest in learning more about imagery. Sarah includes instruction about the use and effects of imagery as part of the plan and makes a note to bring an information sheet about imagery to the next visit. As promised, Sarah will also bring information about energy healing to the next visit with Gary.

Demonstrating a collaborative relationship, when Sarah speaks with Gary's physician, she mentions that Peter seemed exhausted and yet desires to be involved in Gary's care. The physician validates Sarah's observation and concurs with Sarah's plan to refer Peter to practitioners for support in coping with the significant stress he is experiencing. Sarah completes her plan of care by prioritizing the tasks, including the teaching that will be required. She decides that arranging the acupuncture at home is a priority to help reduce Gary's pain, which has not been completely controlled by medication. In addition, Sarah plans to introduce imagery to Gary and Peter by supplying

Continued

them with written information and by conducting a brief imagery session with Gary while Peter observes. This initial imagery session would introduce the process to Gary and his partner, allow Gary to experience a sense of deep relaxation, and assist Gary and Peter with determining how imagery would best serve their needs. In addition, the initial imagery session will allow Sarah to evaluate Gary's response to this intervention. Depending on Gary's response, on subsequent visits Sarah would begin teaching some simple imagery techniques to Gary and Peter so that they could use this whenever needed and especially at night to promote sleep. After evaluating his response to her dietary education aimed at controlling the nausea that was not completely responsive to medication, Sarah may or may not decide to teach Gary and Peter about the acupressure points used for nausea.

On the second visit, Sarah will begin the process of evaluation and ongoing assessment. It is as important for her to evaluate the effectiveness of the complementary approaches she has included in her plan as it is to evaluate the items in Gary's standard plan of care. Sarah decides that she will evaluate the neuropathic pain each visit and asks Gary if he would be willing to keep a pain diary to document the pain he experiences each day. Over time, this diary will give Sarah a valuable tool in her evaluation of the effectiveness of his home acupuncture. She will also reevaluate his nausea and his sleep patterns. Sarah will evaluate Gary's progress with and response to imagery. If acupressure techniques are taught, Sarah will also evaluate Gary's response to that intervention. With Sarah's nursing experience, she knows that much of this evaluation can be accomplished in conversation with Gary during his intravenous care. By using a conversational style rather than a formal style, Sarah can efficiently gather the information she needs while enjoying getting to know her unique client.

ALISON

Harold returns to the office about the same time as Sarah. As he completes the plan of care, Harold realizes that he has been able to address two of Alison's major problems with complementary approaches. He documents his observations of lymphedema and, after consulting with Alison's physician, his referral to a massage therapist trained in manual lymphatic drainage massage. Having identified Alison's anxiety and her documented mild depression, as well as Alison's refusal of medication for this, Harold notes in his plan of care that Alison will be contacting healers and elders of her great-grandmother's tribe. This documentation in the plan of care will help him remember to evaluate whether or not Alison has followed through with her plan, to positively reinforce her plan, and to evaluate the status of her anxiety and depression. Harold tells Sarah about his client's background and his suggestion that contact with her native traditions might be helpful. Sarah is impressed and validates Harold for his creative thinking. She reminds him that if evaluation of Alison's response to the massage treatment does not show improvement, he has properly documented these areas in his plan of care, and he can look for other possible solutions to discuss with Alison's physician.

Harold plans to evaluate Alison's lymphedema at every visit. Although the symptoms of anxiety and mild depression are troubling to Alison, Harold is aware that it likely will take longer than the 3 days until his next visit for Alison to arrange a visit with the healers and elders of her great-grandmother's tribe. He does plan to evaluate her anxiety and depression and ask if she has made plans to contact the healers and elders. It will be easy to discuss this during her intravenous care, and Harold is looking forward to learning more about her native heritage and how she will be using this to improve her well-being.

SUMMARY

Complementary approaches to healing are becoming more widespread in the United States each year. Rich cultural blends of many healing traditions are present in the diversity of the U.S. population, and this diversity is offering new concepts about the meaning of disease and health to all. As home health care professionals, nurses are in a unique position to assess and evaluate clients for use of complementary healing. By maintaining a nonjudgmental attitude toward these healing traditions, nurses can support clients' individuality and cultural diversity, empower clients and their families to participate in their own plan of care, and enrich their own experiences as nurses. As more is being written about complementary healing traditions and as resources for learning expand, it is becoming easier for nurses to obtain the training or certification they need to be knowledgeable in this realm.

REFERENCES

Anselmo J, Kolkmeir LG: Relaxation: The first step to restore, renew, and self-heal. In Dossey BM et al, eds: *Holistic nursing: A handbook for practice,* ed 3, Gaithersburg, Md, 2000, Aspen.

Astin JA: Why patients use alternative medicine: Results of a national study, *Journal of the American Medical Association* 279(19):1548-1553, 1998.

Bach E: *The twelve healers and other remedies,* Essex, England, 1952, CW Daniel.

Brooke E: *Medicine women: A pictorial history of women healers,* Wheaton, Ill, 1997, Quest Books.

Buckle J: *Clinical aromatherapy in nursing,* London, 1997, Arnold.

Chinn PL, Kramer MK: *Theory and nursing: A systematic approach,* St Louis, 1991, Mosby.

Cohen K: Native American medicine, *Alternative Therapies in Health and Medicine* 4(6):45-57, 1998.

Donahue MP: *Nursing: The finest art,* St Louis, 1985, Mosby.

Dossey BM, Guzzetta CE: Holistic nursing practice. In Dossey BM et al, eds: *Holistic nursing: A handbook for practice,* ed 3, Gaithersburg, Md, 2000, Aspen.

Dossey L: How should alternative therapies be evaluated? *Alternative Therapies in Health and Medicine* 1(2):6-10, 79-85, 1995.

Eisenberg DM: Advising patients who seek alternative medical therapies, *Annals of Internal Medicine* 127(1):61-69, 1997.

Eisenberg DM et al: Unconventional medicine in the United States: Prevalence, costs and patterns of use, *New England Journal of Medicine* 328(4):246-252, 1993.

Eisenberg DM et al: Trends in alternative medicine use in the United States, 1990-1997: Results of a follow-up national survey, *Journal of the American Medical Association* 280:1569-1575, 1998.

Eliopoulos C: *Conventional and alternative therapies for the care of chronic conditions,* St Louis, 1999, Mosby.

Ergil KV: China's traditional medicine. In Micozzi MS, ed: *Fundamentals of complementary and alternative medicine,* New York, 1996, Churchill Livingstone.

Ferguson M: *Aquarian conspiracy: Personal and social transformation in our time,* ed 2, Los Angeles, 1987, JP Tarcher.

Henderson VA: *The nature of nursing: Reflections after 25 years,* New York, 1991, National League for Nursing.

Hughes EF: Alternative medicine in family practice: It's already mainstream, *Family Practice Recertification* 19(10):24-44, 1997.

Hutchison CP: Healing touch: An energetic approach, *American Journal of Nursing* 99(4):43-48, 1999.

Jacobs J, Moskowitz R: Homeopathy. In Micozzi MS, ed: *Fundamentals of complementary and alternative medicine,* New York, 1996, Churchill Livingstone.

Krippner S: A cross-cultural comparison of four healing models, *Alternative Therapies in Health and Medicine* 1(1):21-29, 1995.

Marwick C: Alterations are ahead at the OAM, *Journal of the American Medical Association* 280(18):1553-1554, 1998.

Meserole L: Western herbalism. In Micozzi MS, ed: *Fundamentals of complementary and alternative medicine,* New York, 1996, Churchill Livingstone.

Micozzi MS: Characteristics of complementary and alternative medicine. In Micozzi MS, ed: *Fundamentals of complementary and alternative medicine,* New York, 1996, Churchill Livingstone.

Miller T: The value of imagery in perioperative nursing, *Seminars in Perioperative Nursing* 7(2):108-113, 1998.

National Center for Complementary and Alternative Medicine (NCCAM): Fields of practice. In What is CAM? [on-line]. http://nccam.nih.gov/nccam/what-is-cam/2000.

Newman MA: *Health as expanding consciousness,* New York, 1994, National League for Nursing.

North American Nursing Diagnosis Association (NANDA): *NANDA nursing diagnoses, definitions and classification,* Philadelphia, 1995-1996, The Association.

Pizzorno JE: Naturopathic medicine. In Micozzi MS, ed: *Fundamentals of complementary and alternative medicine,* New York, 1996, Churchill Livingstone.

Potter PJ, Guzzetta CE: The holistic caring process. In Dossey BM et al, eds: *Holistic nursing: A handbook for practice,* ed 3, Gaithersburg, Md, 2000, Aspen.

Redwood D: Chiropractic. In Micozzi MS, ed: *Fundamentals of complementary and alternative medicine,* New York, 1996, Churchill Livingstone.

Rogers ME: *An introduction to the theoretical basis of nursing,* Philadelphia, 1970, FA Davis.

Sarter B: *The stream of becoming: A study of Martha Rogers' theory,* New York, 1988, National League for Nursing.

Schaub BG, Dossey BM: Imagery: Awakening the inner healer. In Dossey BM et al, eds: *Holistic nursing: A handbook for practice,* ed 3, Gaithersburg, Md, 2000, Aspen.

Skeet M: *Notes on nursing: The science and the art,* Edinburgh, 1980, Churchill Livingstone.

Skinner S: The world according to homeopathy, *Journal of Cardiovascular Nursing* 10(3):65-77, 1996.

Slater VE: Toward an understanding of energetic healing. I and II. *Journal of Holistic Nursing* 13(3):209-238, 1995.

Stevensen CJ: Aromatherapy. In Micozzi MS, ed: *Fundamentals of complementary and alternative medicine,* New York, 1996, Churchill Livingstone.

Weeks N, Bullen V: *The Bach flower remedies,* Singapore, 1964, Kyodo Printing.

Wright SM: Validity of the human energy field assessment form, *Western Journal of Nursing Research* 13(5):636-647, 1991.

Zysk KG: Traditional ayurveda. In Micozzi MS, ed: *Fundamentals of complementary and alternative medicine,* New York, 1996, Churchill Livingstone.

14 Cultural Competence in Home Care

Carmen J. Portillo

The complexity of the home care environment increasingly challenges home care nurses because of the many factors they must consider in caring for clients from ethnically diverse communities. People from many different backgrounds are being woven into the tapestry of health care delivery, with each cultural thread a different color, shape, size, and texture. From the inner cities to the most rural areas of the United States, home care nurses are caring for clients who no longer resemble the majority population. These nurses need to be mindful of culturally specific assessments and interventions that must be made and implemented. Because rapidly changing demographics in U.S. society enhance cultural diversity, there is an urgent need for culturally sensitive nursing care, especially in the home care environment.

Culture is defined as "that complex whole which includes knowledge, belief, art, morals, law, custom and any other capabilities and habits acquired by man as a member of society" (Tylor, 1992). Home care nurses will continue to face some of the greatest demands for quality and cost-effective services as health care continues to move into community-based settings. For these nurses, the challenges of providing quality nursing care will involve more clients who do not speak English or who are from a different cultural background. For example, in today's economic climate, home care visits and the amount of time a nurse spends per client have been compressed. Therefore the client's cultural beliefs, values, and health practices can no longer be ignored or generalized, but must be integrated in the overall care of the client.

The purpose of this chapter is to provide home care nurses with practical information on cultural competency. A brief overview of cultural competence and its relevance to home care are discussed. *Cultural skill acquisition* is defined, and the importance of cultural information is presented. Specific strategies in communicating with clients who have limited English proficiency (LEP) are outlined. A guide for cultural assessment is discussed, and a case study concludes the chapter. There are many cultural assessment models and tools useful in becoming culturally competent. Covering all of them is beyond the scope of a single chapter. The references listed at the end of the chapter offer additional resources in cultural assessment and competency.

CULTURAL COMPETENCE

Cultural competence is defined as a "set of congruent behaviors, attitudes, and policies that come together in a system, agency, or among professionals and enable that system, agency, or those professionals to work effectively in cross-cultural situations" (Cross et al, 1989). Another definition of cultural competence more specific to nursing suggests that nurses must be sensitive to issues related to culture, race, gender, sexual orientation, social class, and economic situation (Meleis et al, 1995). Just as there are several definitions of cultural competence, there are several ways of referring to health care that are tailored to sociocultural characteristics of a particular client or group: culturally compatible, culturally appropriate, culturally sensitive, culturally responsive, and culturally informed. Some critics argue that a nurse cannot be culturally "competent" if the nurse is not from the same group as his or her client or at least fluent in the client's language. *Culturally competent* implies that the home care nurse is aware and sensitive and has the ability to intervene appropriately and effectively, whereas *culturally sensitive* does not necessarily imply the ability to intervene in a culturally appropriate manner.

CULTURAL NURSING SKILL ACQUISITION

Cultural nursing skill acquisition is a multifaceted process—one that is described from objective, subjective, and contextual views (Lipson, Steiger, 1996). Objectively, the home care nurse focuses on the client's, family's, and community's cultural and social characteristics, including communication patterns and global perspectives. Subjectively, this suggests an internal focus for the home care nurse. What are the nurse's own values, beliefs, and patterns of communication? What does the nurse know about a particular ethnic, religious, or political group? Time is spent on developing internal awareness and discovering the nurse's own cultural baggage and requires time, effort, and guidance. As the learning process begins, guidance from a skilled, culturally competent clinician is often necessary to provide feedback through a "reflection" process.

Contextually, the home care nurse examines the client from a macrosystems level. What are the socioeconomic and political influences affecting the client? These sociopolitical factors are dictated to the home care nurse by the macrosystems of the Health Care Financing Administration (HCFA) and insurance companies. How are those factors related to receiving home care services? Usually, there is an acceptance to go out and do the necessary skills. Another aspect of the contextual process is the immediate environment of the client. Visiting a client in the privacy of his or her own home helps the home care nurse better understand how the client may interpret or respond to delivery of home care nursing.

IS THIS ALL I NEED TO KNOW?

Information about a specific cultural or ethnic group is not all that one needs to know to provide good care, but neither can good care be provided in the absence of information (Lipson, Dibble, Minarik, 1996). The key to delivering quality home care nursing at the client level is being informed about a client's sociocultural background and being competent to integrate preventive interventions and management of health and illnesses for the individual client and for the family. Concomitantly, the essence of promoting high-

quality care indirectly for client aggregates is understanding the multiple facets of the sociocultural background of a group and consulting with other health care providers in the community.

Cultural information by itself can interfere with nursing service if home care nurses use it in a cookbook fashion and indiscriminately apply cultural facts to a client from a particular ethnic group (Lipson, Dibble, Minarik, 1996). Such an approach can be offensive to clients. It can also lead to stereotyping clients if the home care nurse lacks self-awareness, is ethnocentric, or fails to recognize that variability exists within every cultural group.

What is stereotyping? Stereotyping is making an assumption about a person based on group membership without learning whether or not the person fits the assumption. For example, a home care nurse who assumes that primary staples in the diet of the elderly Hispanic/Latino client are beans and corn tortillas is stereotyping. In contrast, generalizing starts with the assumption about a group but leads to learning further information about whether the assumption fits the individual. In the just cited example, the home care nurse may learn that her client's diet does not include beans and corn tortillas if she discovers that her patient's cultural heritage is Puerto Rican, a group that does not have corn tortillas in their diet.

Nurses subscribe to cultural beliefs, values, and practices from their own heritage. Knowing that age, education, and individual personality influence the expression of culture is critical in providing culturally competent home care nursing. Without sufficient knowledge or experience with cultural groups, stereotyping results, with conclusions based on a lack of data and experience with a cultural group. In this instance, it is better to reserve judgment than to make a judgment. The paradox in becoming culturally competent is that there is always much more to learn (Lipson, Dibble, Minarik, 1996).

COMMUNICATING WITH CLIENTS WHO HAVE LEP

Language is an important component of culturally competent care (Villarruel, Portillo, Kane, 1999). It is the foundation for the nurse-client relationship and is the medium for interpersonal and cross-cultural communication. Language is essential for obtaining an accurate comprehensive client and family assessment, formulating and implementing a treatment plan, determining the efficacy and acceptability of nursing care, and evaluating associated outcomes. Differences in language between nurse and client make clear and accurate communication difficult to achieve. The nurse-client relationship is less than optimal, and nursing care, client outcomes, and client satisfaction suffer.

Language differences are a result of demographic changes and immigration trends in the United States. Home care nurses increasingly face the challenge of communicating with LEP clients. Until recently, only a few languages could be heard in the United States. Now there are more than 300 different languages spoken in both rural and urban areas of the United States (Perkins et al, 1998). Spanish is the predominate language spoken by non-English speakers (US Bureau of the Census, 2001). According to the Census Bureau (US Bureau of the Census, 1996), 17.3 million (54%) of all non-English speakers in the United States speak Spanish in the home, and 8.3 million report that they speak English less than "very well."

To communicate effectively with clients who speak limited English, home care nurses must be aware of the different options for addressing language differences and the variable advantages and disadvantages of each approach. There are several approaches for addressing language barriers in home care settings, but it is important to recognize that not all strategies are adequate. The following are only a few approaches available in caring for clients with LEP.

Getting By

Home care nurses and other health care professionals often use gestures, facial expressions, a change in voice volume, or the use of a few key words or phrases in the target language to "get by" when communicating with clients with LEP (Baker et al, 1996; Ginsberg et al, 1995). For example, home care nurses elicit information regarding a client's pain by pointing to an area of the body and making grimaces as if in pain or using the word for pain in the target language.

This method of communicating is often used when there is no one available who speaks the client's language. However, this approach should only be used when basic or uncomplicated information is being exchanged. The risk of miscommunication is high when using this method, particularly if the home care nurse is attempting to elicit extensive and complex information from the client. Home care nurses sometimes use this method of communication inappropriately because of the perceived inconvenience of using other methods of interpretation. Nurses may also overestimate their ability to "get by" in the target language (Ginsberg et al, 1995).

Ad Hoc Interpreters

It is quite common for home care nurses to use an available bilingual family member or friend as an interpreter when communicating with clients with LEP. Advantages of this approach include the availability of a family member or friend when making a home visit. Family and friends also serve as sources of client and cultural information because they are likely to know the client or be from the same sociocultural background, which may be comforting to the client.

However, the use of family members or friends as interpreters can compromise communication and ultimately affect client care. Family members or friends often base their messages to both the client and home care nurses on their own interpretation of the situation and may withhold vital information they believe may embarrass the client. They may lack the ability to speak and understand English well or to understand health care terminology and procedures. The ad hoc interpreter may omit information or add erroneous information; substitute incorrect terms, numbers, names, or interpretation of client concerns; condense information; or inappropriately assume the role of the client (Putsch, 1985; Vasquez, Javier, 1991).

Ethical considerations are important to consider when a family member or friend acts as the interpreter. Since an ad hoc interpreter is not bound by any code of conduct, he or she may interpret, editorialize, or deliberately withhold information perceived as embarrassing or upsetting from either the client or the home care nurse. The interpreter may also breach confidentiality. Situations involving domestic violence or abuse, gynecological problems, reproductive health, and sexually transmitted diseases pose potential limitations for using an ad hoc interpreter. When a family member or friend is used as an interpreter, clients may be unwilling to disclose private information crucial to the delivery of home care nursing.

Home care nurses may have to use a young child as an interpreter because that is the best option at the time. In this case, the nurse should keep to what really needs to be accomplished. A child's developmental level and associated linguistic limitations, the risk of exposure to inappropriate information and misinterpretation of complex information, and the potential of disrupting familial relationships and hierarchies that are deeply rooted in culture strongly suggest that it is inappropriate to use children as interpreters (Woloshin et al, 1995).

Community Volunteers

Home care agencies often use volunteer interpreters from community agencies, church groups, and local neighborhood affiliations (Ginsberg et al, 1995). Advantages of using volunteer interpreters include the low initial costs, familiarity with health-related terminology, and frequently, the assumption of the role of client advocate. Some limitations of using community volunteers include lack of proper medical interpreting skills or ethical training in interpreting, wide variability in the quality of skills, and limited availability of volunteer interpreters.

Professional Interpreters

The term *professional,* as applied to health care interpreters, is loosely defined because there are currently no standards of practice. However, several states, including Washington and Massachusetts, have implemented testing and certification of social service interpreters and practice standards for medical interpreters (Massachusetts Medical Interpreters Association, 1995; Professional Language Certification Examination Manual, 1995).

Hospital-based home care agencies may provide professional interpreters, but prohibitive costs make this approach less used among home care nurses. Professional interpreter services are usually contracted for directly with the home care agency. Although qualifications and quality vary considerably among "professional" interpreters, the caliber of their services is generally higher than that of ad hoc and community volunteer interpreters. Professional interpreters are reliable and are typically bound by a code of conduct.

Telephone Language Lines

Interpreting services are also provided on telephone language lines. Some home care agencies may use telephone interpretation services, such as the AT&T Language Line Services and Pacific Interpreters, Inc., that are equipped to provide access to interpreters in more than 140 languages 24 hours a day, 7 days a week. Language line interpreters have received training in medical interpreting and have been tested for linguistic competency and medical terminology. They are bound by a code of ethics and are usually covered by liability insurance.

Critics of this approach state that telephone interpreting is appropriate only for exchanging basic information and not for conveying sensitive news. The language line interpreter is likely to miss the nuances of body language and facial expression and is forced to depend solely on the content and tone of the conversation (Swaney, 1997).

The high costs associated with this approach may dictate that home care nurses rely on it as a last resort or in an emergency situation. As the national payment rate for home care is reduced and home care visits are decreased, the telephone language line concept may be revisited as a substitution for face-to-face visits.

CULTURAL ASSESSMENT TOOLS

There are multiple cultural assessment tools that have been developed by nurse-anthropologists and nurses interested in culturally competent nursing care. The nursing literature includes the following:

1. Andrews and Boyle's *Transcultural Concepts in Nursing Care* (1995)
2. Campinha-Bacote's *The Process of Cultural Competence in the Delivery of Healthcare Services: A Culturally Competent Approach* (1998)
3. Ferguson's *Case Studies in Cultural Diversity: A Workbook* (1999)
4. Fong's *CONFHER Model for Cultural Assessment* in Fong (1985)
5. Giger and Davidhizar's *Six Cultural Variables Assessment* In Giger (1995)

6. Leininger's *Acculturation Health Care Assessment Tool for Cultural Patterns in Traditional and Non-Traditional Lifeways* (1991)
7. McNeal et al's *Culturally Sensitive Mobile Health Care Services for At-Risk Populations* (1998)
8. Narayan's *Cultural Assessment in Home Healthcare* (1997)
9. Purnell's *Transcultural Health Care: A Culturally Competent Approach* (1998)
10. Spector's *Heritage Assessment Tool* in Spector (1996)
11. Tripp-Reimer's *Cultural Assessment* (1985)

There are many more nonnursing cultural assessment tools, among which are the following:

1. Berlin and Fowkes' A *Teaching Framework for Cross-Cultural Health Care* (1983)
2. Kleinman, Eisenburg, and Good's *Culture, Illness and Care* (1978)
3. Sue's *Counseling the Culturally Different: Theory and Practice* (1981)

CULTURAL SOCIAL RULES AND COMMUNICATION PATTERNS

Even when the home care nurse and client speak the same language, communication may be hindered by specific social rules (Narayan, 1997). This becomes ever more apparent as the home care nurse enters as a guest into the private home and world of his or her client. The home care nurse needs to consider the social customs practiced when visiting a client from another culture. For example, if a home care nurse is visiting a Hispanic client and is offered a refreshment, he or she should accept it. It shows a sign of respect (*respeto* in Spanish) for the client. In another example, if a home care nurse is visiting the home of an elderly Japanese-American client, he or she should ask if shoes are typically removed before entering the home. Typically, shoes are kept outside or by the door, where slippers are stored. Only slippers are worn while in the home because the home is considered sacred. Likewise, in some traditional households, there is one set of slippers worn in the bathroom and another set worn in other rooms in the home.

Cultural-social variables that can influence the perspective of home care clients are listed in Box 14-1. A home care nurse is much more likely to develop a better rapport and credibility with

---

Box 14-1   Cultural Social Roles

Greeting. Is the patient addressed by *Mr.* or *Mrs.?* Is a handshake acceptable?
Social Exchange Period. What kinds of social exchanges are expected before the "nursing work" begins? Refreshment?
Nonverbal Communication. Is direct eye contact acceptable or rude? How is personal space regarded? Do you stand close to the client or do you keep some distance? Is touching acceptable? By whom? Where? What do certain facial gestures mean, such as a nod or a smile?
Tone of Voice. Is a soft or loud tone of voice acceptable in this culture?
Orientation Toward Time. Is time valued? Or is the personal encounter more valuable? Is time orientation present, future, or both?

---

the client if respect is demonstrated in becoming familiar with the client's cultural background. In addition, a culturally congruent plan has much more potential for success in achieving the desired clinical outcomes (Narayan, 1997).

Home care nurses can use a number of techniques in eliciting cultural content from the client and family in a culturally sensitive manner. For example, home care nurses may develop an indirect or conversational approach to assessing the client's background. Home care nurses may consider a conversational remark such as, "What does [family member's name, like mother or wife] think is causing your problem?" According to Buchwald et al (1994), attributing the explanation to another person can help the client in disclosing health beliefs and practices that they feel uncomfortable in expressing directly.

Another technique in conducting a cultural assessment in a culturally sensitive way is to integrate the content into the nursing history. Cultural assessment tools are useful as guides, but the goal is to integrate cultural content into existing home care documents. Achieving this goal would fulfill several intents. First, it would eliminate the notion of "yet one more form to fill out." Second, important client information would be appropriately accounted for in the nursing history and would result in a culturally tailored nursing care plan. Third, culture would not be "singled out"

(Campinha-Bacote, 1995) but appropriately be seen as integral to the home care assessment, plan, intervention, and evaluation.

Integration of cultural information begins in the initial phase of the nursing process: the client's history. Although a cultural assessment can be lengthy, certain questions should be included in the initial home care visit for every client (Lipson, Meleis, 1985). It is important for home care nurses to recognize that as they become competent at conducting cultural assessments, the process of eliciting cultural information from the client will be integrated more easily and be incorporated in every home care visit. This recognition can decrease potential anxiety and frustration that home

care nurses may encounter while developing cultural competence (Campinha-Bacote, 1995). It is also important for home care nurses to understand that their level of cultural competency will vary according to a specific ethnic group. For example, a home care nurse may be more competent in working with Hispanic clients but limited when interacting with Southeast Asians.

The following set of questions and observations is a guide designed to assist the home care nurse in collecting cultural information for the development of a culturally specific plan of care (Lipson, Dibble, Minarik, 1996).

- Where was the client born? If an immigrant, how long has the client lived in this country?

CASE STUDY

Mrs. L, a 70-year-old Mexican-American housewife and retired high school kitchen cook, was referred for home care services for frequent urination and bladder infections and increased thirst. Mrs. L. lives in a predominately Hispanic neighborhood "barrio" with her husband of more than 50 years. She states that she understands and speaks English, but the primary language spoken in the house is Spanish. Mrs. L. is the primary caregiver for herself and her husband. She and her husband have three daughters and one son; none lives at home, but three of the children live a short distance away.

According to the referral, the client has had type II diabetes for approximately 5 years. During the initial medical visit, she began diet management and hypoglycemics. She is currently taking 25 units of 70/30 insulin subcutaneously every morning. A recent laboratory report indicated a hemoglobin A1C greater than 8% and a blood glucose level in the 400s mg/dl. She has had three episodes of urinary tract infection (UTI) in the past 7 months. Mrs. L. usually tolerates UTI symptoms for several days.

CULTURAL ASSESSMENT: PREPLANNING

The home care nurse will want to note the following:
- *As a form of respect, the home care nurse will greet the client by Mrs. or Señora (the Spanish version of Mrs.). A handshake is acceptable but is done lightly because touch by strangers is generally not acceptable.*
- *Since the information provided indicates that the client lives in a predominately Spanish-speaking neighborhood, it may be accurate to assume that this client strongly identifies with her culture. The*

home care nurse could expect to have a period of social exchange with Mrs. L. (e.g., accept a refreshment if offered and make light conversation, perhaps about pictures displayed in the home). This would be an appropriate time to ask the client where she was born and how long she has lived in the current house and in the United States.
- *For Mexican-Americans, it shows respect to communicate with direct eye contact and to smile and nod appropriately. Personal space is generally regarded as private for strangers entering the home. In this instance, the home care nurse would expect to keep acceptable personal distance until the relationship was more established.*
- *The nurse will use a soft, pleasant tone of voice when speaking to Mrs. L. and her family.*
- *Time orientation for Mexican-Americans is generally present oriented. The home care nurse should suspend making a definite judgment about the client until after the first visit. If the client's level of acculturation is higher than assumed, then perhaps the client's orientation toward time may be both present and future.*

CULTURAL ASSESSMENT

- *The client's home is very neat and humble in appearance. There are lots of plants and pictures of children and family, and there is a religious nicho in the living room with candles.*
- *The client was very warm, cooperative, and agreeable during a social exchange period.*
- *The client spoke in English with hesitancy but responded appropriately. She spoke to her husband*

- What is the client's ethnic affiliation and how strong is the client's ethnic identity?
- Who is the client's primary caregiver? Who are the client's major support givers: family members and friends? Does the client live in an ethnic community?
- What are the client's primary and secondary languages and speaking and reading abilities?
- How would you characterize the client's nonverbal communication style?
- What are the client's religion and current practices? What are their importance in daily life?
- What are the client's food preferences and prohibitions?
- What is the client's economic situation, and is the income adequate to meet the needs of the client and family?
- What are the client's customs and beliefs regarding transitions such as birth, illness, and death?

SUMMARY

The chapter has highlighted critical aspects of cultural competency and the importance of incorporating cultural content into home care nursing assessment, planning, intervention, and evaluation. The basic premise of the cultural assessment is that clients have a right to their cultural beliefs, values, and practices. In turn, culturally competent home care nurses must understand their

---

CASE STUDY—cont'd

in both English and Spanish. She appeared more comfortable speaking Spanish.
- *Both the client and her husband were born in Mexico. They immigrated to the United States 25 years ago.*
- *The client's communication style was direct.*
- *The client's food preferences were traditional Mexican dishes. The client has not consumed alcohol since she was diagnosed with diabetes.*
- *The client appeared financially secure. She stated, "We have all we need."*
- *The client believes in Western medicine. She referred to "the medicine my doctor gives me," but she also believes in the use of certain herbs, such as yerba buena.*
- *In the client's own words, her health problems are "too much sugar in my blood."*
- *When the client was asked if she experienced pain with her UTIs, she said, "Yes, but I tried to help myself with drinking teas."*
- *The client also stated, "Sometimes I forget to give myself those injections."*
- *The client's level of acculturation might be assessed as low to medium, based on language ability, health beliefs, and home environment.*

PLAN
The home care nurse formulates the following plan of care for Mrs. L.:
- *Establish a mutual time for another visit.*
- *Refer to dietitian; if possible, home care nurse should be present at meeting with dietitian to provide a smooth transition and introduction; or*

- *Ask permission to invite another* Señora *who also has diabetes or a* promotora *(Spanish-speaking community layperson or community volunteer interpreter, preferably of same gender) to help review diet and medication regimen.* NOTE: *at this point, the home care nurse is not assuming that the client does not understand the regimen, but instead is attempting to provide cultural and educational support. At the same time, the nurse will further assess how much the client understands diabetes and how to manage it.*
- *Inquire if client's husband would be interested in attending a session. The more the family unit understands diabetes and how to manage it, the greater the likelihood of successful clinical outcomes for this case.*
- *Establish weekly goals for the client (short-term).*
- *Develop an educational monitoring (blood glucose level) program.*
- *Teach illness management, such as what happens if the client gets influenza, which will influence insulin levels.*
- *Teach within a cultural context how and when to notify her practitioner about symptoms that she normally does not experience (e.g., urinating frequently).*
- *Investigate whether there are any community programs on diabetes held in Spanish.*
- *Update and confer with the physician or nurse practitioner as needed.*
- *Evaluate outcomes with client and nurse; include the husband when possible.*
- *Discharge the client when goals have been met or diabetic management has been achieved.*

clients' beliefs, values, and practices to render the best possible care. As Meleis (1996) has stated:

> Providing care that is culturally competent care is no longer a luxury; it is a necessity that is being demanded by clients and by those who act as advocates for clients in both hospital and community setting.

Developing and organizing a culturally tailored plan for home care clients demonstrates cultural competency and also a level of expertise that is warranted by both clients and state and federal regulatory systems (see chapter 29). With concerted effort, home care nurses can provide culturally competent care that results in successful, cost-effective outcomes. Changes in the demographics of the country will require not only cultural and clinical competencies in home care nurses, but also ingenious creativity, for which home care nurses have been known from their earliest beginnings.

REFERENCES

Andrews M, Boyle J: *Transcultural concepts in nursing care,* Philadelphia, 1995, Lippincott.

Baker D et al: Use and effectiveness of interpreters in an emergency department, *Journal of the American Medical Association* 275(10):783-788, 1996.

Berlin E, Fowkes W: A teaching framework for cross-cultural health care, *Western Journal of Medicine* 139(6):934-938, 1983.

Buchwald D et al: Caring for patients in a multicultural society, *Patient Care* 28(11):105-123, 1994.

Campinha-Bacote J: The quest for cultural competence in nursing care, *Nursing Forum* 30(4):19-25, 1995.

Campinha-Bacote J: The process of cultural competence in the delivery of health care services: A culturally competent approach, 1998. Available from Josepha Campinha-Bacote, Transcultural C.A.R.E. Associates, 11108 Huntwicke Place, Cincinnati.

Cross T et al: *Towards a culturally competent system of care,* vol 1, Washington, DC, 1989, CASSP Technical Assistance Center, Georgetown University Child Development Center.

Ferguson V: *Case studies in a cultural diversity: A workbook,* Boston, 1999, Jones & Bartlett.

Fong CM: Ethnicity and nursing practice, *Topics in Clinical Nursing* 7(3):1-10, 1985.

Giger JN, Davidhizar RE: *Transcultural nursing: Assessment and intervention,* St Louis, 1995, Mosby.

Ginsberg C et al: Interpretation and translation services in health care: A survey of US public and private teaching hospitals, *A National Public Health and Hospitals Institute (NPHHI) Report,* Washington, DC, 1995, NPHHI.

Kleinman A, Eisenberg L, Good B: Culture, illness and care: Clinical lessons from anthropologic and cross-cultural research, *Annals of Internal Medicine* 88(2):251-258, 1978.

Leininger M: Leininger's acculturation health care assessment tool for cultural patterns in traditional and non-traditional lifeways, *Journal of Transcultural Nursing* 2(2):40-42, 1991.

Lipson J, Dibble SL, Minarik PA: *Culture & nursing care: A pocket guide,* San Francisco, 1996, University of California-San Francisco, School of Nursing.

Lipson JG, Meleis AI: Culturally appropriate care: The case of immigrants, *Topics in Clinical Nursing* 7(3):48-56, 1985.

Lipson J, Steiger NJ: *Self-care nursing in multicultural context,* 1996, Sage Publications.

Massachusetts Medical Interpreters Association, The Education Development Center: *Medical interpreters standards of practice,* Boston, 1995, The Center.

McNeal GJ et al: Culturally sensitive mobile health care services for at-risk populations. In Ferguson VD, ed: *Educating the 21st century nurse: Challenges and opportunities,* New York, 1998, National League for Nursing Press.

Meleis A et al: *Diversity, marginalization, and culturally competent health care: Issues in knowledge development,* Washington, DC, 1995, American Academy of Nursing.

Meleis AI: Culturally competent scholarship: Substance and rigor, *Advances in Nursing Science* 19(2):1-16, 1996.

Narayan MC: Cultural assessment in home healthcare, *Home Healthcare Nurse* 15(10):663-670, 1997.

Perkins J et al: *Ensuring linguistic access in health care settings: Legal rights and responsibilities,* Los Angeles, 1998, National Health Law Program.

Professional language certification examination manual, Olympia, Wash, 1995, State of Washington, Department of Social and Health Services.

Purnell L: *Transcultural health care: A culturally competent approach,* Philadelphia, 1998, FA Davis.

Putsch R: Cross-cultural communication: The special cases of interpreters in health care, *Journal of the American Medical Association* 254(23):3344-3348, 1985.

Spector RE: *Cultural diversity in health and illness,* Stamford, Conn, 1996, Appleton & Lange.

Sue DW: *Counseling the culturally different: Theory and practice,* New York, 1981, John Wiley & Sons.

Swaney I: Thoughts on live vs. telephone and video interpretation, *Proteus* 6:2, Spring 1997.

Tylor EB: Primitive culture: Research into the development of mythology, philosophy, religion, art, and customs. In Helman C, ed: *Culture, health and illness,* Oxford, England, 1992 (1871), Butterworth-Heinemann.

Tripp-Reimer T: Cultural assessment. In Belack J, Bamford P, eds: *Nursing Assessment,* North Scituate, Mass, 1985, Duxbury Press.

US Bureau of the Census: Population projections of the United States, by age, sex, race and Hispanic origin: 1995 to 2050. In *Current Population Reports,* Washington, DC, 1996, US Government Printing Office.

US Bureau of the Census: *The Hispanic population in the United States* (on-line) Washington, DC, 2001, www.census.gov.

Vasquez C, Javier R: The problem with interpreters: Communicating with Spanish-speaking patients, *Hospital Community Psychiatry* 42(2):163-165, 1991.

Villarruel AM, Portillo CJ, Kane P: Communicating with limited English proficiency persons: Implications for nursing practice, *Nursing Outlook* 47(6):262-270, 1999.

Wells MI: Beyond cultural competence: A model for individual and institutional cultural development, *Journal of Community Health Nursing* 17(4):189-199, 2000.

Woloshin S et al: Language barriers in medicine in the United States, *Journal of the American Medical Association* 273(9):724-728, 1995.

Home Care Throughout the Life Cycle

15 Home Care of the New Family

Katherine Camacho Carr

A generation ago, a postpartum stay in the hospital of 7 to 10 days was common. Since 1970, the length of the postpartum hospital stay has decreased by 50%, with the average length of stay decreasing from 4.1 days to 2.6 days overall (from 3.9 to 2.1 days for vaginal deliveries and from 7.8 to 4.0 days for cesarean deliveries) (Centers for Disease Control and Prevention, 1995; Weiner, 1997). This trend toward earlier postpartum discharge has been driven by administrative efforts to decrease hospital costs and by client preference (Gazmararian, Koplan, 1996). Managed-care plans and other third-party payors have placed limits on coverage, resulting in an increase in 1-day maternity stays after vaginal delivery and 2-day stays after cesarean delivery. Clinicians and Congress have rallied with a cry for longer postpartum stays (Declercq, Simmes, 1997) to prevent or facilitate early recognition of maternal or neonatal complications. Both the American Academy of Pediatrics (AAP) and the American College of Obstetricians and Gynecologists (ACOG) have published official guidelines defining adequate stays after delivery and have encouraged follow-up after early discharge (AAP, ACOG, 1992). Managed-care plans have responded in very few cases by providing extensive home care follow-up after early discharge. A recent survey of obstetricians in the United States and Canada reveals that additional postpartum visits are routinely recommended only 39% of the time after vaginal delivery and 68% of the time after cesarean delivery (Britton, 1998). Most practitioners surveyed considered the optimal length of hospital stay to be shorter than those published in the AAP and ACOG guidelines and emphasized the need for follow-up regarding the physical health of the mother, with little emphasis on social or psychological risk. Nationwide, it appears that only a minority of women discharged within 24 hours receive home follow-up care by a nurse or other health care professional (*Maternity Care Appropriate,* 1996).

In response to these "drive-through deliveries," Congress passed the Newborns' and Mothers' Health Protection Act of 1996. This law mandates health insurance coverage for a minimum stay of 48 hours after vaginal birth and 96 hours after cesarean birth and is in sync with the AAP and ACOG guidelines. The law also prohibits care providers from gaining financial incentives if stays are shorter and establishes an advisory panel to conduct studies of the factors affecting length of hospital stay and birth outcomes. Unfortunately, the final version of the bill did not include provisions for follow-up, even if early discharge occurs. This law is primarily concerned with length of stay (LOS), rather than the specific needs of the new family during the immediate postdelivery period, whether these needs occur in the hospital or after discharge.

Nevertheless, home follow-up of the new family will continue to be an important role for nurses and other care providers as health care continues to move from hospital to home and from acute to preventive care and as the real needs of new families are validated through ongoing study and analysis.

OVERVIEW OF DISCHARGE AND HOME HEALTH CARE PRACTICES

Early postpartum discharge is discharge less than 48 hours after vaginal delivery or less than 96 hours after cesarean delivery, as described by federal law, as well as the AAP and ACOG guidelines. Several interesting issues underlie the early discharge debate, such as (1) who should control the decision, (2) whether widespread hospitalization for birth and the immediate post-partum period is desirable, and (3) whether the best way to "mother the new mother" and promote family health in the early postpartum period is to increase the hospital (LOS) or provide some other means of follow-up, including telephone contact, office visits, or home care visits. The federal legislation does not shed much light on these issues. In addition, it is questionable whether women and their care providers share a vision regarding the timing of postpartum discharge and the many and varied needs of new mothers (Britton, 1998; Jones, 1997), and the safety of early postpartum discharge is still under debate (Grullon et al, 1997).

Economics, and not health care needs, had driven the LOS so short that many states and Congress had to take action to ensure adequate time in hospital for new mothers and their infants. In addition, most Americans, although not all, believe that hospitalization for childbirth and the immediate postdelivery period is desirable and necessary. However, home care, and specifically postpartum home visiting, is much more common in European countries, where home birth is also a recognized option for parents. All new mothers receive home visits by midwives up to 10 days after delivery in Great Britain and the Netherlands. With little institutionalized postpartum home care, the average U.S. maternity LOS in the hospital (2 days) is still shorter than most developed countries, including Great Britain (3 days), Sweden (4 days), Norway (4.5 days), and Japan (6.5 days) (U.S. Department of Health and Human Services, 1996). It is clear that a new model of postpartum care—a shorter hospital stay with home follow-up—is emerging in the United States. However, we have chosen to institutionalize the LOS requirement and not the home follow-up component!

ADVANTAGES AND DISADVANTAGES OF EARLY POSTPARTUM DISCHARGE

Early postpartum discharge has potential advantages and disadvantages for the perinatal health care of parents and their infants. Some advantages are (1) earlier reestablishment of family routines, decreased sibling separation, and increased family bonding; (2) decreased incidence of nosocomial infection; (3) emotional and psy-

chological benefits resulting from the relaxed, familiar atmosphere of a client's own home; (4) cost savings of reduced hospital LOS; (5) avoidance of discord associated with signing out against medical advice; and (6) increased self-confidence acquired by learning self-care skills associated with postpartum and neonatal care in a realistic setting.

Some disadvantages are (1) decreased educational opportunities because of early discharge, especially when comprehensive follow-up is lacking; (2) need for increased help at home to provide meals and other home maintenance services; (3) lack of rest as a result of increased neonatal vigilance; (4) lack of nursing help and guidance for breastfeeding and neonatal care (such as diapering, bathing, and cord care); (5) possible occurrence of complications, such as neonatal hyperbilirubinemia, low neonatal temperature, inadequate feeding, sepsis and infection, maternal hemorrhage, excessive maternal pain, and severe nipple damage, some of which will require rehospitalization; and (6) inability to reenter the system for continued care if needed because of a lack of sufficient knowledge and language and cultural barriers.

Continuity of care between hospital and home can also be affected by early discharge. It can be improved with a well-designed postpartum nursing follow-up program, or it can be eliminated or adversely affected by lack of adequate discharge planning. However, most researchers agree that outcome research regarding the advantages and disadvantages of early postpartum discharge is inconclusive (Kessel et al, 1995; Weiner, 1997). It is also unclear whether breastfeeding rates are affected positively or negatively by early discharge.

IMPLICATIONS OF EARLY POSTPARTUM DISCHARGE FOR PERINATAL NURSES

Nurses, as well as doulas and other health care providers, are well aware that the first few weeks of life and the first few weeks of parenting can be crucial to the new family members, who have extensive health care, educational, and psychosocial needs. In some instances, the current health care situation has led to ethical and professional concerns for perinatal nurses, including the maintenance of options for parents who desire very early discharge from the hospital or birthing center and the development of adequate follow-up home care in an atmosphere of increasingly limited resources when these services might be eliminated. On the other hand, the current health care situation has created expanded practice opportunities in the home health care arena (Williams, Cooper, 1996).

Prenatal Preparation and Education for Parents

Early postpartum discharge has many implications for perinatal nursing practice. It places more responsibility on the nurses in the hospital to prepare the family for discharge in a short time. Ideally, families would be prepared during the prenatal period. Prenatal preparation and education for early discharge are usually provided by the perinatal nurse, midwife, or childbirth educator, either through a special class, a prenatal office or home visit, or written material. Prenatal preparation of the parents and the home environment includes (1) gathering appropriate equipment, such as baby's layette and thermometer (Box 15-1); (2) arranging for help at home from family, friends, or a postdelivery follow-up service; and (3) understanding the self-care instructions for mother and infant (Fig. 15-1). In addition, prenatal preparation facilitates the development of rapport between the family and the nurse, midwife, childbirth educator, or doula who will be providing follow-up care.

Screening Criteria

A second critical area for perinatal nurses relates to screening criteria for early discharge. Concern for client safety and medical and legal considerations make it imperative that appropriate screening criteria be developed and strictly followed. Psychological and physical criteria should be

Text continued on p. 216

Box 15-1 List of Equipment for Home Postpartum Care

SUPPLIES FOR MOTHER

Hydrous lanolin for tender nipples
"Peri" bottle
Breast pump
Nursing bra
Nursing pads (if desired)
Extra-large sanitary napkins and small pads
Witch hazel and gauze pads (Tucks)
Clean linens, gowns, and robe

SUPPLIES FOR INFANT

Car seat that meets safety standards (infant will not be discharged without one)
Clothing appropriate for weather. It should maintain infant body temperature. It should be loose, nonirritating, easy to put on and take off, and easy to launder. It should include a hat or bonnet, 6 to 12 blankets, and several pairs of booties.
Diaper wipes
Disposable diapers (or diaper service) for the first few weeks. At least 90 diapers per week will be needed.
Digital thermometer for use under the arm
Bulb syringe (suction bulb)
Bed and 2 to 4 sheets
Large blanket or bunting

SUPPLIES FOR INFANT—cont'd

Washable pads for underneath diaper-changing area
Large plastic tub or clean sink for bathing, washcloths, towels, mild soap (Ivory), cotton balls, cotton-tipped applicators (e.g., Q-tips), and isopropyl alcohol for cord
Toys such as mobiles, stuffed animals, teething rings, rattles, and music boxes
Several 4- and 8-oz bottles and nipples, as needed. Formula if bottle feeding
Pacifier (optional)
Extra-large safety pins, if needed
Nail clippers, small scissors, and nail file
Petrolatum jelly (e.g., Vaseline) (if male is circumcised)
Additional equipment such as bassinet, carriage, rocking chair, stroller, and carrying device (optional)
Chest of drawers and changing table, as desired

GENERAL NEEDS

Watch with second hand
Nourishing food and drink (can be frozen ahead of time)
Reference book on breastfeeding
Reference book on newborns

Postpartum Self-Care Guidelines

The following information will help to guide you in caring for yourself and your baby during your first few days following the birth. IF YOU HAVE ANY QUESTIONS OR CONCERNS, PLEASE CONTACT YOUR PRIMARY CARE PROVIDER.

Important Telephone Numbers
Primary Care Provider/Mother...
Primary Care Provider/Baby..
Home Health Nurse/Breastfeeding Consultant..
Closest Relative/Friend/Doula Service...
Emergency...

Care of the Mother
Vital Signs, Fundus, and Flow

After you return home from the hospital, please check your temperature, pulse, fundus, and flow frequently. Record your findings in the accompanying chart every 4 hours during the first 24 hours and then twice daily over the next 3 days or at intervals identified by your care provider.

	DAY OF BIRTH			DAY #1		DAY #2		DAY #3	
DATE									
TIME									
TEMPERATURE									
PULSE									
FUNDUS									
FLOW									

Temperature
Normal oral temperature range is 97° to 99.4° F (36° to 37.5° C). If your temperature is slightly elevated, drink large amounts of fluids and recheck your temperature in 2 hours. If it is more than 100.4° F (38° C), contact your care provider.

Pulse
Your pulse should be taken while resting and should not exceed 100 bpm. If it is more than 100 bpm, or if it is ever accompanied by heavy vaginal bleeding, call the nurse.

Fundus
Your fundus (the upper portion of the uterus) should feel round and firm and similar to a grapefruit in size and consistency. It is usually felt at, or one to two fingers below, your navel on the first few days after delivery. It should be briefly massaged until firm before each time you get out of bed. You can expect the fundus to involute (get smaller) at a rate of about one fingerbreadth per day below your navel.

Flow
Your flow (vaginal bleeding) should gradually progress from a bright red, heavy flow (during the first 24 hours) to a reddish-pink, lighter flow (within 2 to 3 days of birth). Occasionally, small, 50-cent-size clots and stringy blood are normal for up to 1 week. The normal characteristic odor of your flow, or lochia, is fleshy and resembles the odor of menstrual blood. A foul odor is usually indicative of infection, particularly if accompanied by a fever. If your flow increases significantly, massage your uterus firmly and frequently, increase your fluids and bedrest, and nurse your baby every 2 hours. If the increased flow persists, call your care provider. *Saturation of two or more pads in 1 hour is excessive bleeding.*

Fig. 15-1   Postpartum self-care guidelines.

Breast Care
Breastfeeding Mothers
Some mothers, particularly those with large, pendulous breasts, prefer to wear a well-fitting nursing bra for support. Frequent feedings (every 2 to 3 hours) stimulate the production of milk and usually prevent engorgement. Pure lanolin is recommended for nipple lubrication for sore or cracked nipples. It does not need to be washed off before breastfeeding. Assistance with proper breastfeeding technique is the best solution for sore, bruised, cracked, or bleeding nipples; frequently, the baby is not getting a good, complete grasp of the nipple and areola. Ask for assistance from your care provider, doula, knowledgeable friend or, lactation consultant.

Bottle-Feeding Mothers
Wear a tight-fitting bra or breast binder 24 hours per day for 4 to 5 days. Avoid stimulation of your nipples, and do not massage or empty your breasts. If your breasts become engorged or tender, ice-pack applications and aspirin or acetaminophen may ease the discomfort.

Nutrition
A well-balanced, high-protein diet and 2 to 3 quarts of fluid per day are recommended during the postpartum period. Drink plenty of orange juice and other fluids immediately after the birth of your baby because this will help restore a high energy level. Breastfeeding mothers should be sure to drink adequate fluids and avoid dehydration.

Perineal Care
You may use ice packs on the perineum for the first 6 to 24 hours after the birth to prevent swelling and reduce pain in the vaginal area. You can make a simple ice pack by filling a latex glove with ice and covering it with a small washcloth. After 18 to 24 hours, a sitz bath (sitting in a tub of 4 to 6 inches of clean, hot water or using a portable sitz bath) is strongly recommended for 20-minute periods three to five times per day (to enhance healing process, reduce hemorrhoids, and decrease perineal discomfort). Showers are encouraged before or after sitz baths.

Urination
You must urinate before you will be discharged from the hospital. Remind yourself to urinate every 2 to 4 hours at home, and if you are unable to empty your bladder or if you are only urinating a few teaspoons at a time, contact your care provider. If you have a plastic squeeze bottle, fill it with warm water and rinse off your perineum after each voiding. The perineum should then be blotted dry with toilet paper, always blotting from front to back. A hairdryer may also be used for the same purpose. Witch hazel compresses or Tucks may be applied to the perineum, and sanitary napkins should be changed after each voiding. Plan to use your squeeze bottle until your vaginal discharge has lightened.

Bowel Movements
Most women have a bowel movement within 2 to 4 days after the birth. Continue to eat high-roughage foods (raw vegetables, fresh and dried fruits, and whole grains) and drink large amounts of water and other fluids (at least one 8-oz glass each time you feed your baby). Prune juice may also be used in moderation. In special cases, take stool softeners, laxatives, or enemas if encouraged to do so by your care provider. If you have stitches, you may feel more comfortable applying direct counterpressure over your stitches with a clean pad during the first few bowel movements.

Hemorrhoids
Some women develop painful hemorrhoids (varicose veins of the rectal area) during pregnancy, sometimes aggravated by pushing the baby out during labor. You may apply witch hazel with a small gauze square for relief of the discomfort and use sitz baths and any medication recommended by your care provider. In addition, perform Kegel exercises (vaginal squeezing) to increase blood flow and reduce swelling.

Rest and Relaxation
You may begin to do abdominal tightening and Kegel exercises (vaginal squeezing) within the first few hours after delivery. However, frequent rest periods are highly recommended (naps in the morning, afternoon, and evening); heavy exercise should be avoided until the bright red bleeding stops.

Fig. 15-1, cont'd Postpartum self-care guidelines. *Continued*

Feelings

During the first few days at home, many new mothers and fathers may experience a period of being overwhelmed or depressed. This may be caused by a combination of hormonal changes, fatigue, and expectations of what your baby will be versus reality. These feelings of depression and blues are normal. However, should they persist, call your care provider.

Sexual Relations

Sexual desires during the postpartum period vary tremendously among different couples. If your sex drive is decreased, it will eventually return to normal. You may resume intercourse when both partners feel physically and emotionally ready. However, it is probably best to wait at least 2 to 3 weeks to allow for healing of the uterus and any stitches you may have. Lubrication with a water-soluble lubricant, such as K-Y Jelly (not petroleum jelly), is recommended. Some form of birth control, such as condoms, is also necessary, since breastfeeding is not a reliable contraceptive.

Immunizations

Rh-negative mothers who give birth to Rh-positive babies need to receive an Rh_O (D) immune globulin (RhoGAM) injection within 72 hours of the birth. Rubella-negative mothers also frequently choose to receive rubella vaccine after the birth. Both of these injections are usually administered at the 2- to 3-day visit.

Follow-Up Care

Please call your care provider to make your follow-up postpartum appointment. Any remaining prenatal appointments will be canceled.

Care of the Baby
Vital Signs, Urination, and Bowel Movements

After you return home from the hospital, please check your baby's temperature, pulse, and respirations at least twice daily in the first 3 days. Record your findings in the accompanying chart every 4 hours during the first 24 hours and then twice daily over the next 3 days. Also, record all of your baby's eliminations by noting the time and checking (✓) the appropriate column next to either "urination" or "bowel movement."

	DAY OF BIRTH			DAY #1	DAY #2	DAY #3
DATE						
TIME						
TEMPERATURE						
PULSE						
RESPIRATIONS						
TIME						
URINATION						
BOWEL						
MOVEMENT						

Temperature

Axillary (under the armpit) temperatures are recommended for newborns. For axillary temperatures, hold the bulb of the thermometer high in the baby's axilla (armpit) for at least 3 minutes (or until it beeps, if digital) while pressing the baby's arm gently but firmly against his or her body. At times, especially if the baby appears ill, a rectal temperature might be appropriate. Lightly lubricate the thermometer bulb with K-Y Jelly and then gently insert the thermometer approximately 1/2 in. into the baby's rectum for at least 3 minutes. Axillary and rectal temperature readings are very similar in newborns, and normal range is 97° to 99° F (36.1° C to 37.2° C). Frequently, normal temperatures can be achieved by adding or removing clothing. However, if high or low temperatures persist, contact your care provider.

Pulse

Check your resting baby's pulse by placing two fingertips just to the left of the baby's left nipple. Count for 30 seconds and multiply the number by 2 to give you the number of beats per minute. This rate may be slightly irregular, and the normal range is 120 to 160 bpm. Heart rate may be slightly lower if the baby is sleeping.

Fig. 15-1, cont'd   Postpartum self-care guidelines.

Respirations

Count respirations for 30 seconds by watching the baby's chest as it rises when the baby is quiet. Multiply by 2 to obtain the number of respirations per minute. Respirations will be irregular, but breathing should not appear labored or accompanied by retraction of the sternum (breast bone) or flaring of the nostrils. The normal range is 40 to 70 respirations per minute on the first day and 30 to 50 thereafter.

Urination and Bowel Movements

Your baby should urinate at least one time during the first 24 hours and at least twice during the second 24 hours. The baby should urinate 7 to 8 times per day after the first week of life. Many mothers think that the baby has not urinated because of the absorbency of disposable diapers. Compare the texture of the diaper you take off to a clean one to determine if the baby has voided. The first bowel movement of the newborn is a dark green-to-black meconium stool. Once breastfeeding is established, this will change to a bright yellow, unformed bowel movement. These stools are normal and are not diarrhea.

Bulb Suctioning

If the baby sounds stuffy, has a large amount of mucus, or seems to be choking, use the bulb syringe to remove the mucus from the mouth or nose. Always compress the bulb before placing it gently into the baby's mouth or nose. Be careful of placement; just the tip is inserted.

Positioning for Sleeping

Babies should be positioned on their backs or sides for sleep. Positioning babies on their backs has been found to ease the respiratory efforts of the baby and is related to a decreased incidence of sudden infant death syndrome (SIDS).

Feedings

Your breast milk should begin to come in by the second or third day of nursing. Before that, the baby is receiving colostrum, which is very nutritious and extremely beneficial. Colostrum is not only high in nutrients and antibodies, but it also acts as a natural laxative, thereby increasing the frequency of the meconium stools. *Nurse your baby frequently,* every 2 to 3 hours during the first few days, if the baby is interested. No time limitation is recommended, although 10 to 20 minutes per breast is fairly typical. Water or other supplements are not routinely recommended for breastfeeding babies. However, in special situations, such as when babies are extremely dehydrated, receiving phototherapy, or have other problems, supplementation may be recommended. In these instances, your baby may be supplemented either during or after breastfeeding with the use of an eye dropper.

Umbilical Cord

Triple dye, a purple substance, will be applied to your baby's cord before discharge. Keep the cord dry and exposed to air as much as possible. You may apply alcohol to the umbilical cord with a cotton-tipped applicator or an alcohol pad after each diaper change to aid in drying and healing of the cord. No other care is necessary. The cord clamp will be removed at the hospital or at a 2- to 3-day visit by the nurse or baby's physician. The cord itself usually falls off at 6 to 10 days. If the cord has a foul odor, call your care provider, but you may continue to apply alcohol to the base of the cord to aid in drying the cord and decreasing the odor.

Eyes

Prophylactic treatment was performed on your baby's eyes to prevent gonorrhea and other types of infection. If your baby's eyes appear red and swollen, the symptoms need no treatment and will usually disappear within a week. However, if there is some discharge, gently bathing the eyes with cotton balls and warm water for a day or two will cleanse the eyes without discomfort to the baby.

Jaundice

If your baby's body or whites of the eyes appear to be yellow, or jaundiced, or if the baby is lethargic or eating poorly, call your care provider. A small amount of blood may need to be drawn from your baby's heel to check his or her bilirubin level. If the level is significantly elevated, the baby may need phototherapy. Phototherapy can be done at home or by readmission to the hospital nursery. The baby will be placed under special bright lights, with the eyes protected, to aid in the physiological elimination of the bilirubin before it builds up to a dangerous level.

Fig. 15-1, cont'd   Postpartum self-care guidelines.   *Continued*

Phenylketonuria-Thyroid Test
A phenylketonuria-thyroid (PKU) test is done in the hospital at discharge and repeated at 2 weeks of life at the baby's care provider's office. However, if you choose early discharge, the test is done at the 2- to 3-day visit and repeated at 2 weeks of life.

Immunizations
Vitamin K injections are given to newborn babies within 1 to 2 hours after birth to assist the blood-clotting mechanisms, which are deficient at birth. Your baby will most likely receive the first hepatitis B immunization in the hospital or in the care provider's office at the 2-week check-up.

Circumcision
The AAP has stated that there is no medical indication for routine newborn circumcision. However, if you choose to have your baby boy circumcised, check with your care provider about specific follow-up instructions.

Follow-Up Newborn Care
You need to contact your baby's primary care provider (family physician, nurse practitioner, or pediatrician) to make follow-up appointments for your baby usually at 10 to 14 days of age and at 6 to 8 weeks of age.

Fig. 15-1, cont'd   Postpartum self-care guidelines.

Box 15-2   Criteria for Early Discharge of Mothers and Infants*

MOTHERS	INFANTS
1. Blood pressure >90/60 and <140/90 mm Hg	1. Birth weight >5 lb
2. Temperature <38° C	2. Heart rate 110-150 bpm
3. Lack of significant bleeding	3. Respiratory rate 30-50 respirations per minute
4. Lack of difficulty with ambulation and voiding	4. Temperature 36.1° to 37.2° C (97° to 99° F)
5. Planned assistance at home for at least 2 days	5. Hematocrit 40% to 65%
6. Understanding of self-care instructions for mother and infant and capability to follow them	6. Negative Coombs' test
	7. Parents' demonstration of ability to care for the infant at home
	8. Infant voiding or passing of stool

*Early discharge defined as <48 hr. after vaginal birth and <96 hr. after a cesarean birth.

---

considered. Sample screening criteria are contained in Box 15-2.

NURSING ASSESSMENT AND DISCHARGE PLANNING
Postpartum Discharge Checklist

The application of screening criteria for mother and infant depends on adequate nursing assessment of the family before discharge. An early postpartum discharge checklist (Box 15-3) can be used by the nurse to determine if all criteria for discharge are met. Information regarding follow-up should also be verified with the family. When home follow-up will be done, directions to the home are needed by the nurse. Clear communication between hospital staff and others who may be providing follow-up is needed. Important information such as the date, time of birth, mother's parity, sex of baby, baby's weight and Apgar score, feeding method, and any special concerns or minor complications should be noted on the referral form.

Home or Office Follow-Up

Timing   Home visits are made within established geographical boundaries. Office follow-up, with the family returning to the facility for evaluation, may be done for families living outside the geographical boundaries or when resources for home follow-up are limited. Significant cost

---

Box 15-3   Postpartum Discharge Checklist

MOTHER

☐ Vital signs are stable.
☐ The mother has had nourishment.
☐ The fundus is firm.
☐ Flow is normal.
☐ The perineum is healing.
☐ The mother has voided.
☐ Instructions have been given to the mother:
  1. Self-care instructions for mother and infant
  2. Follow-up appointments for mother and infant
  3. Emergency phone number
☐ Birth certificate information has been completed.
☐ Reliable transportation has been identified.
☐ Discharge orders and notes have been completed.
☐ Supplies have been given or are available at home:
  1. Sanitary pads
  2. Diapers
  3. Squeeze bottle
  4. Bulb syringe
  5. Breast pump, if breastfeeding

INFANT

☐ Vital signs are stable.
☐ The infant has fed successfully.
☐ Eye prophylaxis has been provided.
☐ Vitamin K and hepatitis B prophylaxis has been provided, if appropriate.
☐ PKU and thyroxine testing has been performed or arranged.
☐ Voiding and defecation have been noted.
☐ Cord care has been provided.
☐ A physical examination has been given by the care provider.
☐ The identification process has been completed.
☐ Safety issues have been addressed:
  1. Car seat
  2. Suitable crib or bassinet
  3. Sleeping position
☐ Discharge orders and notes have been completed.
☐ The mother has been given an information sheet regarding circumcision, if appropriate.

---

savings can be demonstrated when families return to a central facility and home visits are not required (Keppler, 1995). The number and timing of follow-up visits are partially determined by the length of postpartum hospital stay. For families discharged within 6 to 12 hours, follow-up within 24 hours is customary. For others, the initial postdelivery follow-up varies from the second to the fourth postpartum day.

Telephone follow-up   Telephone follow-up can also be used to supplement home or office follow-up, but it should not be used as a substitute, especially in very early postpartum discharge (6 to 12 hours) or after home birth.

Nursing assessment   During home or office follow-up, the nurse assesses the physical and psychosocial status of the family and focuses on their educational needs. Nursing assessment of the mother should include the following:

• Vital signs (blood pressure, temperature, pulse, and respirations)
• Concerns or problems

• Breasts, abdomen, fundus (size, location, and consistency), perineum, lochia, legs (edema and Homans' sign), and bowel and bladder function
• Adequacy of nutrition
• Amount of rest and number and helpfulness of visitors
• Feelings
• Rh status and need for immunoglobulin
• Feeding and infant care skills

Nursing assessment of the infant should include:

• Vital signs (apical pulse, respiration rate, and temperature)
• Presence of respiratory distress (excessive mucus, flaring of alae nasae, retractions, or grunting)
• Hydration status (skin turgor, mucous membranes, fontanel, and number of wet diapers)
• Feeding behavior (suck, swallow, and gag reflex and ability to grasp nipple)
• Physical appearance, including color, posture, activity, and eyes (color of sclera and presence of infection)

Home or Office Visit Record: Mother

Name_____ ID No._____ Phone_____

Address_____

_____

Instructions to Home:_____

_____

_____

Date of Birth:_____ Type/Time of Birth:_____

Special concerns or complications:_____

_____

_____

Date: Subjective Data:	Visit #1	Visit #2	Visit #3
Objective Data:			
Temperature, pulse, respirations			
Blood pressure			
Breasts			
Abdomen			
Fundus			
CVA			
Perineum			
Lochia			
Legs			
Bladder			
Bowels			
Other			
Assessment:			
Plan:			
Exam Performed by:			

Fig. 15-2

- Bowel and bladder function
- Occurrence of hyperbilirubinemia (jaundice and lethargy)
- Umbilical cord
- Plans for further neonatal care (PKU, hypothyroid testing, circumcision, and follow-up well-baby care).
- Potential for sibling rivalry

Figures 15-2 and 15-3 depict a typical home or office visit record in which these data are recorded by the care provider. Nursing assessment should also focus on the family unit and in-clude assessment of the integration of the infant into the family and the ability of the family to care for the infant.

Cultural variations and challenges Home health care nurses may frequently encounter families with religious, ethnic, or cultural beliefs about the postpartum period and child care that may be different from their own. Other challenges, including language barriers, poverty, teen or single mothers, lack of education, substance abuse, child or spousal abuse, or lack of a support system, may also be present. Rarely does a

Home or Office Visit-Infant

Name_____ ID No._____

Date of Birth:_____ Type/Time of Birth:_____

Apgar Score:_____ Birth weight:_____

Special concerns or complications:_____

_____

_____

Date: **Subjective Data:** (from parents)	Visit #1	Visit #2	Visit #3
Objective Data:			
Temperature (axillary)			
Apical pulse			
Respirations			
Occipitofrontal circumference			
Signs of respiratory distress			
Current weight			
Skin color, turgor, temperature			
Cord			
Eyes			
Reflexes			
Alertness, responsiveness, tone			
Feeding			
Voiding			
Stools			
Attachment			
Other			
Circumcision			
Assessment:			
Plan:			
Exam Performed by:			

Fig. 15-3

family fit into a "typical" picture. These cultural, economic, educational, and psychosocial challenges call for the nurse to use sound clinical assessment skills, individualized instruction, compassion, and encouragement. Only then can a family's true needs be assessed and met. Special resources, such as interpreters, teen "back-to-school programs," and referrals to various agencies for assistance, may be needed.

It is important for the nurse to realize that in teaching the new mother and family about maternal and infant care, he or she is sometimes treading on cultural, religious, or family beliefs, and resentment can result. An understanding of these various cultural and religious beliefs is helpful, and many excellent articles have been written discussing them (Hutchinson, Baqi-Aziz, 1993). However, when these practices are harmful or do not address the needs of the mother, baby, or family, the nurse might approach the family by pointing out all of the positive practices he or she observes before suggesting something that appears to be critical or culturally foreign. In addition, the nurse should try to integrate her recommendations to meet the physical and psychosocial needs of the family in a way that respects their spiritual and cultural beliefs. Dietary restrictions and fasting requirements, modesty requirements, roles of various family members, and approaches to maternal and infant care, including perineal care, breastfeeding practices, infant bathing, care of the circumcision and umbilical cord, naming of the baby, and decision to circumcise, may all be determined by various religious, ethnic, or cultural beliefs and values.

Self-care guidelines During the first weeks, the educational and emotional needs of the family may be extensive. The follow-up care provider can anticipate reviewing the self-care guidelines with the parents and discussing such topics as breast care, including the need for breast support; proper breastfeeding technique; nutrition and need for continued vitamin or iron supplementation; perineal care, including hygiene and use of a squeeze bottle; application of ice or heat and use of portable sitz baths and medications; the need for rest, relaxation, and limitation of visitors; resumption of normal bowel function; demands of infant care and feelings of fatigue or depression; resumption of exercise; sexual intercourse and contraceptive needs; normal newborn needs and behavior, elimination, and feeding patterns; care of the uncircumcised or circumcised penis for male infants; infant safety (carrying, car seat, head support, sleeping position, choking, household dangers, and so on); infant care (bathing, diapering, and skin, eye, and umbilical cord care); birth certificate information; and continued primary care for mother and infant (follow-up appointments).

An excellent overview of postpartum care, called the Johnson and Johnson Consumer Products, Inc., *Compendium of Postpartum Care* (1996), is available through the Association of Women's Health, Obstetric and Neonatal Nurses. The compendium contains extensive and up-to-date information on postpartum care, helpful diagnostic tools, excellent graphics,

and client education handouts. The development of such a comprehensive resource for nurses recognizes the importance of this critical period for new families. Few women have been exposed to role models for breastfeeding and infant care. Women are unable to retain the overwhelming amount of information presented to them after the birth event and a short hospital stay. With a cesarean birth rate over 20%, many women are recovering from surgical or complicated births and need longer recovery periods. Unfortunately, lack of educational, emotional, and practical support is often the norm after hospital discharge, no matter when it occurs. Nurses are in an ideal position to fill this gap in health care.

Consultation and referral An early postpartum discharge program can be a safe, viable option for parents when continued assessment, teaching, and psychosocial support occur within the home or office setting after hospital discharge. Physician consultation and referral are also essential components, since complications will occasionally arise. The nurse may also provide referrals to other community resources, such as doula services, lactation consultants, postpartum depression hotlines, parenting classes, and mothers' groups.

NURSING STRATEGIES FOR THE MANAGEMENT OF COMMON POSTPARTUM PROBLEMS OF MOTHER AND INFANT

During the early postpartum period, the person providing home follow-up may encounter complications. Once assessed, many of these complications can be managed with nursing interventions and self-care strategies. Occasionally, referral to the physician or midwife will be necessary, and rarely, rehospitalization of the mother or infant will be needed.

Maternal Complications

Maternal complications can include urinary retention, bleeding, pain, breast problems, hemorrhoids, infection, and postpartum affective disorders. Diagnosis, physiological basis, and interventions and therapeutic strategies will be briefly reviewed here for each.

Urinary retention Bladder distention without the sensation of needing to void is a common finding in the immediate postpartum period. The bladder is frequently subjected to trauma during the birth process, which results in edema and diminished sensitivity to fluid pressure. When palpating the abdomen and uterine fundus, the nurse may find the uterus displaced from the midline by an overdistended bladder. Nursing strategies may include (1) prophylactic encouragement to void every 2 to 3 hours to avoid overdistention; (2) encouragement to attempt to void when pouring water over the perineum or to void in water, such as a sitz bath; or (3) straight catheterization. Burning with urination may be an early sign of urinary tract infection and should be followed up by the care provider with a clean-catch, midstream urinalysis.

Bleeding problems Excessive vaginal bleeding can be related to several factors, including retained placental fragments, vaginal or cervical lacerations, rupture of a perineal or vaginal hematoma, or uterine atony. Uterine atony, or failure of the uterus to maintain contraction for hemostasis, is the most frequent cause of early postpartum vaginal bleeding. An enlarged boggy or soft uterus is felt by the nurse during abdominal and uterine assessment. A full bladder can predispose the mother to uterine atony. Nursing strategies for uterine atony include (1) encouragement of frequent emptying of the bladder, (2) gentle two-handed uterine massage in a circular fashion to avoid overstimulation of the uterine muscle, and (3) encouragement of frequent nursing of the infant to stimulate endogenous oxytocin production and resulting uterine contraction. If these methods are not successful, the physician or midwife should be contacted, because an oxytocic agent may be needed to maintain uterine hemostasis.

Retained placental fragments are suspected when placental separation and delivery have not proceeded in the normal spontaneous fashion, although they may also result after a completely normal placental delivery. In many instances, a woman will exhibit uterine atony and will pass the tissue with the administration of an oxytocic agent in the immediate postpartum period. Occasionally, retained placental fragments are not expelled until after discharge from the hospital. If retained placental fragments are not passed, the woman may continue to exhibit uterine atony and excessive bleeding. She may report passing several blood clots or tissue. The nurse should also observe for signs of uterine infection and determine whether the woman needs referral for further evaluation and possible dilation and curettage, if this continues.

Women with unrepaired or disrupted vaginal or cervical lacerations that are bleeding excessively will also need referral for further evaluation and possible repair. Vaginal or perineal hematoma can be identified by the nurse on perineal inspection or by gentle vaginal palpation using a sterile glove. Frequently, the woman will complain of increasing vaginal or rectal pressure as the hematoma grows. Small hematomas will reabsorb. Comfort measures, such as sitz baths and analgesia, can be recommended. Women with large or growing hematomas should be referred to their care providers for further evaluation.

Excessive maternal pain Women frequently experience perineal or uterine pain after normal delivery and episiotomy or laceration repair. Perineal pain can be caused by excessive edema, infection, or hematoma. The nurse should observe the site carefully and with adequate lighting to determine the presence of these complications. The nurse should turn the woman on her side and use a light source, such as a flashlight, to observe the perineum. Comfort measures include ice or heat to the perineum, sitz baths, medication sprays, and use of Kegel exercises. An ice pack can be made by filling a rubber glove with ice and covering it with a clean washcloth. Many women consider a warm sitz bath to be helpful in the relief of perineal pain. A disposable, fit-in-the-toilet sitz bath or simply a small amount of warm water in a clean bathtub can be used. Witch hazel compresses are also analgesic and reduce edema (Varney, 1997). They are made by pouring witch hazel over 4×4 gauze pads so that they are wet but not dripping. They can be applied for 20 to 30 minutes, as needed. Tucks is a commercial variation—pads soaked with witch hazel, glycerin, and water. Aloe vera gel (without preservatives) placed on a pad over the area also provides pain relief. If signs of infection are present, the client should be referred to a physician for further evaluation.

Uterine pain is most frequently associated with afterpains, or the contractions of the uterus to maintain hemostasis. They are worsened when the bladder is full and when the woman is a multipara or has received an oxytocic agent. Comfort measures that can be recommended by the nurse include reminding the client to keep her bladder empty, to use prescribed analgesics, and to position herself on her abdomen for rest. Analgesics and rest should be advised. Motherwort *(Leonurus cardiaca)* tea or tincture is used in many cultures after delivery, including in Chinese traditional medicine. One cup of tea or 5 to 20 drops of tincture in a glass of water may help relieve afterpains (Weed, 1986). Women should be advised that the tea is quite bitter.

Breast problems Engorgement, sore nipples, and infection or mastitis are the most common breast problems in the early postpartum period. Engorgement is due to the overdistention of the breasts with milk, increased vascularity, and congestion. Breast engorgement is not an inflammatory process and does not cause a temperature elevation as was once thought ("milk fever"). For the woman who is breastfeeding, engorgement can be relieved by taking hot showers to release the flow of milk, using heat and massage, frequently nursing her baby, or manually expressing some of the milk and then nursing the baby. Nursing frequently and not missing any feedings is the best prevention and treatment for engorgement in breastfeeding mothers. Applying heat just before nursing may also be helpful. Various poultices, compresses, and soaks have also been used with some relief. Breast engorgement in breastfeeding mothers suppresses milk supply, so it is imperative to relieve it. Frequent (four or five times daily), short (3 to 5 minute), consistent applications work the best (Weed, 1986). A hot compress of parsley or comfrey leaves may relieve engorgement. A supportive bra may also be helpful.

For women who do not wish to breastfeed, lactation can be suppressed with the following measures: (1) wearing a tight-fitting bra or binder 24 hours a day until the breasts become soft again; (2) avoiding stimulation of the nipples or expression of the milk, since this augments milk production; (3) taking analgesics; and (4) using lactation suppressants, if prescribed by the care provider, although these may not be effective, are not without potential side effects, and are not routinely recommended. Ice packs on the breasts may also be used as a comfort measure, but heat should be avoided. Engorgement is usually a temporary condition, but it can lead to plugged ducts,

mastitis, and sore nipples, so it should receive attention.

Sore nipples in the breastfeeding woman are usually caused by inadequate nipple grasp by the nursing baby or delicate maternal skin. The nurse may note red, dry nipples when examining the breasts, and the mother may report nipple soreness or pain during nursing. The nurse should observe the mother nursing and ensure that the baby is grasping the areolar tissue when sucking, not just the nipple tip. Sometimes it is necessary to manually express some milk before feeding the baby if areolar engorgement is preventing a good grasp of the nipple by the infant. After feeding, the mother can be instructed to air dry her nipples and expose them to sun or dry heat. Ice may be applied to the nipples just before feeding, if nipples are extremely painful. Nipple shields can be used as a last resort, since they sometimes make the situation worse. Lanolin, olive oil, or sweet almond oil may be applied lightly to the sore nipples for lubrication after each nursing. Lanolin should not be used if the mother is allergic to wool. Soap, alcohol, and other substances should not be used on the nipples. Deodorant, powder, and cologne should be kept away from the nipples as well. The breasts should be washed with plain water. The mother should be encouraged to experiment with different positions for nursing. Sore nipple treatment and prevention are helpful in avoiding cracked nipples, which are extremely painful and may predispose the mother to breast infection. Cracked nipples are treated in the same manner as sore nipples. Aloe vera gel may be used for healing cracked nipples but should be washed off before nursing. Calendula ointment may also heal and strengthen nipples. Yarrow leaf (poultices or ointment) reportedly relieves pain and heals cracked nipples rapidly (Weed, 1986).

Mastitis is an infection of the breast, usually caused by *Staphylococcus aureus* from the baby's mouth, which produces localized redness, tenderness, swelling, and warmth. Avoidance of plugged ducts or prompt treatment of plugged ducts is the best way to prevent mastitis. It is almost always a sign of inadequate rest and inadequate emptying of the breasts. Symptoms of mastitis include plugged ducts, fever ($>101°$ F), malaise, and breast pain. The mother frequently reports feeling as if she is getting influenza. Bed rest, fluids, analgesics, hot compresses at least four times a day, and massage of the breast promote recovery of plugged ducts and mastitis. Antibiotic treatment must also be sought from the care provider for further treatment of mastitis. Prompt treatment and follow-up are needed to prevent breast abscess.

Hemorrhoids   Hemorrhoids are varicose veins of the rectum. Postpartum hemorrhoids can be quite painful because they may have been traumatized or enlarged with edema and pressure during the second stage of labor. Relief measures, including ice packs, sitz baths, witch hazel compresses, anesthetic or analgesic sprays, and Kegel exercises to reduce edema, should be advised. Medicated suppositories or hemorrhoidal creams may also be used. Constipation should be avoided by drinking plenty of fluids and using stool softeners, if necessary. The nurse may use a lubricated finger cot to gently replace an external hemorrhoid inside the rectum. The woman should then be instructed to tighten her anal sphincter to provide support and to contain the hemorrhoid within the rectum (Varney, 1997).

Infection   Maternal infection is present when the temperature is greater than 100.4° F after the first 24 hours. Before 24 hours, a slight temperature elevation can be related to maternal dehydration. Other maternal symptoms may include tachycardia (>100 bpm), malaise, and pain. An excellent discussion of common postpartum maternal infections and their assessment and differential diagnosis is detailed in Clark (1995). The patient may need a complete blood count with differential, cultures (dependent on site of infection), and urinalysis. To avoid infection, the postpartum woman should be encouraged to drink fluids and eat a well-balanced diet; to keep her environment clean and dry with good ventilation when possible; to stay away from sick people; to promptly dispose of dressings, bed linens, and gowns that are soiled with blood, urine, or feces; to ensure that all equipment used (e.g., bathtub, sitz bath) are clean; to change washcloths, towels, and sanitary napkins frequently; and most of all, to use good handwashing technique.

Urinary tract infection (UTI) is the most common cause of postpartum infection, especially in women who have been catheterized during or after labor. In addition to fever, tachycardia, and malaise, the woman may complain of dysuria, burning, urgency, suprapubic pain, or hematuria. A clean-catch, midstream urine specimen must be obtained for urinalysis, culture, and sensitivity. Women with symptoms should be referred to a physician for further evaluation.

Endometritis or uterine infection results from the invasion of the uterine lining by bacteria. Common symptoms include temperature elevation (101° to 102° F), tachycardia, anorexia, malaise, subinvolution of the uterus, abdominal tenderness, and foul-smelling or scant lochia. Prompt referral for oral antibiotic treatment is indicated. Outpatient management is possible for mild cases. More serious or resistant infections will require rehospitalization. In addition to antibiotic treatment, the client should be instructed to stay in bed, monitor vital signs, drink plenty of fluids, and use analgesics for discomfort.

Postpartum adjustment disorder   Postpartum adjustment disorder (PPAD), including the blues, depression, psychosis, and subclinical presentations of depression or anxiety, affects up to 85% of women (Scharff, 1996). PPAD manifests in a wide range of behaviors, from transient weepiness to extended psychiatric episodes requiring hospitalization. However, only 1 to 4 women per 1000 are diagnosed as psychotic during the postpartum period, and most of these women have a history of schizophrenia. Most women experience some form of postpartum blues (crying, irritability, anger, insomnia, exhaustion, tension, anxiety, restlessness, or emotionality) during the first few weeks, often brought on by fatigue, self-deprecation, concern about the changes in lifestyle brought on by the baby, body image concerns, guilt, conflicting feelings about the baby, stress resulting from change in status, worry about finances or career, and desire to get back to normal. Nursing intervention begins with recognition of the situation, continues with making the correct diagnosis, and extends to counseling and teaching self-help skills or making the referral for additional psychiatric diagnosis and care. Beck (1998) provides an excellent checklist for identifying women at risk for developing postpartum depression. Beck (1995) also conducted in-depth interviews with women experiencing postpartum depression. She describes the aspects of nursing caring that these women found helpful. Sensitivity to maternal (and paternal) concerns and willingness to allow the client to express them in a reassuring, non-judgmental atmosphere was found to be helpful. New mothers have several needs that a nurse could help with, such as a good night's sleep, some help around the house, adequate diet and fluid intake, and resumption of exercise. Lack of communication skills, a poor relationship with a partner, too many visitors, and lack of knowledge can all make PPAD worse. The nurse may need to discuss the normalcy of PPAD and discuss some problem-solving strategies, such as setting boundaries with visitors, making self-care and time-out priorities, discussing beliefs and behaviors that are helpful or not helpful, evaluating self-esteem and the need for help from others, and identifying and dealing with emotions and getting help when needed (mental health professional, crisis intervention, or domestic violence hotline). Continued telephone support by the nurse might be helpful, especially if further home or office visits are not possible. Referrals to support groups, parenting groups, the childbirth educator, a doula service, or a mental health professional may also be useful to the family.

Neonatal Complications

The most common neonatal complications include respiratory difficulty, temperature instability, jaundice, sepsis or infection, feeding difficulty, and dehydration. Diagnosis, physiological basis, and therapeutic strategies will be briefly reviewed here for each.

Respiratory difficulties When respirations are greater than 60 per minute and appear labored or when retractions, nasal flaring, or grunting are present, the infant should be stabilized and referred for immediate evaluation.

Temperature instability Neonates are prone to heat loss because they have a large surface area in relation to their weight, less adipose tissue for insulation, and thinner skin with blood vessels closer to the surface. Loss of heat may occur because of wet blankets or diapers in contact with the infant; because of drafts from windows, fans, or air-conditioning; because of contact with cold surfaces such as changing tables, sheets, or scale; or because of exposure from inadequate clothing. The nurse can observe the home environment for these situations and counsel the parents appropriately. Occasionally, the neonate becomes hyperthermic. This is usually due to excessive

clothing or high environmental temperature. The nurse should counsel the parents to avoid neonatal hyperthermia because of the resultant increase in metabolic rate and oxygen consumption. In general, unless environmental conditions are extreme, parents can be advised to dress the baby in one layer more than they have on to avoid hypothermia or hyperthermia.

Jaundice Because the liver of the neonate is immature, the ability to convert indirect (fat-soluble) bilirubin, a product of red blood cell (RBC) breakdown, to direct (water-soluble) bilirubin, which can be excreted by the kidneys and in stool, is limited. This, coupled with the high RBC count in the neonate and increased lysis of RBCs, frequently results in elevated bilirubin levels, exhibited as jaundice in the newborn between 48 and 72 hours after birth. This physiological jaundice is observed in approximately 50% of newborns. It occurs after 24 hours of life. Pathological jaundice occurs before 24 hours of life. Breast-milk jaundice usually occurs after the first week of life. Jaundice is observed as a yellow-orange color to the newborn's skin and mucous membranes. In observable jaundice, the bilirubin level is at least 6 to 7 mg/dl, but its precise level can be determined only by blood test, not by observation.

Prevention of jaundice should be encouraged by the nurse through teaching parents to avoid neonatal hypothermia, to provide frequent feedings to stimulate stool and urine production, and to avoid dehydration and provide adequate caloric intake. Allowing the infant to be exposed to natural light (sunlight) through a glass window may also help decrease jaundice. If jaundice is observed, blood samples for a bilirubin-level assessment should be drawn by heel prick. Referral for evaluation is needed if lethargy, poor feeding, hypothermia, or sepsis is present. When bilirubin levels indicate need for further therapy, phototherapy may be ordered.

Sepsis or infection The neonate is susceptible to infection as a result of an immature immunological system. The infant can be infected as a result of maternal disease during pregnancy (such as rubella or syphilis); as a result of passage through the birth canal (chlamydia, gonococci, herpes virus, or beta-hemolytic streptococci); or by iatrogenic infection. Early signs and symptoms of sepsis or infection in the newborn are often nonspecific and confusing. Lethargy, poor feeding, vomiting, hypothermia, hypotonia, temperature instability, and color changes (such as mottling, cyanotic discoloration, or graying tone) may be noted. Apnea may also occur. Other signs may indicate the location of the infection: jittery movements and seizure activity may indicate central nervous system infection, diarrhea may indicate gastrointestinal infection, or respiratory distress may indicate pulmonary infection. Infection in the newborn spreads rapidly throughout the bloodstream, and serious, generalized sepsis develops quickly. For this reason, any newborn suspected of having an infection should be immediately referred for physician evaluation and probable septic workup.

Feeding difficulty Feeding difficulties include frequent regurgitation and vomiting, gulping, and inadequate intake. These may occur in the neonate in the early postpartum period for a variety of reasons. Regurgitation and vomiting may be caused by rapid feeding or by too much milk at one time. Parents should be counseled to feed the infant more slowly, decrease the amount of each feeding, or pause more frequently to burp the baby. If vomiting is excessive and continuous or projectile in nature, pyloric stenosis should be suspected. Gulping of milk may also result from rapid feeding. With bottle feeding, this results when the nipple hole is too large or when too many holes are made in the nipple. The infant will swallow a lot of air along with the milk, which produces gas and discomfort. Slow feeding, frequent burping, and holding the infant snugly in an upright position for feeding should help to eliminate this problem. Inadequate feedings may result when milk is offered infrequently, when the baby is sleepy at feeding time, or when maternal breast-milk supply is inadequate. The nurse must assess the source of this problem and counsel parents appropriately. If excessive weight loss (>8% to 10% of birth weight) is observed, parents may need to be educated to feed the baby more or more often. If feedings are infrequent because of maternal-infant separation or other factors, they should be increased. When the baby is sleepy at feedings, the nurse should encourage feeding at times when the baby is awake or suggest ways parents can arouse their baby at feeding time. If maternal milk supply is inadequate, the nurse should encourage additional rest, fluids,

Box 15-4 Conditions and Developments Requiring Immediate Referral

MOTHER
Excessive postpartum bleeding
Large or growing hematoma
Infection
Severe postpartum depression
Wound dehiscence
Maladaptive parenting

INFANT
Respiratory difficulty, distress, or apnea
Jaundice before 24 hr of age or with lethargy, poor feeding, hypothermia, or sepsis
Sepsis or infection
Seizures
Severe dehydration
Excessive diarrhea or vomiting
Persistent hypothermia

food, and relaxation to improve milk production and the let-down reflex.

Dehydration Dehydration can result from excessive emesis (>2 per day), loose stools (>1 in 24 hours), or poor or inadequate feedings. Signs and symptoms of newborn dehydration include poor skin turgor; pale, dry mucous membranes; sunken fontanel; and few wet diapers. Dehydration is treated by correcting the underlying factor that created it and replacing the lost fluids. If diarrhea or loose stools and vomiting continue, the infant must be referred to a physician or nurse practitioner for prompt treatment.

Box 15-4 summarizes the maternal and neonatal conditions that require immediate referral and possible rehospitalization.

POSTPARTUM CARE AFTER CESAREAN BIRTH

Because more than 20% of childbearing women experience cesarean delivery, the nurse at times will be providing postpartum follow-up for these women and their infants. Although LOS is still longer for cesarean mothers and their babies, the trend toward earlier discharge is evident. Mothers and infants who have experienced cesarean delivery have special considerations during postpartum follow-up including (1) a major surgical incision, (2) indications that necessitated surgical delivery, (3) anesthesia effects, (4) maternal pain and limitation of activity, and (5) psychological and emotional considerations.

The surgical incision should be healing well before hospital discharge. However, the nurse providing follow-up should check for signs of infection (tenderness, drainage, and redness) or dehiscence. The REEDA scale may be used to assess the healing of the incision (Table 15-1). The letters in REEDA stand for redness, edema, ecchymosis, discharge, and approximation of the skin edges. Each characteristic is scaled from 0 to 3, depending on the severity, with 0 indicating none (Davidson, 1984). The ratings for the five characteristics are added to obtain the score. Scores should be less than 8 during the first postpartum week. Maternal and fetal indications for surgical delivery vary greatly. Whenever appropriate, the nurse should provide follow-up for these indications. For example, if pregnancy-induced hypertension was the reason for cesarean delivery, maternal blood pressure, reflexes, and urinary protein should be checked. Cesarean mothers and their infants are at greater risk for infection. Therefore they should be observed for a febrile condition or other signs and symptoms of infection. Anesthesia effects on the mother should be minimal by hospital discharge. Gastrointestinal function, bladder function, respiratory function, and venous circulation should be normal. However, careful assessment of lungs, bowel sounds, bladder function, and pelvic and leg veins should be included in the home nursing assessment. Most analgesics given to mothers recovering from cesarean delivery have minimal effects on the nursing baby. When needed, they should be taken 1 to 2 hours before nursing or handling the baby to promote maternal comfort. However, the nurse should be particularly attentive to helping the cesarean mother decrease her discomfort through nonpharmacological means as well. The mother can be shown how to splint her incision to decrease discomfort when moving, how to use pillows for support, and how to change positions. Lying on her side or sitting in a chair with a pillow on her lap may be the most comfortable position for nursing.

Obviously, a woman recovering from a cesarean delivery has special needs for psychological and emotional support during the early postpartum period. Often the prolonged recovery after surgery delays the woman's ability to attend to her infant's needs completely. She may need the help of her partner and others for a longer time. In addition, the woman may have negative feelings about the pregnancy, labor, or birth experience because of disappointment or anger related to the cesarean birth. Body image concerns are also more prevalent after cesarean delivery. These feelings and concerns need to be expressed

Table 15-1   REEDA Scale: Assessment of Incision Healing

Points	Redness	Edema	Ecchymosis	Discharge	Approximation
0	None	None	None	None	Closed
1	Within 0.25 cm of incision bilaterally	<1 cm from incision	Within 0.25 bilaterally or 0.5 cm unilaterally	Serum	Skin separation 3 mm or more
2	Within 0.50 cm of incision bilaterally	1-2 cm from incision	0.25-1 cm bilaterally or 0.5-2 cm unilaterally	Serosanguinous	Skin and sub-q fat separation
3	Beyond 0.5 cm of incision bilaterally	>2 cm from incision	>1 cm bilaterally or 2 cm unilaterally	Bloody, purulent	Skin, sub-q fat and fascial separation
Score	_____	_____	_____	_____	_____
TOTAL	_____				

From Davidson N: REEDA: Evaluating postpartum healing, *Journal of Nurse-Midwifery* 19:6-8, 1984.
sub-q, Subcutaneous.

in a reassuring atmosphere provided by the nurse and other support persons. The nurse should also be particularly sensitive to the promotion of parent-infant attachment for cesarean parents. They have often experienced early separation as a result of a variety of maternal-infant indications. This early separation also affects the establishment of lactation, leading to delayed milk production, increased engorgement, and maternal lack of confidence in her ability to nurse. The nurse can play a supportive and informative role in these situations.

PROBLEMS RELATING TO HOME POSTPARTUM CARE

Some critical problems relating to early postpartum discharge and home follow-up care remain. Nurse reimbursement for home follow-up is not routine by many payor sources. Nurses must support legislative changes that enable autonomous billing by nurses and others for services such as home postpartum care. Another area of concern is that in some hospitals, nurses must go through the physician to make a referral for home follow-up. Hospital policy that facilitates nurse referral should be developed, since the physician (or the managed care organization) may respond negatively to the need for home follow-up.

There is also difficulty in assessing the "success" of early postpartum discharge programs. Review articles have many methodological flaws that make definitive answers about benefits and cost almost impossible (Weiner, 1997). Most programs have used gross measurements of cost savings, whereas others have used client satisfaction criteria. Few have combined maternal-infant outcome and client satisfaction information. Maternal-infant outcome is very hard to measure in any one study because of the rarity of most complications and the need for a very large sample size. More sophisticated cost analyses, maternal-infant outcome assessments, and family satisfaction measures should all be considered in research designed to evaluate early postpartum discharge and home follow-up programs versus longer hospital stays. The cost of a second day of hospitalization may far exceed the cost associated with office or home postpartum follow-up (Weiner, 1997).

Perinatal nurses must continue to research and speak out on this issue to ensure quality, cost-efficient postpartum care that truly meets the needs of today's families. In addition to playing an important role in the prenatal preparation of parents for early discharge, development of screening criteria, and provision of postpartum follow-up care, perinatal nurses need to involve themselves in the formation of health policy to guard against elimination of postpartum inpatient and outpatient services. As the forces of cost containment increase and perinatal care continues to focus on the technological and critical aspects of care (primarily in intrapartum and neonatal care), early postpartum discharge may become the standard. Simultaneously, resources may not be made available for adequate follow-up home care. Clearly, this will be a disadvantage to clients. Postpartum nurses have already identified early discharge as a problem. Lack of time for adequate assessment of mother and infant and decreased teaching time are two of the problems cited. This can lead only to further job dissatisfaction for nurses and inadequate care for clients. Mandating early discharge (even with adequate follow-up) also denies the client's right to care options. It is the ethical responsibility of nursing to guard against such practices. When early discharge is optional and supported, hospital nursing resources can be used more appropriately for families who need to stay longer.

RESOURCES FOR THE NEW FAMILY

During the course of prenatal and postpartum care, parents should be made aware of the various community resources available to them. Primary health care providers and the hospital nursery are the most obvious. Postpartum home health care is available through the visiting nurse service or various public and private agencies, including doula services. The childbirth educator can also be an important source of information, reassurance, and support. Groups concerned with parenting skills, early childhood growth and development, breastfeeding, and cesarean support may also be helpful to new parents. In addition, there are many excellent books on parenting, breastfeeding, well-baby care, infant growth and development, and sick care and safety. These are available in the public library, through the International Childbirth Education Association bookmarks, or in other bookstores, including those on-line, such as Amazon.com. Table 15-2 includes a selected list of resources for the new family.

Table 15-2 Resources for the New Family	
Resource	Comments
Depression After Delivery 91 East Somerset Street Raritan, NJ 08869 1-800-994-4773 http://www.depressionafterdelivery.com	Depression After Delivery, Inc. provides information and support for women (and their families) who have experienced adjustment difficulties, depression, or psychosis after birth.
Doulas of North America Central Office 13513 North Grove Drive Alpine, UT 84004 801-756-7331 801-763-1847 (fax) http://www.dona.com	Doulas of North America refers doulas in your area. Doulas provide labor support, as well as postpartum and breastfeeding help.
ICEA Bookmarks P.O. Box 20048 Minneapolis, MN 55420 1-800-624-4934 or 952-854-8660 http://www.icea.org	ICEA Bookmarks is a comprehensive and reliable source of books on pregnancy, parenting, postpartum period, breastfeeding, and child-rearing.
Harvard Common Press 535 Albany Street Boston, MA 02118 617-423-5803 617-695-9794 (fax)	Harvard Common Press publishes books on childbirth, childcare, and parenting.
La Leche League International 1400 North Meacham Road Schaumburg, IL 60168-4079 847-519-7730 http://www.lalecheleague.org	Local affiliates provide monthly meetings to educate, provide support, and help with breastfeeding. La Leche League publishes books and pamphlets on lactation, infant care, and safety in multiple languages.
National Domestic Violence Hotline 1-800-799-SAFE http://www.ndvh.org	This hotline is a resource for crisis intervention, referrals, information, and support in many languages.
Postpartum depression website: http://www.geocities.com/Wellesley/4665	This website is devoted to mothers and their families who are affected by postpartum depression. It includes a mailing list and chat room.
Postpartum Support International 927 N Kellogg Avenue Santa Barbara, CA 93111 805-967-7636 805-967-0608 (fax) http://www.chss.iup.edu/postpartum	Postpartum Support International promotes awareness of mental health issues related to reproduction.
Postpartum Survival Guide: http://www.whcws.com/articles/oct94.htm	This website has excerpts from the postpartum survival guide.
Single Parent Resource Center 141 W 28th Street, Suite 302 New York, NY 10001 212-947-0221 http://www.singleparentusa.com/index.html	The Single Parent Resource Center is a network of local single parent support groups.
The Best Parenting News on the Web website: http://www.parentstages.com	This website is for parents of all ages.
Baby Center website: http://www.babycenter.com	This is a resource for parents-to-be and new parents from the time of preconception planning through the baby's first year.
Family Network website: http://www.familynetwork.com	This is a membership network for new parents.
Families Like Ours, Inc. http://www.familieslikeours.org	This is a resource for gay and lesbian parents.

SUMMARY

Families, especially the mother and infant, undergo tremendous physical and psychological adaptation during the early postpartum period. Nurses have traditionally been the care providers, whether in the hospital or the home, who assess progress and provide guidance and intervention as women, newborns, and families undergo these complex adjustments. Assessment of needs and anticipatory guidance and teaching range from economic, social, and ethnoreligious concerns to psychological aspects of postpartum adjustment, depression, and maternal-infant bonding. Nurses must be well prepared to intervene and assist families to access appropriate resources when needed. Sometimes this is a struggle in a milieu of controlled costs.

The purpose of this chapter has been to help the caregiver provide the best possible postpartum assessment and support after hospital discharge, recognize common deviations from normal, and refer to a physician or nurse practitioner. It is not intended to be a comprehensive resource on all aspects of the puerperium, the 6-week period between birth and "recovery" from birth. Hopefully, it has helped provide the nurse with some encouragement and education that he or she needs to attend to new families and reminded him or her that as with any relationship, cultural needs and individuality make each situation unique. The close role of the home health care nurse also enables the nurse to act as self care educator. Through the establishment of rapport, the home care nurse enables the mother and family to care for themselves, to promote health, and to prevent complications. A more confident, skillful, and caring parent can result, making these nursing care strategies right on target.

REFERENCES

Beck CT: Perceptions of nurses' caring by mothers experiencing postpartum depression, *Journal of Obstetrical, Gynecologic, and Neonatal Nursing* 24(9):819-825, 1995.

Beck CT: A checklist to identify women at risk for developing postpartum depression, *Journal of Obstetrical, Gynecologic, and Neonatal Nursing* 27(1):39-46, 1998.

Britton JR: Postpartum early hospital discharge and follow-up practices in Canada and the United States, *Birth* 25(3):161-168, 1998.

Centers for Disease Control and Prevention: Trends in length of stay for hospital deliveries—United States, 1970-1992, *MMWR Morbidity and Mortality Weekly Report* 44(17):335-337, 1995.

Clark RA: Infections during the postpartum period, *Journal of Obstetrical, Gynecologic, and Neonatal Nursing* 24(6):542-548, 1995.

Davidson N: REEDA: Evaluating postpartum healing, *Journal of Nurse-Midwifery* 19:6-8, 1984.

Declercq E, Simmes D: The politics of "drive through deliveries": Putting early postpartum discharge on the legislative agenda, *Milbank Quarterly* 75(2):175-202, 1997.

Gazmararian JA, Koplan JP: Length-of-stay after delivery: Managed care versus fee-for-service, *Health Affairs* 15(4):74-80, 1996.

Johnson & Johnson Consumer Products, Inc: *Compendium of postpartum care*, Skillman, NJ, 1996, Johnson & Johnson Consumer Products, Inc.

Jones PM: Patient satisfaction with home care after early postpartum hospital discharge, *Home Care Provider* 2(5):235-243, 1997.

Keppler A: Evergreen hospital postpartum care center: Follow-up care in a hospital-based clinic, *Journal of Obstetrical, Gynecologic, and Neonatal Nursing* 24(1):17-21, 1995.

Maternity care appropriate follow-up services critical with short hospital stays, Pub No GAO/HEHS-96-207, Washington DC, 1996, US General Accounting Office.

Newborns' and Mothers' Health Protection Act of 1996. Public Law 104-204, September 26, 1996, enacted as Title VI of the Departments of Veteran Affairs and Housing and Urban Development, and Independent Agencies Appropriations Act (1997).

Scharff D: Mother to mother telephone support project: Formative evaluation and intervention design, *International Journal of Childbirth Education* 11:26-29, 1996.

US Department of Health and Human Services, Maternal and Child Health Bureau: Maternal and infant health: From insurance to assurance. Paper presented at the annual meeting of the Association of Maternal and Child Health Programs, Washington, DC, 1996.

Varney H: *Varney's midwifery*, ed 3, Boston, 1997, Jones & Bartlett.

Weed S: *Wise woman herbal for the childbearing years*, Woodstock, NY, 1986, Ash Tree.

Weiner J: Beyond meta-analyses and randomized controlled trials: The minimum maternity stay law, *JCOM* 4:16-22, 1997.

Williams LR, Cooper MK: A new paradigm for postpartum care, *Journal of Obstetric, Gynecologic, and Neonatal Nursing* 25(9):745-749, 1996.

16 Home Care of Children

Marsha H. Cohen and Ida M. Martinson

During the 1990s, pediatric home care has become the fastest growing segment of the home health care industry, with more than 50,000 children receiving services daily (Clemans et al, 1997; Goldberg, Gardner, Gibson, 1994). This growth is embedded within a complex and evolving matrix of societal conditions (Samuel, 1991) that includes changes in disease trends, advances in biomedical technology, altered economic conditions, and emerging social imperatives.

TRENDS AND ISSUES AFFECTING PEDIATRIC HOME CARE
Disease Trends

During the first half of the twentieth century, childhood illnesses were largely of an acute, infectious nature with a time-limited and relatively brief course. Children were either cared for in their homes by family members for the duration of the illness or sent home to convalesce after a brief hospitalization. Today, preventive health measures are responsible for a sharp drop in the incidence of such diseases, and diagnostic and pharmacotherapeutic advances have significantly improved morbidity and mortality rates.

Chronic childhood illnesses, however, present a different picture. Although there has been little evidence of a change in the incidence of such diseases since the mid-1900s, biomedical and technological developments of recent years have made it increasingly possible to stabilize physiologically impaired infants, control the progression of many life-threatening illnesses, and repair defects that were previously incompatible with life. The resulting increase in survival rates has contributed to a consequent increase in the prevalence of children with chronic illnesses (Hobbs, Perrin, 1985; U.S. Congress, Office of Technology Assessment,

1987). Unlike previous generations of children with severe or life-threatening chronic illnesses, the majority of today's children can expect to reach adulthood, and a significant number have the potential to lead productive lives despite ongoing medical dependency. For these medically fragile* and technology-dependent† children, home care is a means of normalizing and enhancing the quality of life for them and for their families (Aday, Wegener, 1988).

Technological Trends

Changes in disease trends have encouraged innovative developments in biomedical technology and a corresponding explosive growth in high-tech home care (Arras, 1995). The miniaturization and simplification of equipment permit many types of monitoring and treatment regimens to be carried out at home, and improvements in the portability of equipment have eliminated the need to restrict the child, and hence the family, to the confines of the home. For children whose conditions are relatively stable, it is becoming increasingly possible to deliver almost any type of care in the home that was previously only feasible in institutional settings.

---

*There is no single accepted definition of the term *medically fragile child*. As used in this chapter, it refers to a child with a chronic health condition that is progressively debilitating or that is subject to sudden or frequent fluctuations interspersed with periods of relative stability.

†The most generally accepted definition of *technology-dependent child* was one proposed by the Office of Technology Assessment (US Congress, Office of Technology Assessment, 1987). It is a child who "needs both a medical device to compensate for the loss of a vital body function and substantial nursing care to avert death or further disability. This definition is independent of the setting of care or the particular credentials of the caregiver."

High-tech home care, however, is a double-edged sword. Although it allows the child and family to live together in the more normal environment of the home, it also creates a new set of demands for parents and society that has no historic precedent. Parents must now assume the awesome responsibility of continuously monitoring their child's physiological status and making medical judgments that may have potentially serious consequences for their child's well-being or even for his or her survival. They must learn to operate and maintain an array of medical equipment used in their child's care and develop the skills to perform complex medical procedures that previously fell only within the domain of licensed health professionals.

Society, as well, must respond to the many new demands that this new population of medically fragile and technology-dependent children living in the community place on it. Community-based resources to assist families in caring for their children must be developed, and ways to integrate these children into the life of the community must be found. Currently, the technology to maintain children physiologically far exceeds the capabilities of community-based agencies to provide the necessary support services to the families caring for them (Carson, 1996).

Economic Trends

It has been well documented that the technology is available to provide safe care at home for children who have a broad range of complex requirements, including, but not limited to, electronic monitoring, continuous oxygen administration, mechanical ventilation, hyperalimentation, intravenous drug therapy, and dialysis. The rising cost of hospital care for children requiring these treatment modalities has been one of the major factors responsible for motivating third-party payors to include a home care option for technology-dependent and medically fragile children.

Studies have consistently demonstrated that, with few exceptions, home care is substantially less costly than hospital care. In the early 1980s, when high-tech home care for children was in its early period of growth, it was reported that (1) caring for clients requiring mechanical ventilation was 70% less costly in the home than in the hospital (Faure et al, 1983), (2) the cost of caring for infants with bronchopulmonary dysplasia de-

creased from $627 per day for inpatient care to $14.62 per day for home care (Donn, 1982), (3) home phototherapy versus hospital treatment for term infants with hyperbilirubinemia resulted in a cost savings of approximately $225 per infant per day (Slater, Brewer, 1984), and (4) the cost of home care for dying children was about one half the cost of terminal care received in the hospital (Moldow et al, 1982).

More recent studies report similar findings. In their annual report, the National Association for Home Care (NAHC) (1996) cited studies that compared the cost of home care versus hospital care for low–birth weight infants, oxygen-dependent children, and children receiving chemotherapy for cancer. For these groups, the cost savings were estimated to be $25,860, $6840, and $13,920, respectively, per client per month.

Cost-analysis studies, however, have not gone unchallenged, for although the preponderance of evidence supports the conclusion that home care is less costly for third-party payors, costs to the family and society have not been equally studied. As Feinberg (1991) stated, "Cost shifting to families is a particularly insidious aspect of cost savings to institutions." For example, methodological questions have been raised about the validity of studies that compare the cost of hospital care versus home care since for the latter, studies rarely, if ever, consider the out-of-pocket expenditures of the family for items such as food, equipment, supplies, and increased utility use—items usually included in the estimate of hospital costs. Nor do home care estimates include the costs to the family for home renovations, transportation, respite care, and lost wages if the working parent must remain home with the child (Stein, 1984). When a parent gives up his or her employment to care for a child at home and subsequently becomes a recipient of welfare, the cost of public subsidy must also be considered in determining the ultimate cost of pediatric home care to society.

Finally, estimates of cost savings of home care should consider whether nursing and other supportive services (such as occupational, physical, psychological, or speech therapy) in the home are available and equivalent to those that the child and family would have both access and entitlement to if the child remained hospitalized. Fields et al (1991) reported that the costs of home care for 10 children dependent on respiratory technology were "considerably less than projected" only because of the nonavailability of skilled nursing care. It is misleading to claim that home care is less costly when savings are the result of failing to provide important service.

Although many states have more funding mechanisms today than a decade ago (Petr, Murdock, Chapin, 1995), the home care option for children remains unevenly distributed throughout the country. Some funding sources require assurances from the referring agent that nursing service is required for only a limited time and that independence of the family in the care of the child is a reasonable goal. In fact, authorization for home care nursing by some third-party payors may be contingent on explicit expectations that the service will be time-limited and that the nurse's role will be to train the family to become not only competent, but completely independent. Projections of reduced costs for home care based on the premise of parental responsibility for 24-hour care immediately or shortly after discharge are often unrealistic considering the complex and unremitting nature of the care that some children require.

There continues to be a wide gap between the family-support services that are needed to satisfactorily maintain a medically complex child at home and those that are currently reimbursable by most funding sources. Legislative and policy changes that would permit funding for and access to the full range of services required have been slow in coming.

One roadblock is the concern of funding agencies that without strict eligibility requirements and monitoring, rampant abuses would occur and that home care would become an add-on service rather than a substitute for more costly hospital or institutional care. A second obstacle is the financial disincentive for physicians to support home health care because of loss of income. Physicians who currently charge for visits to hospitalized clients are not paid for clinical management of the child at home under most current reimbursement policies (Goldberg, Gardner, Gibson, 1994). In addition, concerns regarding liability for care delivered in the home, as well as standards of quality for nursing care, have been raised by those who are unconvinced that home care is the best answer to the problem of cost

containment (Kohrman, 1991; McAllister et al, 1986). Clearly, policies regarding funding for pediatric home care must continue to address technology-dependent and medically fragile children whose return home mandates access to long-term, and possibly indefinite, nursing support.

Social Trends

Pediatric home care has also been influenced by a number of emergent social trends, including (1) deinstitutionalization, (2) the increasing number of women in the workforce, (3) changes in family structure, and (4) growing consumer activism.

Deinstitutionalization During the first half of the twentieth century, increasing sophistication of medical and surgical treatment provided the major impetus for transferring the care of the sick from the home to the hospital. A countertrend began in the early 1960s with the discharge of mentally disabled persons from institutions to the community and the establishment of community-based mental health centers that were expected to meet their needs. This trend toward community integration of the disabled now includes many types of proactive and reactive programs that cut across a variety of conditions: from those that attempt to prevent placement of the elderly in institutions to those that propose to return children who had become virtual technological prisoners of institutions to their homes (Zollinger et al, 2000).

Closely related to deinstitutionalization are the concepts of normalization and mainstreaming. Public and professional awareness of the abnormal, and often bizarre, environment that the hospital setting provides for the developing child led to concern that the psychosocial needs of children were being sacrificed in the interest of physiological maintenance.

An important piece of federal legislation was passed by Congress in 1975 that had a significant impact in supporting a home care alternative for hospitalized children. It mandated that all children in the United States were to have available to them a free and appropriate public education in the least restrictive environment. Often referred to as *mainstreaming*, the Education for All Handicapped Children Act (Public Law 94-142) is based on the premise that special education systems or practices are inappropriate if they remove children from their expanded peer group without benefit of constitutional safeguards. Therefore the law requires that impediments to a child's satisfactory progress through school be overcome by the provision of appropriate services whenever possible, including any necessary health services, if this will prevent placing the child in a more restrictive environment. Mainstreaming became a rallying point for those who saw the confinement of children in hospitals as inappropriately restrictive and a violation of the child's right to grow up within his or her own family. In Illinois, the broad definition of home care was adopted from the language of Public Law 94-142 and called for placement of the ill child in the "least restrictive environment for the child and the family" (Kohrman, 1984). Today, increased attention is directed toward normalizing the child's experiences by keeping hospitalization to a minimum.

Women in the workforce   The women's movement, inflation, and other economic pressures have created the conditions for ever-increasing numbers of women choosing or needing to enter the workforce and to remain in it for a longer period of time (Huston et al, 2001). Today over 70% of women in the United States between 20 and 44 years of age work outside the home (U.S. Department of Labor, 2001). Not only are there fewer mothers at home to care for children, but the social value placed on child-rearing as a full-time undertaking has declined. However, despite pervasive economic and social changes that have propelled women into the workforce and changed the way society tends to value full-time parenting, there is still an underlying expectation that parents, particularly mothers, of ill children should remain at home and forgo their career goals or economic aspirations. Thus parents are frequently confronted by a number of competing demands regarding employment and child care. For example, they are likely to experience an increased need to work to maintain their health insurance and meet the additional expenses brought on by the child's medical condition, but if they continue to work, they may find themselves subject to criticism for not choosing to stay at home. Conversely, some parents may have no choice but to resign from the workforce, forfeiting their source of income and health insurance, if adequate funding for home nursing care is not available to them. Home nursing is the single

most critical resource if parents are to be able to remain in the workforce, go to school, or receive job training.

Changes in family structure   Years of decreasing family size and increasing geographic mobility have left many of today's nuclear families lacking in or isolated from an extended family group and often without another adult on whom they can rely for help (Ford-Gilboe, 2000). In addition, there has been a steady increase in the number of single-parent families. Caring for a chronically ill child at home without an adequate family support network overwhelms and exhausts many parents. When they lose their physical freedom and must withdraw from the mainstream of social and occupational activities and when all other roles must be subordinated to that of caretaker, parents are at increased risk for emotional and physical disorders, and their child is at increased risk for institutional placement. Again, the importance of home nursing is a critical factor in maintaining the integrity of the family.

Consumer activism   The trend toward increasing consumer activism in the United States is one that extends to health care as well. Consumers of health care have become more aware of their rights and options, less intimidated by professional authority, and more suspicious of medical advice. Increasingly, parents are demanding access to medical information, forming self-help groups and coalitions, and insisting on being full participants in making decisions that affect their child's care and their family's autonomy. An example of consumer activism is a parent group that organized a continuing-education course to teach physicians how to sensitively present the diagnosis of a child's debilitating condition to families (Lawson, Pierce, 1984).

Public advocacy by parents to obtain needed services for their children when the health care system has been unresponsive is more common today than it once was. Parents have made public appeals via the media for organ donors for their children, brought litigation against third-party payors for denial of benefits, and formed lobbying groups to secure government funding for underserved children. Many have begun to demand that their children's quality of life be given at least equal consideration as the preservation of life, and they have gone to court and to the media for support in either obtaining or discontinuing treatment for their children. A paradigm case of consumer activism is the Beckett family who set in motion a process that resulted in major changes in the scope of Medicaid funding and culminated in the current Medicaid home care option for medically fragile and technology-dependent children.

Katie Beckett was a ventilator-dependent child who had been hospitalized from September, 1978, until December, 1981. After exhausting all avenues for securing funds that would enable them to care for their daughter at home, Katie's parents went public in an appeal to Vice President Bush for an exception to Medicaid policy so that Katie could receive the necessary care at home without losing her Medicaid eligibility. Their appeal was successful and resulted in the establishment of the Katie Beckett Review Board within the Department of Health and Human Services in May, 1982. The function of this board was to consider, on a case-by-case basis, whether clients could be reimbursed under the Medicaid program for services provided in the home rather than in the hospital (Koop, 1983). If home care was approved, waivers were granted on an individual basis. The Katie Beckett Review Board was an interim board set up to function only until states could develop and apply for their own home- and community-based waiver program for Medicaid-eligible clients. The Katie Beckett Review Board was disbanded in December, 1983.

FINANCING PEDIATRIC HOME CARE

The major sources of funding for pediatric home care are private insurance companies, Medicaid, health maintenance organizations (HMOs), and maternal-child health block grants. Other sources include Supplemental Security Income (SSI), special state-funded programs, private voluntary organizations, and the Civilian Health and Medical Program of the Uniformed Services (CHAMPUS). For a comprehensive review of home care financing, see Chapter 6.

Private Insurance

For children, private insurance is provided primarily by group policies that cover dependents of employed parents. Home care benefits from private insurance can vary significantly from policy to policy. Some policies may cover only skilled, intermittent nursing services after hospitalization. Others may limit the total number of nursing visits. Policies that include major medical benefits provide home care nursing and intermittent visits. All require review for medical necessity, and most have lifetime limits. Custodial care, respite for parents, and any care that a parent would be expected to provide for a well child are generally excluded. Insurers may elect to provide coverage on an individual, case-by-case basis outside the parameters of the standard benefit package if the cost effectiveness of home care for a particular child can be documented.

HMOs

HMOs have even greater variation in home care benefits than private insurance companies. Some may not provide any home care, some may authorize nursing and other therapies but no home equipment, and others may provide extensive home care services if they are deemed medically necessary to permit early discharge from the hospital. Some HMOs have established contracts with home care providers, equipment suppliers, and pharmacies and will authorize services only through their contracted provider. These providers may or may not have experience with the needs of children.

Medicaid

Medicaid, also known as *Title XIX of the Social Security Act,* is jointly funded by federal and state governments. The basic Medicaid program requires all states to pay for specified services to categorically eligible groups. One of the mandated services that all states must offer is the early and periodic screening, diagnostic, and treatment (EPSDT) program for Medicaid-eligible children from birth to 21 years of age. The EPSDT program provides screening for health and developmental problems and requires states to pay for all necessary services to remediate or treat the conditions identified through the screening process, even if these services are not covered by the basic state Medicaid plan (Parette, 1993). The EPSDT program is an important benefit to all chronically ill children, including those receiving home care services through other funding mechanisms.

States have the flexibility to determine their own criteria for eligibility in a specific group (e.g., the categorically needy and the medically needy). Therefore criteria for Medicaid eligibility will vary from state to state, but, with few exceptions, eligibility is most often determined by the following factors: (1) the family's income is below the state-determined poverty level, (2) the child is blind or disabled and living in a family with a limited income, or (3) the child's medical expenses are high in relation to family income. Essentially, this means that eligible families are already enrolled in Aid to Families with Dependent Children (AFDC) or SSI or that they qualify under the medically needy option that states may elect to adopt. The medically needy option allows families with dependent children or with one absent, unemployed, or incapacitated parent to qualify for Medicaid if their income is above the Medicaid cutoff but falls below this level when medical expenses are subtracted.

Medicaid also allows states the option to choose to offer any or all of approximately 40 additional services, including case management, hospice services, and transportation (Kinslow, 1996). Therefore not only do Medicaid eligibility criteria vary from state to state, but also the scope of services offered to those who are eligible varies. However, within a given state there must be comparability of services to all members of eligible groups (Kinslow, 1996). Exceptions to the comparability rule are granted through waivers.

States may choose to participate in Medicaid home and community-based care (HCBC) waivers, which came into being as a result of the Katie Beckett appeal, discussed previously. Waivers allow a state not only to include a variety of services generally not covered by Medicaid, such as case management, respite care, homemaker services, and minor modifications to the home (Ahmann, 1986), but also to target specific populations (such as technology-dependent children) and to disregard family income in determining eligibility. Each HCBC waiver is limited to serving no more than 200 individuals; however, states are not limited in the number of waivers that they can request (Kinslow, 1996; Weston, Keefe, 1993).

States may also choose to amend their state Medicaid plan by requesting to provide services to eligible persons under the Tax Equity and Fiscal Responsibility Act (TEFRA) of 1986, rather than by HCBC waivers. TEFRA programs offer additional flexibility, since there is no restriction regarding the number of children that can be served under this program (Haas, 1992).

Maternal-Child Health Block Grants

Title V of the Social Security Act of 1935 established Crippled Children's Services (CCS), a federal and state matching-funds program that enabled states to provide comprehensive services to children with handicapping or crippling conditions. The 98th Congress later changed the name of CCS to Children with Special Health Care Needs (CSHCN). Every state has a CSHCN program, and eligible medical conditions and financial eligibility are determined by each state. Purchase or rental of home equipment, supplies, nursing visits, therapy, and respite care are some of the services that may be provided through a state's CSHCN program. Home nursing care can be provided in some cases to help in the transition from hospital to home, but long-term home nursing is usually not covered by this program.

In the 1980s, federal funding earmarked for CSHCN programs ceased, and states began receiving money in the form of maternal-child health block grants (MCHBGs). MCHBGs combined several categorical programs (e.g., CSHCN, genetic screening, adolescent pregnancy programs) into one grant to the states and left it up to the discretion of each state to determine how the grant money would be allocated among its various maternal-child health programs (Cohen, 1990). Consequently, the extent of CSHCN expenditures for home care varies not only from one state to another but also among the counties within a state.

SSI

The SSI program is a federal income-maintenance program for the aged, blind, and disabled. Disabled children receiving monthly SSI payments may be eligible for attendant care under In-Home Support Services (IHSS). The family is responsible for engaging and training the attendant. Since reimbursement is usually at minimum-wage rates, finding a qualified attendant willing to work can be difficult. However, a family member can act as the child's attendant and be paid the assigned amount.

Special State-Funded Programs

Special state-funded programs may address the needs of a particular group of children, such as those who are developmentally disabled or genetically handicapped. Services are generally not comprehensive but can often be used to augment existing entitlements. For example, respite services or vocational training may be available through state-funded agencies.

Private Voluntary Organizations

There are many private voluntary organizations, such as the March of Dimes, whose main purpose is the support of research or the dissemination of information to the public. Others, however, may provide a variety of services to families who are caring for their children at home. The Muscular Dystrophy Association, for example, provides wheelchairs, orthotic devices, and home equipment. Many voluntary or charitable organizations also operate summer camps for children. Camp not only provides a normalizing experience for the child but also offers the parents at least 1 week of respite from child care that might not be available through other sources.

CHAMPUS

CHAMPUS is the health insurance program of the Defense Department that is available to dependent children of active-duty and retired members of the armed services. It provides a limited home care benefit as well as a program for the handicapped.

Other Potential Sources of Funding

The previous list covers the primary sources of funding for pediatric home care. However, in today's rapidly changing health care arena, it is reasonable to expect that legislative and political changes will continue to alter existing programs, eligibility requirements, and funding mechanisms (Karr, Locke, Leonard, 1993). In this environment of change, nurses should assume an active role in advocating for services and funding to support family-centered, community-based pediatric home care.

Advocacy Role of the Nurse in Securing Funding

Although there are many sources of funding for home care, some medically fragile and technology-dependent children do not qualify for or cannot access any of them. In effect, funding may not be available because the child does not have a "covered disease" or live in a state or county that provides needed services, or the family does not meet income criteria. For some children, fund-

ing is not obtained because there is no person acting on the child's behalf who is knowledgeable enough about all of the existing or potential resources, creative enough to piece together a workable home care program from the limited array of services that are available, assertive enough to compel private and public agencies to work cooperatively, or persistent enough to comply with the tedious and extensive written justifications required by most funding agencies. DeWitt et al (1993) cited delays in the approval of funding for home care as a major obstacle to the timely discharge of stable ventilator-assisted children.

Parette (1993) recommends that nurses develop a "funding portfolio" that contains current and comprehensive information on all potential funding sources for pediatric home care to select those that are likely to be most helpful to clients and their families. Nurses should also keep abreast of any legislation that has the potential to be financially beneficial to families such as the Family and Medical Leave Act (FMLA) of 1993.

The FMLA may allay some financial stress by offering a parent a measure of job security. It allows parents to take 12 weeks of unpaid leave in a 12-month period to care for a family member with a serious health condition (Zink-Pearson, 1997). Since the 12 weeks do not have to be taken at one time but may be used on an intermittent basis, parents can use the time in ways that best meet their child's medical needs.

DISCHARGE PLANNING FOR MEDICALLY FRAGILE AND TECHNOLOGY-DEPENDENT INFANTS AND CHILDREN

A successful transition from hospital to home care begins with discharge planning. A discharge plan that is both comprehensive and acceptable to the child's family is critical for optimizing the safety and well-being of the child, reducing family stress, and determining the resource demands that will be placed on the community (Cohen, 1995).

Facilitating Informed Consent for Home Care

The first step in the discharge planning process is to discuss candidly with the family the full range of known benefits and hardships they may encounter in caring for their child at home, as well as all the posthospital placement options that are available to them. These options will vary based on the child's state and county of residence. In some states (e.g., Michigan), there are no long-term care facilities for infants and young children. In other states (e.g., California), such facilities are quite limited, and those that do exist may be located a considerable distance from the family's home.

The overwhelming majority of children want to go home. Occasionally, however, an older adolescent may express the desire for care at a grandparent's home, an adult sibling's home, or a small group home because of interpersonal conflict with parents.

A few states have developed and licensed prescribed pediatric extended care (PPEC) centers that offer nonresidential day medical care (see Pierce, Lester, Fraze, 1991 for a complete description of PPEC; also Stutts, 1994). There are also a few day-care programs scattered across the country that have been established specifically for servicing medically stable children who require complex treatments and continuous monitoring (Delaney, Zolondick, 1991). Although PPEC centers and medical day-care programs are not a substitute for home care, they reduce the intensity of the home care experience for many families and provide a unique practice site for pediatric nurses.

However, for many children whose parents are unable or unwilling to care for them and whose communities offer limited or no extended-care facilities, the only option may be temporary or extended foster care. If voluntary foster care seems to be the most appropriate placement, families should be advised that they may petition for the return of custody of their child at a later date if their family circumstances change, making care feasible in the parental home (Storgion, 1996).

This review of options with the family is an ethical necessity so that they can make a truly informed choice. Lantos and Kohrman (1991) contend that the complex life-support systems that can now be placed in the home call into question society's traditional values that impose a moral duty on parents to care for their children, judging them acceptable if they provide health care at home and neglectful if they choose not to.

Fear of public censure may make parents reluctant to express any reservations they may have about taking their child home (Arras, Dubler, 1995). Also, conflict among family members who hold differing views about home care stemming from their own personal needs or cultural values may not be readily apparent. Ambivalent or negative feelings about home care may be suspected, however, if the child's designated family caregivers repeatedly do not attend training sessions or seem to have inordinate difficulty mastering the caregiving tasks. It should always be emphasized to families that loving, involved, responsible parents can feel comfortable with the selection of any available option that best meets the unique needs of their child and their family.

A family's willingness to care for their child at home is critical to a decision to send the child home. The presence of involved family members who fully understand the child's condition, the caregiving skills they will need to master, and the hardships and benefits of home care must be ensured. When parents choose home care, it should be made explicit at the outset that they have the right to renegotiate that decision at a later date if caring for the child becomes too great a burden or too destructive to the integrity of the family unit.

Benefits and Hardships of Home Care

There are both hardships and benefits to caring for an ill child at home. Discussion with the family should, at a minimum, include the conceivable effects of home care on (1) the child's growth and development, (2) siblings, (3) family functioning, and (4) family finances.

Growth and development of the ill child   Concern about growth and development is the major reason that health professionals consider home care to be so important. Since the early 1950s, long-term or repeated separation from home and family as a result of hospitalization has been consistently reported to have potentially serious consequences for a child's development. Greater gains in growth and development are expected if hospitalization can be avoided or minimized.

Parents often are more sensitive to cues from their infants and adjust feeding patterns to meet the infant's needs more precisely than is possible even with primary nursing in hospitals. An older child's appetite tends to improve when familiar foods are served, meals are eaten with the family, and favorite snacks are available. Failure to gain weight despite meticulous calculation of nutrients during hospitalization is frequently reversed at home.

Advances in development and growth have been found to progress more rapidly at home. In his presentation before the Senate Committee of Labor and Human Resources in 1983, Perrin stated that social behavior is more normal and gains are more rapid when a child is cared for at home than when a child is hospitalized for a prolonged time. He reported that a three-year study at Vanderbilt University concluded, "Care at home by family members is healthier for both the children and their families. Children develop more soundly, socially and psychologically, when they can participate in family, community, and school life." Children who grow up in the hospital are also likely to have unique cognitive deficiencies that may only become apparent after they leave that environment. For example, one family whose child had been hospitalized since birth reported that when she was discharged to home care, "She couldn't understand why we vacuum the carpet, but we don't vacuum the grass. . . . [she didn't know] that food does not come from a tray. You make food." (University of Illinois at Chicago [UIC], 1986).

On the other hand, it is also important for families to give some consideration to the hardships that home care may pose for a particular child's development. Some communities lack the full range of habilitative or rehabilitative services available in a health care facility that a child may need to optimize his or her developmental potential. Intensive physical, speech, occupational, and psychological therapy may have to be sacrificed if the child returns home to a community where these services are limited, not available, or not covered by the family's home care insurance. When considering home care, long-term developmental goals for the child must be weighed against the regressive effect that hospitalization has been shown to cause (Taylor et al, 2001).

Sibling responses   The needs of siblings are a constant dilemma for parents whose child is hospitalized. Mothers, particularly, report feeling torn between the need to be with their hospitalized child and the need to be with their children at home. As one mother said, "Whichever place I am, I feel guilty that I am not in the other." Sending the child home also sends the parent home!

Disruption of family life when one child is hospitalized is often felt most keenly by the siblings. Reuniting the family can be of great benefit to siblings even though it tends to dramatically change their roles and relationships within the family. This change in role definition is not necessarily harmful and can be a positive factor in the emotional and moral development of siblings. As Siemon (1984) has pointed out, siblings of a chronically ill child often develop an inner strength; show greater maturity, sensitivity, and responsibility; and become more altruistic and tolerant of others. In a videotaped interview, an adolescent sibling of a ventilator-dependent child said the following (UIC, 1988a):

> Having Missy as my sister, it has changed me as far as I have a better attitude toward others and more tolerance with them. And I understand. I have more compassion for not just handicapped kids, but everybody. I'm more sensitive toward their feelings.

Parent-child relationships are often redefined and strengthened as siblings, out of necessity, develop greater independence and more self-reliance and actively participate in the home care program.

In many homes, however, the ill child becomes the centerpiece of family life, particularly if the living room or family room is set up as the care area. When all of the parents' concern, time, and energy seems focused on the medical management of the ill child, siblings frequently become jealous, resent the lenient and inconsistent discipline that parents may impose on the ill child, and feel that they have been given an unfair share of chores and responsibilities. Some parents may not allow siblings to invite their friends home to play because they fear exposing the ill child to infection. Fear of being teased or shunned for having a brother or sister who is "different" may deter siblings from even wanting to invite their friends to their home. The anger and resentment that siblings often feel may be compounded by guilt about having such feelings. Yet despite their emotional turmoil, parents may expect them to be "model" children, doing nothing that will cause any additional family stress. In these circumstances, negative social behavior and poor school performance are not uncommon.

Discussions with families before discharge should address the fact that all parents have limits to their time and energy and that all children feel justified in laying claim to what they feel is their fair share. However, when one child is ill, the realistic consequence is that these limited resources become channeled to that child. Parents may heroically try to continue to spend time with their other children, taking them on outings or attending soccer matches and parents' night at school, but the demands of the ill child or their own exhaustion often make these normal parenting activities extremely difficult or impossible.

Home care for a medically fragile or technology-dependent child has a profound effect on the siblings. A discharge plan that is comprehensive and family centered must always address the needs of siblings and include strategies and resources that can lessen the negative consequences and augment the potential for growth for all children in the family.

Family functioning   A desire to return to a normal family life is the major reason that families request home care. Parents typically anticipate that the child's care demands and the subsequent adjustments in daily routines will be less disruptive to family life than the continued hospitalization of the child. However, complex care requirements that add multiple health care professionals to the household and high-tech equipment that does not come in coordinated colors that blend with the home's furnishings make family life and the home environment far removed from normal. After a period of caring for their child at home, families usually indicate that the adjustments turned out to be greater than they had anticipated and that the expected return to a previous way of functioning as a family never occurred. However, if the child's condition remains relatively stable or improves, a new pattern of family life emerges that becomes normative for each family. Ultimately, despite the numerous added stresses, many families report that home care has strengthened the bonds among family members and added new and important meaning to their lives.

For other families, however, home care has more of a disruptive than a normalizing quality. The presence and demands of the ill child may become detrimental to the well-being of another family member or to the survival of the family

unit. In one case, a mother cared for her severely brain-damaged child for 6 years but made the painful decision to institutionalize him after giving birth to a second child and realizing she was unable to adequately meet the needs of the newborn. In another case, a 58-year-old mother of a 17-year-old quadriplegic, ventilator-dependent child experienced significant deterioration in her own health after 18 months of caring for him at home.

Perhaps the most unanticipated disruption to family functioning is the presence of nurses in the home. Role ambiguity, loss of privacy, and conflicts over authority, especially when the child requires extensive hours of daily nursing care, are common complaints (Murphy, 1997).

In the day-to-day care of a child with complex medical needs, when parents must administer treatments that are painful or distressing to their child and nurses must perform parenting acts such as comforting or teaching social skills, role ambiguity is the natural outcome. One parent, for example, reported that he was troubled by the fact that his 5-year-old well child did not seem to know that the nurse caring for her brother was not a family member and that the child was equally affectionate with the nurse as she was with her parents. Nurses, too, have reported role ambiguity when, for example, they feel the ill child or a sibling needs to be disciplined but the parent is not present when the behavior occurs or does nothing to correct it (Coffman, 1997; Scannell et al, 1993).

The loss of privacy is another hardship that home care creates for many families, particularly in middle- and upper-class nuclear families (see Chapter 16). It affects family functioning by erasing the boundaries that usually demarcate home as a haven from the outside world. When nurses are a constant presence, home is no longer a place where parents can feel free to discuss private issues, yell at their children, argue with each other, walk around in their underwear, enjoy the company of friends, or be intimate. The smaller the living space, the more intrusive the nurse's presence may seem, and the more difficult it may be to share a private moment.

Conflict between parents and nurses over who is in charge is commonly reported. Families have described nurses who disregard the way parents want the child's treatment carried out and, instead, impose their own techniques and schedules (Sharkey, 1995). Some conflicts arise over the mandated "division of labor." As one parent said (UIC, 1988b), "For me to have a nurse in my home to do Wayne's treatment and suctioning so that I can clean my house and wash the clothes was not a good trade off." She described how this arrangement created a sense of alienation from her son and stated she would have preferred a maid instead of a nurse.

Scannell et al (1993) described an incident in which a nurse insisted that she could take care of the child by herself and repeatedly told the mother to go to bed. The mother felt that it was not the nurse's place to tell her what she should be doing in her own home and the next day fired the nurse. Other parents have reported returning home to find that nurses had rearranged the furniture in their house because they found it more convenient for caregiving. As Coffman (1997) stated, " 'Take-charge' skills, which brought success in hospital practice, may lead to failure in the home. . . ."

Family finances   The majority of families with a medically fragile child incur significant out-of-pocket expenses whether the child is in the hospital or at home. Depending on the family's economic status, these expenses may cause a considerable financial hardship. While the child is hospitalized, out-of-pocket expenses include transportation to the hospital, meals, lodging (if the family is from out of town), childcare for siblings at home, and lost time from work. These items can be very costly with a long hospitalization and are not reimbursable. Low-income families reported other expenses during hospitalization that are seldom considered, such as the need to make additional trips to the laundromat to have clean clothes to wear to the hospital every day. An obvious benefit to home care is the immediate reduction in these expenses. Also, for families with private insurance, home care can conserve and extend their lifetime, maximum insurance benefits.

Home care, however, brings about different and even greater out-of-pocket expenses for most families. Benefits for home and outpatient care often vary more than the benefits for hospital care. Since some insurance policies cover hospital costs at 100% and care out of the hospital at 80%, the expense to the family may be greater

when the child is home. Some policies do not authorize equipment, supplies, transportation to and from medical appointments, formula, or special dietary supplements. Special formulas can cost as much as $90 per can. Electricity, gas, and water bills are always considerably higher when life-support equipment is in the home. Wheelchair access may require ramp construction and other costly renovations. Relocation of the family will be necessary if wheelchair access is impossible to achieve. Low-income families may need to purchase or otherwise obtain a variety of non-medical items (e.g., extra towels and bed linens, a refrigerator, or telephone service) before the child can be discharged.

Working parents, particularly mothers, often take a leave of absence or resign from their jobs to care for the child at home. This loss of income can be devastating to some families.

Families who were financially secure before home care may find that extensive expenses have to be incurred before they meet the financial criteria for publicly funded medical care for their child. In the words of one parent (UIC, 1986):

> Funding's degrading. You bring home a child . . . on a $2000-a-month ventilator, which you have to have two for backup, and you have to have all your supplies, and your nursing care. And then they put you on a spend-down. 'Now then, we'll take care of your child, but see, you're making a little too much money here, and we have to have some of that back.' I mean, I'm trying to better myself. . . . 'No, you can't do that now. No, you have a sick child at home.'

Financial issues are one of the greatest stressors of home care, and families, regardless of their financial status, need to be prepared before discharge for the fact that home care will create many out-of-pocket expenses.

Again, just as it is an important function of case management to keep a "funding portfolio" of health care reimbursement options and legislative changes that affect home care economics, it is also important to keep a file of private and public funding sources and programs that can help parents with nonreimbursable home care expenses. For example, the electric company in one community offered low-income families the opportunity to purchase a new, energy-efficient refrigerator for a cost of only $50. The Make-A-

Wish Foundation may purchase electric wheelchairs or home entertainment equipment for eligible children. Church groups may offer families periods of respite or purchase special items for the family. Charitable organizations, such as Saint Vincent De Paul, may be able to provide used furniture or appliances. Potential resources vary greatly from one community to another, but those that do exist to ease the financial burden for families often go untapped because of a lack of awareness of their existence.

DEVELOPING THE HOME CARE PLAN

After the family has been informed of the options for posthospital care and the benefits and hardships of home care and if the family then decides they want to care for their child at home, discharge planning begins. Ideally, the plan is developed with input from all involved members of the hospital health care team, the nursing agency that will provide home care, the durable medical equipment (DME) provider, the insurance carrier, the school district, and, without exception, the family. The child should also be included in the planning process if developmentally able to participate.

The overall goal of pediatric home care is to normalize the life of the ill child and the family by providing the opportunity for the child to return to and remain within his or her own family and community. To realize this goal, it is necessary to locate and coordinate the many services that are needed to ensure the child's safety, contain the effects of the illness, and achieve optimal physical, emotional, and social development. It is equally necessary to plan for adequate family support services to prevent caregiver burnout.

The components of a comprehensive home care plan include the following:

1. Designating a target date for discharge
2. Identifying a stable source of funding for payment of home care services
3. Selecting a home care nursing agency
4. Training at least two family members to be fully competent in each aspect of the child's care, as well as in emergency procedures
5. Ensuring the suitability of the home environment

6. Selecting a DME provider for the delivery, replenishment, and repair of equipment and supplies
7. Notifying the local police, fire, and emergency medical service (EMS), as well as the utility companies, of the presence of a child using vital-to-life equipment in the home
8. Developing an educational plan for the child
9. Establishing a plan for transporting the child home and to and from medical appointments
10. Identifying resources for psychological support services for all family members
11. Developing a plan for periodic and emergency respite care
12. Establishing specific nursing, medical, developmental, and allied health intervention strategies, as well as plans for the child to receive primary (well-child) care
13. Establishing a tentative alternative plan of care if home care does not benefit the child or family

Identification and Training of the Family Caregivers

At the outset of the discharge planning process, the primary and backup family caregivers are identified, and a schedule for teaching is established. A minimum of two adults who are trained in all aspects of the child's care is desirable and, in most cases, required (Wong, 1991). Increasingly, the recommended techniques for performing procedures and for operating, maintaining, and trouble-shooting medical equipment are being videotaped and sent home with the family to allay their fears that they will forget what they have been taught (Baginski, 1994; Bryant, Davis, Lagrone, 1997). Later, parents can use these tapes to orient new home care nurses so that there is greater consistency in the child's care.

Primary responsibility for the child's care is most often assumed by the mother. However, if the mother is absent or unable to assume care, home care is not necessarily rejected as an option if other family members are willing to make the commitment to learning the child's care. With instruction and supervision during the child's hospitalization, fathers, grandparents, aunts, older siblings, or nannies have been able to assume the primary caregiver role successfully (Schoenfelder et al, 2000).

Occasionally, limitations caused by problems such as arthritis or poor eyesight prevent a primary caregiver from carrying out a specific procedure. In these instances, assistance must be obtained from other family members or the community or by the judicious scheduling of home care nursing hours.

Once the primary caregiver is comfortable with the child's care, a home pass is often recommended. The pass, which can be for a few hours or overnight, provides an opportunity to test placement of the equipment in the home, allows the family to determine the most convenient care area, and affords a more realistic experience of the child's care. Often after only a few hours at home with the child, even though a nurse usually accompanies the family, many parents revise their estimate of the amount of help they will need. One family, who resisted having home care nursing because they felt they knew how to care for their child and did not want strangers in their house, called immediately on their return from home pass to request 24-hour care. Although the final plan did not include 24-hour nursing, it did include home care nurses to support family care.

Selecting a Home Care Nursing Agency

The nursing agency that will provide home care should be selected early in the discharge planning process so that the nursing supervisor or designee can meet the family and child in the hospital and participate fully in developing the plan of care that the agency's nurses will be expected to carry out. The remaining time that the child is hospitalized is also an excellent opportunity for home care nurses who may not be familiar with the child's equipment or type of care to receive hands-on experience under the mentorship of the hospital nursing staff. Many home care agencies are now willing to pay their nurses for orientation to the child's care in the hospital setting. Not only can it be very reassuring to the parents and children to be able to meet and observe the skills of the home care nurses before discharge, but also during this initial encounter they can begin to develop a relationship that will help ease the transition from hospital to home. It also offers the family and the nurses an opportunity to assess each other for a "fit" of temperament and caregiving styles so that changes in nursing staff can be made before discharge, if necessary.

Conducting a Community Assessment

An assessment by the hospital discharge planning team of community resources should identify the availability of both primary and specialty medical care, home health nursing agencies, emergency services, equipment and supply sources, pharmacy services, educational facilities, transportation services, and social support groups. The community in which the child lives can vary from a very affluent suburb to a rural farm area to an inner-city, low-income housing project.

If the family lives in a rural area, finding a sufficient number of nurses willing to travel the necessary distance to the child's home can be a problem for many home health agencies. It may also be difficult to find nurses willing to work in an inner-city neighborhood known to have a high crime rate. The issues of accessibility and safety can usually be overcome with adequate planning. When specific pediatric services are not available in a community, innovative use of existing services may achieve the desired outcome, as the following example demonstrates.

In a small, rural community, the only home nursing service was operated by a senior center. However, a call to the director disclosed that one of their supervisors had an extensive pediatric background that included recent neonatal intensive care experience. A discussion with the local pediatrician revealed that his wife was also a former neonatal intensive care nurse. The grandfather of the infant operated the only market in town, and he inquired of everyone who came in for groceries about pediatric nurses in their family. Within 2 weeks, 10 nurses with pediatric skills had been recruited through the efforts of the grandfather, the pediatrician, and the senior center supervisor. Ensuring adequate numbers of appropriately skilled nurses for home care was only the first step.

The senior center supervisor who would be coordinating the home care flew to the hospital and spent three days caring for the premature infant with chronic lung problems while a pulmonary clinical nurse specialist instructed her in tracheostomy care and a rehabilitation clinical nurse specialist instructed her in intermittent catheterization. The infant development specialist and the physical and respiratory therapists also spent time consulting with this nurse. In addition, since the senior center had previously provided only home visits and health aide care, but never shift care, a day at a home health care agency was arranged to familiarize her with billing procedures, the documentation required by insurers, the home health care chart, and a rate schedule. A training program was developed with her for the other nurses in the community.

The family's insurance benefits did not include air ambulance transport. However, negotiation with the insurer resulted in their agreement to pay the cost of ground transportation; family and friends contributed the balance for the air ambulance.

Since any emergency care would have to be at the local community hospital, the baby was transferred there for 48 hours before going home. This enabled the hospital nurses and the emergency room staff to become familiar with her care needs. The family and the nursing supervisor used this time to test the equipment that had been delivered to the home and to set up the care area. When the infant arrived home, the nursing team provided 16 hours of care daily, increasing it to 24 hours per day when necessary to avoid hospitalization.

This example illustrates the extensive and comprehensive community planning that must precede discharge from the hospital of a child with complex care needs if home care is to be successfully implemented and continued.

Conducting a Home Assessment

A predischarge home visit by the home care agency's nursing supervisor should be made to ensure that the home environment is safe and that an adequate area can be set up for care. A working telephone, a refrigerator, and adequate electrical outlets for the required equipment are also verified. If frequent changes of bed linens are to be anticipated, a washer and dryer in the home are a great convenience.

The DME provider should assess wheelchair accessibility and the need for the installation of adaptive devices. Any necessary modifications to the home should be identified and the corrective work completed before discharge.

Most homes can be adapted to provide an adequate environment for home care even if the space is rather small. Children with tracheostomies whose care requires an apnea monitor, a suction machine, a compressor, a nebulizer, oxygen, and other supplies, receive nursing care in studio apartments. In one home, where nine people occupied a two-bedroom apartment, a satisfactory care area was set up in the living room during the day and moved to the kitchen at night.

Occasionally, home care cannot be offered because of the unsuitability of the home. This was true for one ventilator-dependent child whose family lived in an apartment on the fifth floor of a building with no elevator. In another instance, a family was living in an unfinished basement that had only one electrical outlet behind the refrigerator. In both cases, the homes were judged to be unsuitable for the care of the children, and discharge was delayed until more adequate housing was found.

A home without a telephone presents a significant safety problem, since it is impossible to report malfunctioning equipment, obtain medical consultation, or summon emergency help. If telephone service was disconnected because of a delinquent bill, reinstallation often requires full payment of that bill, plus a large deposit. In one case, the back payment and the deposit amounted to $2300, and since no resources could be found to reconcile this bill, the child's discharge had to be postponed. Electrical outlets, safety features, and certain renovations, on the other hand, can often be accomplished with cooperation from the landlord and community resources.

Determining the Level, Amount, and Schedule of Nursing Care

Level of Nursing Care   An assessment of the child's physiological stability and treatment requirements will determine the level of nursing care required: registered nurses, vocational nurses, or a combination of both. Home health aides have also been used satisfactorily for stable children with less complex needs. Alterations in the care plan can also affect the level of care required, as in the following example.

Having depleted a sizable portion of their lifetime maximum benefits, one family was anxious to extend their remaining funds for as long as possible because long-term home care was anticipated. By revising the nursing care plan so that only oral feedings were given during the day and all supplemental gavage feedings were given at night, a vocational nurse during the day and a registered nurse at night could safely meet the needs of the child and were less expensive than 16 hours of care by a registered nurse.

Amount of Nursing Care   The competencies of the designated family caregivers and their usual routines during an average week should also be clarified in determining the amount of nursing care required. Helping the family think through all their ordinary household activities and the errands and obligations that take them away from home, such as driving children to school, going to the laundromat, grocery shopping, and providing assistance to an elderly parent, will provide a more realistic estimate of the hours of care that the family can be reasonably expected to provide for the child. In single-parent households, in which the primary caregiver for the ill child is also the sole person responsible for all household chores and errands, this assessment is even more critical.

Schedule of Nursing Care   The competing demands for the time and energy of the primary caregiver are important determinants in deciding the specific hours that nursing support is most needed. Also important to assess is the availability of others who can participate in the child's daily care, provide intermittent respite, care for the siblings, and assist with errands and housekeeping.

When a child first goes home, it is recommended that the maximum number of hours authorized by the payor be scheduled. As the family gains skill and confidence, the hours can be reduced. Once at home, however, it is very difficult to convince payors to increase the number of hours of care unless there is a change in the child's condition or the plan of treatment.

While the number of hours authorized by the third-party payor is based on medical criteria, scheduling of those hours should be based on the nurses' assessment of the family's needs. Flexibility in scheduling to conform to the family's usual home routines is recommended.

When a child requires constant observation or care and 24-hour nursing is either not desired by the family or not covered by insurance, family caregivers can usually manage more easily with only 16 nursing hours if the family is scheduled to provide two 4-hour periods of care (e.g., from 7 to 11 AM and 7 to 11 PM) rather than 8 consecutive hours. Alternatively, families with school-age children often prefer a 10 + 6 schedule—a 10-hour night shift that allows them to sleep through the night and have enough time in the morning to get other children off to school and a 6-hour shift from 3 to 9 PM to relieve the most hectic time of day when children return from school, dinner must be prepared, and children are bathed and put to bed. Families may prefer a different schedule for weekends than for weekdays. However, if a different schedule is requested each day, it will not be possible for the agency to assign the same nurses who are familiar with the needs of the child and family, and consistency and continuity of care will be lost.

BEGINNING HOME NURSING CARE

The most frightening period of time for families who are bringing a child newly diagnosed with a life-threatening or complex medical problem home from the hospital is the first 24 hours and particularly the first night. This may be true, as well, for families who have been caring for their ill child at home for some time but who are now returning home with new equipment and new care demands or with significant deterioration in the child's physical condition. Home nursing during the first few days at home allows the family time to adjust to the changes required of them, enables them to develop confidence in executing the skills they learned in the hospital, and reduces the number of panic calls to physicians and trips to emergency rooms.

Short-Term Home Care Nursing

For some families, home care nursing may be necessary or desired by the family only until the child's care routines are well established and the family stabilizes. Appropriate home nursing can then be provided by intermittent skilled nurse visits for the purpose of assessment, consultation, and referral if a crisis arises. In the event of a family crisis, such as an illness, hospitalization, or divorce of one of the primary caregivers, the need for home nursing should be reevaluated to prevent rehospitalization or institutionalization of the child.

Once a family is providing total care to a medically dependent child, nurses should be particularly attentive during home visits to indications of family distress and caregiver exhaustion. If either is noted, review and reevaluation of the adequacy of the current home care plan should be undertaken with the family.

The frequent claim that pediatric home care is unique in its complexity and burden is bolstered by a number of findings. For example, it has been reported that nurses who specialize in pediatric home care average less as half the number of home visits per day than home care nurses in other specialties (NAHC, 1996) and that family caregivers of medically fragile children require almost twice as many services as caregivers for the frail elderly (Ostwald et al, 1993).

Long-Term Home Care Nursing

Long-term home care is required for children who have needs that are extensive, complex, and relatively unchanging. Children dependent on sophisticated medical technology such as ventilators often meet these criteria. After a period of supervised practice and total caregiving on a daily basis, families become very competent and independent in the care of their children. They need daily home care nursing, however, because they cannot perform that care 24 hours a day. They must have daily, long-term relief from the caregiving role if they are to be able to care for the child at home.

Flexible Scheduling of Home Nursing

There are also families whose children have demanding care needs but whose conditions are not likely to be affected by short lapses in that care when, for example, they are put to bed for the night. This is true for many families with children with severe developmental disabilities. Although these parents do not need daily home care, they may need intermittent services on a long-term basis so that they may have an occasional rest from the child's care. Telehealth has potential for helping in this way (Farmer, Muhlenbruck, 2001).

Flexible scheduling is also important for families whose home care needs cannot be predicted with any degree of certainty. This situation often occurs in pediatric hospice care, since many children whose death seems imminent when they leave the hospital rally when they get home. A child terminally ill with cancer may feel well enough to go to school or on a trip with the family one day and change so dramatically the next that the care needs overwhelm the family. Agencies must try to be responsive to day-to-day changes in a family's need for supportive nursing care, even though these may be the most difficult arrangements to schedule. If home care is not available on an as-needed basis, families may fear they cannot carry out their wish (or their child's wish) for a home death and see rehospitalization as their only alternative.

PEDIATRIC NURSING PRACTICE IN THE HOME

Caring for the child at home can be a vastly different experience for nurses than providing the same care in the hospital. Nurses from public health departments and visiting nurses associations who routinely make home visits for the purpose of health teaching, health supervision, personal care, and intermittent treatments, as well as nursing students who have had some exposure to making home visits, are generally not prepared for the difference that shift care in the child's home presents.

In the home, family-centered care is not just a nursing concept. It is a reality. The nurse is not just a professional who visits from day to day or week to week, but is a constant presence in the household. Initially, this can be very uncomfortable for the family, as well as the nurse, as they try to establish their respective roles and define their relationships.

Home

Homes will vary as much as the communities in which families live. A home may be a large house with a separate bedroom and play area for the child or a two-room apartment for a family of six. If the nurse is to care for the child during the night, when other family members have gone to bed, it is important to establish a care area that will lessen the intrusiveness of the nurse and provide the other family members with some privacy and quiet. The satisfactory arrangement of space may require more planning and ingenuity than the care itself. Equipment and supplies should be stored as unobtrusively as possible so that the family home does not take on the appearance of an intensive care unit. When supplies and equipment are extensive and the living space is small, a homelike environment may be quite difficult to achieve.

Family

The sociocultural diversity of the lifestyle of families becomes much more apparent in the home than in the hospital. Extended family members and nonfamily people may be permanent or transient members of the household. Grandparents may play a much larger role in the life of the family than had been appreciated by hospital personnel, and they may, in fact, assume major importance in the care of the ill child. In the home, children as young as 4 years of age have been found to be active participants in the caregiving process. Family beliefs about illness and cure may have a much greater impact on family behavior once the child is out of the hospital and living at home. Hospital rules and regulations no longer place limits on or direct parental behavior, and the nurse must acknowledge parental authority in the home. The parents are now the primary caregivers, and it is the nurse who becomes a participant in that care.

Child

Occasionally, a parent may wish to spend extra time with his or her other children or take them on an outing while the nurse is there to care for the ill child. However, the child who has a nurse caring for him or her during all or any part of a day should not be separated or isolated from family activities unnecessarily. Whenever it is congruent with family plans, the nurse should enable the ill child to participate in activities with other members of the family.

Some home health care agencies have very specific policies regarding the extent of the nurses' involvement with other family members. It may be against agency policy to care for any child other than the ill child or to perform any household task that does not directly involve the identified client. The nurse who spends 6 to 10 hours a day with a family in their home may find this policy to be awkward at best and certainly not congruent with family-centered care (Bond, Phillips, Rollins, 1994). It may even be detrimental to family life.

A mother of a child who was receiving home care nursing commented that it was important to her that her children spend time together, yet because of the home care agency's policy, the children were often separated. She stated, "We used to try to keep the nurses happy by separating the children at the expense of sibling jealousy and rivalry. . . . Now we have all come to the agreement to do what's best for Brandon. . . . Now like other brothers and sisters they play, eat, bathe, rest, . . . in a normal type of lifestyle" ("Brandon," 1985).

Socialization with peers is important to every child. When the child is being cared for at home, the nurse and family should plan time for the child to spend with his or her friends or to interact with children in the neighborhood. For the school-age or adolescent child, the nurse may need to make her presence unobtrusive to allow for normal peer interaction.

Nurse

The nurse's role in the home is that of primary resource to the family, but not the primary caregiver. As the primary resource, the nurse coordinates the needed care with the family, other nurses, the physician, and community agencies that may be providing services (see Chapter 4). Because the home care nurse does not have the immediate support of a medical facility, the degree of professional responsibility is, perhaps, somewhat greater. He or she must be able to make independent judgments about the day-to-day status of the child and act with proficiency in any emergency.

The nurse needs to plan for the gradual reduction in the amount or level of nursing services as the child's condition improves and the family becomes more competent and develops more resources. On the other hand, if the child's condition worsens or if the family's ability to provide the needed care decreases, there must be a plan to increase services. The complete withdrawal of nursing care may be seen by the family as a welcome event or a threat. It is important to assure the family that they are competent to carry out the necessary care, that consultation and home visiting will be available to them, and that necessary respite will be provided as needed.

TERMINATION OF NURSING CARE

The termination of home care can be an event that is anticipated with a sense of relief or a feeling of anxiety. Most frequently, care is terminated because of improvement in the child's condition (Agazio, 1997). At other times, termination is due to depletion of funding or at the request of the family. Whatever the reason, families need to be prepared well in advance of the event, preferably by a gradual decrease in the number of nursing hours, rather than sudden termination, and by connecting the family to community resources for respite care if that service is not already being provided (Folden, Coffman, 1993; Mausner, 1995; Sherman, 1995).

SUMMARY

Having a medically fragile or technology-dependent child in the family stresses every family member for an indefinite time. The potential long-term consequences for the family include physical and mental exhaustion, social isolation, increased marital distress, curtailment of family activities, inadequate parental involvement with healthy siblings, and financial strain. In the past, few of these children would have been discharged from the hospital unless they were to enter chronic-care facilities. Today, technological, economic, and social trends have combined to send children who require continuous, and often intense, care and supervision home.

Families who take their children home from the hospital have many needs: one of the most pressing is regular relief from caregiving activities. Unfortunately, the health care system that has committed extensive resources to the development and implementation of biomedical techniques that preserve and extend the life of these children has not yet given equal consideration to planning for their developmental, emotional, or social needs or the long-term needs of their families.

It is imperative that health professionals actively seek ways of ensuring the availability of home health care for all children who could benefit from this service and that they document, through research, the effectiveness of this system of health care delivery.

REFERENCES

Aday LA, Wegener DH: Home care for ventilator-assisted children: Implications for the children, their families, and health policy, *Children's Health Care* 17(2):112-120, 1988.

Agazio JG: Family transition through the termination of private duty home care nursing, *Journal of Pediatric Nursing* 12(2):74-84, 1997.

Ahmann E: *Home care for the high risk infant*, Rockville, Md, 1986, Aspen.

Arras JD: Preface. In Arras JD, Porterfield HW, Porterfield LO, eds: *Bringing the hospital home*, Baltimore, 1995, Johns Hopkins University Press.

Arras JD, Dubler NN: Ethical and social implications of high-tech home care. In Arras JD, Porterfield HW, Porterfield LO, eds, *Bringing the hospital home*, Baltimore, 1995, Johns Hopkins University Press.

Baginski Y: Roadblocks to home care, *Caring* 13(12):18-20, 22, 24, 1994.

Bond N, Phillips P, Rollins JA: Family-centered care at home for families with children who are technology dependent, *Pediatric Nursing* 20(2):123-130, 1994.

"Brandon," *Caring* 4(12):4, 8-10, 1985.

Bryant K, Davis C, Lagrone C: Streamlining discharge planning for the child with a new tracheotomy, *Journal of Pediatric Nursing* 12(3):191-192, 1997.

Carson DP: The socially complex family: New dilemmas for the neonatal social worker, *Clinics in Perinatology* 23(3):609-620, 1996.

Clemens CJ et al: Pediatric home health care in King County, Washington, *Pediatrics* 99(4):581-584, 1997.

Coffman S: Home-care nurses as strangers in the family, *Western Journal of Nursing Research* 19(1):82-96, 1997.

Cohen MH: Ethical issues in discharge planning for vulnerable infants and children, *Ethics & Behavior* 5:1-13, 1995.

Cohen MH: The technology dependent child and the socially marginalized family: A provisional framework, *Qualitative Health Research* 9(5):654-658, 1999.

Cohen SS: Overview of maternal-child health policies. In Natapoff JN, Wieczorek RR, eds: *Maternal-child health policy: A nursing perspective*, New York, 1990, Springer.

Delaney N, Zolondick K: Day care for technology-dependent infants and children: A new alternative, *Journal of Perinatal and Neonatal Nursing* 5(1):80-85, 1991.

DeWitt PK et al: Obstacles to discharge of ventilator-assisted children from the hospital to home, *Chest* 103(5):1560-1565, 1993.

Donn S: Cost effectiveness of home management of bronchopulmonary dysplasia, *Pediatrics* 70(2):330-331, 1982.

Farmer JE, Muhlenbruck L: Telehealth for children with special health care needs: Promoting comprehensive systems of care, *Clinical Pediatrics* 40(2):93-98, 2001.

Faure EAM et al: Home ventilation for high level (C1-C2) spinal cord quadriplegics. Paper presented at the Third World Congress of Emergency and Disaster Medicine, Rome, May, 1983.

Feinberg EA: Ethical issues. In Mehlman MJ, Youngner SJ, eds: *Delivering high technology home care,* New York, 1991, Springer.

Fields AI et al: Home care cost-effectiveness for respiratory technology-dependent children, *American Journal of Diseases of Children* 145(7):729-733, 1991.

Folden SL, Coffman S: Respite care for families of children with disabilities, *Journal of Pediatric Health Care* 7(3):103-110, 1993.

Ford-Gilboe M: Dispelling myths and creating opportunity: A comparison of the strengths of single-parent and two-parent families, *Advances in Nursing Science* 23(1):41-58, 2000.

Goldberg AI, Gardner HG, Gibson LE: Home care: The next frontier of pediatric practice, *The Journal of Pediatrics* 125(5):686-690, 1994.

Haas DL: Historical overview of the development of family-centered, community-based, coordinated care in Michigan, *Issues in Comprehensive Pediatric Nursing* 15(1):1-15, 1992.

Hobbs N, Perrin JM, eds: *Issues in the care of children with chronic illnesses: A sourcebook on problems, services, and policies,* San Francisco, 1985, Jossey-Bass.

Huston AC et al: Work-based antipoverty programs for parents can enhance the school performance and social behavior of children, *Child Development* 72(1):318-336, 2001.

Karr JP, Locke PD, Leonard J: Pediatric home care: Designing unique care for kids, *Caring* 12(12):4,7-8,10,12, 1993.

Kinslow M: Medicaid in 1996: Opportunities and challenges, *Caring* 15(3):36-40,42,44-45, 1996.

Kohrman A: Pediatric home care: A ten-point agenda for the future. In *Home care for children with serious handicapping conditions.* Proceedings of a conference sponsored by the Association for the Care of Children's Health, Houston, May, 1984.

Kohrman AF: Medical technology: Implications for health and social service providers. In Hochstadt NJ, Yost DM, eds: *The medically complex child: The transition to home care,* New York, 1991, Harwood Academic.

Koop CE: Oversight on home care for chronically ill children. Testimony presented at the hearing before the Committee on Labor and Human Resources, US Senate, ninety-eighth Congress, Salt Lake City, Aug 9, 1983.

Lantos J, Kohrman AF: Ethical aspects of pediatric home care. In Hochstadt NJ, Yost DM, eds: *The medically complex child: The transition to home care,* New York, 1991, Harwood Academic.

Lawson C, Pierce P: Continuing education programs for health care providers. In *Home care for children with serious handicapping conditions.* Proceedings of a conference sponsored by the Association for the Care of Children's Health, Houston, May, 1984.

Mausner S: Families helping families: An innovative approach to the provision of respite care for families of children with complex medical needs, *Social Work in Health Care* 21(1):95-106, 1995.

McAllister JC et al: Controversial issues in home health care: A round table discussion, *American Journal of Hospital Pharmacy* 43(4):933-946, 1986.

Moldow DG et al: The cost of home care for dying children, *Medical Care* 20(11):1154-1160, 1982.

Murphy KE: Parenting a technology assisted infant: Coping with occupational stress, *Social Work in Health Care* 24(3-4):113-126, 1997.

National Association for Home Care (NAHC): *Basic statistics about home care, 1996,* Washington, DC, 1996, The Association.

Ostwald SK et al: Caregivers of frail elderly and medically fragile children: Perceptions of ability to continue to provide home health care, *Home Health Care Services Quarterly* 14(1):55-80, 1993.

Parette HP Jr: High-risk infant case management and assistive technology: Funding and family enabling perspectives, *Maternal-Child Nursing Journal* 21(2):53-64, 1993.

Perrin JM: Paper presented at University of Illinois at Chicago, 1986.

Petr CG, Murdock B, Chapin R: Home care for children dependent on medical technology: The family perspective, *Social Work in Health Care* 21(1):5-22, 1995.

Pierce PM, Lester DG, Fraze DE: Prescribed pediatric extended care: The family centered health care alternative for medically and technology dependent children. In Hochstadt NJ, Yost DM, eds: *The medically complex child: The transition to home care,* New York, 1991, Harwood Academic.

Samuel FE Jr: High technology home care: An overview. In Mehlman MJ, Youngner SJ, eds: *Delivering high technology home care,* New York, 1991, Springer.

Scannell S et al: Negotiating nurse-patient authority in pediatric home health care, *Journal of Pediatric Nursing* 8(2):70-78, 1993.

Schoenfelder DP et al: Outcome indicators for direct and indirect caregiving, *Clinical Nursing Research* 9(1):47-69, 2000.

Sharkey T: The effects of uncertainty in families with children who are chronically ill, *Home Healthcare Nurse* 13(4):37-42.

Sherman BR: Impact of home-based respite care on families of children with chronic illnesses, *Children's Health Care* 24(1):33-45, 1995.

Siemon M: Siblings of the chronically ill or disabled child: Meeting their needs, *Nursing Clinics of North America* 19(2):295-307, 1984.

Slater L, Brewer MF: Home versus hospital phototherapy for term infants with hyperbilirubinemia: A comparative study, *Pediatrics* 73(4):515-519, 1984.

Stein REK: Home care: A challenging opportunity. In *Home care for children with serious handicapping conditions.* Proceedings of a conference sponsored by the Association for the Care of Children's Health, Houston, May, 1984.

Storgion SA: Care of the technology-dependent child, *Pediatric Annals* 25(12):677-684, 1996.

Stutts AL: Selected outcomes of technology dependent children receiving home care and prescribed child care services, *Pediatric Nursing* 20(5):501-507, 1994.

Taylor HG et al: Long-term family outcomes for children with very low birth weights, *Archives of Pediatrics and Adolescent Medicine* 155(2):155-161, 2001.

University of Illinois at Chicago, producer: *Only a breath,* Evanston, Ill, 1986, Altschul Group (film).

University of Illinois at Chicago, producer: *Family relationships in home care,* Evanston, Ill, 1988a, Altschul Group (film).

University of Illinois at Chicago, producer: *Parents and nurses: Separate roles, common goals,* Evanston, Ill, 1988b, Altschul Group (film).

US Congress, Office of Technology Assessment: Technology dependent children: Hospital v. home care—A technical memorandum, Pub No OTA-TM-H-38, Washington, DC, 1987, US Government Printing Office.

US Department of Commerce, Bureau of the Census: *Statistical Abstracts of the United States,* ed 116, Washington, DC, 1996, US Government Printing Office.

US Department of Labor, Bureau of Labor Statistics: *Employment and earnings, September, 2001,* Washington, DC, 2001, US Government Printing Office.

Weston BE, Keefe JA: Pediatric home care and public policy, *Caring* 12(12):60-64, 1993.

Wong DL: Transition from hospital to home care for children with complex medical care, *Journal of Pediatric Oncology Care* 8(1):3-9, 1991.

Zink-Pearson EA: Family and medical leave act, *Caring* 16(3):30-35, 1997.

Zollinger TW et al: Children's special health care services program: Impact of administration changes on rural needs, *Children's Health Care* 29(4):295-311, 2000.

17 Home Health Care of the Elderly

Claudia K. Y. Lai

Home health care of the elderly is an important topic because a large proportion of home care clients are older people. It is appropriate that the home health care needs of older people are addressed, since the elderly constitute a section of the population that is considered to be vulnerable. Societal changes are seen not only in the demographic trends related to increasing longevity, but also in changing disease patterns. These factors, together with a change in the philosophical approach to health care, an emphasis on care in the community, increased consumerism, a public demand for greater participation in policy matters, and escalating costs coupled with financial constraints, all point to the need for a greater emphasis on community care. Home health care nurses must face the challenges such fundamental changes bring.

This chapter introduces three key aspects of home health care with regard to gerontological nursing. First, it is important that the principles of care for older people are explored. This must include consideration of the older peoples' perceptions of health. Second, the role of the nurse and care delivery will be discussed using the nursing process as the organizing framework. Third, the role of family caregivers will be examined briefly. An emphasis on the strengths and abilities of older people will form the focus of discussions throughout the chapter. Such an approach is adopted because a successful home health care nurse is capable of helping older individuals capitalize on and mobilize their own resources.

DEMOGRAPHICS AND HOME CARE

Studies on demographics reveal that the country will witness an unprecedented growth in the absolute number of elderly people between 2010 and 2030, when baby-boomers reach 65 years of age and older (Hobbs, Damon, 1996). In 1900, the number of people 65 years of age and older was 3.1 million. By 1994, it had increased to 33.2 million—an elevenfold increase. About 1 in 8 Americans were elderly in 1994. However, the projection is that the number of people 65 years of age and older will reach 80 million by the middle of the twenty-first century (Fig. 17-1).

Within an aging population, the fastest-growing group is those over 85 years of age. Their numbers reached 4.5 million in 1994, representing approximately 10% of the elderly population. The Census Bureau (2000) reported that in 2000 there were 4.1 million people 85 years of age and older in the United States. Although this is considerably less than the 1996 prediction of 5 to 8 million (Hobbs, Damon, 1996), the current projection is that this group will comprise almost 5% of the U.S. population by 2050 (Federal Interagency Forum on Aging Related Statistics, 2000), compared to just over 1% in 1994. Since statistics show that health problems and disability increase with advancing age, health care providers are increasingly challenged to meet the needs of older and frailer clients (Fig. 17-2).

Within the United States, only 5% of older people live in long-term care facilities (Gallagher, 1995). Among the 95% of older people who live in the community, 80% of them have one or more chronic illnesses (Harper, 1988). The number of people requiring home care therefore will rise to a new height with the dramatic growth of the older population, even though the percentage of institutionalized older people may not increase.

Nurses in a variety of settings will become increasingly involved with complex geriatric care, since the majority of health problems experienced by older adults come under the domain of nursing (Eliopoulos, 1990). Traditionally, the

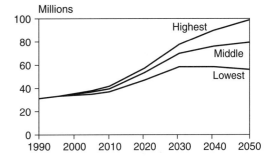

Fig. 17-1 Projected elderly population—alternative series: 1990 to 2050. *(Courtesy U.S. Bureau of the Census.)*

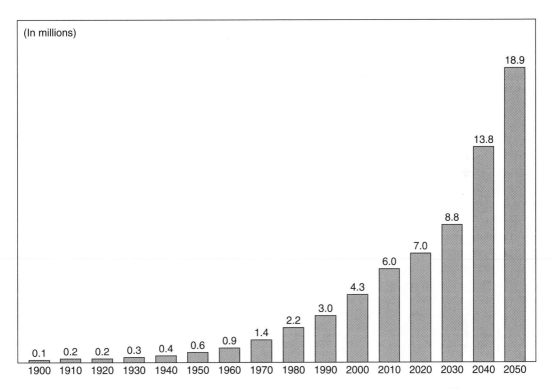

Fig. 17-2 Population aged 85 years and over: 1900 to 2050. *(Courtesy U.S. Bureau of the Census.)*

primary focus of nursing has been on health, rather than sickness. Nurses have a lot to contribute in terms of promoting, restoring, and maintaining health of older individuals. More than 20 years ago, Carnevali and Patrick (1979) stated that nurses are the professional group that has been very much involved in elderly care, primarily because no other discipline has been keen in caring for the elderly. Fortunately, nurses are no longer the professional group closely involved in elderly care by default. Today a multitude of health disciplines show keen interest in elderly care. Together with the increasingly vocal elderly,

professionals and consumers form alliances in providing and developing services.

Older People, Aging, and Health

To many people, even among health professionals, old age is equated with decline, disability, and dependency (Hendricks, 1995). American culture has been regarded as not valuing interdependence, tradition, or the wisdom that comes from having lived many years as much as other cultures (Kagawa-Singer, 1994). In the United States, as well as in other parts of the world, there are notions that elderly people are physically and mentally impaired, unproductive, and a drain on societal resources. The next section will discuss a few concepts that will help guard against biases and stereotypes.

Older people are survivors   It must be remembered that older people have life-long histories of coping. It is therefore important to recognize their strengths and to enhance the use of them. People who live into old age probably have to live with multiple chronic conditions, which means they are survivors and not victims. They are to be respected for their stamina and perseverance in going through life's many challenges. By tapping into their own resources when they require care and promoting the use of these resources, older people can ensure that nursing interventions are appropriate and compatible with their patterns of living.

Many older people are independent   The majority of older people do remain functionally independent despite the increasing prevalence of chronic disease with advancing age. Jette and Branch (1981) interviewed 1654 individuals aged 55 to 84, and found that more than 95% of subjects aged 75 to 84 years were still independent in all activities of daily living (ADLs). Leon and Lair (1990) reported that of subjects 65 years of age and older, only 9% were dependent in bathing, 5% in dressing, and 8% in walking. Over the past 2 decades, the percentage of the elderly population identifying their health as good, very good, and excellent has remained fairly consistent, from 69.8% in 1975 to 71.3% in 1992 (Hobbs, Damon, 1996).

These figures show that home health care nurses must not jump to conclusions concerning the abilities of their clients. Poor health in the elderly is not as prevalent as many believe, especially among the younger elderly (Hobbs, Damon, 1996). Performing an accurate assessment of clients' abilities and expectations is a crucial step in nursing. Being overprotective of older people creates barriers in older people's exploration and restoration of their own abilities. Home care nurses must be cautioned against the urge to "do for." Even well-meaning family and health care providers could promote feelings of dependence and deny older adults needed respect by adopting an infantilizing and patronizing attitude (Sutherland, Murphy, 1995).

Aging is developmental   Most people regard late adulthood as a period of unavoidable decline. However, developmental changes are not necessarily expansive or decremental. They can be both. Psychologists believe that although people are affected by the circumstances in which they find themselves, people could change those circumstances to grow and develop in more beneficial ways (Belsky, 1990). New growth will occur when interactions between older people and their environments produce tension or conflict (Stevens-Long, 1992). If older people were viewed as capable of growing and developing, then services delivered by health disciplines would aim at promoting growth and actualizing potentials, not merely restoring function or maintaining status quo.

Older people are an integral part of society   Older people do not exist in society as an aggregate separate from other age groups. They must be understood as an integral part of the social matrix. Sutherland and Murphy's study on social support among elderly (1995) found that older people obtained strengths from friends and families. Some of them held memories of their deceased loved ones as sources of strength. An appreciation of clients' roles and relationships in the past and present therefore enables nurses to plan and deliver appropriate care. Respecting older people as individuals and at the same time viewing them as part of family and social systems are key to a proper understanding of the care context.

Care must be culturally appropriate   Last, it must be remembered that the world has radically changed with the advent of technology and in particular, informational technology. Younger generations grow up in the global village, where some elements of culture are transcontinental (e.g., wearing jeans, eating fish and chips, or even surfing the internet). English is a major language in worldwide communication, and the number of younger people using English as a communication medium is higher than in the past. When working with older people, it must be remembered that they grew up in a culture that was vastly different from today's culture. When these people were young, technological advances had not yet radically changed the face of the world. Many older people who immigrated to the United States in the early twentieth century may have limited knowledge of the English language. Technology such as computers or discussion of ideas such as euthanasia that seem commonplace may appear threatening to some elderly people.

Health practices that are valued by health professionals may be regarded as irrelevant or harmful to older clients' beliefs. Providing culturally appropriate care is essential if health professionals want their interventions to be effective.

Older Peoples' Perceptions of Health

Home health care nurses need to appreciate that there is no universal norm of health (Jensen, Allen, 1993). Variations in the definitions and perceptions of health can be found not only across cultures, but also among individuals. Older people do not always consider health the absence of disease. The World Health Organization's definition of health, so energetically propagated by health professionals, is not entirely applicable to older people. One commonly cited definition of health for older people is "the ability to live and function effectively in society and to exercise self-reliance and autonomy to the maximum extent feasible, but not necessarily as total freedom from disease" (Filner, Williams, 1979). The value in this definition is that it has room for individual variations. Many older people see health as an integrated concept that involves functional independence, good nutrition, exercise, a positive sense of well-being, social support, and stress management (Davis et al, 1991; Maynard, 1990).

Health is frequently appraised by older people in terms of functional abilities rather than the complete absence of ailments. Older people have a tendency to rate their health as good or satisfactory, in spite of the presence of multiple chronic conditions they experienced (Harper, 1988; Hobbs, Damon, 1996). In particular, the ability to maintain ADLs and to enjoy independence are themes that emerged repeatedly when researchers studied what health means to older people (Ailinger, Causey, 1995; Beneke, 1992; McDougall, 1992). One qualitative study on the oldest elderly's experience of health noted vitality, fulfillment, and rhapsodic reverie as the elements of health (Wondolowski, Davis, 1991). These perceptions of health are quite different from the conventional interpretation of health.

The messages to health professionals are therefore loud and clear. First, it is pertinent to listen to older clients' perceptions of their health and avoid overzealous labels of deficits and dysfunctions. Second, the mission for home care nurses of older clients is to maintain and promote the greatest level of functional independence in the elderly.

MAJOR NURSING ROLES IN HOME CARE

The major roles for home care nurses for older people include the roles of a formal caregiver, a partner in care, an educator, a counselor, a resource person, and a care coordinator. The requirements of the home health nurse's role as a clinician in caring for older people begins with a thorough knowledge base of the biophysical and psychosocial process of aging. In addition, the nurse's assessment, intervention, and evaluative abilities must be specific to the needs of older people.

Home care nurses are described as partners to clients in care because both clients and nurses work toward mutually set health goals. Through understanding older clients as people with strengths and needs, nurses seek to offer care in ways that are acceptable to clients. Older people will be motivated to take an active part in care when they become aware of what they can accomplish. Learning and mastery of basic knowledge and skills in care link closely to the theme of co-participation in home care.

The main goal of home care is to successfully manage a client's health care needs at home. Health promotion therefore should be the focus of home care nurses' activities. The home of the older client, which is a familiar setting and allows a sense of security for the older client, is believed to be more conducive to health restoration and client satisfaction (Voss-Morice, 1996). Because functional independence and self-care abilities are so valued by older clients, it could be said that the nurse's role is to promote and ensure client safety in maintaining self-care. A fall that leads to a fractured hip may have serious consequences for an older person because the mortality rate of older people sustaining hip fractures is high. Teaching plans include topics such as basic accident prevention, use of medications and their side effects, and purposes of various treatment plans.

Many home care agencies use the case-management model in care delivery in which nurses play the coordinator role. Though the part played by nurses in home care is affected by the source of reimbursement and the type of setting, the resourcefulness of the home care nurse does not depend solely on finances. Nurses must work with insurance adjusters to make sure that appropriate care is authorized for clients (Schorr, Farnham, Ervin, 1991). Clients and their families require the nurses' counsel to go through the maze of the health care system. Home care nurses are also useful connections for older clients to link up with community services.

CARE OF OLDER PEOPLE IN THE HOME

In the first section of the chapter, changing demographics and their impact on home care nursing of older people, key concepts in care of older people, the way older people view health, and the roles of nurses in home care have been explored. In the following section, the practice of nursing will be delineated using the nursing process framework. Before each phase of the nursing process framework is explored, discussion of older clients' strengths will be extrapolated.

Older People and Their Strengths

Knowing and appreciating the strengths of older people form the basis for building trust and rapport—priorities in a care relationship. However, today's health care environment has placed an enormous emphasis on problems and dysfunctions. This is contrary to the notion of client empowerment. To empower is to enable people to see their own value and to visualize possibilities and alternatives under constraints and limitations.

Evidence that older people are no less zealous than younger people in taking charge of their own lives is not lacking. Sprizer, Bar-Tal, and Ziv (1996) studied chronically ill older people and found that older people maximized their self-control by not depending on others, but by being self-sufficient in solving their health problems. Many of the older people studied by Clark (1998) were able to correlate the positive actions they took with enhancement of their quality of life.

A problem orientation in nursing practice creates and perpetuates client dependency (Saleebey, 1992). The creation of problem labels such as *dysfunctions, impairments,* and *disabilities* promotes reliance on professional expertise by emphasizing the role of clients as the ones in need. Examples of negative labels can be easily identified in the health care environment. For example, negative labels, such as "noncompliance" and "knowledge deficit," predominate in the North American

Nursing Diagnosis Association's (NANDA) list of nursing diagnoses. The common use of these labels reflects how negative terminology permeates thinking. The power of such a perspective in practice must not be overlooked. The way it molds nurses' ways of thinking would eventually determine nurses' approaches to issues and concerns.

Stolte (1996), on the other hand, encourages the use of a strength approach. Her book, *Wellness: Nursing Diagnosis for Health Promotion,* discusses the need to approach nursing from a perspective that emphasizes wellness. A general strength assessment framework on late adulthood is presented, and nine specific wellness nursing diagnoses are developed. Interventions capitalizing on these strengths to promote well-being are also discussed. It should be noted that adopting a strength perspective does not preclude problem identification. Rather, the method of assessing and building on strengths is incorporated into the use of other approaches (Box 17-1).

Assessment

Other than appreciating the strengths of clients, home care nurses also need to understand the health status of clients from a multitude of dimensions. It is now well acknowledged that older people are subjected to multiple diagnoses and that the physical, mental, and social well-being of an elderly person are very closely interrelated (Kane, Kane, 1981). Multidimensional assessments of health status are therefore necessary to establish a comprehensive database as the foundation of care (Box 17-2). Aspects of health assessment for older clients include the following:

- Comprehensive health history
- Physical examination
- Mental status assessment
- Functional assessment
- Environmental assessment
- Social resources assessment
- Laboratory findings

The overall measurement of older peoples' functioning across a number of dimensions helps to provide a clearer picture of the clients' strengths and abilities, as well as their needs (Kane, Kane, 1981). Baseline information obtained will assist the nurse in formulating an appropriate plan for the care of that client.

Since 1999, home health care agencies have been required to report Outcome and Assess-

Box 17-1 Strengths of Older People

Older people have well-developed ways of dealing with their world. These ways of doing things are their ways of coping—their strengths. Nurses could be more helpful to older clients if nurses were more sensitive to their ways of coping and helped them continue to maintain as many of their usual ways of dealing with the world as possible. Strengths of older people include the following:

1. Relationships with people (e.g., family [children and grandchildren, brothers and sisters and their children], neighbors [both former and current neighbors], friends and acquaintances, church members and ministers, doctors, nurses, delivery people, and store clerks).
2. Basic abilities necessary to cope with life's problems (e.g., wisdom and experience from a long life and the ability to talk with others, to listen to others, to love, to share and enjoy giving to others, to accept love, to care for self and do housekeeping tasks, and to joke).
3. Skills and hobbies (e.g., reading, tending plants, sewing, knitting, collecting, writing, painting, cooking, and playing cards and games). These activities, which differ from person to person, give each one uniqueness and satisfaction.
4. Attitudes (e.g., enjoying new activities, wanting to maintain independence, and anticipating tomorrow and the future). These attitudes are the ways the person views the world. Nurses can help the client in a more satisfying manner if they can appreciate their views.

From Weagant R, Phelps W: Utilization of the older person's established coping skills. In Taber MA et al, eds: *A handbook of practical care for the frail elderly,* Phoenix, 1986, Oryx.

Box 17-2 Issues in Health Assessment

Factors to be considered in health assessment of older people include the following:

1. The relationship between physical illness and psychopathology. Physical illness and psychopathology are closely related in older adults. Conditions such as depression, thought disorders, anxiety, and aggressive behavior have shown to associate with many medical diseases. For example, electrolyte imbalance in dehydration may lead to confusion in the elderly and could be easily overlooked by nurses and mistakenly ascribed as confusion associated with advanced age.
2. The presentation of and response to specific illness. Older people do not experience illness the same way as younger people. An example is that older people often do not experience high fever with pneumonia, as do younger people. The older body may not be able to withstand assault on bodily systems like a younger adult would. Cerebral function in the aged body may then become unable to meet the physiological challenge of illness, which results in the commonly seen confusion in older people in times of stress. Impaired homeostasis in responding to bodily demand explains, in part, the altered presentation of illness in older individuals (Table 17-1).
3. The presence of multiple organ pathological conditions and multiple chronic conditions. Multiple pathological conditions in older people complicate the assessment process. It is easy for practitioners to miss underlying problems in older people. A common example is the misdiagnosis of hypothyroidism as dementia. Multiple organ diseases are frequently being dealt with by the use of multiple medications. In the United States, older clients consume over 30% of prescription drugs and 40% of over-the-counter preparations (Bressler, Katz, 1993). The incidence of adverse drug reaction is likely to increase with the number of drugs used simultaneously. The adverse effects of multiple drug use may cloud the actual clinical picture of clients.
4. Clients' misconceptions that nothing can be done for their ailments, leading to failure to seek help. The next difficulty in assessing clients comes from the clients themselves. One of every eight older Americans said that they needed a primary care physician, but were not seeking medical care (Shanas, Maddox, 1985). A large number of them did not believe that the problems they had were serious enough to need a physician's attention, and they did not think that the physician could do much for them because

Continued

Box 17-2　Issues in Health Assessment—cont'd

of their age. Aches, pains, and physical distress that need treatment are often perceived by older people as a normal part of old age. Believing that deterioration of their conditions is due to old age, that nothing can be done, and that it is not worth mentioning to the nurse hinders timely and accurate diagnosis and treatment.

5. Structured versus unstructured health assessment. To date, health assessment tools are plentiful, and some of them have been introduced in this chapter. However, there are advantages and disadvantages to using both structured and unstructured assessments. Structured tools guaran-

tee consistency in information and can provide useful guidelines to those who have limited experience with client evaluations (Treml, 1996). On the other hand, the disadvantage of using universal data collection tools is that either too much unnecessary information is collected or too much time is spent in gathering information while too little attention is paid to a client's unique health status and needs. It cannot be underscored enough that regardless of whether a nurse is using standardized or less structured approaches, the client should be the one who determines what is the most important for him or her.

Table 17-1　Altered Presentations of Specific Illness in Older Persons

Problem	Classic Presentation in Young Patient	Presentation in Elderly Patient
Urinary tract infection	Dysuria, frequency, urgency, nocturia	Dysuria often absent, frequency, urgency, nocturia sometimes present. Incontinence, confusion, anorexia are other signs.
Myocardial infarction	Severe substernal chest pain, diaphoresis, nausea, shortness of breath	Sometimes no chest pain, or atypical pain location such as in jaw, neck, shoulder. Shortness of breath may be present. Other signs are tachypnea, arrhythmia, hypotension, restlessness, syncope.
Pneumonia (bacterial)	Cough productive of purulent sputum, chills and fever, pleuritic chest pain, elevated white blood count	Cough may be productive, dry or absent; chills and fever and/or elevated white count also may be absent. Tachypnea, slight cyanosis, confusion, anorexia, nausea and vomiting, tachycardia may be present.
Congestive heart failure	Increased dyspnea (orthopnea, paroxysmal nocturnal dyspnea), fatigue, weight gain, pedal edema, night cough and nocturia, bibasilar rales	All of the manifestations of young adult and/or anorexia, restlessness, confusion, cyanosis, falls.
Hyperthyroidism	Heat intolerance, fast pace, exophthalmos, increased pulse, hyperreflexia, tremor	Slowing down (apathetic hyperthyroidism), lethargy, weakness, depression, atrial fibrillation and congestive heart failure.
Depression	Sad mood and thoughts, withdrawal, crying, weight loss, constipation, insomnia	Any of classic, plus memory and concentration problems, weight gain, increased sleep.

From Harper MS: *Home Health Care Services Quarterly* 9(4):61-124, 1988.

ment Information Set (OASIS) data to their respective states for their clients. The OASIS is a tool that was derived in the context of a funded national research program by the Centers for Medicare and Medicaid Services (CMS) (formerly known as HCFA) and Robert Wood Johnson Foundation to develop a system of outcome measures for home health care. The purpose of the OASIS is to develop outcome-based quality improvement measures for home health care. Since the summer of 1999, home health care agencies have been required to integrate the OASIS into their own comprehensive assessments. There are several useful websites, and the following are two in particular:

http://www.hcfa.gov/medicaid/oasis/oasis hmp.htm

http://www.hcfa.gov/medicaid/oasis/hhnew. htm

Readers will be able to review OASIS' home page, which contains an overview of the tool, specifications, most frequently asked questions (FAQs), and current information.

Comprehensive health history   Quality care begins with thorough and accurate assessment of client's conditions. When obtaining a health history from older people, it is important to understand that older people may not have the energy to sit through a lengthy interview. It may be more realistic to obtain key data during the first interview and other data through several shorter attempts. A number of gerontologists use a biographical approach in obtaining histories and perspectives from their clients and subjects (Brunner, 1990; Strickland, 1994). Such an approach would not be new to nurses working with older people. Home care nurses who are adept at working with the elderly would likely appreciate the richness of data they collect while listening to older peoples' stories about themselves. These data offer insights regarding clients' views of health and life and ways they cope with life's many challenges.

Physical examination   Home health care nurses should be knowledgeable about normal age-related physiological changes found in older people (Table 17-2). Such knowledge enables a nurse

Table 17-2   Common Aging Changes and Care Adaptations

Changes	Adaptations
Sensory	
Decreased pupil size	Provide direct, adequate lighting
Narrowing of visual fields	Avoid monochromatic color schemes
Yellowing, opacity, rigidity of lens	Provide educational materials in large print
Presbyopia (farsightedness)	Address safety concerns in the environment
High-frequency hearing loss	Correct use of glasses and hearing aids
Tone discrimination loss	Lower the pitch of your voice
Increased production of cerumen	Face the patient at eye level
Decreased elasticity of tympanic membrane	Check for and remove cerumen impaction
Integumentary	
Epidermis thins and atrophies	Assess risk of pressure ulcers
Increased vascular fragility	Use appropriate pressure reduction devices
Loss of subcutaneous fat	Avoid the use of tape on fragile skin
Decreased perception to touch, pain, etc.	Avoid frequent bathing; use emollients
Slower wound healing	Maximize nutrition to promote wound healing
Cardiovascular	
Decreased stroke volume and cardiac output	Frequent small meals
Decreased ability to increase heart rate in response to stress	Avoid extremes and sudden changes in temperatures
Increased amount of collagen and fat	Provide frequent rest periods
Thickening and rigidity of heart valves	Be aware of effect of fever, stress on limited cardiac reserve

From White SJ. In Adkins RB Jr, Scott HW Jr, eds: *Surgical care of the elderly,* ed 2, Philadelphia, 1998, Lippincott-Raven.

Continued

Table 17-2   Common Aging Changes and Care Adaptations—cont'd

Changes	Adaptations
Respiratory	
Decreased elasticity and number of alveoli	Schedule rest periods with activities
Decreased vital capacity	Careful assessment of respiratory status
Decreased mobility of bony thorax	Aggressive pulmonary toilet postoperatively
Weakening of respiratory muscles	Monitoring of pulse oximetry
Decreased ciliary action	—
Gastrointestinal	
Poor dentition	Careful assessment of nutritional status
Decreased taste sensation and appetite	Minimize dietary restrictions
Decreased emptying time	Encourage upright position for meals
Decreased gastric acid and hepatic enzymes	Appropriate texture and consistency of meals
Increased incidence of malnutrition	Consider need for bowel regimen
Genitourinary	
Decreased blood flow to kidneys	Encourage adequate fluid intake
Decreased number of nephrons	Investigate incontinence for cause
Decreased creatinine clearance	Monitor for atypical presentation of fluid and electrolyte imbalance
Bladder capacity decreased from 500 to 250 ml	Monitor medications closely, especially those cleared through the kidneys
Decreased bladder tone and elasticity	Avoid diapers
Musculoskeletal	
Decreased muscle strength and symmetrical muscle wasting	Avoid bedrest, promote early mobilization and involvement of physical therapy
Demineralization of bones with loss of height (2 in between 20 and 70 years)	Initiate fall prevention strategies when appropriate
Decreased flexibility and mobility	Proper fitting and use of assistive devices
Increased risk for falls	Proper fitting and use of shoes; proper nail care
Changes in gait	Modify the environment for safety
Neurologic	
Decreased number of neurons	Assess baseline cognitive function
Decreased size and weight of brain, but dementia is not normal aging	Teach in multiple, short sessions
Change in sleep patterns	Adjust care to avoid disturbing sleep
Slower response to stimuli	Use schedules and memory aids as needed
Decreased sensation	Change positions frequently

From White SJ. In Adkins RB Jr, Scott HW Jr, eds: *Surgical care of the elderly,* ed 2, Philadelphia, 1998, Lippincott-Raven.

to differentiate between normal and abnormal findings and facilitates the evaluation of treatment effectiveness. However, the fact that aging is heterogeneous needs to be underscored. Patterns of aging in one person cannot be generalized to another. While appreciating general age-related physiological changes, the nurse must not lose sight that aging is an individualized phenomenon. Lueckenotte's *Pocket Guide of Physical*

Examination of Older Adults (1994) is a good resource on the topic of physical examination.

Mental status assessment   *Mental status* refers to the client's current emotional, intellectual, and perceptual functioning (Keene, 1997). Mental status assessment therefore includes a number of different dimensions. Clients' orientation, mood, memory, attention span, general knowledge, language abilities, thought processes, judgment, and insight all need to be assessed. Two particular aspects of mental status assessment are highlighted in this chapter—cognitive abilities and mood.

Cognitive abilities are essential for maintaining independence in living. They have been found to be significantly related to self-care ability (Little, Hemsley, Volans, 1986). Cognitive ability is an important indicator in assessing a client's ability to avoid accidents and injuries at home. When cognitive impairment is identified, the nurse should consult with the physician or the nurse practitioner for further diagnostic evaluation. The nurse also needs to confer with other disciplines, such as the occupational therapist, to assess in better depth the ability of the client to maintain self-care and explore measures that could be instituted to ensure client and family safety. Alterations in cognitive status, such as confusion in the elderly, are not normal and must not be attributed to age changes. The home care nurse should be proficient in assessing the cognitive status of the elderly to initiate prompt treatment.

Another dimension that warrants attention from home care nurses is the mental health of older people in the community. Depression is the most common psychiatric disorder in later life (Matteson, Bearon, McConnell, 1997). Estimates of depressed older adult populations in combined community and institutional settings range from 5% to 65% (Blazer, Hughes, George, 1987; Matteson, Bearon, McConnell, 1997; St Pierre, Craven, Bruno, 1986). Although the prevalence of depressive disorders in older adults varies considerably in different findings, most epidemiological studies show that the occurrence of depressive disorders in older people is too frequent to be ignored (Anthony, Aboraya, 1992).

Health care providers often fail to notice signs and symptoms of mental disorders (Borus et al, 1988; Bowers et al, 1990; Larson, Kukull, Katzman, 1992). To provide quality care, the nurse needs to be well informed in this area. The nurse needs to master the skills in differentiating between acute confusional state (delirium), dementia, and depression.

Functional assessment   As discussed earlier, many older people define their health in relation to their functional abilities. Home health care

nurses therefore need to understand this aspect of care. In the United States, 46% of people aged 65 and over were found to experience some kind of activity limitation (Felton, 1990).

Many factors can account for such a phenomenon. Reduced ability to respond to stress, increased frequency and multiplicity of loss, and physiological changes associated with normal aging operate simultaneously to put clients at higher risk for the loss of functional ability (Lueckenotte, 2000).

Functional health is usually measured by the ability of the client to perform ADLs. Although there is no universally accepted agreement on what constitutes ADLs, comprehensive functional assessment generally covers self-care, leisure, work, and instrumental activities of daily living (IADLs) (Shah, Cooper, 1993).

The IADLs (Lawton, Brody, 1969) assess functional abilities essential for independent living. The concept of IADLs includes a much more complex range of activity than basic ADLs. The IADLs assess the ability of an individual to use the phone, to go shopping, to cook, to handle finances, and to do other activities pertinent to independent living. In the OASIS, however, IADLs also include aspects of medication management and health care–related equipment. The rationale is that home care clients are attended to for health-related issues.

Measurement of functional status provides valuable information as to how clients manage self-care at home. It may also be used as an indicator of the quality of care received. Deterioration of functional status provides warning signs that the nurse must note so that both the plan of care and the care delivery process can be reevaluated.

Environmental assessment   Observing how clients live their lives at home provides a realistic picture of how clients and caregivers are managing in the place they live. It also provides a good opportunity to understand family dynamics in the home environment. Family assessment in home care is discussed in Chapter 7 and therefore will not be dwelled on in this section. However, it must be emphasized that the evaluation of the home for safety hazards and correction of such hazards play an important role in care of older people. Appraisal of the environment also forms part of the OASIS data. The initial assessment conducted in the home may not necessarily follow a specific protocol unless difficulties are suspected (Treml, 1996). For instance, the nurse can bring in the expertise of the occupational therapist to perform more in-depth environmental assessment when needed. Older clients can maintain safe and independent living in their homes for the longest possible time when problem areas have been rectified.

Social resources assessment   One of the key concepts in the care of older people is that people are social beings. The value of social support in helping individuals to maintain health, reduce susceptibility to disease, and avoid institutionalization has been well documented for over 25 years (Sutherland, Murphy, 1995).

Variables such as the size and diversity of the client's social support system, the availability of financial support, and the presence and use of community resources constitute part of the client's social resources. These data will provide the nurse with the information required for formulating a holistic, as well as a realistic, plan of care.

However, it must be remembered that for the most part, nurses meet their clients in a limited span of time in the home setting. Even though the visit is made in the client's home, observation of the individual's interaction with the environment is not necessarily reflective of his or her usual way of living or dealing with situations. An understanding of the client's resources and lifestyle provides the information necessary for the nurse to plan nursing interventions accordingly.

It is essential to determine in advance how much reimbursement will be available for a particular service for the older client. Payment sources must be a part of each client assessment to enable the agency to continue to provide adequate services to the client in the home and maintain the client in a safe environment. The nurse must be cognizant that older people, whether they live in rural or urban areas, are at risk for not receiving adequate medical care and necessary social services (Corbin, Cherry, 1997). Around 3.4 million elderly people were below the poverty level in 1996 (American Association of Retired Persons, 1997). Therefore financial assessment is important. Again, this is also included in the OASIS.

Laboratory findings   Although officially, home care nurses do not evaluate laboratory findings, laboratory findings form an integral part in health assessment of older people. Understanding the meaning of laboratory values facilitates communication with clients and other members of the home care team (Table 17-3).

When interpreting laboratory findings of older people, it must be remembered that there are no health and illness norms in the older age group. The effect of aging varies among individuals, rendering it extremely difficult to establish normative values for physiological parameters in older people. Latent or overt disease, dysfunction of multiple organs, effects of diet and exercise, and individual age-related changes are some variables that make the interpretation of laboratory values in the client a daunting task (Abrams et al, 1995). One of the most useful techniques for determining if a health problem exists is to compare current laboratory values with baseline data obtained when the client did not experience any disorder. Therefore baseline information should be established whenever possible.

Understanding of the client definitely involves more than capturing all information according to specified forms and tools. Thorough understanding is possible only through the progress of time and with the development of trust and rapport between the nurse and the client. Obviously, there is a time constraint on the completion of such a long and comprehensive assessment with multiple components. Assessment, in fact, could be simplified in accordance with the needs of individual agencies, since each may have its own care philosophy and focus. The assessment process and the building of a client database could also be a coordinated function among different members in the home health care team. Moreover, a home care agency can adopt a standardized assessment protocol specially designed to serve its need, as well as in accordance with the requirements of the CMS.

Common Health Problems in the Elderly

The older population experiences the greatest proportion of chronic illness. In a report by Guralnik et al (1989), 70% of the women and 53% of the men among those 80 years of age and older had 2 or more of the 9 common conditions studied. The common conditions include arthritis, cataracts, heart disease, varicose veins, diabetes,

Test	Unchanged/Same as Younger Reference	Decrease with Older Subjects	Increase with Older Subjects
Table 17-3 Interpretation of Laboratory Values in Older Adults			
CBC			
RBC	Unchanged	or Slight decrease	
Hgb	Unchanged	or Slight decrease	
Hct	Unchanged	or Slight decrease	
RBC indices	Unchanged		
WBC count	Unchanged		
Differential			
Basophils	Unchanged		
Eosinophils	Unchanged		
Myelocytes	Unchanged		
Bands	Unchanged		
Monocytes	Unchanged		
Lymphocytes	Unchanged	or Slight decrease	
Platelets	Unchanged		
ESR			Slight increase
Folate/folic acid		Decrease	
TIBC/transferrin	Unchanged		
Serum Fe	Unchanged		
Blood Chemistry			
Electrolytes			
Na	Unchanged	or Slight decrease	
K	Unchanged		or Slight increase
Cl	Unchanged		
Ca	Unchanged	or Slight decrease	
P	Unchanged		
Mg		Decrease	
Glucose			
FBS	Unchanged		or Slight increase
PPBS			Increase
OGTT			Increase
HgA$_{1c}$			Increase
End products of metabolism			
BUN	Unchanged		or Slight increase
Creatinine	Unchanged		or Slight increase
Creatinine clearance		Decrease	
Bilirubin	Unchanged		
Uric acid			Slight increase

From Metillo KD: Interpretation of laboratory values in older adults, *Nurse Practitioner* 18(7):59-67, 1993.
CBC, Complete blood count; *RBC,* red blood cell; *Hgb,* hemoglobin; *Hct,* hematocrit; *WBC,* white blood cell; *ESR,* erythrocyte sedimentation rate; *TIBC,* total iron-binding capacity; *Fe,* iron; *Na,* sodium; *K,* potassium; *Cl,* chloride; *Ca,* calcium; *P,* phosphorus; *Mg,* magnesium; *FBS,* fasting blood sugar; *PPBS,* postprandial blood sugar; *OGTT,* oral glucose tolerance test; *HgA$_{1c}$,* hemoglobin A1C; *BUN,* blood urea nitrogen; *ALAT (SGPT),* alanine aminotransferase (serum glutamic pyruvic transaminase); *AST (SGOT),* aspartate aminotransferase (serum glutamic-oxaloacetic transaminase); *LDH,* lactate dehydrogenase; *LDL,* low-density lipoprotein; *HDL,* high-density lipoprotein; *T$_4$,* thyroxine; *T$_3$,* triiodothyronine; *TSH,* thyroid-stimulating hormone.

Continued

Test	Unchanged/Same as Younger Reference	Decrease with Older Subjects	Increase with Older Subjects
Table 17-3 Interpretation of Laboratory Values in Older Adults—cont'd			
Liver function tests			
ALAT (SGPT)	Unchanged		
AST (SGOT)	Unchanged		
LDH	Unchanged		or Slight increase
Alkaline phosphatase			Gradual increase
Total protein	Unchanged	or Slight decrease	
Albumin		Decrease	
Globulin	Unchanged		
Lipoproteins			
Total cholesterol			Gradual increase
LDL			Increase
HDL	Unchanged	or Slight decrease in women	or Slight increase in men
Triglycerides			Increase
Thyroid function tests			
T_4	Unchanged	or Slight decrease	
T_3		Decrease	
TSH			Slight increase

From Metillo KD: Interpretation of laboratory values in older adults, *Nurse Practitioner* 18(7):59-67, 1993.
CBC, Complete blood count; *RBC,* red blood cell; *Hgb,* hemoglobin; *Hct,* hematocrit; *WBC,* white blood cell; *ESR,* erythrocyte sedimentation rate; *TIBC,* total iron-binding capacity; *Fe,* iron; *Na,* sodium; *K,* potassium; *Cl,* chloride; *Ca,* calcium; *P,* phosphorus; *Mg,* magnesium; *FBS,* fasting blood sugar; *PPBS,* postprandial blood sugar; *OGTT,* oral glucose tolerance test; *HgA$_{1c}$,* hemoglobin A1C; *BUN,* blood urea nitrogen; *ALAT (SGPT),* alanine aminotransferase (serum glutamic pyruvic transaminase); *AST (SGOT),* aspartate aminotransferase (serum glutamic-oxaloacetic transaminase); *LDH,* lactate dehydrogensase; *LDL,* low-density lipoprotein; *HDL,* high-density lipoprotein; *T$_4$,* thyroxine; *T$_3$,* triiodothyronine; *TSH,* thyroid-stimulating hormone.

cancer (except nonmelanoma skin cancer), osteoporosis or hip fracture, and stroke. The multiple chronic conditions of older people result in a number of very common health concerns such as difficulties in mobility, problems in maintaining skin integrity, incontinence, and inappropriate management of medication regimens. These are but a few of the areas in which home care nurses need to maintain expertise in their practice.

Arthritis is the most prevalent of physical problems bothering older people, and heart disease is the leading cause of death. Strokes, pneumonia and influenza, and chronic obstructive pulmonary diseases remained the other major causes of death of the elderly population. Cerebrovascular disorders, such as stroke, are common, and the prevalence of cancer has increased among the elderly since 1960. Neurodegenerative disorders, such as Parkinson's disease, are also common in older people. Falls and hip fractures have fairly high prevalence among older people and frequently result in increased morbidity and mortality.

Multiple chronic conditions can require a combination of several medical regimens, leading to an increased potential for adverse drug reactions. Declining vision and hearing, decreased energy and mobility, and limited dexterity complicate older peoples' ability to manage their chronic conditions (Kane, Ouslander, Abrass, 1994). Any or all of these factors affect older peoples' ability to follow treatment instructions and therefore increase the possibility of medication errors.

Hearing and vision impairments, which increase rapidly with age, have an important impact on older peoples' safety and self-care abilities. Hearing and vision deficits are also correlated with increased incidence of mental health problems for older people (Belsky, 1990). They can lead to social isolation, depression, and loss of social support systems. Both mental illness and sociobehavioral problems become more prevalent with age (Harper, 1988).

It is worth mentioning that the rates of severe mental illness and suicide (Kennedy, 1996) are much higher in those 65 years of age and older than in any other age groups. Loneliness may be a constant feature of some older people, with the home care nurse as the only connection to the outside world. A common problem for many older people is the social isolation and loneliness that may occur as a result of a loss of friends and family, as well as loss of functional ability (Moneyham, Scott, 1997). Unfortunately, older people do not always seek counseling and help for their mental health concerns. To some of them, consulting a psychiatrist shows weakness of the mind. To many others, the signs and symptoms of depression or dysthymia present in an unconventional manner. It is because older people are noted to somatize their unhappy or depressed feelings. They may consult their physician reporting poor appetite or insomnia while in fact attention to their emotional state may be a better treatment option.

Although good mental health and adequate support often aid the client in coping, many social and emotional problems associated with the maintenance of the chronically ill client in his or her home are being ignored. Medicare and Medicaid cover treatment plans based only on accepted medical diagnoses. It points to the necessity for nurses to be advocates for clients, not only on day-to-day operational issues, but also on broader issues of care, to bring about policy changes in the health care system.

The implication for home health care nursing practice is that nurses should be proficient in nursing people with altered health statuses as a result of these commonly seen health problems. Home care nurses need to be skillful in the assessment of biopsychosocial symptomatology so that treatment for clients can be mobilized in a timely fashion.

Planning of Care

Nurses take a leading role in home health care because they are responsible for writing and carrying out clients' plans of care. The needs of the older person form the basis of planning. Good planning is also necessary because of the importance of securing reimbursement from Medicare and Medicaid for service coverage.

The older person's plan of care is usually written and coordinated by the registered nurse (RN), although orders are prescribed by the physician. Needs of the clients form the basis for determining the kind of services required. Some older persons may need assistance in stabilizing and improving their functional status. For example, a client who suffered a stroke would go through rehabilitative processes. In other situations, the client may just require support and guidance for a brief time (e.g., wound care after minor surgery). Still, there are those who need long-term care, as in the case of a paraplegic client who requires periodic catheter change. In all instances, the client must be an active partner in care.

To date, professionals still occupy positions in which they judge the client's life situation and potentials. The power relationship in most health care settings is hardly balanced. However, in the final analysis, clients maintain the responsibility for determining the quality of their own lives and must be facilitated to do so. Studies reveal that clients do have the interest to do the best they can for their own health, given the opportunities (Baltes, Baltes, 1990; Oudt, 1988). According to Baltes and Baltes, there is a growing body of knowledge on the reserves of the elderly and their potential for change to facilitate successful aging.

Healthy People 2000 had been promulgated as a comprehensive health agenda with concrete objectives and priority areas since 1990, and the development of a national health objective for 2010 has begun. The aim of Healthy People 2010 is to develop a new holistic health policy based on the concepts of equity and solidarity, emphasizing the individual's, the family's, and the community's responsibility for health and placing health within the overall development framework (Office of Disease Prevention and Health Promotion, 1999). Older people who need care in the home should enjoy the same kinds of rights and responsibilities in this national agenda.

Client education is an integral part in the plan of care. Client education equips clients with the required skills and knowledge for self-care and independence. In the planning of what older clients need to master, adult learning principles apply. An important yet basic principle of adult education is that adults learn best when the focus is on issues that are relevant to their current situation instead of on remote topics. Contents of the teaching need to be practical and directly applicable. Clients are more likely to become actively engaged in the learning process when their own interests are met. Teaching dietary planning and management immediately after discharge from the hospital for poorly controlled diabetes would likely interest the older client more than teaching him or her matters pertaining to home hygiene. Goals must be realistically set and preferably be broken down to several small goals. For example, the mastery of safe transfer techniques can be delineated into components: (1) from bed to chair, (2) from chair to bed, and (3) from standing to sitting on the toilet seat. The older person's commitment to achieving self-care can be better sustained through small incremental gains than a remote achievement.

The frequency of home visits is determined by the client's condition and must be endorsed by the physician to ensure that services provided will be reimbursed. Initially, for a client newly discharged from hospital for an acute illness, visits may be daily. The frequency of visits will likely decline as the client's condition improves. It must be noted that though nurses may focus on preventive care, regrettably Medicare will not pay for services if they are directed toward prevention. For example, Medicare does not reimburse skilled nursing (RN) visits for general health maintenance, preventive care, or emotional or socioeconomic needs. However, these services can be incorporated when providing the following: (1) teaching of the client or caregiver to carry out appropriate treatments for an acute or new treatment, (2) client assessment for an acute process or for a likely change in condition, and (3) direct care services requiring the professional skills, knowledge, ability, and judgment of the RN (Morgan, McClain, 1995).

Health care must be planned around personal financial constraints, since health care is increasingly costly. Older people need assistance in monitoring their chronic conditions and in determining the appropriate time to obtain medical services before symptoms become severe and more costly medical treatment is warranted (Scott, Moneyham, 1995).

Learning to navigate the reimbursement systems for both Medicare and Medicaid is not easy. Medicaid and Medicare bear about two thirds of the health care costs for the elderly (Moneyham, Scott, 1997). However, they are often criticized for addressing only problem-oriented, physical, or medical needs of the elderly. Services that help older people remain in the community, prevent illness, or maintain the highest level of health possible are insufficiently reimbursed under these two policies (Moneyham, Scott, 1997). For instance, some prescription drugs are not covered under Medicare.

Nurses need to provide information and counseling for clients and their families about the mechanisms for obtaining services so that clients and families can plan around their personal resources. If an older person has private insurance, such as a health maintenance organization (HMO), it is appropriate for the agency to review the request for home care with the insurer in advance. A number of community organizations, such as churches, senior centers, and retirement communities, are interested in funding services for older adults, and they could be the other source of funding.

Implementation

A plan of care that is capable of enlisting client partnership is already heading toward success. Essentially, there are a few things the nurse must take into consideration when implementing care. These include the value of the clients' strengths, good coordination of services, the maintenance of open communication between clients and professionals and among professionals themselves, flexibility in carrying out the plan, and proper documentation of care delivered and client outcomes. Sensitivity toward the ethnic background and cultural practices of clients is also a variable that affects the successful implementation of care.

When interventions are planned and implemented, the older person needs to be viewed as an active participant whose wishes, preferences, and aversions strongly affect the course and outcome of the interaction. In the implementation stage, nurses have a better chance to see the strengths of clients in action. With encouragement from nurses and other members of the care team, a client's positive image of self can be promoted. A positive image can further motivate older people to develop and use their own resources. It would be most satisfying for clients to see that by following through with the plan of care devised with the nurse, they are capable of attaining the highest level of self-care abilities in accordance with their own potentials.

The gerontological nurse needs to be an expert in communicating, negotiating, and mediating (Morse, 1991), since communication is the key to implementing and maintaining continuity of quality care (Santamaria, 1990). Regular communication with the client's primary physician is important in keeping the physician aware of progress and the need for adjustments to the plan of care. Communication with other professionals and agencies involved with the client is beneficial in ensuring consistency of goals and approaches and avoiding duplication of services.

Communication with older people and their families should be ongoing with each visit. Their feedback on care would inform the nurse as to how satisfied they are with the service, how they are coping, and what could be done to improve care. Without active participation from clients, pertinent information is missing and the outcomes are less than desirable (Morse, 1991). In communicating with older people, the nurse needs to remember that they perform better in cued recall than free recall of information. Older people should be taught to write down or use simple markings in a personal diary or calendar to remind themselves of pertinent health-maintenance data. Large and legible writings should be used when written language is used to communicate with older clients. Information needs to be given repeatedly to facilitate memorization. When older people are taught mnemonic strategies, their performance on recalling information has been found to improve (Belsky, 1990).

The giving of service information and making of referrals are important aspects of care. However, interventions designed to help older people and their family members to promote self-care often require more than information sharing and referrals (Moneyham, Scott, 1997). The RN may intervene in numerous ways, including doing for and doing with older people and their families, while at the same time using a variety of communication skills, such as modeling and teaching self-care, negotiation, and self-advocacy.

In implementing care, nurses need to be sensitive to the decreased ability of older people to maintain homeostasis under stress. Some older clients may not have the stamina to withstand a concentrated period of intense interventions. Intense physical therapy or very lengthy teaching may produce adverse effects rather than promote wellness. In short, planning and implementation of actions must be well suited to the individual's needs.

Other than for administrative and legal purposes, documentation is also a form of communication between members of the care team. Each agency has its own nurses' or therapy progress forms on which visits are documented. Proper documentation informs the home care team members of a client's most current health status and treatment plan. This is of particular significance if the older client has a failing memory or is unable to provide reports on what care has been delivered because of, for instance, hearing or speech impairment. Continuity of care therefore can be maintained with timely and consistent information sharing among members of the home health care team.

Another point to note is that nurses must be culturally sensitive when delivering care. The United States is a multicultural nation. Nurses need to be prepared to work with older clients from a variety of cultural groups and to understand the ways in which cultural factors influence health and illness behaviors. For older clients to accept services, health care should be presented in ways that are appropriate to each individual client. Chapter 14 of this book will provide a more thorough discussion on this aspect.

Supervision of home health care aides warrants attention in home health care delivery. Home care invariably involves the use of aides, since they provide personal care at low costs. They work according to the directives of professional staff in various aspects of personal care (e.g., assisting the client in bathing, supervising the client in exercises, and encouraging clients to perform self-care functions such as toileting and changing simple dressings). They also need to provide feedback on the client's status to the care team. Advanced technology has not been used widely for in-home care of the elderly. Often, many personal care items are relegated to the health care aides for follow-up by the RN. The older clients therefore most probably would spend a lot of time with this group of unregulated care providers. Nurses must develop a plan for the aide to follow and ensure that the aide understands the plan in terms of the unique care requirements for the older client. The nurse may need to visit periodically to supervise care being provided by the aide.

Evaluation

In home health care, evaluation of care is indispensable in that it helps clinicians to monitor the outcomes of care, to look for ways that would improve outcomes, and to be accountable for their own practice. Evaluation is a collaborative process with the client too. One requirement for participation in Medicare is to submit a periodic review of client status and treatment plans to the HCFA. Invariably, the home health care nurse has the major responsibility of evaluating the ordered plan of care. This is why home health nursing is such a challenging and exciting practice for nurses. Evaluation of home care could be done in terms of client outcomes (i.e., the resolution of health problems). In Medicare's framework, it refers to the restoration of bodily dysfunctions. Another indicator for the quality of care provided is the measurement of functional status. Systematic and regular evaluation of functional health would provide early warning signs to the nurse or the case manager with regard to the effectiveness of the plan of care. The managed care model in case management, which is becoming a very popular trend in health care, also plays a significant part in home health care services. These topics are dealt with in the beginning of this book. Readers are suggested to refer to Chapters 1, 2, and 5 for integration of these concepts in home health care practices for older people.

With the emphasis on cost containment and cost effectiveness, health care is driven more to identifying objective and concrete outcome measures. Measurable and observable outcomes are no doubt important in justifying the care being provided. However, objective data should be supplemented by subjective variables, such as the older clients' and families' satisfaction. Similar to care planning and care implementation, clients' appraisal of care must be solicited. Once again, the nurse should be cognizant of the delicate balance of power between older clients and practitioners in a care relationship. An older adult who is sick with multiple diseases, who is financially disadvantaged, or who is cognitively impaired is at particular risk of losing his or her autonomy in decision making.

In home health care practice, the nurse works independently, yet there is a great deal of nurse-to-nurse collaboration on a daily basis, such as seeking advice in team meetings and coordinating care among one another. This informal but effective mechanism ensures the best approach to client care, and it serves as a form of peer review. When complex care problems occur, the nurse can consult with the nurse specialist of the agency or the nurse specialist that affiliates with the agency. Such a process of referring and seeking expert advice when needed ensures safe, effective, and quality care. Given the complexity and multiplicity of disorders in older clients, service provided by a nurse specialist or a nurse practitioner is invaluable.

The length of time a client stays on service is determined by many individual factors, as well as by general practice within the area or the state, which indicates how long certain types of clients may receive care (Johnston, Clark, 1994). Discharge from home health care may be judged appropriate when the older client can perform ADLs and fulfill special care needs independently or with family assistance. Nurse visits can also be made as long as those visits are reasonable and necessary to the treatment of the person's illness or injury. Unfortunately, to date, the necessity for treatment is appraised according to medical need, and preventive care is not covered by Medicare and Medicaid. Still, certain clients can be seen for a long time if they meet the requirement for intermittent skilled nursing care (e.g., clients with urinary catheters or feeding tubes or clients requiring repeated blood tests, such as for monitoring blood warfarin levels). In all situations, the plans for care are directed toward a gradual increase in clients' and families' ability to take over care provided by the team.

Discharge of clients from services must be well planned. Before discharge, the older client and family need to be reassessed for further needs not present on admission to home care.

Any unresolved issues must be explored and addressed to bring service to a satisfactory closure. Linking older persons and families with community resources and providing phone numbers for consultation are important so that clients and families know what to do and whom to approach after discharge from home health care services. With proper management and support, older people can be helped to keep their chronic conditions stable or to regain stability after complications (Corbin, Cherry, 1997). Considerable quality of life can be regained despite aging and illness in older people. Krach et al (1996) studied the functional status of the oldest elderly. Their findings indicate that many of the oldest elderly, particularly those with adequate social support, are content into the last years of life.

FAMILY CAREGIVER TO OLDER PEOPLE

It has been estimated that the number of older people living in the community requiring assistance to maintain their ADLs varies from 1.8 million to about 6.7 million (Guralnik, Simonsick, 1993; Hing, Bloom, 1990; Stone, Cafferata, Sangl, 1987). The lack of uniformity in measuring functional disability across surveys clearly has produced a wide range in the estimates of the size of the population with disabilities (Hobbs, Damon, 1996). Nonetheless, studies showed that family members, friends, neighbors, and volunteers provided almost 80% of the home care assistance needed by older people (Nelson, 1982).

Indeed, families play an important role in caregiving to older people. Findings by researchers persistently indicate that families in general have not abandoned their caregiving responsibilities to elderly members. Rather, the more realistic picture is that families are the ones who follow through with the professionals' plans of care. They perform many direct care activities and even learn to master some skilled nursing actions (e.g., monitoring intravenous feedings and ventilators) to take care of their loved ones at home. Therefore support, education, and assistance to the entire family are some of the ways to ensure that health goals for older people are achieved.

Since families provide the essential support of older people to help them stay in the community, families must be supported too. Family education and support can promote family health and help to prevent the occurrence of elder abuse. Support can be provided in an informal manner through daily or intermittent interactions, or families can be encouraged to attend formal programs available in the community. Some useful topics for family education include promotion of intergenerational relationships and stress-reduction techniques. Educational interventions are particularly useful for older people and their families because a wide variety of formats can be used. When they are conducted in the home, more personal examples can be used. The program can be customized to the older person and the family and therefore can be more relevant. Educational programs for families can also be found in diverse settings, such as community agencies, churches, schools, and hospitals. Family education programs are beneficial too, because learning in a group enables families to draw support from each other and learn from each other. Moreover, they are usually offered in an atmosphere that is free from labeling or stigmatization (Giordano, Beckman, 1985). Various models of community support, such as respite care and geriatric day centers, are important services in helping families to take care of their senior members and to stay home for the longest possible time.

Emotional support for families is often needed, especially when caregiving is a long process. In these situations, counseling of both older clients and families may be required. Although home health nurses may not be able to offer counseling on a continuous basis because of practice constraints, they can link clients and families with available resources, such as social workers, counselors, or self-help groups. Self-help groups are also a substantial source of emotional support developed to assist people in the community.

In ethnic families, family caregiving may have a somewhat different picture. Informal caregiving is proportionally more evident in ethnic families (Sokolovsky, 1990). This is not to say that ethnic families do not require the same kind of support that is needed for the demanding job of caregiving. Formal support, such as respite and day care programs, can also be very useful in helping ethnic families take care of their elders in the community. However, it must be emphasized that perceiving ethnic families as having infinite abilities to care for their own elders would be a grave mistake. Assumptions must not be made that ethnic families are different from the rest of the society in terms of their needs and abilities. Nurses should regularly confer with families and explore with the team regarding long-term care possibilities of older clients to avoid physical, emotional, and financial exhaustion. Leininger's theory of transcultural nursing (1994) can provide clear directions on this aspect. Ebersole and Hess (1998) present two different models of cultural status assessment, and Lueckenotte (2000) has a succinct summary introducing how different religious beliefs affect nursing care. These are helpful as references.

One chapter cannot possibly address the care of older people adequately. The practice of gerontological nursing is a highly specialized field. Rather, this chapter intends to orient readers to salient aspects of home care of the elderly. Readers are recommended to consult textbooks and references on gerontological nursing for in-depth discussion of the care of older people.

FUTURE DEVELOPMENT OF HOME CARE NURSING FOR OLDER PEOPLE

The world has not witnessed such a rapid expansion of the number of older people in human history. As average life expectancy increases and more people live into advanced age, the cost of health care provisions, as well as the quality of their later life, become important concerns. The future that lies ahead for home health care nurses is full of challenges and opportunities. Home health care services for older people are expanding rapidly in response to increasing demand. Societal and market factors have been the main driving forces behind service expansion. They include the growing number of single or childless older adults, the simultaneous aging of family members along with their frail relatives, and the shrinking pool of women caregivers as a result of more work opportunities for women. These factors, together with the shifting focus of providing care in the community, will inevitably lead to delays in admission to long-term care (Monk, Cox, 1991). As a consequence, there will be tremendous expansion in home health care in the health service sector.

Nurses who are committed to health promotion and restoration are required in the home care setting. There is also a need for expert clinicians in high-acuity care, since more and more clients are being discharged from hospitals at a very early stage of recovery from acute illness. Home health care nurses who are highly skilled in complex care will be required to meet client care needs. With the ever-growing diversity and complexity of caseloads, home health care nurses must be committed to maintaining competency through continuing education. More than ever, home health care nurses are required to be self-directed in developing proficiencies to deliver high-quality services. The capacity for self-directed growth and the ability to master added and advanced skills with changing requirements of care will be essential qualities for home health care nurses.

Now and in the future, technology will have a tremendous impact on the practice of home health care nursing. The rapid advance in medical treatment, including the development of new technology that allows certain types of services and equipment to be used in the home, has supported the high-tech home health care boom. In this respect, nurses will need to assimilate the use of advanced technology and improve their ability to provide new information to clients. High-tech home care is generally classified in two categories: (1) medical services, treatment, and equipment and (2) home adaptations and environmental designs (Kaye, Davitt, 1995). Services such as artificial nutrition and hydration, cardiac monitoring, and novel home adaptations (e.g., personal emergency response systems and telecommunications systems) are becoming more commonly used to support older people at home. In terms of practice areas that will become significant parts of home care services, nurses will increasingly need to be highly skilled in palliative care, pain control, chronic care monitoring, and case finding and surveillance (Buerhaus, Staiger, 1997).

Accelerated developments in home health care deliver great opportunities for nurses to become more visible in the work they do. Although many disciplines are involved in home care, nursing is the focus. Santamaria (1990) called nurses "the backbone of home health services." Because of the shift to community care and the need to use more cost-effective practitioners in health service delivery, home health care nurses will be given more power by the society they serve to fulfill their designated roles and functions. Admittedly, the assessment, planning, implementation and coordination, and evaluation of care fall within the responsibility of the nurse. It will be up to nurses to show the pubic that the profession is ready to take up the challenge of home health care in the future. Home health care has created the most new growth in nursing jobs, and the trend will likely continue. Expanding roles and settings will require a new breed of home health care nurses who are proactive, highly flexible, and independent and who have strong interpersonal skills, making them skillful team players and case managers.

CASE STUDY

Mrs. Campbell is an 81-year-old woman who has diabetes mellitus (DM), hypertension, arthritis in both knees, and a history of ischemic heart disease. She has been widowed for over 40 years. She lived in a retirement apartment in the same large city as one of her daughters, and had been managing very well on her own. A month ago, she broke her left hip and required surgery. She was transferred to a rehabilitation facility after an uncomplicated surgery. Mrs. Campbell is considerably frailer than she was before the operation. She now often forgets her medicine and sometimes neglects personal grooming. She is unsteady on her feet and is often incontinent. After 6 weeks at a rehabilitation facility, she was discharged home and referred to a home care nurse for home care and support.

On Mrs. Campbell's admission to the home health care program, the nurse finds Mrs. Campbell's blood pressure to be fairly stable. She has experienced no chest discomfort lately. However, her blood-glucose level is not well controlled, and she has been put on an oral hypoglycemic since admission. Before the operation, she required only dietary control. She is not very steady on her feet, and she is well aware of her unsteadiness. Whereas many older people become wary of walking and going out after falling, having had an operation and being unsteady on her feet do not seem to bother Mrs. Campbell at all. She is most happy to return to her own place, and at the first home visit, the nurse found Mrs. Campbell to be very active and moving around in her own apartment by holding on to furniture. She is most upset, however, because of her urinary incontinence. She is unable to get to the toilet in time and is extremely embarrassed that she soils her clothing and linens. She verbalizes that she was forced to put on incontinence briefs in the rehabilitation facility and hated it. She is frustrated to find herself incontinent even at home, since she believes that she was incontinent in the hospital because the place was too crowded and awkward. The

nurse observes that Mrs. Campbell actually knows her medication but cannot recall whether she has taken the tablets accordingly throughout the day. She is confused about her follow-up appointments and refuses to follow the instruction of the physiotherapist to continue with the prescribed exercise program, stating that she is now well. A neighborhood Meals On Wheels program brings her a hot meal every day during the week and leaves her with some light snacks and sandwiches for the evenings. Mrs. Campbell seems to be managing other ADLs well. Some friends and acquaintances in the apartment building help her with her IADLs. The nurse identifies areas in which Mrs. Campbell requires assistance as (1) better control of DM; (2) dietary and medication management; (3) prevention of falls; and (4) maintenance of continence.

The nurse is also aware that Mrs. Campbell has strengths that would enable her to cope with her current difficulties. First, Mrs. Campbell is a well-adjusted older individual who has been leading an active lifestyle throughout her life. She has lived in a retirement complex for over 15 years, and over the years she has cultivated many friendships. Second, the nurse observes that Mrs. Campbell has a strong sense of independence and is determined not to be a bother to anyone. The nurse realizes that she is so determined to regain her lost self-care abilities that she probably will cooperate in any way with the home health care team to achieve that end. Third, Mrs. Campbell has a close relationship with Dorothy, her daughter who lives in another state, although she refuses to let her daughter, Mary, who lives in the same city, to participate in her care. Whenever Dorothy calls, Mrs. Campbell is happy for the entire week.

Because of Mrs. Campbell's sociable nature and her long years of residency at the retirement home, it is fairly easy for the nurse to solicit help from one of Mrs. Campbell's friends to check on her medication after lunch and in the evening. Meanwhile, the nurse

Continued

contacts Mrs. Campbell's physician and has the medication regimen simplified as much as possible.

Prevention of falls is a major concern for Mrs. Campbell at this moment because of her unsteady gait. Wanting an in-depth assessment of the home situation, the nurse arranges for the occupational therapist on the home health care team to visit. Some concrete suggestions are made regarding the rearrangement of furniture to make room for a larger obstacle-free area so that Mrs. Campbell can move about her apartment easily. Grab bars are to be installed in the bathroom, and the nurse needs to get in touch with Mary to help with negotiating with the management at the retirement home. Though initially Mrs. Campbell objects to contacts with Mary, she finally agrees with persuasion from Dorothy.

Unable to maintain urinary continence has been a big concern for Mrs. Campbell. Since her problem is functional, the nurse suggests that Mrs. Campbell try to maintain a scheduled toileting routine. Mrs. Campbell is taught to observe her frequency pattern. After the initial assessment of her voiding pattern, she is advised to follow a routine of toileting every 3 hours. The routine seems to work very well for her and before long, Mrs. Campbell is able to get rid of all incontinence products.

An important area to address is Mrs. Campbell's unstable DM. As the nurse and Mrs. Campbell get to know each other better, it comes to the nurse's knowledge that Mrs. Campbell is not eating properly. Sometimes she skips meals, and when she is hungry, she simply fills herself up with biscuits and cookies. Though feeling fairly excited about coming back to her own place after staying in different hospitals for almost 2 months, she finds it fairly lonely to face all

these recent challenges by herself. Her relationship with Mary is poor, and Dorothy calls only weekly or biweekly. Later, the nurse finds out that Mrs. Campbell was born and brought up on a farm. She loves to work with her hands, and whenever the topic of farm work comes up, her face lights up. Luckily, the nurse is able to find a volunteer through a community center in the neighborhood who is from the same state as Mrs. Campbell and who will pay her friendly visits. The two seem to have endless conversations concerning farm life. It greatly boosts Mrs. Campbell's spirit to know someone from outside the retirement home who is from the same home state. She is now more motivated to look after her own health and to maintain her appearance. Gradually, as her eating habits and her overall health improve, her blood glucose level becomes more stabilized. Her morale is good, and her occasional confusion and forgetfulness become less prominent.

After a few weeks in the home health care program, Mrs. Campbell is very well adjusted to her own established routines. She joins the morning exercise programs in the retirement complex instead of following the prescribed physiotherapy regimen. Apparently, she is happier exercising with others than doing exercises on her own. The nurse encourages Mrs. Campbell to stay with the group but not to forget the exercises that are important to her arthritic knees. Soon, Mrs. Campbell reports that she does her knee exercises after the group session while chatting to people, and nobody seems to mind. Capitalizing on the strengths of Mrs. Campbell, the home health care nurse is able to help Mrs. Campbell reestablish her own pattern of living. She is well and ready to be discharged from home health care.

SUMMARY

The rapidly expanding older population creates many opportunities for the development of home health care nursing. Home health care nurses need to be prepared for the exciting challenges ahead. In the future, home health care nurses are expected to be able to use advanced skills and technology in delivering and coordinating care. They are also expected to be self-directed learners who are able to cope with increasingly complex geriatric care.

The home health care nurse who works with

older people needs to be highly competent, caring, independent, and flexible. This role includes the duties of a clinician, educator, counselor, care coordinator, and resource person. It also has the responsibility to teach, delegate, and supervise home health care aides, since much basic care is provided for older clients by aides in the home care setting.

Aging is a developmental process that is heterogeneous in nature. Gerontological nurses need to recognize and appreciate the uniqueness of older individuals to provide truly individualized care.

Though older people face multiple losses as they grow old, old age does not necessarily result in significant loss of functional abilities. A large percentage of older people are capable of looking after themselves and require only some form of assistance from families and friends to maintain independent living in the community.

Older peoples' appraisal of health focuses mainly on their ability to maintain self-care and independence. Existing chronic conditions do not preclude older peoples' pursuance of health or enjoyment of life.

Multidimensional assessment is required in home health care of older people to understand the strengths, abilities, and health problems of older people so that an appropriate plan of care can be designed.

The plan of care for older people in home health care should evolve around the strengths of older people, rather than merely focusing on their dysfunctions and disabilities. By doing so, home health care nurses can capitalize on the existing strengths of their clients. Care and services rendered will more likely be compatible with the life-long pattern of living of their clients.

When implementing the plan of care, it is of utmost importance to maintain good communication among clients and families and the home health care team. Good communication is a key component in continuity of care. Maintaining cultural sensitivity is also vital for the home health care nurse to develop trust and rapport with clients.

Data collected for the evaluation of care provide feedback as to the effectiveness of care and the quality of the service. Evaluation, similar to assessment, planning, and implementation, is an integral and collaborative process in home health care.

Most older people are able to stay at home and remain in the community because they have large networks of family and friends to help meet their needs. Since family caregiving plays a crucial role in maintaining older people in the community, families need to be supported too.

Older people are an integral part of society and must be understood as such. Myths and stereotypes about old age must be dispelled. Home health care nurses are older peoples' advocates in this respect.

REFERENCES

Abrams WB et al: *The Merck manual of geriatrics,* ed 2, West Point, Pa, 1995, Merck Research Laboratories.

Ailinger RL, Causey ME: Health concept of older Hispanic immigrants, *Western Journal of Nursing Research* 17(6):605-613, 1995.

American Association of Retired Persons: *A profile of older Americans,* Washington, DC, 1997, The Association.

Anthony J, Aboraya A: The epidemiology of selected mental disorders in later life. In Birren J, Sloane R, Cohen G, eds: *Handbook of mental health and aging,* ed 2, San Diego, Calif, 1992, Academic Press.

Baltes PB, Baltes MM: Psychological perspectives on successful aging: The model of selective optimization with compensation. In Baltes PB, Baltes MM, ed: *Successful aging: Perspectives from the behavioral sciences,* Cambridge, UK, 1990, Cambridge University Press.

Belsky JK: *The psychology of aging: Theory, research, and interventions,* ed 2, Pacific Grove, Calif, 1990, Brooks/Cole.

Beneke DA: *Life goals in elderly women: A phenomenological study,* doctoral dissertation, Ann Arbor, 1992, Texas Woman's University.

Blazer D, Hughes DC, George LK: The epidemiology of depression in an elderly community population, *The Gerontologist* 27(3):281-287, 1987.

Borus JF et al: Primary health care providers' recognition and diagnosis of mental disorders in their patients, *General Hospital Psychiatry* 10(5):317-321, 1988.

Bowers J et al: General practitioners' detection of depression and dementia in elderly patients, *The Medical Journal of Australia* 153(4):192-196, 1990.

Bressler R, Katz M: *Geriatric pharmacology,* New York, 1993, McGraw-Hill.

Brunner J: *Autobiography and self: Acts of meaning,* Cambridge, Mass, 1990, Harvard University Press.

Buerhaus PI, Staiger DO: Future of the nurse labor market according to health executives in high managed-care areas of the United States, *Image: Journal of Nursing Scholarship* 29(4):313-318, 1997.

Carnevali D, Patrick M: *Nursing management for the elderly,* Philadelphia, 1979, JB Lippincott.

Clark CC: Wellness self-care by healthy older adults, *Image: The Journal of Nursing Scholarship* 30(4):351-355, 1998.

Corbin JM, Cherry JC: Caring for the aged in the community. In Swanson EA, Tripp-Reimer T, eds: *Advances in gerontological nursing: Chronic illness and the older adult,* New York, 1997, Springer.

Davis DC et al: An interactive perspective on the health beliefs and practices of rural elders, *Journal of Gerontological Nursing* 17(5):11-16, 1991.

Ebersole P, Hess P: *Toward healthy aging: Human needs and nursing response,* ed 5, St Louis, 1998, Mosby.

Eliopoulos C: *Caring for the elderly in diverse care settings,* New York, 1990, JB Lippincott.

Felton BH: Coping and social support in older people's experiences of chronic illness. In Stephens MAP et al, eds: *Stress and coping in later life families,* New York, 1990, Hemisphere.

Filner B, Williams R: Health promotion for the elderly: Reducing functional dependency. In *Healthy People 2000,* Washington, DC, 1979, US Government Printing Office.

Gallagher RM: *Community-based long term care: Agenda for the 21st century,* Washington, DC, 1995, The American Nurses Association.

Giordano JA, Beckman K: The aged within a family context: Relationships, roles, and events. In L'Abate L, ed: *The handbook of family psychology and therapy,* vol 1, Homewood, Ill, 1985, Dorset Press.

Guralnik JM, Simonsick EM: Physical disability in older Americans, *The Journal of Gerontology* 48(Spec No):3-10, 1993.

Guralnik JM et al: *Aging in the eighties: The prevalence of comorbidity and its association with disability,* Pub No 170, Washington, DC, 1989, US Department of Health and Human Services.

Harper MS: Behavioral, social, and mental health aspects of home care for older Americans, *Home Health Care Services Quarterly* 9(4):61-124, 1988.

Hendricks J: The social construction of ageism. In Bond LA, Cutler SJ, Grams A, eds: *Promoting successful and productive aging,* Thousand Oaks, Calif, 1995, Sage.

Hing E, Bloom B: *Long-term care for the functionally dependent elderly,* Series 13, No 104, DHHS Pub No (PHS)90-1765, Hyattsville, Md, 1990, Public Health Service.

Hobbs FB, Damon BL: *65+ in the United States,* 1996, US Bureau of the Census (on-line) http:www.census.gov/prod/1/pop/p23-190.html.

Jensen L, Allen M: Wellness: The dialectic of illness, *Image: Journal of Nursing Scholarship* 25(3):220-224, 1993.

Jette A, Branch L: The Framingham disability study: II. Physical disability among the aging, *American Journal of Public Health* 71(11):1211-1216, 1981.

Johnston JE, Clark BR: Orientation to home care: Maximizing Medicare reimbursement. In McHann M, ed: *What every home health nurse needs to know: A book of readings,* Memphis, 1994, Consultants in Care.

Kagawa-Singer M: Diverse cultural beliefs and practices about death and dying in the elderly, *Gerontology and Geriatrics Education* 15(1):101-116, 1994.

Kane R, Kane RL: *Assessing the elderly: A practical guide to measurement,* Lexington, Mass, 1981, Lexington.

Kane R, Ouslander J, Abrass I: *Essentials of clinical geriatrics,* New York, 1994, McGraw Hill.

Kaye LW, Davitt JK: The importation of high technology services into the home, *Journal of Gerontological Social Work* 24(3/4):67-94, 1995.

Keene AM: Health assessment. In Black JM, Matassarin-Jacobs, eds: *Medical-surgical nursing: Clinical management for continuity of care,* ed 5, Philadelphia, 1997, WB Saunders.

Kennedy GJ: *Suicide and depression in late life: Critical issues in treatment, research, and public policy,* New York, 1996, John Wiley & Sons.

Krach P et al: Functional status of the oldest old in a home setting, *Journal of Advanced Nursing* 24(3):456-464, 1996.

Larson EB, Kukull WA, Katzman RL: Cognitive impairment: Dementia and Alzheimer's disease, *Annual Review of Public Health* 13:431-439, 1992.

Lawton MP, Brody EM: Assessment of older people: Self-maintaining and instrumental activities of daily living, *Gerontologist* 9(3):179-186, 1969.

Leininger MM: *Transcultural nursing: Concepts, theories, and practices,* Columbus, Ohio, 1994, Greyden.

Leon J, Lair T: *Functional status of the noninstitutionalized elderly: Estimates of ADL and IADL difficulties,* DHHS Pub No PHS 90-3462, Rockville, Md, 1990, Public Health Service.

Little AG, Hemsley DR, Volans PJ: Cognitive ability as a predictor of self-care performance and change in the elderly, *International Journal of Geriatric Psychiatry* 1:109-117, 1986.

Lueckenotte AG: *Pocket guide of physical examination of older adults,* St Louis, 1994, Mosby.

Lueckenotte AG: *Gerontologic nursing,* ed 2, St Louis, 2000, Mosby.

Matteson MA, Bearon LB, McConnell ES: Psychosocial problems associated with aging. In Matteson MA, McConnell ES, Linton AD, eds: *Gerontological nursing: Concepts and practice,* ed 2, Philadelphia, 1997, WB Saunders.

Maynard M: Two groups of elderly residents' health attitudes and behaviors: Implications for health promotion, *Physical and Occupational Therapy in Geriatrics* 9(2):43-54, 1990.

McDougall LS: *Health: The experience of healthy seniors,* doctoral dissertation, 1992.

Moneyham L, Scott CB: A model emerges for the community-based nurse care management of older adults, *Nursing and Health Care: Perspectives on Community* 18(2):68-73, 1997.

Monk A, Cox C: *Home care for the elderly: An international perspective,* New York, 1991, Auburn House.

Morgan KS, McClain SL: Role of the registered nurse in home care. In Morgan KJ, McClain SL, eds: *Core curriculum for home health care nursing,* Gaithersburg, Md, 1995, Aspen.

Morse J: Negotiating commitment and involvement in the nurse-patient relationship, *Journal of Advanced Nursing* 16(4):455-468, 1991.

Nelson G: Support for the aged: Public and private responsibility, *Social Work* 27(2):137-142, 1982.

Office of Disease Prevention and Health Promotion: *Healthy People 2010: Fact Sheet,* (on-line), http://web.health.gov/healthypeople/2010fctsht.htm.

Oudt BM: *Self-reported health status and health behaviors of women aged 85 years and older,* doctoral dissertation, Ann Arbor, Mich, 1988, Rush University College of Nursing.

Saleebey D: Introduction: Power in the people. In Saleebey D, ed: *The strengths perspective in social work practice,* ed 2, New York, 1992, Longman.

Santamaria B: Home health care. In Eliopoulos C: *Caring for the elderly in diverse care settings,* New York, 1990, JB Lippincott.

Schorr JA, Farnham RC, Ervin SM: Health patterns in aging women as expanding consciousness, *Advances in Nursing Science* 13(4):52-63, 1991.

Scott CB, Moneyham L: Perceptions of senior residents about a community-based nursing center for older adults, *Image: Journal of Nursing Scholarship* 27(3):181-186, 1995.

Shah S, Cooper B: Issues in the choice of activities of daily living assessment, *The Australian Occupational Therapy Journal* 40(2):77-82, 1993.

Shanas E, Maddox GL: Health, health resources and the utilization of care. In Binstock RH, Shanas E, eds: *Handbook of aging and the social sciences,* New York, 1985, Van Nostrand Reinhold.

Sokolovsky J, ed: *The cultural context of aging: Worldwide perspectives,* New York, 1990, Bergin & Garvey.

Sprizer A, Bar-Tal Y, Ziv L: The moderating effect of age on self-care, *Western Journal of Nursing Research* 18(2):136-148, 1996.

Stevens-Long J: *Adult life: Developmental processes,* ed 4, New York, 1992, William C Brown.

Stolte KM: *Wellness nursing diagnosis for health promotion,* Philadelphia, 1996, JB Lippincott.

Stone R, Cafferata GS, Sangl J: Caregivers of the frail elderly: A national profile, *The Gerontologist* 27(5):616-626, 1987.

St Pierre J, Craven R, Bruno P: Late life depression: A guide for assessment, *Journal of Gerontological Nursing* 12(7):5-10, 1986.

Strickland L: Autobiographical interviewing and narrative analysis: An approach to psychosocial assessment, *Clinical Social Work Journal* 22(1): 27-41, 1994.

Sutherland D, Murphy E: Social support among elderly in two community programs, *Journal of Gerontological Nursing* 21(2):31-38, 1995.

Treml LA: Accessibility and safety. In Emlet CA et al: *In-home assessment of older adults: An interdisciplinary approach,* Gaithersburg, Md, 1996, Aspen.

United States Census Bureau: *Population 65 years and over and 85 years and over, region, and state: 1998,* 2000, US Department of Commerce, http:www.census.gov.

Voss-Morice S: *Geriatric outline series,* Albany, NY, 1996, Skidmore-Roth/Delmar Thompson Learning.

Weagant R, Phelps W: Utilization of the older person's established coping skills. In Taber MA et al, eds: *A handbook of practical care for the frail elderly,* Phoenix, 1986, Oryx.

Wondolowski C, Davis DK: The lived experience of health in the oldest old: A phenomenological study, *Nursing Science Quarterly* 4(3):113-118, 1991.

18 Home Care of the Dying

Joyce V. Zerwekh

B efore the twentieth century, death was a common event in everyday life. Emotional and spiritual comfort was provided by a large extended family, and physical suffering was considered inevitable. This chapter describes the challenges and possibilities of relieving physical, emotional, and spiritual suffering at home in contemporary America. The sections that follow discuss death in the United States, those able to die at home, self-care for the hospice nurse, the pathophysiological processes and nursing process when death is imminent, palliative practice guidelines, priority preterminal diagnoses, and impending death.

DEATH IN THE UNITED STATES

In contemporary America, death is unfamiliar because the dying person is quietly lost behind institutional doors. There is a common delusion that we can somehow avoid the touch of death, and people feel powerless to face the dying of a loved one. Physical suffering is now controllable, but emotional and spiritual comfort are generally not provided by an extended family. Let us examine the contrasting deaths of two men named Jacob, one dying in 1800, and one dying in 2000. The remainder of the chapter will then explore how skilled nursing can improve the circumstances of contemporary dying.

WHO DIES AT HOME?

After the twentieth-century movement toward medicalization and institutionalization of human problems, the dying person has been transported from his or her own bed at home into the hospital and the nursing home. Institutionalization of dying has been determined by cultural "death avoidance," contemporary faith in medical answers to escape mortality, fragmentation and

mobility of families, and health care reimbursement that historically has been a disincentive to home care of the dying. The pendulum is now slowly reversing its swing because of the parallel forces of the self-help consumer movement, the hospice movement, and changing financial incentives. This section examines the forces determining who actually can be cared for at home and under what circumstances: client and family choices, support network characteristics, the disease and type of dysfunctions, and characteristics of available health resources.

Choices and the Support Network

Dying people and their families frequently seek home care for the security of being "at home." The familiar bed, homemade food, the children playing, the cat curled at their feet, normal household sounds, and "Star Dust" on the stereo are all comforting. People feel in charge, and life can be normalized. Family and friends are active participants in continuing daily home life and providing personal one-to-one attention. Loved ones can express their caring and commitment, and meaningful closure of relationships becomes possible.

As dependency needs increase, however, the strengths and human limitations of the family support network determine whether a dying person can continue to be at home. In this chapter, the contemporary family is broadly defined as whomever the dying person considers "family" and includes the traditional spouse and blood relatives as well as nontraditional significant others, such as friends and lovers. Families will cope with a dying member just as they have with other stresses in their history. The strongest caregivers are those who communicate about problems in a straightforward way, who plan and problem

JACOB (1800)

Jacob Youngblood died at an average age for his time—35 years. He was sick for less than a year with progressive weakness, weight loss, abdominal pain, ascites, and jaundice. With the assistance of his two sons, he continued work as a shopkeeper until severe vomiting and pain forced him to his bed. He knew he was dying, as did his entire family. He and his wife, Dorothy, had planned his burial and purchased mourning clothes for the family. In an effort to remain strong as long as possible, he had used multiple herb teas prescribed by the village herbalist. For a while, he had anointed his belly with a vile-smelling ointment "to draw out the tumor." Toward the end, a university-trained physician bled him twice daily into a large pewter cup. Soon after a powerful laxative was given to move his obstructed bowels, he lapsed into a fitful coma. He cried out often; his fever rose. Dorothy and the children and his sister, Sarah, kept vigil around the clock, bathing his body and praying. He died as the family was united together reading the 23rd Psalm, "Even though I walk through the valley of the shadow of death, I fear no evil; for Thou art with me. . . ."

JACOB (2000)

Jacob Oldfellow died at 80 years of age. He had survived three heart attacks, and his failing heart had been controlled by digitalis and diuretics. Approximately 9 months before his death, carcinoma of the large bowel and liver was diagnosed. Jacob had been divorced for 6 years from his second wife, Suzanne. He was renting a one-bedroom city apartment in a senior citizens' retirement building. His sister and one granddaughter lived within an hour's drive; two sons and another grandchild lived in other states. He told no one about his diagnosis. The focus of discussion with doctors and nurses was on the chemotherapy and its side effects. After 6 months, his condition began to deteriorate. He began to look and feel sick with progressive weakness, weight loss, abdominal pain, ascites, and jaundice. One October day, he was admitted to the hospital with uncontrolled vomiting and severe abdominal pain. He received hydrating fluids and morphine intravenously; a nasogastric tube was inserted.

Family gathered at the hospital bedside, but they felt totally helpless; they were shocked at his appearance and had no idea what to say. Jacob was too tired and overwhelmed to say anything much. After visiting hours, his sister and children went out for a drink. The hospital called his sister in the morning to say that Jacob had just died.

Since Jacob had not been a religious man and had expressed no known views on funerals or burial, he was cremated. His daughter-in-law's minister performed a short memorial service, after which everyone hurried back to work or to make their flights. His former wife's arthritis flared up, and his sister could not get rid of her feelings of guilt at "not doing anything for my only brother." They tried to forget the whole experience but were immobilized by chronic depression.

Jacob of 1800 actively planned his last days and received physical and emotional comforting. Family and friends stayed by him and kept that sense of power and survivors' self-esteem that comes from living through crisis and caring for the suffering. Jacob of 2000 gave up his active role, as did his family. Though he received capable medical care, he became a helpless victim by ignoring death and thus denying himself any choice about how he wanted to live and die. He died alone and out of touch. Family had no opportunity for gathering, reconciling, or caring. His death was an unfortunate event in a life estranged from human community.

solve instead of withdraw under stress, and who give help to others, receive help from others, and work as partners with community resources and health professionals.

The presence of a caregiver in the home is essential. The strength of bonds between client and caregiver and the actual number of caregivers help determine who dies at home. A caregiver who has the breadwinner responsibility will become exhausted with multiple roles and cannot be physically present when client deterioration mandates constant attention. Likewise, there often comes a time when around-the-clock availability of one caretaker is not enough, especially when dying is drawn out over months or years. Many American individuals and nuclear families expect themselves to tough it out alone and may have weak connections with the outside world. In contrast, the exhausted nuclear family that reaches out to mobilize friends, neighbors, church members, the Elks, and the Friday-night bowling gang is going to do well. The strength of the family social support network predicts family capacity to care for sick members.

A growing number of Americans of middle and old age are living alone. Lacking primary caregivers, their care becomes a demanding challenge for hospice teams when they can no longer be left alone. The hospice team consists of nurses, social workers, chaplains, therapists, and volunteers making periodic home visits. Around-the-clock care is not provided. Agencies have responded innovatively by creating a patchwork of paid caregivers, volunteers, and professionals; by planning for admission to a facility when the client's condition requires it; by developing hospice day care programs; by using technologies such as lock boxes for access, personal security alarms, and smoke alarms; and by developing supportive community residences (Carter, 1996).

Disease and Dysfunctions

A planned death at home is most likely in the case of chronic illness with a limited predictable duration of end-stage dependency. Shorter-term, irreversible illness is less likely to exhaust client and caregiver coping skills. Longer-term dying with unpredictable trajectory, which may include treatment of reversible processes, is very difficult to manage over years. Thus progressive metastatic cancer is more likely to be managed at home with an anticipated short-term dying trajectory than the decades-long decline associated with Alzheimer's disease.

Terminal cardiopulmonary, hepatic, and renal diseases lend themselves to some general predictions related to the trajectory of death and suitability of home care. They are characterized by unpredictable courses; acute medical treatment can temporarily stabilize processes such as cardiac decompensation, respiratory acidosis, esophageal varices, and renal failure. There is generally something more that can be tried to turn each physiological crisis around. Although medical treatment may be only "buying time," these clients are seldom labeled *terminal*. Death remains likely to occur in an acute care setting during yet another high-tech effort to stabilize the client's condition. With a prolonged course resulting in severe disability after the best medical care, some clients will die at home if the family

network can manage, and many will die in a nursing home. The National Hospice Organization (1996) has published guidelines to determine the prognosis in heart disease, pulmonary disease, and dementia. These continue to be refined, but prognostication remains a subjective and challenging art (Christakis, 1998).

Terminal neurological diseases generally have a slow downhill course. Death in these conditions is frequently precipitated by profound immobility with resulting urinary or lung infections. Again, the ability to die at home is determined by the strength of the support system, which often has had to endure many years of chronic illness.

Hospice care for dementia is hindered by unpredictable survival time. However, the presence of advanced dementia (inability to communicate and to engage in purposeful activities) combined with serious medical complications (such as severe urinary tract infection, decubiti, septicemia) predicts death drawing near. Using such criteria, hospices can enroll clients with end-stage Alzheimer's with the expectation that the duration of care will be limited (Hanrahan, Luchins, 1995).

Cancer clients are most likely to die at home and are the group with whom the hospice movement has had the most experience. For cancer, the clinical course varies on a continuum extending from total cure at one end to far-advanced disease at diagnosis and rapid deterioration at the other end. Some people have an initial remission in response to treatment, but then malignancy recurs. Others do not respond to treatment and progressively deteriorate. Length of the terminal course is commonly not so long as to exhaust home caregivers. The following commonly cause cancer death: infections, organ failure, infarction of lungs or heart, and hemorrhage.

Available Health Resources

Resources in the available health care system must be mobilized to the maximum to enable home care of the dying. Interdisciplinary collaboration and palliative expertise, as well as more time available for each client, are necessary to respond to client and family needs. (See "A Homecare System to Enable Dying at Home" at the end of this chapter.) The beliefs of trusted professionals about the best place to die will strongly influence the locus of death. Availability of homemaking and personal care assistance to supplement the caregiving family network can make or break success.

Insurance limitations A growing number of Americans have no health insurance. For the insured, the provisions and reimbursement of health insurance affect the place of death. Medicare, Medicaid, and private insurance limit choices. The question used to be whether to admit a loved one to the hospital when he or she became "really sick"; now Medicare expects those people to stay home or go to nursing homes. Under prospective Medicare hospital reimbursement, there is no diagnosis related group (DRG) for "terminal care." Families are appalled that their relative is dying but not "sick enough" to be in the hospital. In addition, most dying people cannot qualify under Medicare's narrow guidelines for reimbursable "skilled nursing care" in nursing homes. Their symptoms can be reasonably well controlled, and they seldom require complex technical procedures. Rather, the dying need help to meet their basic human needs as they become progressively more dependent on others. Families must realize that out-of-pocket payment and Medicaid pays for most nursing home care. Unless health consumers are encouraged to purchase nursing home insurance policies that cover what is termed *custodial,* as well as skilled nursing care, many people may be able to die only in second-class nursing homes as welfare clients. Some families will ultimately care for their dying relatives at home because there literally is no institutional option.

Insurance for home care and hospice The home health and home hospice provisions and limits of Medicare, Medicaid, and insurance coverage are discussed in Chapter 6. Private insurers are extending their coverage of home care of the dying, both through expanding home care benefits through designated hospice benefits. Families need assistance to understand the provisions of their coverage and options that may or may not be possible.

Need to expand hospice services Hospice home care programs have generally been unsuccessful in serving people from nonwhite communities (Crawley et al, 2000). Contributing factors include programs' failure to publicize services in the minority community, minority members' cultural values related to death and dying that contrast with hospice philosophy, dis-

trust and unfamiliarity with mainstream professionals, inadequate access to health care as a whole, and limitations in providing home care from lack of economic resources (Gordon, 1995; Harper, Gordon, 1995). The National Hospice Organization has sought to systematically identify barriers and increase access to hospice care for minorities.

In summary, a complex interplay of forces, including support available, responses to the illness itself, and existing services and financing, determine the possibility of dying at home.

CARING FOR THE CAREGIVER: THE HOSPICE NURSE

To constructively face extreme human suffering and constant dying, expert hospice nurses learn to sustain themselves by discovering ways to continually express their grief, letting go of their personal agendas about how much they can accomplish with each client, believing that working with the dying is an extraordinary gift, and deliberately choosing ways to replenish their energy and maintain their own health (Zerwekh, 1995). The greatest stresses reported by home hospice nurses are troubling organizational issues, such as lack of control over their practice, lack of support from colleagues, inadequate resources, and work overload (Vachon, 1995). Continual work with suffering brings up personal suffering related to a variety of unresolved emotional issues, including lack of support in a nurse's personal life. Ongoing focused caring may bring a sense of "emotional flooding" and "attentional fatigue" that requires carefully planned rest and restoration. Organizational strategies to sustain hospice nurse well being include deliberate efforts to increase staff autonomy, strategies to enhance colleague support, identification and resolution of the most troubling deficits in resources, creative efforts to celebrate life, and ongoing staff-support meetings with provision for individual counsel as needed. Staff may need straightforward individual encouragement to seek health in their personal lives.

PATHOPHYSIOLOGICAL PROCESSES OF IMMINENT DEATH

The physical problems common to dying are caused by failure of vital body organs. Failure of the respiratory, cardiac, hepatic, and renal systems is summarized in Table 18-1. Further

Table 18-1	Pathophysiology of Dying Organs		
Basic Processes	Contributing Pathological Processes	Signs and Symptoms	Palliative Nursing Diagnoses
HEART			
The heart with myocardial damage is more likely to fail to contract adequately, but previously undamaged myocardium may fail as a result of workload imposed at end of life.	Preexisting congestive heart failure Myocardial infarction Arrhythmias Anemia Hypoxia Hypovolemia	No endurance Lethargy Reduced mentation Diminishing level of consciousness Tachycardia Arrhythmias	Alteration in thought processes Impaired physical mobility
Left ventricular function is diminished so that blood pools in ventricle and cardiac output is reduced.	Hemorrhage Sepsis Intracranial pressure on medullary circulatory centers	Angina Oliguria Hypotension	Alteration in comfort related to pain and other symptoms
Reduced cardiac output reduces perfusion of vital organs, particularly brain, kidney, and myocardium. Sympathetic nervous system responds with compensatory peripheral vasoconstriction.	—	Dusky nail beds Fleeting or absent peripheral pulses Cyanosis and mottling of extremities	Impending death
Blood backs up into pulmonary veins and capillaries to cause pulmonary edema.	—	Crackles and bubbles on auscultation Dyspnea, tachypnea, orthopnea	Impaired gas exchange/ineffective airway clearance and ineffective breathing pattern
Blood backs up into right atrium, vena cava, jugular vein, hepatic vein, and general circulation, especially abdomen and lower extremities.	—	Distended neck veins Ascites Pitting peripheral edema	Alteration in comfort related to swelling
LIVER			
Impaired detoxification of ammonia and other metabolites correlates with development of hepatic encephalopathy.	Cirrhosis Hepatitis Malignancies	Weakness Lethargy Reduced mentation Diminishing level of consciousness	Impaired physical mobility Alteration in thought processes

Table 18-1   Pathophysiology of Dying Organs—cont'd

Basic Processes	Contributing Pathological Processes	Signs and Symptoms	Palliative Nursing Diagnoses
LIVER—cont'd			
Resistance to blood flow into liver forces excess fluid to escape into lymphatic channels and then into peritoneal cavity. Reduced hepatic detoxification of aldosterone and antidiuretic hormone causes sodium retention to further extravascular fluid accumulation. Reduced synthesis of albumin reduces colloidal osmotic pressure so that fluid moves out of blood vessels.	—	Ascites Peripheral and pulmonary edema Oliguria, renal failure	Alteration in comfort related to swelling
Diminished function of hepatic Kupffer cells reduces filtration of intestinal blood so that more bacteria survive.	—	Peritonitis Sepsis Subacute bacterial endocarditis	—
Portal hypertension causes distention of venous channels in esophagus, stomach, or intestines. Rupture causes slow bleeding or massive hemorrhage.	—	Hematemesis Melena Bleeding esophageal varices Shock	Impending death
KIDNEYS			
Nitrogenous wastes accumulate to cause azotemia.	Hypovolemia reducing renal perfusion Glomerulonephritis Pyelonephritis Renal malignancy	Lack of endurance Lethargy Reduced mentation Pruritus, uremic frost Neuromuscular irritability	Impaired physical mobility Alteration in thought process Alteration in comfort related to pruritus and other symptoms
Inability to excrete hydrogen ions causes metabolic acidosis.	Polycystic kidney Renal vascular disease Collagen disease	Nausea and vomiting Pericarditis Deep and rapid respirations	—
Inability to excrete potassium causes hyperkalemia.	—	Bradycardia and cardiac arrest	Impending death
Kidney retains sodium, and consequent fluid overload produces peripheral and pulmonary edema.	—	Dependent pitting edema Pulmonary edema	Alteration in comfort related to swelling

Continued

	Table 18-1	Pathophysiology of Dying Organs—cont'd		
Basic Processes	Contributing Pathological Processes	Signs and Symptoms	Palliative Nursing Diagnoses
LUNGS			
Hypoventilation, increased airway resistance to expiration, and airway obstruction caused by pulmonary secretions result in low oxygen and sometimes elevated carbon dioxide levels. Hypercapnia and hypoxemia have dramatic cerebral effects. Heart works harder to circulate diminishing amount of oxygen.	Pneumonia Emphysema Chronic bronchitis Pulmonary infarction Pulmonary edema Atelectasis Pleural effusion Pulmonary or tracheal tumor Neuromuscular disease or disease of chest wall preventing lung expansion Pulmonary fibrosis Collagen disease Sarcoidosis Silicosis Asbestosis	Lack of endurance Lethargy Reduced mentation Diminishing level of consciousness Reduced breath sounds Inability to remove excretions Bubbles, crackles, wheezes Tachypnea Bradypnea Arrhythmic breathing Dyspnea, orthopnea Pursed lips Uses of accessory muscles Tachycardia Angina	Impaired physical mobility Alteration in thought processes Ineffective airway clearance and breathing pattern; impaired gas exchange Impending death

research is needed to elucidate terminal pathophysiological processes. Multiorgan failure is likely as death draws near. Nurses prepared to guide clients through a home death need a solid grasp of predictable pathophysiological processes to be able to anticipate the dying course and to be able to explain developments to the client and family in clear, concrete language. Note that many signs and symptoms are predictable events regardless of the specific organ involved. Palliative nursing diagnoses focus on determining alterations in comfort and diagnosing impending death, not on alteration of physiological function.

NURSING PROCESS FOR TERMINAL CARE AT HOME
Palliative Philosophy

Palliative principles focus on the alleviation of suffering and the promotion of comfort. Since these are subjective experiences, it is essential to pay close attention to the experience reported by the client and family and to respect the choices that come out of that experience. Palliative study seeks to understand individual perception of suffering and quality of life. Palliative goals seek to use the most appropriate therapies to relieve the suffering experience. Table 18-2 contrasts philosophies when dying is approached as a medical process and when it is approached as a human process. The palliative nursing process is grounded in ongoing systematic assessment, delineation of nursing diagnoses that focus on comfort and client and family coping, determination of goals by mutual agreement, and implementation of approaches that use the most up-to-date knowledge base.

Assessment and Diagnosis

Holistic physical, psychosocial, and spiritual assessment is ongoing in the developing nurse-patient relationship. Attention to the dying person's humanity and understanding of family and friends are central to assessment. Developing

Table 18-2 Contrasts in Philosophy of Conventional Medicine and Palliative Care	
Conventional: Focus on Medical Processes	Palliative: Focus on Human Process
Denial of dying	Dying as part of life cycle
Attention to technology	Attention to human experience; participation
Attention to disease	Attention to whole person
Attention to quantity of life—maintaining physiological systems	Attention to quality of life—therapies to comfort and meet personal goals
Medical defeat	Human growth
Silence; paternalistic withholding of facts	Open communication as chosen; teaching to empower
Withdrawal from the dying	Gathering around the dying
Avoidance of narcotics and sedatives	Careful adjustment of narcotics and sedatives to promote comfort and optimal function

rapport leads nurses to focus first on their perceived needs and priorities.

Physical investigation is systematic and determined by considering what information has palliative purpose. When about to draw blood, do a rectal examination, or even take a blood pressure, the nurse asks how the information gathered will be used to benefit the dying person's quality of life. Will treating the results of the investigation bring comfort? Good judgment should be exercised about what needs regular monitoring and how intrusively to assess new complaints. An uncomfortable diagnostic procedure is usually considered worthwhile if the person can look forward to eventual improvement in quality of life. In the period immediately preceding death, investigation only heightens suffering with no long-term gain possible.

Palliative psychosocial assessment is discussed in the sections on priority preterminal diagnoses. The nurse investigates the reciprocal supportive relationships in the community that have been used in prior difficulties or could be invoked in the present.

Dying occurs at the mysterious articulation between life and death. Questions about the meaning of life and suffering and universal and divine purpose are integral to "living on the edge." Spiritual assessment is difficult because contemporary Americans lack the common language for discourse about spiritual matters. We so easily feel intruded on or threatened by each other's beliefs. Sensitive spiritual assessment "opens the door" to enabling the client to explore old and new meanings and to reach out for understanding from others. Spiritual care is discussed in the section on diagnosing fear and spiritual distress.

With a client's multiple system failure and overwhelming loss in interpersonal functioning, a long list of nursing diagnoses is potential or actually present. However, listing them in a care plan is an intellectual exercise. The priority nursing diagnoses focus on threats to comfort and to client and family coping.

Determining Goals of Care

Goals are determined by merging professional judgment with choices that come out of client and family experience. Garland, Bass, and Otto (1984) have studied contrasting caregiver and hospice nurse perception of needs. From a review of the death and dying literature, they identified 5 need categories for primary caregivers and 10 need categories for clients (Box 18-1). Both nurses and caregivers perceived "respect for wishes" as the most important client need and "open communication with professionals" and "assistance to cope with providing care" as the top two needs of caregivers. When clients are interviewed to identify goals for themselves, desires such as increasing strength or fighting illness may contrast with caregiver and nurse perceptions of needs.

Negotiating goals   Dialogue and negotiation among caregivers, client, and nurse are essential to determine the initial contract and refocus the partnership at each visit. Commonly, each has some overt or covert goals that may be mutually

Box 18-1   Client and Primary Caregiver
            Needs

CLIENT NEEDS RANKED BY CAREGIVERS
  1. Respect for wishes
  2. Pain control
  3. Maintenance of normal family relations
  4. Open communication with professionals
  5. Assistance to cope with illness
  6. Knowledge that family has help to cope
  7. Financial assistance
  8. Discusson of spiritual concerns
  9. Preparation for death
 10. Assistance with household tasks

CAREGIVER NEEDS RANKED
BY CAREGIVERS
  1. Open communication with professionals
  2. Assistance to cope with providing care
  3. Legal assistance
  4. Discussion of spiritual concerns
  5. Assistance with household tasks

Modified from Garland TN, Bass DM, Otto ME: *The American Journal of Hospice Care* 1(3):40-45, 1984.

exclusive. The nurse encourages each person to speak his or her view, summarizes each position, discovers common ground that recognizes each person's position, and maintains the focus on respecting the wishes and comfort of the dying person.

Questioning goals   When the focus is indeed a comfortable death that respects client wishes, many conventional life-sustaining nursing goals must be scrutinized. Respect for choice is counterbalanced with concern that some choices may hasten death or further suffering. Nurses must be conscious of how they coerce people to do what they think is best, yet they must know their own "bottom line" in evaluating the hurtful effects of client choices on themselves, significant others, and the professional team. For instance, a nurse may respect a client's right to maintain complete denial of his or her own death but draw the line at tolerating client choice of alcoholic binges as a way of coping.

Palliative goals are different from life-sustaining goals   As death draws near, palliative treatment is very different from restorative treatment. Physically mobilizing the client and implementing

vigorous measures to prevent immobility complications are usually not appropriate. Physical therapy switches from promoting activity to implementing comfort-giving modalities. Occupational therapy may assist adaptation to perform those activities the client perceives as meaningful. Therapies to monitor or sustain bodily systems may not promote comfortable dying.

Forcing a dying person to eat and drink is cruel and inappropriate at the end of life. More controversial is the use of tube feeding, intravenous fluids, and total parenteral nutrition. Artificial hydration in the presence of multisystem shutdown can actually cause discomforting symptoms, such as accumulating edema, ascites, accumulating pulmonary and pharyngeal secretions, and vomiting of increased gastric volume (Zerwekh, 1997a). Though practitioners conventionally worry about the "suffering" they fear will occur because of dehydration, hospice physician and nurse observers actually find the most troublesome consequence is thirst. However, no clear correlation between thirst and level of dehydration has actually been demonstrated. Dry mouth is seen consistently in dehydrated people near death, but other factors, such as mouth breathing and medication side effects, contribute to it. Symptoms of dehydration in healthy people, such as headache, nausea, vomiting, and cramps, are not documented when people are dying. The blood chemistry tests of dehydrated dying people have been reported to be strikingly normal, with consistent elevations in urea, uric acid, and creatinine. The physiological processes of dying need further study, but observation reveals that people may be more comfortable in a dehydrated state than when hydrated. Intravenous technology may also be a source of distress, causing localized pain, restraining movement, and diverting attention of caregivers. The palliative nursing role includes helping the client and family clarify values, articulating the burdens and benefits of hydration in each individual case, and guiding a negotiated decision.

PALLIATIVE PRACTICE GUIDELINES
Palliative Relationships

Reaching out to meet the fear of dying people and their families, expert nurses describe the empathetic process of connecting through developing empathetic relationships. Connecting involves deliberately developing trust, hearing the stories that need to be told, asking difficult questions that no one else has the courage to ask, and being present and available in a way that goes beyond words. Speaking truth and encouraging end-of-life choice are integral to expert hospice nursing (Zerwekh, 1994a, 1995). Advocacy for the client begins with the nurse's trust in the client's ability to choose what is best for himself or herself. Nurses inform people that they have the option to choose, encourage the problem-solving process, and advocate for choice.

Collaboration

All of hospice nursing is collaborative and interdisciplinary; teamwork means letting go the idea of being the most important caregiver for the family and accepting that many perspectives are better than one in finding solutions for challenging problems. Each team member needs all the help the others can provide. The interdisciplinary approach with the nurse as case manager is a highly effective model. Nurse case managers assess multidimensional needs in the home environment, orchestrate referrals to other professionals, and take responsibility for ongoing evaluation of the interdisciplinary plan.

Strengthening Family Caregivers

Families are strengthened by the nurse's active listening to their life stories and encouragement to reminisce. Nurses can foster client and family power and identity by listening, giving feedback about behaviors and patterns observed, clarifying values, encouraging reflection, and affirming strengths. Through teaching, nurses enable people to care for themselves. Translating medical knowledge to human experience empowers the client and family to be in control. Nurses need to assess activities that caregivers rely on for support and to focus their interventions to strengthen them. The nurse's definition of *essential supports* expands to encompass the family definition. Hairdressing or waxing the floor may be frivolous extras to the nurse but they may be of incredible support to some caregivers. The need for support from other people intensifies greatly with progressing invalidism of the dying person. The nurse teaches the family to systematically identify caregiving helpers and organize them to be of maximal assistance. Some families' choice of privacy and independence precludes depending on others, and they will handle it alone as long as possible, often precipitating crisis. This is their choice.

If families choose to prepare themselves, anticipatory guidance begins at the first visit. Nurses must teach them what to expect with the progression of disease and how to manage expected difficulties. Most people express a desire to plan ahead but have some turmoil about consciously preparing for the harsh reality of death. It usually takes many visits to prepare a family adequately. Information must be given in small portions that they can assimilate and accept. By assessing family history of coping with stress, nurses can predict a family's ability to take control versus their being overwhelmed by changes and controlled by intense emotionalism.

When coping mechanisms are overwhelmed by alarming episodes in home terminal care, 24-hour call enables the nurse to respond immediately. With the family immobilized, the nurse assigns concrete tasks and teaches new coping strategies that are needed immediately. Crisis intervention mandates a directive manner to reestablish order. With the situation stabilized, the nurse shifts out of controlling style to help the family mobilize their existing resources. The family self-concept is reframed in terms of the competencies they do possess and the nurse's faith in their future ability to cope. With crisis comes opportunity.

Comforting

Expert hospice nurses practice comforting by providing hands-on care, anticipating comfort needs, trying multiple options, balancing pharmacological effects and side effects, organizing and reorganizing drug regimens, making major changes in those regimens, trying nontraditional complementary therapies, and realizing the limits of comforting (Zerwekh, 1995).

Palliative management of symptoms to promote comfort is based on the following principles, which should be consistently woven into the fabric of caregiving:

- Attention to client and family perception, not nurse assumption
- Ongoing assessment and documentation of symptoms and the effectiveness of therapy
- Inclusion of measures to alleviate psychosocial, spiritual, and physiological dimensions of suffering

Table 18-3 Useful Drugs for End-Stage Symptoms		
Representative Drug	Uses for Terminal Symptoms	Significant Side Effects

Phenothiazines
  Prochlorperazine (Compazine)
  Chlorpromazine (Thorazine)
	Antianxiety in small doses
	Antiemetic
	Enhancing pain relief
		Sedation
		↓ Mentation
		Hypotension
		Extrapyramidal effects

Haloperidol (Haldol)	Antipsychotic Antiemetic Enhancing pain relief	Sedation ↓ Mentation Hypotension Extrapyramidal effects

Antihistamines
  Hydroxyzine (Vistaril)
  Diphenhydramine (Benadryl)
	Antianxiety
	Antiemetic
	Enhancing pain relief
	Control of acute dyspnea
		Sedation
		↓ Mentation (less common)
		Anticholinergic effects
		Convulsant at high doses
		Sometimes hypotension

Benzodiazepines
  Diazepam (Valium)
  Chlordiazepoxide (Librium)
  Lorazepam (Ativan)
	Antianxiety
	Not antiemetic
	Can intensify pain perception
		Sedation
		↓ Mentation
		Paradoxical excitement
		Antianalgesia
		↓ Respirations
		Physical dependency

Metoclopramide (Reglan)	↑ Gastrointestinal motility
	  (stomach, small bowel)
	↑ Gastroesophageal sphincter
	  tone
	Antiemetic
		Sedation
		Extrapyramidal effects
		Diarrhea

Corticosteroids
  Dexamethasone
  Prednisone
	↓ Inflammatory response,
	  ↓ edema → relief of compres-
	  sion, obstruction, bronchospasm
	Lymphatic suppression
		Adrenal insufficiency with sudden
		  withdrawal
		Hyperglycemia
		Hypokalemia
		Risk of infection

Atropine and scopolamine	Anticholinergic → ↓ saliva and
	  respiratory secretions
	For "death rattle"
		Dry mouth, constipation, blurred
		  vision, urinary retention,
		  tachycardia

Tricyclic antidepressants Amitriptyline (Elavil)	Mood elevation Direct analgesic effect	Excessive sedation Orthostatic hypotension Anticholinergic effects
Antiseizure drugs Gabapentin (Neurontin)	Neuropathic pain	Fatigue, dizziness

↓, Decreased; ↑, Increased

- Prevention of symptoms through regularly scheduled use of medication (Table 18-3)
- Frequent readjustment of medication to minimize side effects and maximize comfort
- First choice of oral, sublingual, and rectal routes and cautious use of parenteral routes
- Active pursuit of uncontrolled symptoms

PRIORITY PRETERMINAL DIAGNOSIS
Fear and Spiritual Distress

Dying is traveling toward the unknown in a materialistic, know-it-all society that fears what it cannot prove or control. Immobilized by dread of annihilation at death, contemporary humans lie to themselves about their own mortality. The ideal becomes death in sleep, without warning, so that they don't have to think about it. "Thank goodness he went so quickly. He never knew a thing." The dying and the bereaved are socially quarantined lest they be visible reminders that technological society has limits (Aries, 1981). Thus it is that dying people fear losing themselves, losing control, and being abandoned. Spiritual distress underlies the struggle through fear to find meaning.

Dying people fear the loss of their known selves, gradually experiencing small losses, and, ultimately complete loss of identity as they have known it. "Little deaths" include deterioration in body structure and function, diminishing control, and loss of roles and relationships. One great fear of people dying at home is uncontrolled suffering at the moment of death. Other paramount worries are about the responses and well-being of family members and fear of the experience of death itself. People want ongoing anticipatory guidance and around-the-clock crisis availability of home care teams to help control problems. Family and friends are commonly at a loss to know how to respond to the dying person, and, reminded of their own mortality, they may withdraw. Those recently bereaved will often tell you how many friends and relatives "disappeared" during their loved one's dying. Thus a significant way to reduce fear for the dying is to facilitate their staying home with loved ones and encouraging the loved ones. Those without such support will indeed be faced with dying as a stranger among strangers.

Frankl (1963) described the search for meaning while suffering the extreme horrors of Nazi concentration camps. Victims facing death found meaning in the realization that there was unfinished business in life and tasks remaining to be fulfilled. Likewise, for those who are terminally ill, acknowledging death's approach allows the person to find meaning in completing life's tasks and choosing his or her legacy. Encouraging reminiscence and conscious decision-making fosters this goal.

Spirituality has been described as the longing for meaning, the essence of being a person, the experience of God or ultimate reality, or trust in the transcendent. The goal of spirituality is connection with a reality that lasts beyond individual identity (Zerwekh, 1993). Spiritual distress occurs as the individual struggles to find meaning in suffering and inevitable death. Many people do not express concerns in spiritual terms, yet it is easy to see that they are dispirited. Recurrent conversational themes that may be indicators of spiritual distress include estrangement and feeling unloved, inability to forgive oneself or others, hatred, feelings of guilt and worthlessness, purposelessness, and intractable agitation. Those who express being dispirited in religious language may have a religious identity, estrangement from past identity, or a personal belief system that is not identified with a group. They may express rejection, uncertainty, fear, anger, or guilt, or they may wish for more faith and experience of a supreme being.

Derrickson (1996) describes four dimensions of dying people's spiritual struggle to answer the deepest questions of their lives: remembering, reassessing, reconciliation, and reunion. Remembering is a life review. Reassessing requires new definitions of worth and identity. Reconciliation requires healing broken relationships. Reunion involves disconnection with earthly reality and reconnection with spiritual reality. Zerwekh (1993) has described hospice nurses' expert practice in helping dying people "transcend life." Nursing competencies that address transcendent needs include guiding letting go and caring spiritually. Guiding letting go involves helping people let go of all aspects of life as they have known it. Caring spiritually is rooted in a personal grounding to replenish personal energy, understand caring as giving and receiving, and continually learn from experience. Other spiritual caring skills include identifying spiritual issues, being there (the practice of human presence), dialoguing, fostering reconciliation and integration of life experiences, and sharing nearing-death mystical experiences.

Whenever possible, referral should be made to clergy or others with special training in spiritual counseling. People committed to a specific religion will find comfort in traditional ministry of teachings, scripture, prayer, and rituals. Those estranged from a religious past or without a religious identity will do best with counselors specially trained in nondogmatic spiritual counseling.

Grieving Related to Loss

Grief is the intense emotion that floods life when a person's security is shattered by an acute loss, most severe when the loss is death itself. The grieving process involves letting go of life as it has always been, facing the unknown, and reengaging in life for survivors. Grief is accompanied by changes in thought, behavior, social interaction, physical well-being, and ability to go about everyday life. The more engaged in life and the more vigorous we are, the more likely are everyday losses: friends leave; the cat dies; the car gets a dent or a death rattle in the transmission; a knee injury prevents jogging; or vacation plans fall through. At the highest level of engagement and commitment, we love life and love other people.

Dying initiates grief at the expected loss of one's own life or the expected loss of a loved one. Grief permits resolution and reconciliation in relationships, a chance to say goodbye, and completion of unfinished business. However, prolonged grieving can be exhausting, particularly if the disease course includes periods of reprieve and improvement.

Normal grief   The nurse teaches the client and family about normal grief and helpful responses. Grief reactions do not necessarily progress in predictable sequential stages, and people shift back and forth in their emotional responses until they can let go. Shock and denial are a natural buffer to reality and occur initially as well as intermittently over weeks, months, or years. As a prolonged coping style, denial immobilizes feelings and blocks energy to go forward. Nurses cannot force people to walk through the doorway into open awareness; they can only open the door and offer attentive listening for the person to explore reality at his or her own pace. Many people die denying their own death, and many relatives also never acknowledge anticipated death. Frequently we must attend to the frustrations of those who wish to speak openly, but are blocked by their loved one's denial.

Anger is a common emotion of grieving. It may be directed at the loved ones or oneself, at illness and treatment, at health professionals, or at God. Nurses should encourage identifying and expressing anger through talking, crying, screaming, and yelling when alone and through strenuous activities, if possible. When anger is a prolonged coping style, people become estranged from each other at a time of great need. The nurse reminds those involved that anger is an emotion secondary to grief. Grief needs to be ex-

pressed and explored. Restlessness and disorganized and absentminded behavior are common. Decision making is difficult, and carrying on life's ordinary business is a struggle. Nurses can help the grieving set priorities and limits and understand their everyday functional difficulties as normal, not "crazy."

Depression and despair are expected with grieving. The grieving person becomes immobilized and withdrawn without any sense of pleasure, hope, or meaning. Dependency is great. Self-destructive thoughts may arise. The opportunity to share his or her life story may be healing. Addressing spiritual issues may bring relief, as may surrounding the grieving depressed person with love and inviting reengagement in meaningful life. Antidepressants may lift the dark cloud enough to permit choice of reengagement. However, some people will literally turn their faces to the wall and await death. The bereaved are at high physical and emotional risk in this state, and a more structured approach must be taken to facilitate their reengagement. Many times dying people will be able to move through depression to acceptance with peaceful closure and letting go of life.

Dysfunctional grief   The diagnosis of potential or actual dysfunctional grief in survivors can be the responsibility of the home care nurse. Danger signs include lack of emotional affect; severe hostility toward helpers; excessive guilt; self-destructive behavior, including drugs and alcohol; reclusive behavior; and prolonged antisocial acting out in children. History of unresolved losses predisposes grief. The newly bereaved experience a higher rate of both physical and emotional disorders. Recent studies actually document suppression of immunity in those who are mourning; morbidity and mortality increase with bereavement. For this reason, hospice programs include bereavement counseling as an integral element of service. Any long-range health plan to maintain consumer health and reduce acute psychiatric and medical intervention should include bereavement services for the high-risk candidate.

Alteration in Family Processes Related to Terminal Illness

Dying is a normal developmental process in the multigenerational family system. Family equilibrium is disrupted, with the risk of physical, emotional, and social dysfunction of members determined by the characteristics of the family system. The smoothest transitions occur in families with high member self-worth, clear communication between members, flexible roles, and reciprocal relationships with outside support networks. The roughest occur in families with low member self-worth, indirect communication with unspoken rules, rigid roles and resistance to change, and refusal to accept outsider help. Families with a history of living from crisis to crisis will continue to do so. Even families who manage everyday life with adequate communication and problem solving may decompensate when someone is dying and have difficulty with planning. Small, short-term nursing goals are most attainable.

Family caregiver burden Family caregivers frequently report physical difficulties in providing care, primarily lifting and moving the dependent client, and experience extreme stress in witnessing their loved one's physical and emotional suffering. They have great need to have time for themselves and for rest and sleep (Steele, Fitch, 1996). Caregiver health should be an ongoing concern; physical and mental well-being should be continually assessed, with intervention provided as necessary. Respite for family caregivers may occasionally require brief client admission to hospital or nursing home or paid caregivers coming into the home.

Stetz and Brown (1997) have described the tasks of families taking care of people with life-threatening illness to include managing the illness, facing and preparing for dying, managing the environment, coming to know their own strength, personal suffering, responding to family relationship issues, and struggling with the health care system.

Shifting family responsibilities Dying elicits the need to reshuffle all family roles. First, physical disability prevents a dying person's complete functioning in the full spectrum of roles such as breadwinner, bowler, gardener, parent, lover, or friend. The nurse can propose role modifications to maximize the person's contribution within his or her energy limits. To continue the family system, other members must gradually assume new responsibilities. Caring for the loved one is balanced precariously with the needs of others. Economic survival of the family can be threatened by the loss of the breadwinner, by the burden on another breadwinner who also may be expected to be caregiver, and by the accumulation of med-

ical bills. Essential household tasks such as shopping, cooking, child care, and laundry must continue. Individuals need to maintain normality and rest, exercise, worship, and have fun. Children need to be informed; to express themselves; to feel involved; and to be allowed to act like children, which includes testing limits. They need to be assured that they will be cared for after the death. Problem solving and networking enable the family to accomplish these tasks.

Family nursing The nursing role with families of dying people is strengthening the family by continually assessing them to understand their unique family experience, developing their ability to care, strengthening communication between family members, and realizing family limitations. Assessment requires attunement to family dynamics and history and the effects of dying on all aspects of family life. Developing caregiving ability requires teaching that attends to readiness to learn and the reality of intense emotions that challenge the ability to learn. Teaching requires dialogue, repetition, and role modeling of what to say and do. The family's ability to care needs to be continually validated and encouraged. Fostering communication between family members, hospice nurses encourage them to say the words that need to be said to one another. Avoidance and denial still dominate family-member discussion until hospice team members can mediate to move them beyond customary small talk (Beach, 1995). Nurses often suggest that family members gather around the bed or kitchen table to talk truthfully to each other.

Facing limitations of family caregiving ability is an everyday home hospice nursing experience. The expert nurse learns to recognize dysfunctional patterns and adversities that require reducing goals to what is achievable. For instance, reconciliation is unlikely to occur in a life-long abusive relationship. Facing limitations also requires setting limits on antisocial and destructive behavior that the nurse will permit in his or her presence.

Physicians and nurses depend on family caregivers' reports of the severity of symptoms clients experience at home, yet research demonstrates that client and family ratings of symptoms and quality of life are quite divergent. Family members rarely know the intensity, quality, or pattern of their loved one's pain (Madison, Wilkie, 1995). Therefore family caregivers can be taught to use objective, straightforward symptom assessment tools, such as number ratings from 0 to 10 or visual analogue scales or vertical graphic scales (Weitzner, Moody, McMillan, 1997).

Impaired Physical Mobility and Self-Care Deficit

An inevitable consequence of progressing terminal illness is impaired physical movement related to diminishing endurance, muscle weakness, movement restrictions imposed by discomfort, and reduced motivation. The person will take first to his or her chair and sooner or later to bed. Problems with dressing, bathing, toileting, and self-feeding can be anticipated. The family will need to assist partially and then totally in meeting basic needs. The plan to respond to reduced mobility and self-care must be consistent with client and family goals. On one end of the continuum, there may be an effort to maximize function and capability for a time. At the other end of the continuum, there is a time for withdrawal and dependency at the end of life. The nurse clarifies valued activities and choices. Where does the client wish to focus diminishing energy? Teaching energy conservation is helpful. Acceptance of immobility and dependency is tantamount to accepting defeat, so there are often conflicting goals among client, family, and professionals that need to be resolved. For instance, the decision to rent a hospital bed may be a practical one from the nurse's point of view to ease caregiver back strain and workload. The client may, however, see this as the final symbol of defeat, and the husband may choose an aching back rather than give up his last days of sleeping with his wife. Anticipatory guidance focuses on planning for that expected time when dependency mandates frequent or constant bedside attendance by loved ones, paid caregivers, or in an institutional setting. Such anticipation is threatening, but careful advance planning empowers people to be in control.

Alteration in Thought Processes

Review of the symptoms of the pathophysiology of dying organs in Table 18-1 reveals anticipated mental-status changes. In addition to the pathophysiological consequences of organ failure, other factors impairing mental status include drug side effects, fever, depression, cerebral le-

sions, and electrolyte imbalances. Impairment ranges from mild, with diminishing concentration and judgment, to severe, with disorientation, delusions, and hallucinations. In the last days of life, the level of consciousness drops gradually or rapidly before death. Antipsychotic medications are used to diminish hallucinations and paranoia; haloperidol has the least sedative and anticholinergic side effects. Terminal restlessness in the days before death is effectively managed by benzodiazepines, particularly sublingual lorazepam or rectal diazepam (March, 1998) or antipsychotics, particularly haldoperidol (Ferrell, Coyle, 2001).

Loss of the "mind" can be more dreaded than loss of the ability to move. The practical consequence is increasing dependency on others and threatened safety because of lack of judgment. Eventually, the dying person may not be able to be left alone at home. Workup should be considered to identify and reverse likely causes. Drug regimens must be scrutinized and perhaps readjusted.

Family members are taught to use reorientation tactics, structure the environment, plan bedside attention, and eliminate safety hazards. Many may anticipate caring for a comatose client. Some individuals will say that their "bottom line" of personal limitation is caring for their loved one if he or she becomes noncooperatively disoriented or goes into a coma. Help will be needed either from an expanded caregiver network or from hospital or nursing home admission.

Pain

Pain management demands considerable palliative expertise. Pain is the most prevalent physical problem for dying cancer clients (Weitzner, Moody, McMillan, 1997) and affects a significant number of people dying from other causes. Knowledge of the assessment and effective control of terminal pain is now well established but too often remains unlearned and therefore not practiced (Ferrell, McCaffery, 1997). Uncontrolled pain dominates consciousness and extinguishes possible attainment of all other end-of-life goals—physical, psychosocial, and spiritual. Therefore it is imperative that nurses explore their own knowledge and beliefs that may prevent them from seeing and responding to suffering.

The compassionate presence of the nurse ameliorates the emotional and spiritual dimensions of pain. In addition to human presence, the mainstay of terminal pain control is medication. Opioids are often used with appropriate selection of antianxiety agents, antidepressants, anticonvulsants, antiinflammatories, and acetaminophen. All measures to relieve pain are grounded in systematic assessment—location and character of the pain as reported by the client, intensity of the pain using a scale or visual indicator (such as a smiling or frowning face), variability of the pain, and factors that intensify or relieve it. In hospice care, it is essential to believe and pay careful attention to the client's subjective report; pain is considered to be whatever the client says it is. Because pain relief is so often peripheral to the attention of contemporary professionals who have not been held accountable for pain management, investigation of pain is now proposed as the "fifth vital sign."

Morphine Carefully titrated opioids are highly effective for terminal pain resulting from tissue damage, but neuropathic pain is only partially responsive. Morphine is the standard strong opioid used for terminal pain. Morphine mimics the actions of endogenous opioids to provide analgesia and sedation. Physical dependence occurs with long-term use. Addiction, which involves compulsive drug seeking, is a separate phenomenon that was found in a classic study to involve only 4 of 12,000 medical clients taking opioids. Side effects of morphine initially include sedation, which subsides in a few days, and nausea and vomiting, which respond to antiemetic drugs. Constipation is a predictable consequence of long-term use and must be persistently countered with concomitant laxative administration. Respiratory suppression is seen only when an excessive dose is initially administered in an opioid-naive client or when the drug dose is dramatically increased without cautious incremental titration to level of pain. For maintenance analgesia in terminal clients who can still swallow, long-acting morphine tablets are now the opioid of choice. MS Contin and Roxanol SR are sustained-release tablets lasting approximately 12 hours. When swallowing becomes a problem, unusually high concentrations of morphine solution (20 mg/ml) are available; dosage must then be every 4 hours.

Other opioids Although morphine is considered the opioid of choice, other opioids are quite

effective and commonly used for terminal pain. Particular mention needs to be made about the effectiveness of oral high-dose oxycodone. Now that it is available in a plain preparation as a tablet or solution, oxycodone is found to be as effective as oral morphine with oral dosages equivalent in potency (Zerwekh, 1994b). It is now available in short-acting form, as well as OxyContin, which provides 12-hour relief. Methadone is much less expensive than the long-lasting new opioid preparations and well absorbed orally, with a duration of 6 to 8 hours. It must be chosen carefully because of its tendency to accumulate and cause over-sedation (Kemp, 1999). Hydromorphone (Dilaudid) is an effective alternative to morphine, particularly useful because it can be highly concentrated in solution. Oxymorphone (Numorphan) is available in a practical rectal suppository form.

Alternatives to oral dosing Inability to swallow and nausea and vomiting are the most common reasons to use other routes for opioid administration. Rectal, oral transmucosal, transdermal, and subcutaneous medication routes are all effective low-tech palliative interventions (Mercadante, 1998). Since the beginnings of home hospice care, nurses have taught families to insert medication rectally when the client could no longer swallow. Rectal opioids are usually well absorbed with a 4-hour duration; this route is inexpensive and requires no technology. The main objection is the embarrassment and unpleasantness associated with rectal insertion; however, for many people, this is not a concern. Likewise, sublingual and buccal administration of liquid morphine or morphine tablets with moisture added was an early home hospice strategy that continues to be widely used today. However, morphine is not as well absorbed through the oral mucosa as methadone and fentanyl are. Fentanyl citrate is now available as a lozenge on a handle; it is rapidly absorbed and highly effective for break-through pain (Chandler, 1999b). Transdermal fentanyl patches (Duragesic) provide continuous absorption for 3 days. They are most appropriate for clients with stable pain who are no longer able to take opioids by mouth. Their cost can be prohibitive. After application, it takes 12 to 24 hours for fentanyl levels to stabilize. After the patch is removed, it takes 17 to 36 hours for the drug effects to wear off (Ferrell,

McCaffery, 1997). Effectiveness is limited when cachexia limits the fat depot through which fentanyl is absorbed.

Intramuscular and subcutaneous injections should be avoided because of the suffering caused and the discontinuous nature of pain control. An indwelling subcutaneous route is a recent successful palliative approach to administering bolus opioid injections for break-through pain. When pain is extreme and lower-tech routes have failed, continuous subcutaneous infusions keep a constant high level of narcotic in the blood. Home care involves the cost and maintenance of an infusion pump and subcutaneous access but not the complications and level of skilled supervision associated with maintaining an intravenous line.

Break-through pain Clients receiving around-the-clock narcotics should have sublingual or oral short-acting immediate-release opioid tablets or solution prescribed as rescue doses for break-through pain. The dose should be 5% to 15% of the total equivalent 24-hour narcotic dosage (Ferrell, McCaffery, 1997). Bolus intravenous injections of narcotics should be reserved for severe break-through pain; they are not suitable for maintenance analgesia because of the frequent injections needed (intravenous morphine has a duration of 1½ to 2 hours) and resultant roller-coaster pattern of suffering and relief. In the home, subcutaneous bolus injections into an indwelling plastic cannula or butterfly needle can provide effective relief of severe break-through pain for up to 4 hours.

Pain that responds poorly to opioids Some types of pain are best treated with other drugs or approaches. In particular, the pain of bone metastasis is most effectively managed first with palliative radiation and nonsteroidal antiinflammatories such as ibuprofen. The pain of increasing intracranial pressure should be managed with corticosteroids and opioids. Likewise, neuropathic pain, particularly common in people with acquired immune deficiency syndrome (AIDS), is most challenging to control. It results from nerve injury that causes nerves to fire spontaneously, producing burning or shooting pain, often imposed on dull aching. Neuropathic pain requires adjuvant analgesics, such as tricyclic antidepressants (particularly amitriptyline) and anticonvulsants (Kemp, 1999).

Nausea and Vomiting

Nausea and vomiting result when the vomiting center in the medulla is stimulated by visceral input from the vagus nerve, emotional input from higher brain centers, and drugs or metabolites affecting the chemoreceptor trigger zone in the brain. At the end of life, comfort is the goal, not better nutrition. Nausea and vomiting should be approached in the terminally ill by medical assessment to find and treat reversible causes. Pharmacological intervention includes use of phenothiazines (prochlorperazine [Compazine]), dopamine antagonists (haloperidol [Haldol] and metoclopramide [Reglan]), antihistamines (diphenhydramine [Benadryl]), benzodiazepines (lorazepam [Ativan]), anticholinergics (scopolamine), corticosteroids (dexamethasone [Decadron]), cannabinoids (dronabinol [Marinol]), or serotonin antagonists (ondansetron [Zofran]) on a scheduled basis and in combination if vomiting is uncontrolled (Rousseau, 1995).

As death approaches, the client normally first stops taking in food and then fluids. Food and fluid are essential to life but not essential for a comfortable death. However, they represent love and the sustenance of life to loved ones, and letting go of nutritional hopes means acceptance of death approaching. Families need considerable active listening and teaching about the normal dying process to work through this. Without artificial alimentation or hydration, there is diminished gastric content and thus less vomiting. (See the discussion of dehydration in the section on determining goals of care.)

Bowel and Bladder Alterations: Constipation, Diarrhea, and Urinary Incontinence

The likelihood of constipation increases with diminishing mobility and reduced intake of fluids and dietary fiber. Narcotics have three effects on the gastrointestinal tract: decreased secretions causing delay in food digestion; decreased gastrointestinal peristalsis; and increased water absorption from stool from the delay in passage, causing dryness and hardening. For clients unable to consume adequate fiber, bulk laxatives and increased fluids can be tried to maintain a soft stool. Anorexic or nauseated clients generally find bulk laxatives intolerable. Stool softeners should always be administered with narcotics, but may only soften feces without stimulating propulsive peristalsis. Therefore the standard senna tablet (Senekot) may be used routinely to stimulate colon peristalsis when narcotics are used routinely. Bowel stimulants such as senna or bisacodyl (Dulcolax) must be titrated to the frequency and softness of stool.

Daily records of bowel movements are essential to palliative care. If many days pass without elimination, cathartics and enemas become an inexcusable torture. In that case, gentle means such as milk of magnesia and oil-retention enemas should be used with persistence and patience before resorting to methods that cause severe abdominal cramping. Analgesics should be used before any disimpaction procedure.

Inoperable malignant bowel obstruction can be effectively managed at home. When obstruction is incomplete, metoclopramide (Reglan) promotes emptying of the stomach and small bowel peristalsis and is also antiemetic. Stool softeners may be useful. When obstruction is complete, narcotics are used to slow the painful peristaltic waves, and antiemetics may be tried. The dehydrated client with a complete bowel obstruction may vomit only once or twice daily. Antiemetics such as prochlorperazine (Compazine) and haloperidol are used when emesis is frequent and distressing. Ondansetron and octreotide may be useful when nausea and vomiting remain uncontrolled (Baumrucker, 1998). Transdermal and parenteral scopolamine are useful for relaxing smooth muscle when there is colicky pain. A nasogastric tube is used only if it is chosen by the client as less distressing than vomiting.

Diarrhea is an uncommon problem in the terminally ill. However, it is a major challenge in terminal AIDS (see Chapter 25). In the case of intractable diarrhea, antidiarrheal medications, particularly diphenoxylate and atropine (Lomotil) and loperamide (Imodium) are scheduled regularly. Octreotide (Sandostatin) may diminish intestinal secretions. The perianal area is cleansed with squeeze bottles and protected with a petroleum-based ointment. Stomahesive is an effective barrier for broken skin. Enterostomal therapists should be consulted to preserve the perianal area from breakdown in cases of persistent refractory diarrhea (Kemp, Stepp, 1995).

Urinary incontinence is likely with diminishing level of consciousness at the very end of life. However, with diminishing fluid intake, the urine volume is so small that incontinence may occur only once or twice daily. Caregivers should be prepared for the possibility of loss of urinary control. They will need to protect the mattress, have absorbent pads or towels, and understand the importance of frequent perineal hygiene. Clients who have been well hydrated will produce a large urinary volume, and the use of a retention catheter may be difficult to avoid. A catheter is also indicated if urinary retention is causing discomfort. The choice to catheterize is based on client comfort and the family's capacity to manage frequent linen changes and bathing.

Ineffective Breathing Pattern and Ineffective Airway Clearance

Alterations in respiratory function are predictable with progressive cardiopulmonary disease and are also present at the very end of all lives when cardiopulmonary failure begins as a result of other end-stage system failure. End-stage processes that impair pulmonary circulation or movement of gases at the alveolar level will cause hypoxia and hypercapnia with subjective report of shortness of breath and fatigue and objective signs, including pursed lip breathing, use of accessory muscles, orthopnea, reduced breath sounds, abnormal breath sounds (wheezes, crackles, and bubbles), cyanosis, and impaired mentation. Ineffective airway clearance is due to viscous secretions and impaired cough.

Interventions at home to reverse the underlying processes are discussed in Chapter 19. Since alteration in comfort is the focus in this chapter, recommended home care approaches focus on alleviating the distress associated with shortness of breath and profuse secretions.

Dyspnea is a subjective experience that can be effectively assessed by asking the client to rate breathlessness on a scale of 1 to 5 or 1 to 10. A visual analogue scale may be easiest to understand. A horizontal line is labeled with "no problem breathing" on one end and "terrible difficulty breathing" on the other end. Like pain, dyspnea is a subjective experience with social, psychological, and spiritual dimensions. It is best understood as being whatever the client reports (Zeppetella, 1998). Shortness of breath is relieved by an upright position, a fan circulating air, oxygen blowing into the nostrils even if there is little objective hope of improving oxygen pressure, human presence during periods of desperate air hunger, and selected medication. Long-acting morphine (MS Contin or Oramorph) every 12 hours with immediate-release morphine as needed every 3 hours controls shortness of breath. High-dose sublingual morphine has been used when people can no longer swallow. Benzodiazepines, particularly lorazepam (Ativan) sublingual or by mouth, frequently are adjuncts in the relief of restlessness and shortness of breath. Diuretics may continue to be palliative in end-stage chronic obstructive pulmonary disease (COPD) and cardiac disease. Corticosteroids are useful in COPD and pulmonary malignancy, as is unrestricted use of inhalants and nebulizers (Stephany, 1996a, 1996b). Phenothiazines are useful when anxiety and agitation are associated with breathlessness. There is much anecdotal evidence of the effectiveness of nebulized morphine for severe end-stage dyspnea; controlled studies have not been conducted (Chandler, 1999a).

Secretions and cough are minimized by side-lying position, narcotics, and dehydration. Atropine 0.4 to 0.6 mg subcutaneously or intramuscularly or scopolamine patches are occasionally needed to reduce the accumulation of pulmonary and pharyngeal secretions (death rattle). The anticholinergic effect reduces saliva and respiratory secretion production. The other anticholinergic effects are irrelevant in the hours immediately preceding death, when body systems are shutting down. The risk of unacceptable side effects, such as neuroexcitability, blurred vision, urinary retention and constipation, and tachycardia, increases if use is prolonged to days or weeks. Suctioning is usually unnecessary, discomforting, and traumatic at home. Oral suctioning with an infant bulb syringe may be helpful and readily learned by family.

IMPENDING DEATH AT HOME

The nurse assists the family to recognize signs that death is likely within hours or days, to be ready for the anticipated caregiving needs, and to prepare for death's immediate aftermath. The nurse recognizes death approaching when the person with known irreversible terminal disease develops indicators that the heart or lungs are failing. Common predictable symptoms of the last 48 hours, which the family can readily be taught to recognize and manage, include the following:

- Diminishing level of consciousness, confusion, and restlessness
- Consumption of little or no oral fluids
- Labored, irregular breathing; periods of apnea; and dyspnea
- Bubbling in throat and chest
- Progressive cyanotic mottling in lower extremities
- Oliguria or incontinence

Some families may want to learn to take vital signs to recognize changes such as weak or irregular pulse, hypotension, irregular breathing, or fever. For some, having this information permits a greater sense of control. Others may worry about what they find. Families are taught to make a definitive determination when death occurs by noting the absence of breath and heartbeat. Many will appreciate having a stethoscope and will practice listening to the heartbeat.

Final Preparations

Home management of impending death is possible with caregiver knowledge of what to expect and how to manage, a capable caregiver network, and necessary equipment and drugs on hand to manage predictable symptoms. The nurse defines the situation as the "final stretch" of the terminal course and encourages the final stage of mobilizing resources. It is wise to plan for the long haul, longer than it is anticipated the person will live. The nurse strongly recommends a plan to bring in reinforcements at the bedside. Exhaustion is a severe problem threatening the caregiver's ability to cope. Sleep is precious, and sleep deprivation can be the undoing of the home care plan. Primary caregivers must have a network to help them help the client.

Decisions regarding where the client will die and whether to initiate cardiopulmonary resuscitation must be made before this final stretch so that caregivers have clear direction and matters are not resolved by default. When the caregiver remains ambivalent about his or her comfort level in just letting the client die without calling the paramedics, conflict and crises are predictable, and the nurse is in the middle trying to respond to contradictory cries for help. The stressed family must understand that if they call 911 for emergency help from trained paramedics, they can expect aggressive resuscitative measures to be initiated. Instead, it is important to call the hospice nurse instead of 911.

Despite quality anticipatory nursing guidance, a vital component to enabling home death is the 24-hour availability of skilled professionals to call for emergency help. Many times the needed intervention is telephone counseling and recommendations, but the changeable and not always predictable condition of people near death demands emergency availability of nurses who can go to the bedside.

Death and the Immediate Aftermath

Anticipatory guidance includes helping the family to prepare a checklist of whom to call in the period immediately after death. The nurse prepares the family to comply with the legal ramifications of dying at home in their community. Sometimes police and the medical examiner must be involved. If this is so, plan ahead with these officials to reduce trauma for the family. Urge the family to choose in advance a trustworthy funeral home to provide responsible guidance through the maze of legal, social, and religious expectations at the end of life.

As family members gather for vigil at the bedside, the following specific psychosocial approaches are particularly helpful:

- Urging loved ones to say what they need to say to the dying person and assuming that hearing is possible. What is said should not demand a response.
- Encouraging reminiscence by loved ones.
- Encouraging a peaceful environment with the person surrounded by what he or she would enjoy.
- Acknowledging the ordeal of "lingering on the brink" when everyone is exhausted and ready for the death
- Exploring the unfinished business that might be preventing a person from letting go of life. People can put all of their will into surviving if there is an unresolved matter or relationship that needs closure.
- Fostering worship, prayer, and other spiritual rituals at the bedside that are consistent with client and family belief.

To demonstrate the effect palliative home care can have on a client and his or her family, the scenario for Jacob Oldfellow's death changes. He is discharged in stable condition to the home of his sister, Sarah, and her husband, with the granddaughter, Heather, helping on weekends. With family caregivers present, the home care team skilled in palliative care can make a significant change in the quality of Jacob's last days.

Although Jacob acknowledges his dependency in the presence of progressive physical deterioration, he is not able to discuss his dying directly. However, his family explores their grief and unresolved past emotional pains with the home care team. They develop problem-solving skills and mobilize a network for themselves that they had never known existed. Jacob quietly participates in several family gatherings and reminisces about old times with children, other relatives, and friends. All are astonished when he accepts a bowling buddy's offer to come and read Psalms to him. In bereavement, the family is proud of their accomplishment and all agree, "It is hard to watch Jacob passing away, but the Oldfellows are a strong family. We're tough, and we stick up for each other, even in hard times."

Jacob's symptoms require extensive anticipatory guidance to manage at home. Opioid dosage and route are continually modified with increasing abdominal pain and vomiting. The family needs extensive teaching to understand the disease process, accept the need to not force food and fluids, provide total hygiene and bedside attention when Jacob becomes bedridden, and manage his increasing restlessness and disorientation shortly before death. With the assistance of only one nursing emergency visit, the family is able to keep him comfortable without resorting to emergency hospital care. He receives high-quality, high-tech care at much lower cost than an institutional option. The key is skilled palliative home care support of a mobilized family network.

HOME CARE SYSTEM TO ENABLE DYING AT HOME

What system most effectively enables palliative home care as described? Table 18-4 contrasts the emphasis of contemporary hospice programs with the emphasis of home health programs. The hospice movement is now being mainstreamed into the existing illness care agencies, with many attending issues related to quality of care, ethics, regulations, and reimbursement. Those planning to integrate hospice concepts into home care of

Table 18-4 Hospice Contrasted with Home Health	
Hospice	**Home Health**
Primary focus on quality of life and palliation	Primary focus on rehabilitation and restoration
Focus of care on whole family; active counseling for family	Focus of care on client with family issues addressed only as they affect client care
Client and family choices governing care	Medical condition governing care chosen
Intermittent visits intensifying in frequency until death	Intermittent visits decreasing in frequency until the client is medically stable
Home care for medical crises and death if client and family choose	Hospitalization for medical crises
Nurse as case manager until client dies	Nurse as case manager during period of admission to home care
Emphasis on living in a way chosen by the client and seen as comforting	Priority on maintaining physical systems: eating, activity, vital signs, diagnostic monitoring, correction of imbalances, etc.
Expertise in managing terminal symptoms; active effort to try alternative comforting approaches	Common symptoms of terminal illness seen as inevitable and up to the physician to control
Sedatives and opioids carefully adjusted to maximize client comfort	Sedatives and narcotics used with hesitance to reduce but not eliminate suffering
Terminal course of events anticipated; crises avoided	New problems tending to be seen as medical crises, not as a normal expectation with dying
Spiritual dimension of dying as the focus of entire team	Client with religious affiliation supported by own clergy
Bereavement care for survivors	No further contact after death
Staff support process built in	Staff isolation in caring for terminally ill

the dying without actually setting up a separate hospice program should do the following:

1. Develop palliative care expertise by existing home health team members. Consider hiring a hospice or oncology clinical nurse specialist for staff training, client and family assessments, and ongoing consultation.
2. Assign caseloads so that nurses with terminal cases have more time to visit.
3. Seek supplementary resources to make individual and family counseling and spiritual care available.
4. Seek supplementary funding to permit on-call services for dying people.
5. Collaborate with community organizers interested in developing a network of trained volunteers to provide practical and emotional support before and after death.

SUMMARY

As home health care professionals develop increasing knowledge of how to provide home pal-

liative care, the limiting forces will be family and community resources. When these are shrunken and disorganized, institutionalization will be necessary before death. When there is a strong network of loved ones and when society nurtures well-funded resources to sustain the needy, the disabled, and the dying, people will be able to live their final days at home if they wish. The American public must choose to affirm quality of living at the completion of life and pay for life-affirming services. Home care nurses need to take an active role in advocating for these services and to discuss relevant issues in appropriate settings so that the public, politicians, and third-party payors are aware of the compelling need for community-based services at the end of life.

REFERENCES

Aries P: *The hour of our death,* New York, 1981, Knopf.
Baumrucker S: Management of intestinal obstruction in hospice care, *American Journal of Hospice and Palliative Care* 15(4):232-235, 1998.

Beach DL: Caregiver discourse: Perceptions of illness-related dialogue, *The Hospice Journal* 10(3):13-25, 1995.

Carter J: Can hospice care be provided to people who live alone? *Home Healthcare Nurse* 14(9):710-716, 1996.

Chandler S: Nebulized opioids to treat dyspnea, *American Journal of Hospice and Palliative Care* 16(1):418-422, 1999a.

Chandler S: Oral transmucosal fentanyl citrate: A new treatment for breakthrough pain, *American Journal of Hospice and Palliative Care* 16(2):489-491, 1999b.

Christakis N: Predicting patient survival before and after hospice enrollment, *The Hospice Journal* 13(1-2):71-87, 1998.

Crawley L et al: Palliative and end-of-life care in the African American community, *Journal of the American Medical Association* 284(19):2518-2521, 2000.

Derrickson BS: The spiritual work of the dying: A framework and case studies, *The Hospice Journal* 11(2):11-30, 1996.

Ferrell B, Coyle N: *Textbook of palliative nursing,* New York, 2001, Oxford.

Ferrell, BR, McCaffery M: Nurses' knowledge about equianalgesia and opioid dosing, *Cancer Nursing* 20(3):201-212, 1997.

Frankl V: *Man's search for meaning,* New York, 1963, Washington Square Press.

Garland T, Bass D, Otto M: The needs of hospice patients and primary caregivers, *American Journal of Hospice Care* 1(3):40-45, 1984.

Gordon K: Deterrents to access and service for blacks and Hispanics: The Medicare hospice benefit, healthcare utilization, and cultural barriers, *The Hospice Journal* 10(2):65-83, 1995.

Hanrahan P, Luchins DJ: Feasible criteria for enrolling end-stage dementia patients in home hospice care, *The Hospice Journal* 10(3):47-54, 1995.

Harper BC, Gordon AK: Report from the national task force on access to hospice care by minority groups, *The Hospice Journal* 10(2):1-10, 1995.

Kemp C: Terminal illness: *A guide to nursing care,* ed 2, Philadelphia, 1999, JB Lippincott.

Kemp C, Stepp L: Palliative care for patients with acquired immunodeficiency syndrome, *American Journal of Hospice and Palliative Care* 12(6):14-27, 1995.

Madison JL, Wilkie DJ: Family members' perceptions of cancer pain: Comparisons with patient sensory report and by patient psychologic status, *The Nursing Clinics of North America* 30(4):625-646, 1995.

March PA: Terminal restlessness, *American Journal of Hospice and Palliative Care* 15(1):51-53, 1998.

Mercadante SG: When oral morphine fails in cancer pain: The role of the alternative routes, *American Journal of Hospice and Palliative Care* 15(6):333-342, 1998.

National Hospice Organization: Medical guidelines for determining prognosis in selected non-cancer diseases, *The Hospice Journal* 11(2):47-64, 1996.

Rousseau P: Antiemetic therapy in adults with terminal disease: A brief review, *American Journal of Hospice and Palliative Care* 12(5):13-18, 1995.

Steele RG, Fitch M: Needs of family caregivers of patients receiving home hospice care for cancer, *Oncology Nursing Forum* 23(5):823-828, 1996.

Stephany T: Low-tech hospice home care for end-stage heart disease, *American Journal of Hospice and Palliative Care* 13(2):35-36, 1996a.

Stephany T: Palliative nursing care during end-stage COPD, *American Journal of Hospice and Palliative Care* 13(5):20-21, 1996b.

Stetz KM, Brown MA: Taking care: Caregiving to persons with cancer and AIDS, *Cancer Nursing* 20(1):12-22, 1997.

Vachon M: Staff stress in hospice/palliative care: A review, *Palliative Medicine* 9(2):91-122, 1995.

Weitzner M, Moody LN, McMillan SC: Symptom management issues in hospice care, *American Journal of Hospice and Palliative Care* 14(4):190-195, 1997.

Zeppetella G: The palliation of dyspnea in terminal disease, *American Journal of Hospice and Palliative Care* 15(6):322-327, 1998.

Zerwekh JV: Transcending life: The practice wisdom of hospice nursing experts, *The Hospice Journal* 10(5):26-31, 1993.

Zerwekh JV: The truth tellers: How hospice nurses help patients confront death, *American Journal of Nursing* 94(2):30-34, 1994a.

Zerwekh JV: What's new in the journals about palliative use of octreotide and high dose oxycodone? *Fanfare VIII* (2):2-3, 1994b.

Zerwekh JV: A family caregiving model for hospice nursing, *The Hospice Journal* 10(1):27-44, 1995.

Zerwekh JV: Do dying patients really need IV fluids? *American Journal of Nursing* 97(3):26-31, 1997a.

Clients
with Specific
Disorders

19 Pulmonary Compromise in Home Care

Tony Hilton, Tammy Young, Philip M. Gold, and Ronald M. Perkin

One of the most frightening experiences a nurse can encounter, whether in the hospital or home setting, is a client in respiratory distress. The nurse must use all resources available, including experience, education, skill level, technology, and outside resources. The purpose of this chapter is to provide an overview of the most common pulmonary problems a client or nurse may encounter in the home care setting. It is important to remember that pulmonary compromise may stem from the respiratory system itself or from a secondary pathological condition, such as neuromuscular, cardiac, or other systemic failure. Suggestions and guidelines will be provided for the treatment and management of pulmonary-compromised clients to ensure safe and competent care outcomes.

This chapter will review (1) accurate health history and physical assessment; (2) diagnoses and disease management, including lung disease, neuromuscular disease, spinal cord injuries, and sleep disorders; (3) resultant complications, such as pneumonia, upper respiratory infections, hypoventilation, and airway-clearance problems specific to pulmonary compromise; (4) pulmonary rehabilitation; (5) home mechanical ventilation; and (6) interdisciplinary-team functioning, ethical and legal considerations, and related case studies.

Chronic obstructive pulmonary disease (COPD) and its associated or related conditions rank fourth and pneumonia and influenza rank sixth as the leading causes of death in the United States (Marx, Majersky, Wiseman, 1998; National Center for Health Statistics, 1998). Care in the home environment encompasses the following three domains: (1) palliative care (e.g., terminal lung cancer), (2) rehabilitative and habilitative care to maintain and optimize physical condition (e.g., spinal cord lesion), and (3) transitional care with the goal of complete recovery from a reversible acute condition (e.g., bronchopulmonary dysplasia or asthma). A nurse must be familiar with the pulmonary-compromised client population and the associated technology, must understand the components of care involved, and must work toward the outcomes and goals developed by the client, family, and other members of the health care team. Management of this high-risk, high-liability population can be costly and, if inadequate, can lead to frequent readmissions to emergency departments and acute care settings. Third-party payors are alarmed by the expense of inpatient care and continuously evaluate alternative methods, such as home care, to deliver quality health care to this population. It is imperative that early intervention and disease management in the home care setting be provided with in-depth knowledge, skill, efficiency, and understanding.

HEALTH HISTORY AND PHYSICAL ASSESSMENT

The nurse must be aware of the client's past and present health and perform a comprehensive physical assessment. A thorough history, a review of medical records, and an in-depth interview with the client and family are necessary to establish a sound treatment plan. The initial history taking should include past and present pulmonary data (Table 19-1). This information includes lung and airway disorders, neuromusculoskeletal disorders, signs and symptoms of respiratory disorders, family history, allergies, immunizations, activities of daily living (ADLs), psychosocial history, past and present treatment and diagnostic procedures, nutritional history,

Table 19-1	Past and Present Pulmonary History
Historical Data	Related Conditions
Lung and airway disorders	COPD, asthma, pneumonia, chest surgery, and malignancy
Neuromusculoskeletal disorders	Amyotrophic lateral sclerosis (ALS), multiple sclerosis (MS), spinal cord injury, sleep disorders, and muscular dystrophy
Signs and symptoms of respiratory disorders	Dyspnea, shortness of breath, coughing, sputum, chest pain, wheezing, use of accessory muscles, orthopnea, tachypnea, bradypnea, cyanosis, pallor, pain, fatigue, exercise intolerance, wheezing, jugular venous distention, bronchospasm, and hypoxemia
Family history	Respiratory disorders (acute and chronic) and neuromusculoskeletal disorders
Allergies and effects	Medications, animals, pollens, and foods
Immunizations	Pneumonia, influenza, tuberculosis, respiratory syncytial virus, age and condition specific
ADLs	Exercise tolerance, self-care, mobility, sleep disturbances, snoring and positioning
Psychosocial	Tobacco, alcohol, caffeine, anxiety, adaptation, home and occupational environment, and childhood pulmonary problems
Past treatments and diagnostic procedures	Hospitalizations and emergency department visits, medications, diagnostic procedures and results, pulmonary rehabilitation, desensitization therapy, sleep study, radiology tests, blood gas analysis, pulmonary function tests (PFTs), electrocardiogram (ECG), complete blood count, blood chemistry panel, exercise stress test
Nutritional history	Fluid intake, weight loss or gain, and gastroesophageal reflux
Sexual function	Fears, concerns, previous patterns, and counseling needs
Spirituality	Belief system and religious preference

sexual function, spirituality, and most important, the client's knowledge of the disease process and home treatment program. When the initial history is taken, a physical assessment, including a review of pulmonary symptomatology, should be performed. Guidelines for obtaining a thorough physical assessment are illustrated in Table 19-2.

DIAGNOSES AND DISEASE MANAGEMENT

Chronic conditions that directly impair the respiratory system include (1) airway disease (e.g., asthma, bronchitis, bronchiectasis, bronchiolitis, and cystic fibrosis), (2) lung tissue disorders (e.g., tumors, pneumonia, emphysema, bronchopulmonary dysplasia, pulmonary fibrosis, and COPD), and (3) cardiovascular disorders (e.g., pulmonary hypertension, cardiomyopathy, and

heart failure). Conditions that impact the performance of the respiratory system and interfere with normal functioning, even though there may be no inherent pathological problem, include (1) neuromusculoskeletal disorders (e.g., Duchenne's muscular dystrophy, spina bifida, Werdnig-Hoffmann disease, Guillain-Barré syndrome, congenital myopathy, multiple sclerosis, amyotrophic lateral sclerosis, scoliosis, kyphosis, and tumors of the brain and spinal cord), (2) spinal cord dysfunction (e.g., compression, spinal cord lesions), and (3) sleep disorders (e.g., obstructive and central sleep apnea).

Table 19-3 lists the most common diagnoses and treatment options, Table 19-4 summarizes disorders of respiratory neuromuscular function, and Table 19-5 illustrates conditions that impact the performance of the respiratory system and treatment options for them.

Text continued on p. 308

Table 19-2 Physical Assessment and Pulmonary Symptoms	
Physical Assessment	Pulmonary Signs and Symptoms
Lung diseases and disorders Pulmonary evaluation 　Inspection 　Palpation 　Percussion 　Auscultation	Subjective 　Dyspnea on exertion or at rest 　Cough 　Sputum production 　Fatigue 　Anxiety 　Decreased appetite 　Chest tightness 　Ability to perform ADLs Objective 　Tachypnea or bradypnea 　Increased use of accessory muscles 　Decreased diaphragmatic excursion 　Periods of sleep apnea 　Increased anteroposterior (AP) diameter of chest 　Crackles and wheezes 　Fever 　Weight loss 　Symptoms of hypoxemia
Neuromusculoskeletal disorders 　Neurological evaluation 　　Cranial nerves 　　Sensory and motor deficits 　　Deep tendon reflexes 　　Spasticity 　　Rigidity, tremors, bradykinesia, cognition, 　　　awake state, muscle strength or weakness, 　　　and paralysis 　Language 　Mobility 　Pulmonary evaluation 　Skeletal evaluation (e.g., kyphosis 　　and scoliosis) 　Developmental evaluation	Subjective 　Increased shortness of breath 　Fatigue 　Anxiety 　Weak cough 　Decreased appetite 　Restless sleep 　Morning headaches 　Anxiety or panic Objective 　Periods of sleep apnea 　Tachypnea or bradypnea 　Cyanosis 　Increased use of accessory muscles 　Inability to expectorate secretions 　Weight loss 　Muscle wasting 　Documented sleep apnea 　Inability to be independent in self-care or physical 　　conditioning 　Atelectasis

Table 19-3	Common Conditions that Impair the Respiratory System with Treatment Options
Condition	**Treatment Option**

AIRWAY DISEASE

Condition	Treatment Option

Asthma: A lung disease characterized by airway inflammation with intermittent airway narrowing from various causes; it is usually accompanied by a wheezing sound or a dry cough during an episode of airway narrowing.	Medications
	  Bronchodilators
	  Anticholinergics
	  Corticosteroids
	  Mucolytics
	  Oxygen therapy
	Pulmonary rehabilitation

Bronchitis: A lung disease characterized by chronic cough and excess production of sputum.	Medications
	  Mucolytics and expectorants
	  Antibiotics
	  Bronchodilators
	Smoking cessation
	Pulmonary rehabilitation

Bronchiectasis: A structural distortion of the bronchial tubes caused by damage to the cartilage and muscle tissue. The damage is almost always the result of a severe lower respiratory-tract infection occurring early in life.	Medications
	  Mucolytics
	  Antibiotics
	  Oxygen therapy
	Increased fluid intake
	Pulmonary rehabilitation

Bronchiolitis: An acute or a chronic inflammatory process affecting the bronchioles.	Medications
	  Mucolytics and expectorants
	  Antibiotics
	  Bronchodilators
	Pulmonary rehabilitation

Cystic fibrosis: An inherited disorder of the exocrine glands causing those glands to produce abnormally thick secretions of mucus.	Medications
	  Antibiotics
	  Mucolytics
	  Oxygen therapy
	  Pulmonary hygiene
	Fluid and hydration management
	  Increased fluid requirement
	  High caloric needs
	Pulmonary rehabilitation
	Surgical correction: lung transplantation
	Noninvasive ventilatory support

LUNG TISSUE DISORDERS

Condition	Treatment Option
Tumors: A spontaneous new growth of tissue forming an abnormal mass that performs no physiological function and interferes with the respiratory system.	Surgical intervention Chemotherapy and radiation Palliative care

Pneumonia: An inflammation of the lungs caused by bacteria, viruses, chemical irritants, dust, and allergies.	Medications
	  Antibiotics
	  Bronchodilators
	  Oxygen therapy
	  Antipyretics

Table 19-3	Common Conditions that Impair the Respiratory System with Treatment Options—cont'd

Condition	Treatment Option
LUNG TISSUE DISORDERS—cont'd	

Emphysema: A lung disease characterized by destruction of the air sacs.	Medications
	  Bronchodilators
	  Antiinflammatory agents or corticosteroids
	  Oxygen therapy
	Pulmonary rehabilitation
	Surgical correction: lung transplantation (American Thoracic Society, 1995)

Bronchopulmonary dysplasia (BPD): A syndrome characterized by the triad of oxygen dependence, radiographic abnormalities, and respiratory symptoms that persists beyond 28 days of life in infants with respiratory failure at birth. It is now the most common chronic lung disease of infants (Hazinski, 1998).	Medications
	  Bronchodilators
	  Anticholinergics
	  Antiinflammatory agents or corticosteroids
	  Mucolytics
	  Oxygen therapy (oximetry may be required)
	  Diuretics
	  Chest physical therapy
	  Digitalis
	  Vasodilators
	  H_2 blockers
	Fluid and hydration management
	  Fluid restriction
	  Electrolytes
	  High caloric needs
	Long-term mechanical ventilation

Pulmonary fibrosis (restrictive): A disease in which small amounts of scar tissue form in the lungs, resulting in stiff lungs and inability to oxygenate.	Medications
	  Corticosteroids and other antiinflammatory drugs
	  Oxygen therapy
	Palliative care
	  Comfort measures
	  Medications to facilitate relief of shortness of breath
	Lung transplantation

Chronic obstructive pulmonary disease (obstructive): A disease process that causes decreased ability of the lungs to perform their function of ventilation. Diseases include chronic bronchitis, emphysema, chronic asthma, chronic bronchiolitis, and bronchiectasis.	Medications
	  Bronchodilators
	  Antiinflammatory agents or corticosteroids
	  Oxygen therapy
	  Diuretics
	Pulmonary rehabilitation
	Pulmonary hygiene

CARDIOVASCULAR DISORDERS	

Pulmonary hypertension: A condition in which the pulmonary vascular resistance is elevated. The cause may be known or unknown.	Medications
	  Pulmonary vasodilators
	  Vasodilators
	  Oxygen therapy
	  Anticoagulants (selected cases)
	Cardiopulmonary rehabilitation
	Lung transplantation

Continued

Table 19-3	Common Conditions that Impair the Respiratory System with Treatment Options—cont'd	
Condition	**Treatment Option**

CARDIOVASCULAR DISORDERS—cont'd

| Cardiomyopathy: A primary myocardial disease, either of specific or unknown etiology, resulting in mild to severe ventricular dysfunction. | Medications
    Cardiac drugs (dopamine [Intropin], angiotensin-converting enzyme inhibitors, and other vasodilators)
    Oxygen therapy
Cardiopulmonary rehabilitation
Fluid and nutrition management and monitoring
    Electrolyte testing
    Daily weights
Surgical intervention |
| Heart failure: An abnormality of cardiac function. Systolic heart failure occurs when the heart fails to contract normally, and diastolic heart failure occurs when the contraction is normal but the relaxation is abnormal. The most common syndrome of heart failure is caused by left ventricular systolic dysfunction. | Medications
    Cardiac drugs
    Oxygen therapy
Cardiopulmonary rehabilitation
Fluid and nutrition management
    Electrolyte testing
    Daily weights
Surgical intervention |

Table 19-4	Disorders of Respiratory Neuromuscular Function	
Level of Dysfunction	**Diagnoses**
Brainstem	Spina bifida with Arnold-Chiari malformation Encephalitis Trauma Central alveolar hypoventilation
Upper motor neuron	Spinal cord lesion
Lower motor neuron	Poliomyelitis ALS Spinal muscle atrophy
Peripheral neuron	Guillain-Barré syndrome Polyneuropathy Lupus Werdnig-Hoffmann disease
Muscle	Muscular dystrophy Congenital myopathy
Skeleton	Scoliosis or kyphosis

Table 19-5	Conditions that Impact the Performance of the Respiratory System and Their Treatment Options
Condition	Treatment Options

NEUROMUSCULAR AND SKELETAL

Condition	Treatment Options

Duchenne's muscular dystrophy: A genetic condition of males characterized by progressive muscle weakness starting generally in the lower extremities and eventually affecting the muscle tissue throughout, particularly respiratory muscles and cardiac function.	Noninvasive and invasive ventilatory support
	Pulmonary hygiene
	  Chest physiotherapy
	  Mechanical cough
	Medications
	  Oxygen therapy
	  Cardiac drugs
	Nutrition management
	  High caloric needs
	  High-fiber diet
	Bowel and bladder program
	Skin care program
	Palliative or rehabilitative care

Spina bifida: A congenital neural-tube defect characterized by a developmental anomaly in the posterior vertebral arch resulting in severe neurological dysfunction, including hydrocephalus and Arnold-Chiari malformation.	Noninvasive and invasive ventilatory support
	Pulmonary hygiene
	  Chest physiotherapy
	  Mechanical cough
	Bowel and bladder program
	Ventriculoperitoneal or ventriculoatrial shunt management
	Nutrition management
	Medications
	  Anticonvulsants
	  Antispasmodics
	  Antibiotics
	Skin care program

Werdnig-Hoffmann disease: A genetic disorder beginning in infancy or early childhood, characterized by progressive atrophy and skeletal muscle weakness.	Noninvasive and invasive ventilatory support
	Pulmonary hygiene
	  Chest physiotherapy
	  Mechanical cough
	Medications
	  Bronchodilators
	  Oxygen therapy
	Bowel and bladder program
	Skin care program
	Nutrition management
	Palliative or rehabilitative care

Guillain-Barré syndrome: A reversible idiopathic peripheral polyneuritis resulting in symmetrical pain and weakness affecting the extremities; and causing possible paralysis.	Noninvasive and invasive ventilatory support
	Pulmonary hygiene
	  Chest physiotherapy
	  Mechanical cough
	Medications: Antiinflammatory agents
	Pain management
	Bowel and bladder program
	Nutrition management
	Rehabilitative care: limited muscle-strengthening program
	Plasmapheresis

Continued

Table 19-5	Conditions that Impact the Performance of the Respiratory System and Their Treatment Options—cont'd

Condition	Treatment Options
NEUROMUSCULAR AND SKELETAL—cont'd	

ALS: A degenerative disease of the motor neurons characterized by atrophy of muscles of the hands, forearms, and legs, spreading to involve most of the body.	Noninvasive and invasive ventilatory support
	Pulmonary hygiene
	   Chest physiotherapy
	   Mechanical cough
	Medications: antispasmodics
	Pain management
	Bowel and bladder program
	Nutrition management
	   Artificial feeding devices
	   Nutritional support
	Airway protection (aspiration)
	   Artificial airway (tracheostomy)
	   Alternative communication devices
	Palliative care

Congenital myopathy: A genetic disorder beginning in infancy or early childhood characterized by progressive atrophy and skeletal muscle weakness.	Noninvasive and invasive ventilatory support
	Pulmonary hygiene
	   Chest physiotherapy
	   Mechanical cough
	Medications
	   Bronchodilators
	   Oxygen therapy
	Bowel and bladder program
	Skin care program
	Nutrition management
	Palliative or rehabilitative care

MS: A neuromuscular disorder with progressive deterioration of the nerve cells resulting in sclerotic plaques and paralysis.	Noninvasive and invasive ventilatory support
	Pulmonary hygiene
	   Chest physiotherapy
	   Mechanical cough
	Medications: Muscle relaxants and agonists
	Pain management
	Bowel and bladder program
	Nutrition management
	   Artificial feeding devices
	   Nutritional support
	Airway protection (aspiration)
	   Artificial airway (tracheostomy)
	   Alternative communication devices
	Palliative care

Scoliosis or kyphosis: Abnormal curvature of the spine resulting in cardiopulmonary dysfunction. *Scoliosis* is an abnormal right or left thoracolumbar or pelvic curvature of the spine greater than 70%. *Kyphosis* is an exaggeration of angulation of normal posterior curvature of the spine. *Kyphoscoliosis* is a lateral curvature of the spine accompanying anteroposterior hump. It may be a result of congenital anomaly, disease (tuberculosis or syphilis), malignancy, compression fracture, faulty posture, rickets, or rheumatoid arthritis.	Noninvasive and invasive ventilatory support
	Pulmonary hygiene
	   Chest physiotherapy
	   Mechanical cough
	Medications
	   Bronchodilators
	   Oxygen therapy
	Bowel and bladder program
	Skin care program
	Nutrition management
	Palliative or rehabilitative care
	Surgical correction

Table 19-5 Conditions that Impact the Performance of the Respiratory System and Their Treatment Options—cont'd

Condition	Treatment Options
SPINAL CORD DYSFUNCTION	

Compression: An abnormal and often serious condition resulting from pressure on the spinal cord (e.g., spinal fracture, vertebral dislocation, tumor, hemorrhage, and edema associated with contusion).	Relief of compression
	   Surgical correction
	   Radiation therapy
	   Traction
	Medications
	   Corticosteroids
	   Muscle relaxants and agonists
	Noninvasive and invasive ventilatory support
	Pulmonary hygiene
	   Chest physiotherapy
	   Mechanical cough
	Pain management
	Bowel and bladder program
	Nutrition management
	Palliative or rehabilitative care

Spinal cord lesion: Traumatic disruptions of the spinal cord often associated with extensive musculoskeletal involvement (e.g., spinal fractures, dislocations, and trauma).	Noninvasive and invasive ventilatory support
	Pulmonary hygiene
	   Chest physiotherapy
	   Mechanical cough
	Medications: Antispasmodics
	Pain management
	Bowel and bladder program
	Skin program
	Autonomic/vascular support
	Nutritional management
	Rehabilitative care

SLEEP DISORDERS	

Obstructive sleep apnea: A disorder characterized by physiological or structural obstruction of the airway (e.g., obesity, craniofacial abnormalities, laryngomalacia, and hypertrophic airway tissues, including tonsils and adenoids), resulting in apneic events during sleep.	Surgical correction (e.g., tonsillectomy, adenoidectomy, or tracheostomy)
	Weight management (Pickwickian or Prader-Willi syndrome)
	   Restricted caloric intake
	   Exercise regimen
	Noninvasive ventilatory support: continuous positive airway pressure (CPAP) via full-face or nasal mask

Central sleep apnea: A condition characterized by dysfunction of the respiratory center of the brainstem resulting in apneic events (e.g., Arnold-Chiari malformation, central alveolar hypoventilation, tumors, stroke, and central hypoventilation syndrome).	Noninvasive and invasive ventilatory support
	   Bilevel positive airway pressure (BiPAP) ventilation with back-up rate
	   Negative-pressure ventilation (e.g., Porta-Lung, chest cuirass, or negative extrathoracic ventilation)

PULMONARY COMPLICATIONS

Home care nurses should be familiar with the more common complications that affect the respiratory system and specific disease entities. Table 19-6 illustrates complications that may occur with common pulmonary diseases.

NURSING DIAGNOSIS

A nursing diagnosis involves identifying client problems and understanding the etiology of the disease, as well as assessing subjective and objective information to make appropriate decisions for the care of the high-technology–dependent

Table 19-6 Common Complications of Pulmonary Diseases	
Condition	Potential Complications
CHRONIC LUNG DISEASES	
Asthma	Pneumothorax
	Atelectasis
	Severe hypoxemia
	Side effects of bronchodilator therapy
	Respiratory failure (hypercapnic and hypoxemic)
Emphysema	Pneumonia
	Upper respiratory infections
	Respiratory failure or distress
	Cor pulmonale
Chronic bronchitis	Airway obstruction
	Pneumonia
	Respiratory failure
	Cor pulmonale
Bronchiectasis	Airway obstruction
	Severe hypoxemia
	Hemoptysis
	Atelectasis
	Cor pulmonale
Bronchopulmonary dysplasia	Severe hypoxemia
	Pneumonia
	Airway obstruction
	Respiratory failure
	Apnea (central and obstructive)
	Aspiration
	Pulmonary hypertension and right-sided heart failure
Cystic fibrosis	Airway obstruction
	Pneumonia
	Severe hypoxemia
	Atelectasis
	Hemoptysis
	Recurrent bronchitis
	Respiratory failure
	Cor pulmonale
Pulmonary fibrosis	Respiratory failure
	Cor pulmonale
COPD	Pneumonia
	Respiratory failure
	Cor pulmonale
	Side effects of bronchodilator therapy

patient. Collecting information includes assessing laboratory findings, implementing nursing interventions and priorities (e.g., observation, treatment, education), and evaluating outcome criteria (Jennings, 1988). The most common problems experienced by pulmonary clients include (1) ineffective breathing patterns, (2) ineffective airway clearance, (3) decreased ability to perform ADLs, (4) poor nutrition, (5) sleep-pattern disturbance, (6) dehydration related to diminished fluid volume, (7) excess fluid volume, (8) depression, (9) airway irritability,

Table 19-6 Common Complications of Pulmonary Diseases—cont'd	
Condition	Potential Complications
NEUROMUSCULOSKELETAL DISEASES	
Duchenne's muscular dystrophy	Pneumonia
	Airway obstruction (upper and lower airways)
	Atelectasis
	Upper respiratory infections
	Respiratory distress or failure
Spina bifida	Pneumonia
	Airway obstruction
	Atelectasis
	Upper respiratory infections
	Central sleep apnea
	Respiratory distress or failure
Werdnig-Hoffmann disease	Atelectasis
	Pneumonia
	Upper respiratory infections
	Airway obstruction
	Respiratory distress or failure
Guillain-Barré syndrome	Pneumonia
	Atelectasis
	Upper respiratory infections
	Respiratory distress or failure
ALS	Pneumonia
	Atelectasis
	Upper respiratory infections
	Respiratory distress or failure
SPINAL CORD DYSFUNCTION	
Compression	Pneumonia
	Atelectasis
	Respiratory distress or failure
	Upper respiratory infections
Spinal cord injury	Pneumonia
	Atelectasis
	Respiratory distress or failure
	Upper respiratory infections
SLEEP DISORDERS	
Obstructive sleep apnea	Hypoventilation
	Cor pulmonale
Central sleep apnea	Hypoventilation

(10) impaired physical mobility, (11) diminished or poor self-concept, (12) knowledge deficits, (13) impaired sexual functioning, and (14) spiritual distress. Each client is an individual, and a care plan should reflect specific client needs (Zorn, Lareau, Della Bella, 1984). The use of nursing diagnoses is demonstrated in the two case studies found in this chapter.

PULMONARY REHABILITATION PROGRAM

Pulmonary rehabilitation is defined as an art of medical practice wherein a diagnostically specific interdisciplinary program of therapy, emotional support, and education is formalized for individual clients. The goal is to stabilize or reverse both the physiopathological and psychopathological processes of the pulmonary disease and return the client to the highest possible functional capacity allowed by the pulmonary disability and overall life situation. In 1994, the National Institutes of Health consensus conference on pulmonary rehabilitation developed the following definition to describe the process: "A multidimensional continuum of services directed to persons with pulmonary disease and their families, usually by an interdisciplinary team of specialists, with the goal of achieving and maintaining the individual's maximum level of independence and functioning in the community" (Marx, Majersky, Wiseman, 1998).

The desired outcomes and goals of pulmonary rehabilitation are outlined in Box 19-1. This section will describe documented outcomes and essential components of the pulmonary rehabilitation program. Sample guidelines on the initial assessment, pursed-lip breathing, and home exercise prescription are described in the *Guidelines for Pulmonary Rehabilitation Programs* by Marx, Majersky, and Wiseman (1998).

Pulmonary rehabilitation has traditionally focused on clients with COPD; however, it can also benefit clients with other conditions, including asthma, alpha 1-antitrypsin deficiency, cystic fibrosis, interstitial lung disease, neuromuscular disease, neurological disorders, pulmonary hypertension, and lung cancer; clients undergoing lung-volume surgery and lung transplantation; clients who require ventilatory support; and clients with pediatric pulmonary disease (Marx, Majersky, Wiseman, 1998). Pulmonary rehabilitation programs function in a variety of settings, including (1) rehabilitation facilities, (2) outpatient rehabilitation programs in acute care facilities, (3) clinic settings, and (4) home care settings. A client must be physically capable of leaving his or her home to participate in the outpatient and clinic settings. Clients must have access to transportation, be physically able to endure the journey, and have insurance coverage to participate. A rehabilitation program may begin in a home care program and can transition into an outpatient pulmonary rehabilitation program (Rice, 1996). It is beneficial to work with clients in the home setting to better assess limitations, restrictions, and benefits of the treatment process. Goals remain the same regardless of the rehabilitation setting; however, a program may be modified to accommodate a client based on his or her limitations.

Box 19-1 Demonstrated Outcomes of Pulmonary Rehabilitation

Reduced hospitalizations and use of medical resources
Improved quality of life
Reduced respiratory symptoms (e.g., dyspnea)
Improved psychosocial symptoms (e.g., reversal of anxiety and depression and improved self-efficacy)
Increased patient knowledge of pulmonary disease and its management

Increased exercise tolerance and performance
Enhanced ability to perform activities of daily living
Increased survival in some patients (e.g., use of continuous oxygen in clients with severe hypoxemia)
Return to work for some patients

From Marx J, Majersky LW, Wiseman S: *Guidelines for pulmonary rehabilitation programs: American Association of Cardiovascular and Pulmonary Rehabilitation,* Champaign, Ill, 1998, United Graphics.

MEDICAL HISTORY

A 61-year-old Hispanic man with COPD presented to pulmonary rehabilitation for evaluation because of progressive shortness of breath on exertion.

He was in good health until age 51, when he noticed symptoms of breathlessness with exertion and was diagnosed with COPD and congestive heart failure. He began treatment with a beta-2 sympathomimetic metered-dose inhaler (MDI), digoxin, furosemide (Lasix), and potassium. He had a history of smoking a pack of cigarettes a day since age 13. He gradually cut down on his tobacco use to a pack of cigarettes per week and at age 60, quit completely. There was a history of occupational exposure to asbestos at age 25. He had no significant childhood illnesses, asthma, or allergies. The family history was unremarkable for pulmonary disease. He was first hospitalized at age 60 for an exacerbation of COPD with a partial arterial carbon dioxide pressure (PaCO$_2$) of 52 mm Hg and a partial arterial oxygen pressure (PaO$_2$) of 41 mm Hg on room air. His most recent pulmonary function test (PFT) revealed severe expiratory flow obstruction with marked hyperinflation of static lung volumes. Chest radiograph indicated hyperinflation and flattening of the diaphragm. He did not require mechanical ventilation or intubation. He was treated with intravenous antibiotics, corticosteroids, and theophylline, as well as respiratory care modalities. After 5 days, he was discharged on 1.5 L/min continuous oxygen therapy; prednisone 40 mg daily, tapering as directed; theophylline 300 mg by mouth 3 times a day; and albuterol MDI two puffs every 3 to 4 hours.

Most recently, the client complained of a chronic productive cough persisting since hospitalization, as well as increasing breathlessness and fatigue. He expressed concern about his change in function and described himself as depressed and anxious. He is able to walk less than a block, and he sleeps with two pillows. He continues to take the same medications with the addition of ipratropium MDI two puffs 4 times a day. He is using oxygen therapy at 3 L/min continuous. During assessment, the client showed significant signs of respiratory distress and was admitted to the medical intensive care unit (ICU), where he was intubated and placed on mechanical ventilation for treatment of respiratory failure. After 12 days, he was weaned and later was transferred out of the ICU and continued to show signs of recovery. Because of the client's increased weakness and a reduced ability to ambulate resulting in a severely deconditioned state, referral was made to a home health care agency, and arrangements were made for support after discharge.

The client would benefit from outpatient rehabilitation; however, he was unable to tolerate outpatient therapy.

CURRENT DISCHARGE ORDERS TO HOME

- *Theophylline 300 mg twice a day (xanthine/ bronchodilator for asthma, chronic bronchitis, and emphysema)*
- *Albuterol MDI two puffs every 4 hours and as needed (beta-2 agonist for bronchospasm, asthma)*
- *Ipratropium MDI two puffs every 4 hours (anticholinergic for bronchospasms associated with chronic bronchitis and emphysema)*
- *Beclomethasone MDI four puffs 4 times a day (steroid for asthma requiring chronic corticosteroid therapy)*
- *Furosemide (Lasix) 20 mg once a day (loop diuretic for edema)*
- *Potassium chloride 15 mEq once a day (electrolyte supplement)*
- *Digoxin 0.25 mg once a day (cardiac glycoside for mild to moderate heart failure)*
- *Alprazolam (Xanax) 0.25 mg once a day (benzodiazepine for anxiety with or without depression; panic disorder)*
- *Oxygen therapy 2 L/min continuous (supplement to maintain oxygen saturation)*
- *Activity as tolerated, to encourage independence*
- *Diet 2-g low-sodium diet to decrease fluid retention*
- *Fluid restriction 1200 ml/day (fluid control management)*
- *Daily weights, to monitor fluid balance*
- *Referral to home care nursing to initiate home pulmonary rehabilitation program and management of COPD (self-care management)*
- *After initial assessment was made, referral to physical therapy, occupational therapy, and social work for therapy, training, and counseling*

PULMONARY REHABILITATION EVALUATION

The client revealed he had a mild case of polio at age 5 but showed no pulmonary or neuromuscular residual. He had worked in an asbestos factory for 6 months at the age of 25. He has no allergies and no history of hypertension, cardiac disease, diabetes, or bone or joint problems.

He was born in Pennsylvania and moved to the west coast in 1963 with his family. He was married for 38 years and has four grown children who are alive and well. He worked for Boeing as an engineer for 25 years and retired this past year for health

Continued

reasons. He was current on his influenza and pneu-mococcal immunizations.

ASSESSMENT

During the initial home care evaluation, the following problems were identified:
- *Ineffective breathing and coughing techniques*
- *Poor knowledge and understanding of disease process, management, and treatment*
- *Inability to recognize and report worsening symptoms*
- *Use of elevated bed and two pillows for sleeping*
- *Poor compliance with continuous oxygen therapy*
- *Incorrect use of MDI*
- *Anxiety and panic episodes*
- *Dyspnea with all ADLs*
- *Ability to walk for only 2 minutes before complete exhaustion*
- *Deconditioned with decreased exercise tolerance*
- *Decreased strength in upper and lower extremities*
- *Lack of energy-saving and pacing skills*

Based on this assessment and identification of client problems, an interdisciplinary-team treatment plan was developed to achieve the following client outcomes (Table 19-7):
- *Optimized and stabilized pulmonary status at maximum level of function*
- *Basic understanding of the disease process, complications, risks, symptomatology of exacerbations, and treatment (Meyers, 1997)*
- *Understanding of medications, including proper use, side effects, and actions*
- *Ability to recognize and report worsening symptomatology early in an exacerbation to avoid acute care intervention*
- *Increase in exercise and tolerance of ADLs*
- *Ability to control dyspnea through correct use of breathing techniques in coordination with ADLs*
- *Ability to pace activities*
- *Ability to mobilize secretions effectively*
- *Ability to control panic attacks and episodes of anxiety*
- *Improved compliance with oxygen therapy*

Table 19-7	Nursing Care Plan	
Client Problem	Nursing Intervention	Desired Outcomes
Ineffective breathing pattern	Administer pharmacological agents. Teach pursed-lip breathing. Teach energy-conservation techniques. Reteach relaxation techniques.	Observable improvement in dyspnea, fatigue, anxiety Improvement in respiratory rate and rhythm and exercise tolerance; increase in oxygen saturation Ability to perform breathing exercises and relaxation therapy
Ineffective airway clearance	Perform chest physiotherapy and coughing. Encourage use of positive expiratory pressure therapy. Administer humidifying agents, including aerosolized bronchodilators and mucolytics. Teach fluid hydration. Teach symptomatology of infection and bronchospasm.	Decreased symptoms of dyspnea, cough, and sputum production Improvement in sputum mobilization; decrease in wheezing and rales Early recognition of signs and symptoms of respiratory infection and intervention Maintenance of adequate hydration Ability to perform pulmonary hygiene techniques

Table 19-7	Nursing Care Plan—cont'd	
Client Problem	Nursing Intervention	Desired Outcomes
Decreased ability to perform ADLs	Administer oxygen therapy as ordered. Maximize pharmacological treatment program as ordered (e.g., bronchodilators). Provide muscle strengthening and conditioning exercises as tolerated. Provide adaptive equipment (e.g., tub bench, shower, hose). Instruct in energy-conservation techniques. Teach pacing of activities and work simplification.	Decreased fatigue and dyspnea with ADLs; oxygen use as ordered Independence in self-care Improvement in physical conditioning and exercise tolerance Energy-conservation and work-simplification techniques
Poor nutrition	Plan more frequent, smaller meals to facilitate less difficulty with work of eating and indigestion. Arrange medication or treatment program so that optimal bronchodilation is facilitated at meal times. Avoid large meals at bedtime. Review elements of balanced diet and proper nutrition.	Maintenance of recommended weight, caloric, and nutrient intake Daily weights to determine fluid balance Decrease in complaints of shortness of breath during and after meals and during sleep Identification of signs and symptoms of poor nutrition
Depression and anxiety	Assist client in setting up a structured daily schedule of activities. Spend time with client reviewing his assets and building on them. Assist client in identifying long- and short-term realistic, achievable goals. Teach signs and symptoms of depression and treatment.	Identification of signs and symptoms of depression and the relationship to dependent behavior Knowledge of physical limitations of the disease process but recognition of personal assets Conversation that reflects feelings of self-reliance and self-worth Organized social interaction
Impaired sexual functioning	Optimize scheduling medications to allow for maximum bronchodilation during sexual activity. Teach client to plan for sexual activity. Teach energy-conservation techniques for sexual activity, including planning and recommended positioning. Recommend medication changes of agents contributing to sexual dysfunction. Explore alternate methods of sexual enjoyment and expression.	Subjective improvement of sexual function Ways to reschedule medication and treatment program to maximize benefit of sexual activity Identification of certain drugs as potential source of problems contributing to sexual dysfunction Satisfaction in sexual relationship
Spiritual distress	Refer client to chaplain, clergy, or other religious representative as requested. Provide privacy for worship. Support discussion on spiritual concerns. Inform staff of client's religious preferences.	Verbalization of concern about resolving issues in belief system exacerbated by present illness or suffering Seeking of assistance in resolving spiritual crisis Achievement of a new or higher level of resolution through present crisis Verbalization that faith is clarified, reaffirmed, and strengthened, yielding a more effective resource for the client

HOME MECHANICAL VENTILATION PROGRAM

Mechanical ventilation developed in ICUs in the 1960s for acute life-threatening illnesses. The treatment of chronic disease was expensive. The need to justify major expenditures had stimulated greater interest in outcome studies (Tarlov et al, 1989; Wenberg, 1990). In the late 1970s, this technology moved to the home setting for the treatment of chronic respiratory failure. Home mechanical ventilation (HMV) became an important option for the long-term management of clients (Gilmartin, 1991). Although many clients were housed in long-term care facilities, many were also discharged to the home setting.

However, in the 1980s, when diagnostic related groups (DRGs) came into effect and the technology was made available for home care, the majority of acute care hospitals explored HMV programs. To set up a standard of care for HMV programs, a group of professionals developed guidelines for health care providers to use in preparing the client for home care (O'Donohue et al, 1986).

The literature continued to focus primarily on the cost effectiveness of HMV for invasive ventilation (Rosen, Bone, 1988). The trends for use of noninvasive ventilation (tank, cuirass, mouthpiece, and rocking beds) moved to invasive ventilation (endotracheal and tracheostomy tubes) (Rosen, Bone, 1988). Traditional outcome studies have focused on morbidity and mortality; however, increased interest has been in the quality-of-life issues in the home setting (Testa, Simonson, 1996). Numerous studies show that HMV is beneficial in relation to morbidity and mortality in clients with chronic respiratory failure and that it is cost effective when compared with long-term institutional care (Moss, 1996; Plummer, O'Donohue, Petty, 1989). There are currently over 14,000 clients who require ventilator management in the home setting in the United States alone (Sevick, Braham, 1997).

The programs in use across the United States consistently use an interdisciplinary-team approach from hospital to home care (Sevick, Braham, 1997). The team members may include physicians, nurses and respiratory therapists, and additional professionals, including physical, occupational, and speech therapists; social workers; and insurance case managers. The primary focus is to move the client from an acute care hospital to a less expensive level of care, such as the home setting (Capen, Dedlow, 1998). Clients are screened for potential candidacy in HMV programs. Outcomes focus on maintaining successful home care and reducing readmission rates, as well as improving quality of life for the client and family.

The remainder of this section focuses on several aspects of an HMV program, including noninvasive and invasive ventilation, advantages and disadvantages of HMV, the home environment, the definition of caregiver competence, home equipment and supplies, and emergency breathing techniques.

Noninvasive Ventilation

A new generation of ventilators may be used in the home. These deliver BiPAP and CPAP by nasal or face mask for clients with obstructive sleep apnea, central sleep apnea, chronic lung diseases, neuromuscular diseases, and numerous other chronic respiratory problems (Abou-Shala, Meduri, 1996; Simonds, Elliott, 1991). This modality of care is particularly attractive to clients and families, managed care providers, and health care professionals because of the significant clinical and economic advantages, including (1) shortened length of hospital stay; (2) lower costs for BiPAP and CPAP compared to conventional technology; (3) ease of learning and maintaining the technology by clients and families; (4) increased comfort to the client, thereby improving the quality of life for the client and caregiver; and (5) avoidance of tracheostomy tubes.

Invasive Ventilation

Invasive ventilation is defined as ventilatory support provided through an artificial airway, most commonly in a tracheostomy tube. Ventilation is initiated in the ICU setting and transitioned into the home-care setting or alternative sites. Charges for care in an ICU, basic-care unit, or home or subacute setting are remarkably high. Average charges for ICU care are approximately $100,000 per month; basic care is $60,000 per month; skilled-nursing facility and subacute care range from $12,000 to $15,000 a month; and home care ranges from $3,000 to $35,000 per month, depending on the number of hours of nursing and licensed vocational nurse (LVN) or licensed practical nurse (LPN) versus registered nurse (RN) care. Nursing care in the home represents the highest cost factor (Hilton et al, 1993; Sevick, Braham, 1997).

Clients are selected for the HMV program based on the following criteria: (1) diagnosis of chronic respiratory failure, (2) client and caregiver compliance with treatment regimen, (3) reasonably good prognosis for improvement, (4) availability of community support systems, and (5) funding to provide care in the home setting (O'Donohue et al, 1986). Client selection is always ethically difficult and is the most crucial factor in the success of HMV. Most programs exclude long-term ventilation to severely neurologically impaired clients. A checklist is useful in assisting the coordinator in enrolling a new client in an HMV program. It is also important to obtain a caregiver-team program agreement.

A client must meet the following criteria to enter the program:
- Interest in and willingness to participate in the program
- Need for ventilatory assistance for at least 8 hours a day (fractional inspired oxygen concentration [FiO$_2$] <40%, positive end expiratory pressure [PEEP] 0 or <5 cm/H$_2$O)
- Medical stability on ventilator
- Financial resources to support medical care at home
- Suitable home environment
- Access to professional and community resources, such as physicians, health care providers, home health agency, durable medical equipment providers, and pharmacists who are competent in this level of care (American Association of Respiratory Care, 1995)

In addition, the primary caregiver (usually a family member) has the following responsibilities:
- Participating in and assuming responsibility for client care
- Maintaining or obtaining financial resources to support the client at home
- Participating in all teaching sessions and conferences as scheduled
- Communicating effectively with the team

Advantages

- Clients are in their own home environment, with potential for improved quality of life.
- Clients have more control of their lives, rather than being confined to a regimented system in an institution or hospital setting.

- Clients have potential for medical improvement.
- Respite care (8 to 16 hours a day, 7 days a week) may be available to help relieve caregiver burden.
- Costs for home care are reimbursed by most third-party payors as a covered benefit.
- Clients have the potential for a longer life to share with significant others.
- Maximal developmental potential for children is at home.

Disadvantages

- Home and respite care are perceived by some families as an invasion of privacy and loss of control.
- Emergency medical care is not readily available as in the acute care setting
- Caregiver burden is a significant problem that, in many cases, leads to burnout and family dysfunction.
- Costs of care not covered by insurance may affect a family's financial status.
- Quality of home care nursing and respite care is often inconsistent.

The goals of long-term ventilation are to (1) extend life, (2) enhance quality of life, (3) provide an environment that will enhance the potential for medical improvement, (4) reduce morbidity, (5) improve physiological function, and (6) be cost effective (O'Donohue et al, 1986). In rare cases, the goal for long-term ventilation as per client or caregiver request is to provide palliative care in the home setting in a hospice approach. Team members evaluate and develop a specific plan of care individually and in conjunction with each member to achieve the goals for HMV. The most recent guidelines developed for the HMV program are the American Association of Respiratory Care Clinical Practice Guidelines (1995). Noninvasive ventilation programs follow the same guidelines for the home care setting (Leger et al, 1989, 1994).

Home Environment

It is crucial that the home environment is safe and capable of supporting the client and family requiring home ventilation. This includes working electricity, heating and cooling systems, and gas; clean running water; and telephone and emergency services (e.g., fire department and emergency medical services). The home utility service systems are notified before a client's entry into the community, and requests are made for priority of services in the event of a disaster that may be life threatening.

It is very important that HMV health care providers determine home safety before discharge by completing a home evaluation. Factors evaluated include (1) size and number of rooms in the home; (2) entry and exit access for safety of client and equipment mobility; (3) electrical systems, including number of grounded outlets; and (4) availability and working order of kitchen and bathrooms.

Caregiver Competence

The following categories of safety are required to manage a client in the home setting, including (1) caregiver competence, (2) the medical stability of the client, and (3) a safe home environment. The competence of clients, family caregivers, and health care providers is a requirement before discharge to the home setting, and maintaining competent and compliant care in the home environment is necessary to achieve successful outcomes (Abou-Shala, Meduri, 1996). Documentation is required to demonstrate competence of both the family caregivers and home care nurses. Most clients are managed by a family member as the primary caregiver and have 8 to 16 hours a day of nursing (RN, LVN, or LPN) in the home, generally night shift and day shift. Other health care providers participating in the management of care include RNs, respiratory therapists, physical therapists, occupational therapists, speech therapists, dietitians, clinical psychologists, and social workers. All caregivers are required to be competent in the care needs of the client (Gold et al, 1989).

Home Equipment and Supplies

The following section describes the most common equipment and supplies needed for a client in the home setting, including ventilator equipment and supplies, airway equipment and supplies, pulmonary hygiene, monitoring devices, mobility equipment, and ADL equipment. There are multiple home-care products from which to choose, and the final decision will depend on the client's specific needs, the physician's and team members' personal preferences, specific types of technology available in the community, and equipment appropriate for the home environment.

Ventilators used in the home environment may be used invasively and noninvasively. In most cases, clients who require full-time ventilation use invasive positive-pressure ventilators. However, either negative or positive devices can be used for invasive or noninvasive ventilation. The current trend and client preference, when possible, is to use noninvasive ventilatory devices for nocturnal ventilation, thereby avoiding tracheostomy tubes and the complications and risks involved. The criteria used to determine if the client is a candidate for noninvasive bilevel ventilation include (1) the ability to breathe spontaneously and use the device to augment ventilation, (2) the ability to mobilize secretions effectively, and (3) the ability to effectively maintain normal respiratory function as evidenced by stable blood gases, normal sleep patterns, and adequate energy level. There is also a trend to transition clients from invasive to noninvasive ventilation if a client can tolerate decannulation and can be effectively ventilated via nasal or face mask. An additional trend is to wean clients from mechanical ventilation in the home setting rather than in the institutional setting, which may result in improved clinical outcomes and increased cost effectiveness (Plummer, O'Donohue, Petty, 1989; Rothkopf, Askanazi, 1992).

The most common complications encountered in the home care setting depend largely on the type of ventilatory support provided. For example, complications associated with invasive ventilators relate to airway obstruction (e.g., mucous plugs), accidental disconnections, or alarm failure. Accidental disconnections are the most common cause of death in the stable ventilator client (Gilgoff et al, 1988). In the case of noninvasive ventilation, common problems include skin breakdown (e.g., over nasal bridge), sinus congestion, alarm failures, and power-source limitations.

Positive-pressure ventilators LP-6 and LP-10 ventilators are commonly used for clients who require positive-pressure ventilation with tidal volumes of 100 to 2200 cc and respiratory rates of 1 to 38 bpm (Fig. 19-1). The PLV-100 and PLV-102 ventilators have volumes that can be set digitally between 50 and 3000 cc, with the respiratory rates between 2 and 40 bpm, which enable this equipment to be used for pediatric clients (Fig. 19-2). These ventilators require external

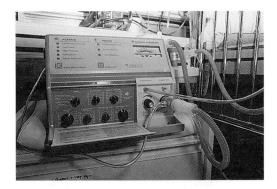

Fig. 19-1   LP-10 ventilator.

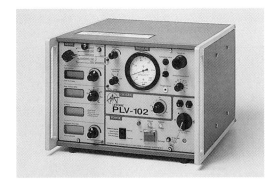

Fig. 19-2   PLV-100 ventilator.

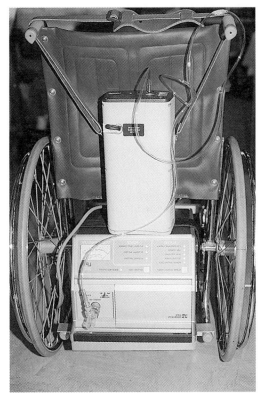

Fig. 19-3   LP-10 ventilator mounted on a wheelchair with liquid oxygen.

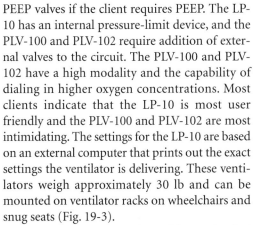

PEEP valves if the client requires PEEP. The LP-10 has an internal pressure-limit device, and the PLV-100 and PLV-102 require addition of external valves to the circuit. The PLV-100 and PLV-102 have a high modality and the capability of dialing in higher oxygen concentrations. Most clients indicate that the LP-10 is most user friendly and the PLV-100 and PLV-102 are most intimidating. The settings for the LP-10 are based on an external computer that prints out the exact settings the ventilator is delivering. These ventilators weigh approximately 30 lb and can be mounted on ventilator racks on wheelchairs and snug seats (Fig. 19-3).

The most common mode used for mechanical ventilation is assist control so that clients may initiate a breath if desired. The synchronized intermittent mandatory ventilation mode is not advised on the LP-10, PLV-100, or PLV-102 because the work of breathing is dramatically increased compared with the use of acute care ventilators. The newest generation of ventilators,

such as the LTV-1000 or Achieva ventilators, can deliver intensive care capability in the home environment. In most cases, weaning is accomplished by "sprinting" clients off the ventilator using a "T-piece" device starting at 5- to 10-minute intervals and gradually increasing to the client's tolerance while documenting effective ventilation (stable parameters such as blood gas levels, oxygen saturation level, and carbon dioxide level). Other criteria used to indicate a client's tolerance for successful sprinting include good skin color, maintenance of energy level, absence of fatigue and drowsiness related to increased work of breathing, and baseline mental status.

Airway leaks can result in hypoventilation. The source of the leak could be nasal, oral, or stomal. Therefore knowing where and when the leak occurs is important to the method to correct the problem. Methods to manage airway leaks include (1) increasing tidal volume to compensate for the leak to maintain acceptable peak inspiratory pressures with added pressure limit for

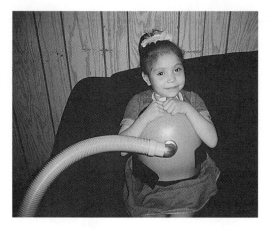

Fig. 19-4   Chest cuirass.

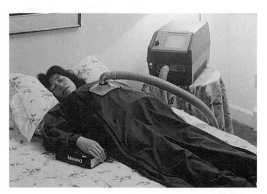

Fig. 19-6   Nu-Mo suit.

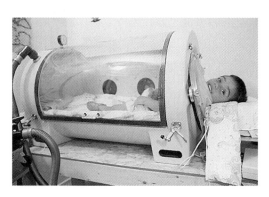

Fig. 19-5   Porta-Lung.

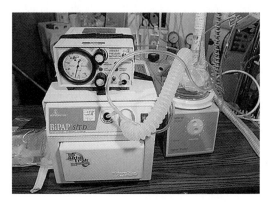

Fig. 19-7   Respironics BiPAP ST/D-20.

safety, (2) increasing the site of the tracheostomy tube, (3) using a chin strap or jaw bra for nasal and oral leaks, (4) changing nocturnal ventilator settings to compensate for leaks occurring primarily at night with added pressure limit (undesirable), and (5) using cuffed tubes (least desirable) (Mason, 1993).

Negative-pressure ventilators   In the early 1950s, negative-pressure ventilators, such as the chest cuirass (Fig. 19-4), Porta-Lung (Fig. 19-5), and Nu-Mo suit (Fig. 19-6) were devices used for respiratory failure, primarily for polio victims. However, these devices have been redesigned today for clients requiring noninvasive ventilation and particularly those with neuromuscular disease (Oppenheimer, Myers, 1993). The primary characteristic of these devices is that the torso is covered and a pump creates a negative extrathoracic pressure. This forces the chest cavity to en-

large, resulting in inspiration. Clients are fitted with a specific device based on the shape and size of the chest, torso, and body. These devices are used primarily for clients who do not have tracheostomy tubes or cannot tolerate nasal or facial mask. Limitations include the fact that clients' positioning during sleep throughout the night can contribute to skin breakdown (e.g., Porta-Lung), the devices are not easily portable, and they possess no external battery power source or alarm system.

Noninvasive ventilators   Common CPAP devices include the Quantum, Virtuoso, Good-Knight, Remstar, BiPAP ST/D-20 (Fig. 19-7), Bi-PAP ST, VPAP, and Puritan-Bennett 300 and 335. CPAP is indicated for clients who require such support because of obstructive sleep apnea and craniofacial disorders (Simonds, Elliot, 1991; Teague, Fortenberry, 1995) (Box 19-2).

Box 19-2   List of Equipment and Supplies for Noninvasive Ventilation

BiPAP STD-20 with auto track
Circuits (2) (reusable)
Airway pressure monitor (1)
Humidifier (Oasis/Fischer & Paykel)
Mask/interface
External battery
Battery recharger

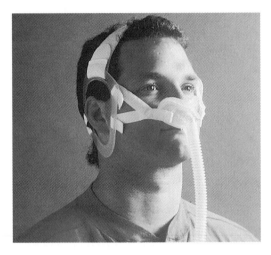

Fig. 19-8   Nasal mask.

Some bilevel devices are the BiPAP, ST/D, VPAP, and Puritan-Bennett 335. Indications for use of bilevel devices are (1) intolerance to CPAP, (2) required back-up rate (e.g., central sleep apnea or respiratory muscle fatigue), (3) increased comfort with pressure ventilation rather than volume ventilation, (4) client ability to support his or her own breathing, (5) potential to be weaned from ventilator, and (6) client requirement of continuous flow. Bilevel noninvasive ventilation has proved particularly beneficial for clients with bronchopulmonary dysplasia (BPD), COPD, and neuromuscular and skeletal disorders (Leger et al, 1994).

Bilevel devices are used in conjunction with individualized mask and circuit supplies. Different manufacturers have developed numerous types of nasal and facial masks. The masks come in a variety of sizes, can be disposable or reusable, can be custom made, and can be latex free (Fig. 19-8). The success or failure of noninvasive ven-

tilation is contingent on client compliance, a correctly fitting mask, and proper use of the noninvasive device (MacIntyre, 1997).

Table 19-8 summarizes the modes of ventilatory devices and common products used in the home environment. Volume ventilators, such as the LP-10 and PLV-100, are rarely used noninvasively via masks. Pressure-support ventilators, such as the BiPAP ST/D-20, may be used invasively.

Emergency breathing   Glossopharyngeal breathing (GPB), also called *frog breathing,* and neck breathing enable clients to learn breathing techniques for emergency purposes or to sprint off the ventilator. Clients who require full-time ventilation should be evaluated and, if possible, trained for emergency breathing techniques in case there is an accidental disconnection. Clients who have learned to use GPB or neck breathing have an increased sense of security in the event of ventilator failure. It also facilitates personal care such as showering, transfer, tracheostomy tube changes, and circuit changes, if the client can tolerate this type of breathing technique (Bach et al, 1987; Gilgoff et al, 1988).

Airway equipment and supplies   A variety of airway equipment and supplies are required for clients who use ventilators invasively or noninvasively. Equipment includes tracheostomy tubes, tracheostomy dressings, suction machines (alternating current [AC] and alternating current/direct current [AC/DC]), suction catheters, hand resuscitators, and speaking devices.

Tracheostomy tubes   A variety of tracheostomy tubes are available (Fig. 19-9). They fall into the following categories: (1) stainless steel metal tubes, (2) silicone tubes, (3) cuffed and uncuffed tubes, (4) fenestrated tubes, (5) disposable inner cannulas, and (6) custom tubes. Pediatric tracheostomy tubes are uncuffed and range in size from neonatal 0 to pediatric size 5. It is best that all pediatric and adult clients use uncuffed tracheostomy tubes at home to prevent compromise of tracheal-wall integrity and to enhance the ability of clients to vocalize. A principal exception is the client with ALS who has developed vocal-cord paralysis and loss of neck muscle function and is at risk of aspiration. When uncuffed tubes are used, the ventilator should be pressure limited, and the tidal volume should be increased to compensate for air leaks. Fenestrated tubes are rarely used in the home environment on a long-term

Table 19-8 Ventilatory Devices	
Mode	Product
Positive-pressure ventilation/volume *(used invasively)*	LP-6, LP-10, PLV-100, PLV-102
Negative-pressure ventilation *(used noninvasively)*	Chest cuirass, Porta-Lung, Nu-Mo suit, NEV-100 extrathoracic ventilator
Pressure-support ventilation *(used noninvasively)*	BiPAP (ST, ST/D, Duet LX), CPAP (Quantum, Puritan-Bennett 335)
Volume/pressure ventilation *(used invasively and noninvasively)*	LTV900, LTV950, or LTV1000 (Pulmonetic Systems) Achieva (Mallinckrodt)

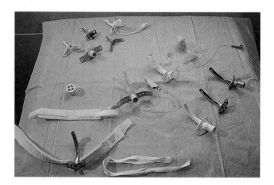

Fig. 19-9   Tracheostomy tubes.

basis, since tissue can grow into the fenestration, causing airway damage and bleeding, resulting in surgical intervention. Some clients require a custom tracheostomy tube when standard tubes are not suitable because of obesity, tracheomalacia, or unusual neck and tracheal anatomy. Ear, nose and throat (ENT) specialists will measure the client for a custom device. The manufacturer will make the tube based on client specifications. Cleaning and reusing tracheostomy tubes, inner cannulas, and other supplies help decrease the cost of care.

Tracheostomy dressings   Most clients use some type of dressing around the tracheostomy stoma to keep the stoma dry and to prevent skin irritation. Dressings are available in precut and foam and come in a variety of sizes. Gauze dressings are not recommended because of the risk of abscess or infection caused by microfibers. Tracheostomy tube ties are also available in a variety of sizes and materials such as drawstrings, foam,

Velcro, or padding. Some clients are very creative in designing their own collars for comfort, ease of use, and attractiveness. Tracheostomy tube ties and collars can be washed and reused. It is vital that the tracheostomy tube be secure to reduce potential for disconnection or extubation.

Commercial disposable tracheostomy cleaning kits are available, or the client may only need components of the kit that may be purchased separately. Kits include brushes, ties, solution containers, gauze, and gloves. It is usually more cost effective to use separate components, since these can be washed and reused. Tracheostomy care procedures can be found in any client education manual or in a home care agency's policy and procedure manual (Gold et al, 1989).

Suction catheters and machines   Clients should have a minimum of three methods of suctioning available in the home setting. They should include (1) an AC suction machine, which remains at the bedside; (2) an AC/DC suction machine (Fig. 19-10), which is kept in the client's travel bag and used for transport, and (3) the DeLee suction device, used when a power source is not available.

There are a variety of suction catheters available, from size 6 to 14. The internal diameter of the tracheostomy tube and the external diameter of the suction catheter usually determine the size of the catheter. To prevent complete airway occlusion while suctioning, the suction catheter should not exceed half the size of the internal diameter of the tracheostomy tube. It is helpful to use clear suction catheters to observe the consistency, color, and amount of secretions.

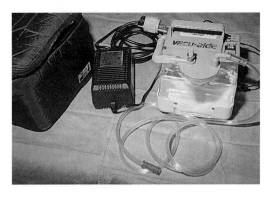

Fig. 19-10   AC/DC suction machine and airway accessories.

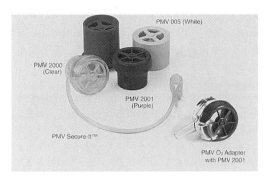

Fig. 19-11   Passy-Muir tracheostomy and speaking valve.

Practice standards require that equipment and accessories be kept clean according to manufacturer's guidelines and infection-control protocols. Clients tend to colonize their own bacteria found in the home environment, and unless they require frequent admission to the acute care facility, they are not exposed to nosocomial infections (methicillin-resistant *Staphylococcus aureus* [MRSA]/vancomycin-resistant *Enterococcus* [VRE]). There is a limited number of caregivers in the home environment. Therefore the chances of acquiring infections are reduced. Routine cleaning of equipment and accessories reduces infection rates.

There are a variety of ways to clean and reuse airway care supplies and ventilator accessories. For example, suction kits are available, or supplies may be obtained separately. Most kits include a suction catheter, gloves, and a box for the solution. The choice of whether to use a kit or individual supplies depends on individual client and caregiver needs and financial resources. The most common cleaning solutions are mild soap and water, vinegar and water, or Control III solution. Boiling of equipment and accessories is an option based on durability of material.

Hand resuscitators   A variety of types, sizes, and complexity of hand resuscitators are available. Selection depends on the client's specific medical needs. In the home care setting, the most basic type of hand resuscitator is used for the purpose of hyperinflating the lungs during procedures, both nonemergency and emergency ventilation. All hand resuscitators should have the capability of adding oxygen in-line in the event the client is oxygen dependent or during an emergency. The size of the bag will depend on the age, weight, and lung compliance of the client. Primary and back-up hand resuscitators, adapters (tracheostomy tube), and interfaces (masks) must be available at all times in the event the client requires ventilation. Hand resuscitators should be cleaned and reused.

Speaking devices   Speaking devices have become commonplace in the home care environment. The most common type is the Passy-Muir speaking valve (Fig. 19-11). These devices are lightweight, one-way valves directly attached to the tracheostomy tube or placed in-line in the ventilator circuit. To use speaking valves, a client must (1) be awake and responsive, (2) be medically stable, (3) be able to tolerate an uncuffed tube, (4) be able to mobilize secretions, and (5) have upper airway patency. The valve should be maintained, cleaned, and reused. Secretions from the tracheostomy should be cleared to avoid obstruction of the valve and upper airway. Use is recommended during waking hours. The speaking valve should not be worn continuously. Advantages of using a speaking valve include (1) improved coordination of swallowing and vocalizing, (2) increased airway protection against aspiration pneumonia, and (3) natural humidifying and filtering device.

Pulmonary hygiene devices   There are two devices that are frequently used in the home care setting when conventional pulmonary hygiene treatments, such as chest physiotherapy and suctioning, are not effective in mobilizing secretions and preventing chronic atelectasis. These include intrapulmonary percussive ventilation (IPV) and the inexsufflator (Fig. 19-12). IPV combines aerosol therapy with intraairway positive-pressure and chest physiotherapy (Birnkrant et al, 1996). It delivers high-flow minibursts of air to the lungs at rates of 100 to 300 times per minute. Each treatment lasts about 15 minutes and is administered three or four times a day. The IPV is used primarily in conjunction with nebulizer treatments, whereas the inexsufflator is strictly a cough device. IPV is generally ordered in combination with bronchodilators, steroids, and normal saline to total 15 cc volume and is prescribed up to four times a day as necessary.

The inexsufflator assists clients in clearing retained bronchopulmonary secretions by gradually applying a positive pressure to the airway, then rapidly shifting to negative pressure. This rapid shift in pressure via a mask or tracheostomy produces a high expiratory flow rate from the lungs, stimulating a cough (Bach, 1993, 1995). Inexsufflator treatments are used by setting inspiratory and expiratory pressures appropriate to the client's age, size, and weight. Expiratory pressures are generally 10 cm H_2O higher than inspiratory pressures to facilitate an effective cough. Treatments are given in four to five cycles per treatment, four times a day and as needed. Inexsufflator treatments can be given by face mask or by tracheostomy tube.

Monitoring devices Monitoring devices are essential in establishing the safety and treatment of client care in the home setting. These devices include pulse oximeters, capnography monitors, apnea monitors, and pressure-alarm monitors. Pulse oximeters are used to trend oxygen saturation, and capnography monitors are used to trend carbon dioxide levels noninvasively. These devices are also used to trend, document, evaluate, and facilitate the appropriate plan of care. Noninvasive monitoring devices are used exclusively for establishing trends, and clients must be assessed before initiating a change in treatment plans. Most pulse oximeters have the ability to measure heart rate as well and are useful when a life-threatening cardiac event occurs and requires immediate action. Some monitors have the capability of downloading data to a computer for interpretation.

Airway-pressure monitors are used as back-up alarm systems for the internal ventilator alarms or in the absence of ventilator alarms. They indicate that a client has been disconnected from the ventilator or that pressure is low as a result of decreased volume. It is imperative that pressure alarms be used for all clients who require HMV and who are totally dependent on life-support equipment.

Apnea monitors are used to detect when a client has temporarily or permanently suspended breathing. They may also serve as back-up alarm systems in the event of ventilator failure, internal alarm failure, or accidental disconnection. Apnea-monitor data can be downloaded to retrieve information about the characteristics of previous events.

Rehabilitation equipment Rehabilitation equipment is used primarily to increase independence and to provide comfort, ease, and safety for clients and caregivers. Such equipment includes bathing devices (e.g., EZ-Bathe), hospital beds and specialty mattresses, bedside commodes, bath chairs, mouth sticks, eye-gaze–activated and voice-activated computers, and environmental-control units. A client mechanical lift is imperative when transferring adult-sized immobile clients. In most cases, a specialized sling with head and neck support is required for ventilator-dependent clients.

Mobility For clients to be transported, various devices, including power or manual wheelchairs, are helpful. These are usually custom-made to accommodate the client's size and equipment. Infants use snug seats, which are custom-made.

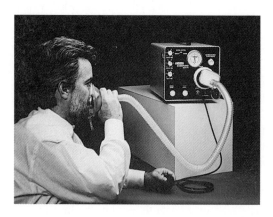

Fig. 19-12 Intrapulmonary percussive ventilator.

Clients should be evaluated for appropriate seating, since most of their day is spent sitting in a chair. Vehicle transportation is based on the client's wheelchair and equipment needs. A customized van designed to transport clients to school, work, clinic, and other outings is ideal. It is not uncommon for the ceiling of the van to be raised or the floor to be lowered to accommodate a wheelchair and a hydraulic-lift system. It is advisable to have portable ramps for access to buildings that are not handicap accessible. Multiple sources of transportation, including nonmedical emergency transport, city bus, school bus, or taxi, can be explored. If the client is a child, special principles and car-seat safety laws must be ensured if a car is the method of transportation. Safety issues include securing the client with restraints in the appropriate car or snug seat and securing equipment, such as the ventilator and oxygen tanks, next to the child. It is imperative that clients have a travel or "go bag" available at all times. The travel bag should include an AC/DC suction machine, a DeLee suction device, a hand resuscitator, extra tracheostomy tubes and dressings, suction catheters, gloves, and saline for lavage. Other items, such as feeding tubes, urinary catheters, enteral supplies, and medications, can be included in the travel bag.

Collaborative services Multiple ancillary services including intravenous therapy (e.g., central lines, peripherally inserted central catheters [PICC lines], Port-a-Caths) and diagnostic testing (laboratory and radiology), can benefit technology-dependent clients in the home. These services may be helpful in assessing early development of problems, allowing for prompt intervention. These services allow clients to remain in the home setting and can be timesaving and cost effective. Physicians can use this information to determine whether treatment can be accomplished in the home or whether clients need to be admitted to the acute care setting for complicated medical management.

Periodic evaluation HMV providers are beginning to realize the benefits of having periodic evaluations to determine if the client's current treatment plan is appropriate and effective. This may include an overnight stay in the acute care setting to revise and update the current treatment plan. A bronchoscopy may be performed to evaluate upper and lower airways for granulation, ob-

struction, tracheostomy tube sizing, and malacia. Chest radiographs are obtained to determine atelectasis and tracheostomy tube placement. Ventilation is evaluated by measuring end tidal carbon dioxide and oxygen saturation levels during the day and night. Ventilator settings are adjusted at night to maintain the patient's carbon dioxide range that was trended during the day. Blood gases are obtained to compare carbon dioxide levels. Evaluations by the dietitian, rehabilitation specialist, physical therapist, speech therapist, occupational therapist, child-life specialist, and social worker are obtained to update and revise the plan of care. The younger the client, the greater the need for frequent evaluations (e.g., age newborn to 3 years-every 6 months and as necessary; age 4 to 18 years-annually and as necessary; adults-every 1 to 2 years and as necessary).

Technological capacity does not ensure or equate with benefit to clients or their families. Health care professionals and families are obligated to make difficult choices in the care of ventilator-dependent clients. Survivability and available technology should not be the only criteria by which the choice for long-term ventilatory support is made.

A decision to provide long-term ventilation in the home must be based on adequate and thorough information provided to clients and families. Once the information is provided and understood, a decision based on the collective best interests of client and family should be sought. The decision must weigh benefits and burdens primarily to the client, but also to the family members. Investigation of the family's ability to provide the environment, as well as the many duties required of technology-dependent clients, must be conducted. This investigation is concerned with psychological, social, or cultural barriers to effective care.

The client's general condition, including associated handicaps and other medical problems, and ability to participate in social and academic activities need to be weighed in the light of the natural history of the disease process to decide about benefits of long-term support. This judgment is fundamentally subjective, but it requires consideration by both clients and caregivers. In this situation, informed consent must be seen as a dynamic process whereby the caregiver, client, and family benefit from one another's thinking, not as a finite moment in time. The home care process must allow decisions to be reviewed and revised and must take into account the family's quality of life. Without a process to change decisions, families may resort to making their own decisions, implementing privately sanctioned "do not resuscitate" orders that are later explained as equipment failures or accidents. The home care movement must advocate a system of continuing assessment of the client and the family. High-tech home care contracts should be renegotiable throughout the course of the client's care.

The very notion of appreciating benefit to clients implies consciousness. It could be argued that the permanently unconscious client cannot appreciate the benefit of long-term ventilatory support and that long-term ventilatory support is contraindicated in these clients.

Ethical issues in home care of the technology-dependent client may also include many of the following: (1) resolution of conflict between caregiver and client and family; (2) health care in adverse environments; (3) client abandonment, neglect, or abuse; (4) management of role changes (e.g., families become professionals or professionals become parents); (5) decisions at the end of life; (6) response to acute change in client condition; (7) inadequate or incompetent care; (8) availability and adequacy of equipment; (9) adolescent decision making: (10) noncompliant clients or families; (11) termination of home care services; and (12) financial problems faced by families and health care agencies.

In conclusion, home care should be endorsed as one reasonable option in a continuum of alternatives to acute hospitalization. Home care should be seen as a beneficial choice when both the client and the family desire it. However, home care cannot mean abandonment of the family by health care professionals. Central features of the care plan must include supportive services, a continuing mechanism for evaluating and monitoring the initial goals, opportunities for reassessment of the site of treatment, and changed directives when there is alteration in client status or wishes or when the family can no longer provide the necessary care.

LEGAL IMPLICATIONS

The liability concerns are great among technology-dependent clients because of the complex nature of their condition and the reliability and limitations of technology. The health care team and client must evaluate all aspects of the individual care process to determine benefits and burdens.

Issues associated with liability involve standard of the delivery of care and equipment failure. Standards of care must be determined and defined by providers and regulatory agencies (Baldwin-Myers et al, 1992). Safety of equipment and supplies should be determined by evaluating reliability, user friendliness, and incidence of product failure. Other liability issues are the qualifications, competence, and impairment of staff. Informed consent, including refusal of treatment or limitation of treatment, must be thoroughly documented. Suit-prone clients are often immature, insecure, hostile, and uncooperative and express unrealistic expectations, lack of confidence in the staff's judgement, and co-dependent behavior. From a home health care agency perspective, high-risk problems include medication errors, impaired staff, incomplete documentation, unclear lines of authority, uncoordinated efforts among multiple providers, lack of emergency standards of care, and inappropriate transfer, discharge, or discontinuation of services.

Methods that reduce liability exposure include "going the extra mile," focusing on the underlying problem, maintaining a nonjudgmental attitude, acknowledging client and caregiver feelings, documenting thoroughly, anticipating needs and feelings of the client, avoiding negligence, knowing the standards of care, fostering good client relationships, practicing in area of expertise only, being alert, and providing ongoing client education.

SUMMARY

Management of the pediatric and adult pulmonary-compromised client can be challenging and rewarding. Current availability of medical home technology and community resources has made it possible for the client to be managed successfully in the home-care setting. The focus of care should be to maintain medical stability in the home or provide for palliative care in the event a cure is not an option or is not available.

The nurse should demonstrate competence in the management of the client requiring pulmonary rehabilitation, HMV programs, or palliative care by (1) providing sound clinical as-

MEDICAL HISTORY

J.D. was an 8-year-old Hispanic boy in good physical health until 1991, when he was hit by an automobile, causing a C1-C2 spinal cord lesion and resulting in quadriplegia and ventilator dependence. A computed tomographic (CT) scan revealed multiple intracranial areas of bleeding, brain edema, and separation noted at C1-C2. A fracture of the left superior pubic ramus with a hematoma in the left internal obturator muscle was noted on a pelvic CT scan. He underwent decompression laminectomy at level C6-C7. He was unresponsive with reflexive eye opening for 5 to 6 months, after which time he began to vocalize and to recognize significant people in his life. He had a gastrostomy tube and a tracheostomy placed 1 month after his initial injury. He never regained spontaneous respiration or movement below the face.

While hospitalized, he had multiple episodes of fever, various episodes of left lower-lobe atelectasis, and three episodes of ear infections that were all treated. He was started on a physiotherapy and occupational-therapy program that enabled him to sit with the assistance of a collar and corset. He had no control of his head or neck and no neck muscles. He had a laminectomy from C6 to T1. He was at high risk for developing scoliosis. He had spasticity and spasms of all four extremities, with increased reflexes of both upper and lower extremities with clonus bilaterally. He did not develop pressure sores while hospitalized. He follows a routine bowel and bladder program and is catheterized intermittently. He successfully completed the acute spinal cord injury rehabilitation program and was discharged to home under the care of his parents with 16 hours per day of LVN care 7 days a week.

He recently presented to the hospital in respiratory distress with a change in mental status, diminished breath sounds bilaterally, and hypothermia.

DISCHARGE ORDERS TO HOME

- Pseudoephedrine (Actifed) 10 ml orally or in the gastrostomy tube, three times a day as necessary for thick nasal secretions
- Baclofen 25 mg orally or in the gastrostomy tube three times a day
- Diphenhydramine (Benadryl Elixir) 1½ tsp every 6 hours as necessary for rash or hives
- Phenylpropanolamine (Dimetapp Elixir) 5 ml every 4 to 6 hours as necessary for congestion
- Bisacodyl (Dulcolax) suppository at bedtime followed by manual evacuation

- Ear drops or mineral oil, over the counter for removal of ear wax 2 to 4 drops three times a day as necessary
- PLV-100 ventilators with cascades, 2
- Vent settings: PLV-100. Assist control—FiO_2—21%, tidal volume—1750 cc; back-up rate—12, pressure limit—36
- Low-fat diet
- Bulb syringe to remove wax (Do not use cotton-tipped applicators inside the ear.)
- Hydrocortisone cream 1% to skin rash three times a day as necessary
- Intrapulmonary percussive ventilation treatments may give 3 to 4 puffs MDI albuterol with ipratropium (Atrovent) every 6 hours and increase to every 4 hours as necessary.
- Multivitamin 1 tablet every day through the gastrostomy tube or orally
- Normal saline drops 1 or 2 per nostril as necessary to thin secretions
- Nystatin ointment to the tracheal or gastrostomy tube site as necessary for redness
- Guaifenesin (Robitussin) 1 tsp orally every 6 hours as necessary for upper respiratory infection
- Robitussin CF 5 ml every 4 hours as necessary for congestion
- Phenylephrine (Rynatan) 1 tablet orally or through the gastrostomy tube as needed for rhinitis
- Triamcinolone cream 0.1% to tracheal or gastrostomy tube site as needed for redness
- Acetaminophen (Tylenol) 325 mg 2 tablets orally every 4 to 6 hours as necessary for temperature over 101° F or pain
- Beclomethasone (Vancenase) nasal spray 1 to 2 puffs per nostril at bedtime or during the night as needed for rhinitis
- Oxygen therapy 1 to 2 L/min as needed
- Activity as tolerated

ASSESSMENT

During the initial home evaluation, the following problems were identified:
- Deconditioned and decreased strength and endurance
- Poor compliance with continuous oxygen therapy
- Limited knowledge and understanding of disease process, management, and treatment
- Inability to recognize and report worsening symptoms
- Anxiety and panic episodes

Based on this assessment and identification of client problems, the following interdisciplinary-team

Continued

CASE STUDY—cont'd

treatment plan was developed to achieve the following outcomes:

- *Stable and optimal pulmonary status at maximal level of function*
- *Basic understanding of the disease process, complications, risks, and symptoms of complications*
- *Ability to verbalize an understanding of medications, including proper use, side effects, and actions*
- *Ability to recognize and report worsening symptoms early in the exacerbation to avoid acute care intervention*

- *Improvement in muscle strength and endurance (e.g., sitting tolerance)*
- *Ability to control dyspnea through correct use of breathing techniques in coordination with ADLs*
- *Ability to pace activities*
- *Ability to mobilize secretions effectively*
- *Ability to control panic attacks and episodes of anxiety*
- *Compliance with oxygen therapy*

---

sessment and treatment skills, (2) facilitating compliance and competency of home caregivers, (3) maintaining basic and advanced pulmonary care skills to prevent unnecessary hospital admissions or life-threatening events, (4) delivering cost-effective and efficient care, (5) addressing quality-of-life issues, (6) understanding and demonstrating standard of care for this client population, (7) understanding technology and teaching the client to use the technology safely, (8) evaluating and making recommendations for current and potential clinical and management problems, (9) verbalizing an understanding of ethical and legal implications, (10) developing an appropriate plan of treatment for the client, (11) working with an interdisciplinary team and third-party payors, and (12) using professional and community resources.

REFERENCES

Abou-Shala N, Meduri GU: Noninvasive mechanical ventilation in patients with acute respiratory failure, *Critical Care Medicine* 24(4):705-715, 1996.

American Association of Respiratory Care: Clinical Practice Guidelines: Long-term invasive mechanical ventilation in the home, *Respiratory Care* 40(12):1313-1320, 1995.

American Thoracic Society: Standards for the diagnosis and care of patients with chronic obstructive pulmonary disease, *American Journal of Respiratory Critical Care Medicine* 152(suppl):93-94, 1995.

Bach J et al: Glossopharyngeal breathing and noninvasive aids in the management of post-polio respiratory insufficiency, *Birth Defects: Original Article Series* 23(4):99-113, 1987.

Bach J: Mechanical insufflation-exsufflation: Comparison of peak expiratory flows with manually assisted and unassisted coughing techniques, *CHEST* 104(5):1553-1562, 1993.

Bach J: Respiratory muscle aids for the prevention of pulmonary morbidity and mortality, *Seminars in Neurology,* 15(1):72-83, 1995.

Baldwin-Myers A et al: *Standards of care for the ventilator-assisted individual,* Loma Linda, Calif, 1992, Loma Linda University Medical Center.

Birnkrant D et al: Persistent pulmonary consolidation treated with intrapulmonary percussive ventilation: A preliminary report, *Pediatric Pulmonology* 21(4):246-249, 1996.

Capen C, Dedlow ER: Discharging ventilator-dependent children: A continuing challenge, *Journal of Pediatric Nursing* 13(3):175-183, 1998.

Gilgoff IS et al: Neck breathing: A form of voluntary respiration for the spine-injured ventilator-dependent quadriplegic child, *Pediatrics* 82(5):741-745, 1988.

Gilmartin M: Long-term mechanical ventilation: Patient selection and discharge planning, *Respiratory Care* 36(3):205-216, 1991.

Gold P et al: *The ventilator-assisted patient: Preparing for home,* Loma Linda, Calif, 1989, Loma Linda University Medical Center.

Hazinski MF: *Nursing care of the critically ill child,* ed 2, St Louis, 1992, Mosby.

Hazinski TA: Bronchopulmonary dysplasia. In Chernick V, Boat TF, eds, *Kendig's disorders of the respiratory tract in children,* Philadelphia, 1998, WB Saunders.

Hilton T et al: End of life care in Duchenne muscular dystrophy, *Pediatric Neurology* 9(3):165-176, 1993.

Jaffe M, Skidmore-Roth L: *Home health nursing: Assessment and care planning,* ed 3, St Louis, 1997, Mosby.

Jennings M: *Nursing care planning guides for home health care,* Baltimore, 1988, Williams & Wilkins.

Jones DJ et al: Nasal pressure support ventilation plus oxygen compared with oxygen therapy alone in hypercapnic COPD, *American Journal of Respiratory Critical Care Medicine* 152(2):538-544, 1995.

Leger P et al: Home positive pressure ventilation via nasal mask for patients with neuromuscular weakness or restrictive lung or chest wall disease, *Respiratory Care* 34(2):73-79, 1989.

Leger P et al: Nasal intermittent positive pressure ventilation: Long-term follow-up in patients with severe chronic respiratory insufficiency, *Chest* 105(1):100-103, 1994.

MacIntyre N et al: Consensus Conference IV: Noninvasive positive pressure ventilation, *Respiratory Care* 42:362-449, 1997.

Marx J, Majersky LW, Wiseman S: *Guidelines for pulmonary rehabilitation programs: American Association of Cardiovascular and Pulmonary Rehabilitation,* Champaign, Ill, 1998, United Graphics.

Mason M: *Speech pathology for tracheostomized and ventilator-dependent patients,* Newport Beach, Calif, 1993, Voicing.

Meduri GU et al: Noninvasive positive-pressure ventilation via face mask, *Chest* 109(1):179-193, 1996.

Meyers D: *Client teaching guides for home health care,* ed 2, Gaithersburg, Md, 1997, Aspen.

Morgan K, McClain S: *Core curriculum for home health care nursing,* Gaithersburg, Md, 1993, Aspen.

Moss AH: Patients with amyotrophic lateral sclerosis receiving long-term mechanical ventilation, *Chest* 110(1):249-255, 1996.

National Center for Health Statistics: *Monthly vital statistics report,* vol 48, Hyattsville, Md, 1998, Division of Data Services.

O'Donohue WJ et al: Long-term mechanical ventilation: Guidelines for management in the home and alternate community sites, *Chest* 90(1):1s-37s, 1986.

Oppenheimer E, Myers A: *Ventilator alternatives for long-term and home use,* Los Angeles, Calif, 1993, Regional Kaiser Foundation Hospital.

Plummer AL, O'Donohue WJ, Petty TL: Consensus conference on problems in home mechanical ventilation, *American Review of Respiratory Diseases* 140(2):555-560, 1989.

Rosen LR, Bone RC: Economics of mechanical ventilation, *Clinics in Chest Medicine* 9(1):163-169, 1988.

Rothkopf M, Askanazi J: *Intensive home care,* Baltimore, 1992, Williams & Wilkins.

Sevick MA, Braham DD: Economic value of caregiver effort in maintaining long-term ventilator-assisted individuals at home, *Heart & Lung* 26(2):148-157, 1997.

Simonds AK, Elliott MW: Use of BiPAP ventilators for noninvasive ventilation: Advantages and limitations, *American Review of Respiratory Diseases* 143:A585, 1991.

St Coeur M: *Case management: Practice guidelines,* St Louis, 1996, Mosby.

Tarlov AR et al: The Medical Outcomes Study: An application of methods for monitoring the results of medical care, *Journal of the American Medical Association* 262(7):925-930, 1989.

Teague WG, Fortenberry J: Noninvasive ventilatory support in pediatric failure, *Respiratory Care* 40:86-96, 1995.

Testa MA, Simonson DC: Assessment of quality of life outcomes, *New England Journal of Medicine* 334(13):835-840, 1996.

Zorn E, Lareau S, Della Bella L: *Guidelines for nursing care of the pulmonary patient,* 1984, California Thoracic Society.

20 Cancer

Barbara Germino and Ida M. Martinson

For years, people with cancer and their families have dealt with the experiences of their illness and treatments on their own between any necessary hospitalizations and outpatient visits for diagnosis, treatments, and follow-up monitoring. More recently, these families have faced even more of a challenge, since health care systems in which cancer is diagnosed and treated have responded to the national mandate for cost containment by limiting hospital admissions, shortening hospital stays, and discharging people with cancer earlier and earlier. Those who have been hospitalized for treatment of cancer or complications still require a great deal of direct and indirect care, including teaching, support of various kinds, monitoring, and help managing side effects of treatment and symptoms of their cancer. Managed care, in affecting not only hospitals, but also home and community health care agencies, has profoundly impacted cancer care. These agencies are being called on to meet the needs of more acutely ill clients with cancer and their frequently overwhelmed families. They are also dealing with more technological interventions in the home setting, more stringent requirements and limitations on reimbursement, and more stringent guidelines for care.

CURRENT TRENDS IN HEALTH CARE POLICY: IMPACT ON CANCER CARE IN THE COMMUNITY

The recent history of home care reflects current health care trends. The underlying issue is cost containment and the cost-containment movement. Managed care is having an impact on all aspects of home care for those with cancer and their families. The changes resulting from managed care include changes in funding and payment methods, changes in the type of agencies providing home cancer care, changes in the needs of the client and family population served, increasing acuity of clients at home during all stages of their illness, and more use of complex technology in the home. These changes have precipitated the need for creative, well-planned approaches to cancer care in the home.

New Models for Cancer Care in the Community

New models for cancer care delivery in community facilities and at home are developing across the United States. Community hospitals, private practices, and clinics are providing some of the diagnostic, treatment, and follow-up services once offered only by regional cancer centers and major tertiary-care institutions. Cost-effective strategies for delivering specialized care to clients and families dealing with cancer at home have emerged. Many formerly tertiary care centers have become part of huge health care networks including home health, hospice or palliative care, and long-term care services. Liaison services are increasingly common, in both cancer centers and community hospitals. Such services provide a continuing person, usually a nurse, who maintains contact with and availability to the client, the family, and the home health care providers. The liaison nurse may have the primary responsibility of working in an outpatient oncology clinic or inpatient oncology unit but has as part of this role the provision of continuity and personalized contact with the caregiving institution or agency. Some nurses in liaison roles provide this contact primarily by telephone, seeing the client and family when they return for follow-up appointments or readmission. Others are able to make visits with nurses in home health care agencies, both to provide continuity of care and to assist home health care nurses with the increasingly common high-tech aspects of care for people with cancer.

Transition services for people with cancer and their families are one innovative model for community nursing practice, designed to offer personalized services and continuity of care to clients and their families dealing with the ongoing changes imposed by progressive, deteriorating illness at home (Tornberg, McGrath, Benoliel, 1984). This practice model is built around the belief that facilitating autonomy for the dying person is a primary goal and mandates the provision of optimal information for informed decision making. In this model, the nurse operates in two interrelated ways to provide a problem-focused support system for the client and family and to serve as a communication link between the client-family system and the larger health care system providing care. Each role has specific goals for practice. Examples of goals are shown in Box 20-1.

Although the transition-services model is appropriate for those whose cultural values include individual autonomy, it may not be appropriate for others for whom autonomy is not an impor-

tant value. For care to be culturally appropriate and respectful of the specific value system of the client and family, assessment and understanding of their value system are crucial in planning and implementing care.

Models for cancer-care delivery are changing in other ways as well. There has been movement to take such services from tertiary cancer centers to the community. This has been especially crucial for populations who experience barriers to care, such as costs of transportation, physical and functional limitations, environmental threats, and even distance and weather barriers. Mobile specialty-unit services are being used in a number of communities in an attempt to overcome these barriers. Such services usually involve a specially outfitted motor home and a multidisciplinary team that travels from a hospital center to the community, either to a central location or to individuals' homes. Teams may provide home chemotherapy, on-the-spot laboratory tests, or monitoring and care of infusion pumps or venous access devices. Mobile services such as those described are designed to bring specialized cancer-care services to those unable to leave their homes to obtain such services at a community hospital or tertiary care center. Home health care services of the level and intensity needed by such homebound clients and their families may not be available in the community, or the financing for such care may not be possible. Many poorly insured lower-middle- and middle-income persons under 65 years of age may fall through the cracks of the system of reimbursement for home care. Specialized mobile units may provide a more efficient way of bringing specialized home care services to such families.

EPIDEMIOLOGY OF CANCER

Approximately 1,268,000 new cancer cases were projected for 2001 in the United States. About 553,400 people were expected to die of cancer, the second leading cause of death in the United States, exceeded only by heart disease (American Cancer Society [ACS], 2001). Males are more commonly affected, with 643,000 new diagnoses projected for 2001; females diagnosed with cancer were estimated to number 625,000 (ACS, 2001). About 33% of all living Americans will eventually have cancer. The 5-year relative survival rate for all

---

Box 20-1	Examples of Roles and Specific Goals for Practice

ROLE: PROBLEM-FOCUSED SUPPORT

Goals:
1. Maintaining the client's integrity through attention to that client's stated goals, needs, and desires
2. Identifying and using various support resources needed by the client and family

ROLE: PROMOTING CONTINUITY OF CARE

Goals:
1. Ensuring that the cancer client and family members are informed about what is happening, who is involved, and what services are available to assist them
2. Facilitating coordination of services to client and family through planning with other care providers and coordination of client-family-provider expectations from mutually understood and accepted goals (Tornberg, McGrath, Benoliel, 1984)

kinds of cancer is 60% (ACS, 2001). Relative survival rate takes age and life expectancy into account. Survival rates have improved over time from 1 in 5 people in the 1930s to 3 in 5 people in 2001 (ACS, 2001).

In the United States, lung, breast, prostate, and colorectal cancers are the cancers with the highest incidence. For 2001, it was estimated that there would be 169,500 new cases of lung cancer, 193,700 new cases of breast cancer, 198,100 new cases of prostate cancer, and 135,400 new cases of cancer of the colon or rectum (ACS, 2001).

For lung cancer, the incidence rate in the United States is declining in men, from a high of 86.5 per 100,000 in 1984 to 69.1 per 100,000 in 1997. In the l990s, the increasing rate of lung cancer among women leveled off, with incidence rates near the 1997 rate of 43.1 per 100,000 (ACS, 2001) Decreasing lung cancer incidence and mortality rates most likely result from decreased smoking rates in the United States over the past 30 years. However, decreasing smoking patterns in women lag behind those for men. While there have been declines in adult tobacco use, tobacco use among youth increased considerably during the 1990s (ACS, 2001). Efforts to discourage smoking in the young and to provide resources for smoking cessation must be developed (Wynder, 1998). Recent settlement terms between major tobacco companies and state governments in the United States have included plans to prioritize youth-focused advertising for tobacco products. Whether monies will actually be expended in this way remains to be seen. In addition, legislation has either been passed or is in process in many states to make it illegal to sell tobacco to minors and illegal for minors to purchase tobacco.

The 5-year survival rate for women with localized breast cancer has increased from 72% in the 1940s to 97% today. If the cancer has spread regionally, the 5-year relative survival rate is 77%, and for women with distant metastases, the rate is 21%. Survival of breast cancer declines over time, is stage dependent, and is best for women diagnosed with early-stage disease (ACS, 2001). Breast cancer has become a highly visible disease. Its visibility has probably been very positive in informing women and encouraging them to get mammograms and learn self breast examination. It has also created some anxiety among women about their risk. Some of that anxiety is made

worse by questionable mammography findings that require repeat or follow-up testing. A recent study (Lowe et al, 1999) concluded that women who were recalled to follow-up after abnormal findings experienced an increase in their level of concern regarding breast cancer; higher levels of concern about breast cancer were sustained even after a negative result had been determined.

Counseling women about their risk factors is made more difficult by the fact that there is still limited definitive information about risk factors for breast cancer. The role of dietary fat and obesity in the causation of breast cancer has not been clearly determined. The role of alcohol consumption in breast cancer is being studied, and the theory that hormone replacement therapy is a risk factor has recently garnered more support. The effects of other closely related factors such as weight gain, caloric intake, and physical activity are hard to separate (Greenwald, 1999). There is some evidence of increased risk of breast cancer related to perimenopausal weight gain, and some researchers have suggested the importance of avoiding middle-age weight gain and accumulation of central body fat (Stoll, 1999).

Prostate cancer incidence rates continue to be significantly higher in black men than in white men. Between 1988 and 1992, prostate cancer incidence rates increased dramatically because of earlier diagnosis in men without any symptoms through increased use of the prostate-specific antigen (PSA) blood test. Subsequently, prostate cancer incidence rates declined and have leveled off (ACS, 2001). In 2001, an estimated 31,500 deaths occurred from prostate cancer, the second leading cause of cancer death in men. Although mortality rates are declining among white and black men, rates in black men remain more than twice as high as in white men (ACS, 2001). The 5-year relative survival rate for men whose tumors are diagnosed in the local or regional stages is reported to be 100%. Over the past 20 years, the survival rate for all stages combined has increased to 93% from 67%. After 5 years, survival rates decline, though recent data indicate that 72% of men diagnosed with prostate cancer survive 10 years, and 53% survive 15 years (ACS, 2001).

Colorectal cancers are the third most common cancers in men and women. Incidence rates have slowly but steadily decreased from 1985 to

1997 because of increased screening and polyp removal, preventing progression of polyps to invasive cancers (ACS, 2001). The overall 5-year relative survival rate for colorectal cancers detected at an early, localized stage is 90%. Unfortunately, only 37% of colorectal cancers are discovered at that stage. For colorectal cancers that have spread regionally, the survival rate is 65% (ACS, 2001). Clearly, colorectal cancer is highly curable when detected early; however, many Americans over age 50 are either not aware or unwilling to be screened for this type of cancer, perhaps because of the discomfort and expense of sigmoidoscopy or colonoscopy, the most effective screening tools. Genetics plays a role in 15% of colorectal cancer cases; those people with personal or family histories that put them in the high-risk category should be followed and screened more frequently than recommended for those of average risk.

Other kinds of cancers with high incidence rates in the United States are cancer of the urinary tract in men (>59,000 estimated for 2001) and cancer of the uterus (>38,000 estimated for 2001) and ovaries (>23,000 estimated for 2001) in women. Survival rates for these three kinds of cancers are high if the cancers are diagnosed in the localized stages. In the United States more than 31,000 cases of leukemia were projected for 2001, with only slightly lower numbers for cancers of the stomach, pancreas, and oral cavity.

About 8600 new cases of cancer in children were expected in 2001. About 1500 cancer deaths were expected to occur in children aged 0 to 14 in 2001. Cancer is relatively rare in children, but is the chief cause of death by disease in children ages 1 to 14. Mortality rates have decreased 50% since 1973 (ACS, 2001).

In the United States, black men are at greater risk for cancer than black women and men or women of any other ethnic group. In particular, they are more likely to develop colorectal, lung, or prostate cancer. Black women have the highest incidence rates of colorectal and lung cancers of women in the United States. Blacks are about 33% more likely to die of cancer than whites in the United States (ACS, 2001). Similar data for other ethnic groups are only recently available, and it is important to note that differences in cancer incidence and mortality for ethnic groups should be interpreted with caution, because mis-

classification of race on medical records, death certificates, and in census data can reduce accuracy (ACS, 2001). In addition, new categories of ethnicity that are unrepresented in much legal documentation are emerging. Some studies indicate that ethnic differences are really socioeconomic; poor people have higher overall cancer rates. It has been suggested that access to care is limited for the poor and that they may be diagnosed later and have fewer treatment options if uninsured or underinsured. The issue of late diagnosis is a complex one. The daily priorities of those who have to worry about such basic essentials as food, shelter, and being able to pay for utilities and medicines must also be considered. Transportation to care may be an issue, as may safety of the environment.

CONCEPTUAL FRAMEWORK FOR HOME CARE OF CLIENTS WITH CANCER AND THEIR FAMILIES

The way in which a nurse conceptualizes people with cancer and their families has a direct effect on all aspects of care, from assessment to intervention and evaluation. Health care systems in which nurses practice have made it difficult to view clients and families as individuals living and operating in family contexts. In home care, for instance, people have been referred to agencies for assistance with disease or treatment-related tasks such as dressing changes, catheter irrigations, and pulmonary toilets. Nurses have made a distinction between the client's disease and the human responses of the client and family, which are parts of a larger illness experience. Nurses have worked hard to focus not only on the disease and its symptoms, but also on the impact of the illness on the day-to-day living of the ill person and family.

Family-systems theory continues to provide a perspective on clients and families that can prevent fragmentation of care and guide the nurse in working with the client and family in a way that considers their environment. Family systems are more than just groups of individuals in ongoing interaction with one another and with their environment. Families, however defined, share some common commitment and goals, common values, a history, and significant bonds, whether blood, marriage, adoption, or emotional and practical commitment. Any event or change that occurs for one person in the family system, because of its unitary nature, has some impact on the entire family. These basic principles of family-systems theory can inform the nurse's understanding of the implications of problems experienced by clients and their families. They may also assist in examining the implications of relationships with care providers, both individuals and agencies (Germino, O'Rourke, 1996; McCorkle, 1992; McCorkle, Germino, 1984).

Dealing with the impact of cancer is as much an ongoing process of adaptation for families as it is for clients (Lewis, 1992, 1997). When one member of a family is affected by illness, all members will be affected in some way. For a family unit to survive, it must adapt to pressures, both from its members and from the larger social system. The family must struggle to maintain some sense of order while making decisions about how to deal with the many changes an illness such as cancer may impose (McCorkle, Germino, 1984). When nurses are assessing the needs and strengths of an individual client, they must also consider how these needs and strengths may relate to the family as a unit (Zahlis, Lewis, 1998).

Comprehensive care for family problems precipitated by an illness such as cancer cannot be offered by any one discipline in isolation, but rather depends on the availability of a variety of disciplines with providers who bring different resources and skills to bear on complex problems. Thus the provision of home care for clients and families living with cancer must be planned and implemented using multiple resources and systems of care (Given et al, 1997; Kurtz et al, 1996; McCorkle, 1992).

Nursing services in the home are client and family centered and are designed to assist clients and families to cope effectively with the effects of the disease and treatment. Home care is an intermediary service, the essential component of which is assistance by professional nurses for families making transitions. Care encompasses two types of transitions—the passage of the client and family through different states or aspects of illness and the passage of the client through different health care settings as the illness changes. The purpose of such care is to provide continuity by explicitly establishing the nurse as a communication link between the client and the client's established social network. The nurse also links the client with the physician and other health care providers who constitute the complex social network of health care agencies involved in treatment and care (McCorkle, Germino, 1984).

Underlying this framework is a belief that people with cancer have a right to participate in the choices and decisions affecting their illness and treatment, as well as the circumstances surrounding how they will live. Home care for people with cancer can be viewed as a special model of care delivery in which nurses are pivotal as facilitators of personalized care (McCorkle, Germino, 1984).

SPECIAL NEEDS OF CLIENTS WITH CANCER AND THEIR FAMILIES

The person with cancer lives with its impact or the fear of its potential recurrence throughout life. Those with cancer are living longer and may thus experience a wide range of acute and chronic disabilities, some of which will persist and others that are transitory. Cancer has become recognized as a chronic illness. Chronic illnesses have the following particular characteristics: (1) they are permanent and nonreversible, (2) they often leave residual disability, (3) they require special efforts at rehabilitation, and (4) they may require a long period of observation, supervision, or direct care (Feldman, 1974). Chronic illness involves losses and threats to which people respond in many ways. These include threats to bodily integrity, to the view of self, to relationships, and to every aspect of meaningful functioning (Germino, 1998; Penman et al, 1992). Adaptation to the illness can be influenced by family, friends, and professionals, but much of it requires management of the many transitions that change the client's reality in profound ways (Corbin, Strauss, 1988; Germino, 1998).

Timing of Home Care Services

The impact of cancer and cancer treatment for a client and family changes over time; therefore needs for particular kinds of care and services must be assessed on an ongoing basis. The following are periods of high risk for difficulty in dealing with cancer and its sequelae: (1) between the onset of symptoms and diagnosis, (2) at the time of diagnosis and soon after, (3) during treatment, (4) at recurrence, and (5) in advanced illness (Holland, 1989; Pasacreta, McCorkle, 1996). Home care referrals are more likely to be made at times when the client is dealing with recovery from surgery, significant side effects of treatment, and symptoms of advancing disease. All of these have the potential to create self-care limitations and serious complications, or they may interact with other ongoing illnesses.

It is important for the nurse to understand the range of responses to cancer at various points during the illness. Once an initial diagnosis has been made and some staging and prognostic information is available, clients' and families' fears often focus and accelerate. This was described in a classic study as an "existential crisis"—a time during which the ill person has questions about why this is happening to him or her, what the meaning of this illness is for his or her life, what the future holds, and whether he or she may die from the cancer (Weisman, Worden, 1976-77). As clients go through treatment, they often experience disruption of their daily lives, a sense of loss of control, and uncertainties about the treatment outcomes and side effects (Mishel, 1984, 1988). Clients and families deal with these feelings in a variety of ways. One common response is to work at keeping at least some aspect of their lives as normal as possible and taking one day at a time. The need for information is crucial at this time—information about the treatment, the way it affects the body, side effects to be expected, length of time until such effects appear and their duration, possible impact of treatment side effects on the client's functioning, and strategies for managing these things. The home care nurse needs to assess client and family needs and desires for information in these areas throughout the time they are working together to manage side effects, prevent complications, and maximize functioning.

Living with Cancer Over Time

People with cancer and their families deal to some extent with the effects and impact of that cancer throughout the rest of their lives. Clients may experience a variety of acute or temporary and long-term disabilities. Cancer fits the definition of a chronic illness as an impairment or deviation from normal that has one or more of the characteristics described earlier. More than ever

before, initial treatment for many types of cancer is followed by adjuvant therapy of a different modality. Periods of time between a mastectomy and a course of adjuvant chemotherapy, for instance, may be relatively short, bombarding the client with a series of physical symptoms and changes in activity, sexuality, and energy. The client will have more new information to absorb and a new set of logistics, such as arranging time and transportation to treatment or rearranging the family routines and habits or their environment to accommodate treatment at home. During this time, home care services may be needed for treatment or for assessment and management of symptoms and symptom distress, client and family teaching about treatment, and the effects and impact of treatment and how to manage them. Information about resources, financial assistance, and support services may be relevant. The nurse, as an ongoing care provider who knows the family, can be extremely helpful in providing support to them during these difficult times. What may be reimbursable, however, is postoperative wound care, assessment for surgical complications, and home chemotherapy administration, leaving the home care nurse with the challenge of addressing the client's and family's many other needs in the context of limited visits.

In the example of a woman with breast cancer who has both a mastectomy and adjuvant chemotherapy, the course of her illness may involve a long period of remission, even 5 years or more. Many women consider themselves "cured" after such a long period of freedom from the disease and its stressful accompaniments, even though there is a growing body of evidence that fears of recurrence persist even for women who are doing well, and those fears are reactivated when they have mammograms, breast examinations, or unexplained symptoms. When a recurrence of the illness comes after such a long remission, women and their spouses have reawakened feelings of uncertainty about the future and feelings of shock, anger, and injustice. This may occur even after several recurrences (Chekryn, 1984). The home care nurse can use this opportunity to assist the client and family to deal with the effects of another course of treatment or to help them strengthen or find new sources of support as they face the impact of the recurrence.

In advanced cancer, there is a high risk of multiple distressing symptoms, major individual and family life changes, and the stresses dealing with an illness now considered terminal. For clients and families who choose home care or home hospice care, the need for such care is best determined as early as possible. In this way, planning for anticipated needs and problems can take place in a contractual manner among the professional caregiver involved, the client, and the family. Crises may be prevented or at least minimized. For instance, the progression of symptoms can be anticipated, avoiding extremely stressful, energy-consuming periods of wondering what is going on and how to access available resources (Germino, 1995).

ASSESSMENT OF THE KINDS OF HOME CARE SERVICES NEEDED

Assessments of clients and families dealing with cancer should include all major areas of assessment for home care needs in addition to some that are particular to cancer. Accurate information about the cancer diagnosis, staging, treatment, history, disease and treatment symptoms, and side effects is crucial. In addition, information about the client's other health problems, particularly chronic illnesses and their treatment, is crucial for appropriate planning and symptom management (Box 20-2). For instance, pain-

Box 20-2 Specific Areas for Client Assessment
Ability to function independently, especially with activities of daily living (ADLs)
Physical condition (symptoms, strength, and stamina)
Symptom distress
Nutritional status
Cognitive functioning (mental status)
Feelings and mood, outlook on life, and behavior and communication with others
Interpersonal competence in making needs and wishes known to others
Personal goals and values
Ability to carry out job and family roles
Relationships with others
Understanding of illness, treatment, and prognosis
Ways of coping with the cancer and its impact

management strategies for the person with cancer pain who also has rheumatoid arthritis should take the latter information into account. If the client and family are referred for home care, such information should be included in the referral. If it is not, it is well worth the home care nurse's time to obtain it.

Assessment of the Client and Family

Like others in need of home care services, families dealing with cancer may identify at least some of the particular problems with which they are dealing but may not be able to identify all the areas in which home care services could help them, because they are not aware of either the kinds of services available or the existence or potential of some problems related to the cancer and its impact. To identify how the client and family are dealing with the illness and whether they are in need of further information or clarification about what's going on, the nurse must explore information about their perceptions of the illness, its treatment, and its effects. The nurse doing an initial home care assessment with a family dealing with cancer needs to plan the time to hear the account by client and family members of their experiences related to the cancer diagnosis and treatment. Providing client and family members the opportunity to "tell their story" accomplishes several purposes. Reviewing the experiences and their impact helps the client and other family members process and deal with the cancer's effects on their lives. Nurses' requests to hear such stories and interest in them communicate to the client and family the importance of their unique experience and may help to initiate a strong, positive, caring relationship between the nurse and family. For the nurse, the stories provide important insights into the impact of the cancer on each person and on the family unit. The client's story, for instance, may reveal a variety of issues, such as wondering how and why this happened to him or her, the sense of his or her life spinning out of control, concerns about physical and functional changes, and worries about the future (Germino, Funk, 1993). On the other hand, family members' stories, although containing a theme of concern about what is happening to the client, reveal many other issues, shaped by their role and relationships in the family, the fears and concerns precipitated for them by the client's illness, and their worries about themselves and other family members (Germino, Funk, 1993). Hearing more than the client's or any one family member's perspective on their experiences is crucial to the nurse who must begin working with this family based on their identified understandings and interpretations of what is going on. Family members' accounts can provide important cues about family relationships, family functioning, and areas of concern or uncertainty. Different views and different information result from different family members' perspectives. The "truth" about the family is the melding of all of these perspectives as they affect the daily lives of the family and its functioning as a unit.

Specific Areas for Family Assessment

In addition to the information revealed in individual family members' stories about the cancer experience, there are specific areas about which the nurse needs to learn (Table 20-1). Assessment is an ongoing process for several reasons. Practical constraints on the nurse's time, the complexity of information needed for family-focused home care, changing needs and priorities during the illness, and the availability of family members all require that assessment continue throughout the process of care. Specific areas for family assessment are discussed in the following sections.

Immediate priorities   As in any other home care situation, the nurse assessing the client and family

Table 20-1	Client and Family Assessment Guide		
	DATA SOURCES		
Area for Assessment	Client	Family	Other
Immediate priorities	X	X	HCP
Environment	X	X	
Family resources	X	X	
Family roles and relationships	X	X	
Family functioning	X	X	
Social support	X	X	
Family goals and values	X	X	
Impact of cancer on the family	X	X	

HCP, Health care provider.

for the first time needs to identify and begin with areas of care that are urgent priorities from the client's, family's, and nurse's perspectives. Control of distressing symptoms, the need for information and teaching, and respite care are common immediate priorities in families dealing with cancer. Asking the client and family members about their most urgent needs for home care services conveys the clear message that care will be personalized and responsive and that the client and family have ultimate control. To the extent that the nurse can deal with immediate priorities to the client's and family's satisfaction, that nurse's credibility will have a strong foundation.

Environment   The physical environment of the home, including safety and comfort factors related to the client's current and future care, needs to be assessed. The social environment of the family, including relationships with and support from extended family, friends, place of worship, and community, may be an important resource for the family over time. An environment that is supportive of home care for a person with cancer is one that has human and physical resources needed by that person and family. Such care does not necessarily require a large, loving family or any particular kind or size of home. It does require at least one family member or significant other who is able and willing to assist basic safety and comfort factors. Preferably, there are community resources such as equipment services, family support groups, respite care services, and programs to supplement availability and reimbursement of care for those with limited insurance, lower incomes, and fewer economic resources.

Family resources   The adequacy of economic resources may be a major area of concern for families dealing with cancer. Major expenses may be incurred for cancer treatment, even without hospitalization. Even with insurance coverage for most aspects of care, many families will have difficulty stretching their economic resources to pay for the uncovered balance. In addition, clients and family members may lose income because of illness or time required to care for the ill family member. Expenses such as travel to and from treatment, meals in restaurants, and extra child care are less obvious expenses that can accumulate and quickly unbalance a modest family budget.

Family caregiving   Family caregiving was, for a long time, seen as women's work and a potential burden on caregivers (Braithwaite, 1992); the focus was on avoiding negative outcomes, such as compromised physical and psychological health from the stresses and strains of caregiving (Braithwaite, 1992). More recently, as knowledge about caregiving has increased, it has become clear that family caregiving is done by husbands, wives, adult children, siblings, parents, and other family members, as well as close friends and significant others who function as family for the client (Walker, Pratt, Eddy, 1995). In spite of the fact that family caregivers, if giving extensive care or supervision, may have those responsibilities added to their ongoing roles and responsibilities, caregiving has been found to have positive as well as negative outcomes for family members. Positive outcomes include satisfaction at being able to keep the client at home and have his or her care meet the family's standards and values, a sense of meaning in a difficult situation, increased closeness with the person being cared for, and a sense of satisfaction in being able to give a significant "gift" to the ill person. Nurse researchers have been developing and testing strategies to assist families to provide high-quality care for their ill member, to have positive rewards from doing so, to learn ways of coping effectively with the stresses and strains of caregiving, and to maintain physical and psychological health during and after the caregiving experience (Archbold et al, 1995; Given, Given, 1992; McCorkle et al, 1993; O'Rourke, Germino, 1998).

Resources for providing care for the client should be explored with the family. In particular, the nurse needs to talk with the primary caregiver to assess that individual's age and state of health, relationship with the client, and other roles and responsibilities. The availability of other caregivers, their ages and health status, and their willingness and ability to provide some of the client's care and respite to the primary caregiver should be determined. Part of the examination of family resources is the exploration of other family stressors that are ongoing and may have existed before the client's cancer was ever diagnosed. For instance, financial problems, developmental changes such as children leaving home and getting married, and problems with relationships may make the cancer an additional rather than the primary stressor. Caregiving may be stressful because of the context in which it occurs when that context is characterized by ongoing family strains and problems.

Family roles and relationships Exploration of family members' relationships with one another and their roles can help the home care nurse assess current and future alterations that may be disrupted and negatively influenced by the experience of cancer (Germino, Funk, 1993; Lewis, 1993). Family roles, particularly in low-income, nonwhite families, may be changed by cancer, and this has the potential for creating strains in the family and for having adverse effects on a client's ability to function as parent, companion, homemaker, or breadwinner (Sales, Schulz, Biegel, 1992). The amount of flexibility in a family system, in terms of family members being able to shift roles and responsibilities as needed, may be important in how well the family deals with changes imposed by the cancer.

Family functioning Families have patterns of functioning in day-to-day situations and in stressful times such as cancer may impose. Assessment of usual family functioning, including ways of dealing with household, child care, financial, and social aspects of family life, provides useful insights for the nurse in planning home care that will be most acceptable and effective for a particular family. The daily routines of the family, family rules about communication inside and outside the family, and areas of functioning particularly important to maintain at a normal level are all part of such information.

Social support The availability of human resources for the family and their adequacy during difficult times are key areas for assessment in home cancer care. The support of others has repeatedly been found to influence a client's psychosocial adjustment to cancer (Penman et al, 1986) and is likely to be as important for families dealing with the disruptions of cancer in one of their members. Living with cancer over time means having periods of great stress and difficulty, as well as periods of relative stability. The support of others is most often an important factor in how families cope with the impact of cancer. The availability of extended family members and friends does not guarantee their willingness or ability to provide support to the client and family dealing with cancer. Assessment of who is available, able, and willing to assist is essential. The kinds of support desired by the client and family should be explored as well. Concrete support services, such as assistance with transportation, errands, cooking, and child care, may provide major relief for families at difficult times. In addition, support may be provided by the visits or telephone calls of caring people who can allow the client and family to express their fears and concerns, to maintain some semblance of normality in their lives, or to distract themselves by focusing on other aspects of life.

Family goals and values   The family's goals and values should be major factors in planning home care. Goals and values for any particular client and family are affected by religious, spiritual, and cultural beliefs and norms, as well as by the social and community context in which the family is living. However, knowing that a client and family belong to a particular ethnic group or have a particular religion or spiritual belief is clearly not sufficient. There is tremendous variability within ethnic and religious populations, and such factors as educational background, socioeconomic status, and individual personal and family values all operate in any single situation. It is dangerous and unfair to impose the caregiver's stereotypes and assumptions on a particular client and family. Cancer is itself a devastating experience, and there is a strong mandate for care that respects and takes into account client and family values at a time of great stress. A major illness such as cancer may cause the family to strengthen already existing values or to reexamine its goals and values and reevaluate its priorities. For care to be personalized, the nurse must understand what is important to the client and family and how those values may be related to the cancer experience and to dealing with it.

On occasion, client and family values conflict, and the nurse working with the family at home may become a mediator or problem solver with the family to negotiate the management of such conflict. For example, a terminally ill woman with breast cancer whose pain is under control has reached the point where she no longer has any appetite and does not wish to eat. Preparing food for the client and having her eat it to "keep up her strength" is very important to her husband and sister who are caring for her. They get very upset with her "stubbornness" in refusing to eat and continue to ply her with food. The client gets angry and withdraws from her family; the husband and family get frustrated, frightened, and upset as well. The nurse in this situation can help the client maintain her autonomy and control by assisting the husband and sister to understand that loss of appetite is part of the natural progression of the client's illness. It will become clear that forcing her to eat will not accomplish anything except to make her feel that she cannot control her life and that allowing her such choices is allowing her to live as she chooses in the time remaining. At the same time, the family's frustration and need to feel they are doing something to help can be acknowledged as legitimate and important. The nurse can provide opportunities for them to care for the client in other ways and to express their feelings of grief as they watch the client die.

Impact of the cancer on the family   The client's illness and the changes it imposes on the family affect the family as a unit and affect each family member individually. To deal with family as well as client needs, the nurse must assess the impact. A number of ways in which cancer may affect the family have been identified from published research (Lewis, 1986) (Box 20-3). Cancer may create emotional strains in the family related to fears of the future, fears of the impact of the disease and treatment, unresolved or ongoing relationship issues, and disrupted communication. If the client requires direct hands-on care at times during the course of the illness and especially if the family is already experiencing stressors and is not prepared to take on this difficult task, the demands of caregiving may be very difficult to address. Depending

---

Box 20-3   Effects of Cancer on the Family

Emotional strain
Physical demands of direct care
Uncertainty about the client's health
Fear of the client dying
Altered household roles and lifestyle
Financial stress
Concerns about providing comfort for the client
Perceived inadequacy of support services
Concerns about the purpose and meaning of life
    and about death
Sexuality
Differences in family and patient perceptions and
    needs

on the client's prognosis, it is common for family members to experience uncertainty about the client's current and future health. Family members will have uncertainties about what current symptoms and problems mean, what causes them, how long they will last, and whether they will be permanent. The future is even more uncertain, and family members worry about the client's future health and limitations, about the increasing demands of the client's illness, and about the possibility that the client may die from this illness.

If the client either has physical limitations related to disease or treatment or is limited in his or her activities by fatigue, household roles and lifestyle may be altered. Even without such limitations, having to receive treatments and go to check-ups is disruptive to household routines and usually involves some arrangements with others. Lifestyles may be altered temporarily or permanently because of the client's fatigue, pain, susceptibility to infection, financial limitations, or other factors. Financial stress is common for families who have limited or no insurance coverage and who are attempting to pay out of pocket for treatment. Even with adequate coverage, other expenses during treatment and recovery can burden families with lower incomes or those with little savings. Transportation costs, child care, time lost from work for client or family members, medications, and other factors can devastate a family's budget.

One of the key concerns of families with a member having cancer symptoms or treatment side effects is being able to provide comfort for that person. Education and support to facilitate comfort are crucial aspects of home care. In particular, the management of pain and nausea is challenging because seeing a family member suffering with these symptoms is so difficult. Home care nurses who work with clients who have cancer and their families are likely to be faced with these problems after surgery, during chemotherapy, and as the disease progresses.

A major problem for families in rural areas or in smaller towns may be the limitations of available support services. In these situations the home health nurse is challenged to use his or her creativity to find substitute resources for the family by working with health care providers, clergy, social workers, voluntary organizations such as the ACS, and even local hospitals.

The threat of a major illness such as cancer, whether realistic or not, is related to fears of death and disabling symptoms, especially pain. Such a threat raises concerns for family members, as well as the client, about the purpose and meaning of life (O'Connor, Wicker, Germino, 1990). Spiritual beliefs may assist each family member in addressing these questions, but for some, finding meaning in the cancer experience is a process not easily accomplished and one that takes time.

The client's sexuality, and therefore that of his or her partner, may be temporarily or permanently affected by a variety of kinds of cancer treatment. Sexuality encompasses the individual's view of him or herself as a man or woman; his or her perceptions of appeal or potential desirability to a partner or, if unpartnered, to others; and his or her sexual desire and sexual functioning. It also encompasses reproductive potential for those who desire to have children. Sensitivity to these issues is part of assessment in working with clients and families with cancer, and although these issues are more difficult to discuss than others, the home care nurse may be an invaluable resource.

Finally, it is important to reiterate a point made earlier in this chapter—that each family member is both part of the family unit and a unique individual. Therefore clients' and family members' perceptions and needs may differ from one another, and consideration of those differences is as important as consideration of the needs of the family unit.

These areas can serve as a guide for the assessment of cancer's impact on the family. Clearly, there may be other areas of difficulty, and any given family may or may not have problems in the areas identified.

Specific Areas for Client Assessment

Since the focus of many of the home care services provided is on the person with cancer, it is essential for the nurse to have detailed information about that person's problems and needs. As mentioned earlier, specific information about the client's cancers, including the type and stage of cancer, evidence of metastasis, past and current treatment, and prognosis, provides an essential baseline for care. The client assessment, then, can focus on the client's responses to the cancer, including physical, functional, psychosocial, emotional, and cognitive responses. See Table 20-1 for criteria that may be useful in assessing the cancer client for home care needs. Criteria for specific focused assessments related to age groups, type of cancer, and type of treatment are beyond the scope of this chapter but may be found in cancer nursing texts, journals, and guidelines cited at the end of this chapter. Increasingly, cancer care is being given on an outpatient basis, and home care nurses are dealing with highly technical aspects of care, such as implanted infusion ports and pumps for chemotherapy and pain management and central venous catheters for chemotherapy or hyperalimentation. A recent phenomenological inquiry (Tarzian et al, 1999) identified the experiences of clients with autologous bone-marrow transplantation and the need for a range of information. It was clear in this study that health care providers differed in matching client needs with information. Giving information to clients is complex since they vary in the amount of information they desire. Nurses need to also teach the client's family. They also wish to talk with a breast cancer survivor. The recommendations of the investigators, based on their findings, included being realistic, as well as viewing the client education as a process to individualize according to each client's needs. State-of-the-art information on the monitoring and care of clients receiving treatment may be found in recent cancer nursing journals and in educational materials provided by drug and medical product companies who manufacture devices to assist in cancer care. Oncology nurses in inpatient, clinic, and home care settings have been able to use these resources effectively.

PLANNING FOR HOME CARE

In planning for home care of clients with cancer and their families, the nurse must consider client and family goals and needs in relation to their fit with available services. According to the conceptual framework described earlier, personalized home care services for people with cancer and their families are based in part on the idea that the consumers of these services have the right to participate in decision making. Client and family goals and values should be the primary guide for professional caregivers planning home care. Nurses and others working with cancer clients and their families need to be aware of their own beliefs about client and family choice and autonomy and ways that those beliefs affect their choice of interventions. For instance, a client with a poor prognosis who is receiving chemotherapy at home may reach a point where he or she decides to discontinue treatment. If that decision is an informed one in which the client has reviewed options and their consequences, the nurse who supports the client's right to make decisions about living and dying may have to deal with personal values and feelings to continue to support the client and family by shifting the plan of care to fit their changed goals and wishes.

The issue of personal control in caring for cancer clients and their families is neither simple nor clear. Not all clients and families desire a great deal of control over and participation in decision making about care. Some find it more comfortable to put themselves in the hands of experts and have choices made for them on such matters. Again, fitting plans for home care to the client's and family's values and goals requires the understanding that goals and even values may be reexamined during life-threatening illness and that responsive home care can only be achieved through effective, ongoing communication among client, family or significant others, and caregivers (Germino, 1987).

NURSING INTERVENTION

Specific nursing interventions depend, in part, on the kind and site of cancer, the stage of disease, and the treatment, but they depend primarily on the human responses to the illness, including the distressing symptoms of the physical and physiological manifestations of the cancer, the need to live with the feelings these precipitate, and the changes the illness demands for all those involved.

Information

Since cancer care in institutions is highly specialized and often fragmented, clients and their families may have gaps in the information they need and wish to have about the cancer, treatment, and symptoms, and their responses to these. One of the initial and important interventions that the home care nurse can provide is assistance in obtaining and understanding needed information. This part of care needs to be based on individual family member assessment, since the client and different members of the family may want and need different kinds and levels of information. Individualizing responses to client and family information needs requires more than just answering a few questions or providing pamphlets. For instance, some clients and families may react against the word "hospice"; the development of the concept of palliative care is part of the response to the negative reaction to the term hospice (Aranda, 1999). Providing a climate in which people feel comfortable asking questions and in which the nurse can individualize the response is essential to personalized care.

Nurses caring for clients and families are fortunate to have a variety of resources for cancer information, both for professionals and for clients and their families. A number of these are listed at the end of this chapter. The ACS provides a variety of written, audiovisual, and internet resources related to cancer and all aspects of cancer care. As well, the ACS has a national toll-free hotline from which anyone can get answers to their general and specific questions about cancer and resources for care and support. The National Cancer Institute also publishes written materials, provides a variety of computerized databases for professionals involved in cancer care, and maintains a frequently updated website for professionals and the public to obtain accurate information. Regional cancer centers are sites where oncology professionals from a variety of disciplines provide the most current and advanced cancer care, but many community hospitals have expanded that network, and most have resources as well. Professional books, journals, and a growing variety of internet resources (see list at end of chapter) report cancer-related research and model programs for the delivery of services, as well as information for clients and families.

Basic Physical Care

Much of the physical care for cancer clients during treatment and as the disease progresses is geared to three goals: comfort, maintenance of maximal possible function, and prevention of complications. This involves not only helping the client and family learn, as necessary, new ways of bathing, toileting, ambulating, and exercising, but also monitoring nutritional status and watching for early symptoms of disease or treatment-related changes that can be managed or alleviated.

Anticipation of such problems can sometimes prevent crises and emergencies and may make it easier to deal with problems such as hypercalcemia, intestinal obstruction, and infection early in their courses. Physical care for the cancer client at home may include postoperative wound care, observation, and progressive exercise to regain strength and stamina. Since some cancer surgery does cause significant bodily changes, the nurse has an important role in helping the client and family understand these changes and find ways of adapting to them. The needs of clients who have had ostomies, head and neck dissections, mastectomies, and amputations are likely to be assessed and dealt with, since those bodily changes are visible and known to be difficult for many clients initially. The needs of individuals whose surgery is not visibly disfiguring may not be as obvious but still may require nursing intervention. The woman who has had a total hysterectomy, for example, and the man who has experienced a radical prostatectomy may need the opportunity to talk with a knowledgeable professional about the physical changes and their implications for sexuality and for the clients' feelings about themselves. Specific strategies for dealing with changes can be explored with clients and their families, and highly specialized resources may be obtained through referral. Surgery is the oldest treatment for cancer, followed by radiotherapy, which celebrated its hundredth anniversary in 1998, and these have been followed by a continuous development of chemotherapy (Kearney, 1999). One client, a nurse, has stated on several occasions for the past 5 years after metastases from breast cancer that as long as one new drug keeps coming out before the last one is no longer totally effective, she will continue her life.

Nutritional Support

Maintenance of an optimal nutritional state is crucial to supporting the best possible response of the cancer client to the disease and its treatment. Many oncologists are now recommending various combinations of vitamins for clients as they go through treatment and recovery. Ongoing research is testing the impact of various dietary strategies and vitamin and mineral supplementation on clients' responses to treatment and on the progress of their diseases. In addition to preventive nutritional strategies, adequate fluid, nutrient, and vitamin intake can best be promoted by careful monitoring of clients who have difficulties with dysphagia, anorexia, nausea and vomiting, diarrhea, and loss of body fluids and nutrients through lesions. Nutritional problems, as with many other complications of cancer and cancer treatment, are best identified early to prevent serious problems that require hospitalization and possible hyperalimentation. Serious oral pain and mucositis can develop, and close attention must be paid to mouth care (McGuire et al, 1998). Many home care agencies, some health departments, and certainly the majority of hospitals have nutritionists who can provide the home care nurse assistance in both monitoring nutritional state and providing nutritional supplementation and support. Many communities also have nutritionists in private practice who may be resources for nurses, clients, and families. Again, resources are fairly readily available in all but the most rural areas, and even where they are not, a telephone consultant can be quite helpful. For more information on nutrition in home health, see Chapter 12.

Home Chemotherapy

Until fairly recently, prolonged chemotherapy was done only in the hospital setting, primarily because of the monitoring needed for safe administration. Advances in technology have made home chemotherapy safer and therefore more available at lower costs (Brown, 1990; Steinheiser, 1995). Implantable pumps, continuous drug delivery systems, venous access devices, and peripherally inserted central catheters (PICCs) have provided the client and family with the mandate to avoid unnecessary hospitalizations and receive safe treatment at home. Such devices are associated with decreased toxicity and more client comfort, although they do require special training of nurses, clients, and families to avoid complications. Clearly defined policies and procedures and effective coordination of services are also essential because home infusion therapy is often performed by nurses from agencies designed specifically to provide infusion services, rather than a broad range of services (Steinheiser, 1995).

The home care nurse administering chemotherapy for cancer should be aware of the criteria for client selection and of safety considerations. Care in transport, preparation, and administra-

tion of chemotherapeutic drugs, as well as dealing with spills and disposal according to current OSHA policies, must be addressed (Grace, Tomaselli, 1995; McNally, 1996). The dangers of handling antineoplastic agents are documented in research literature. Guidelines for the handling of such agents are also published and have become widely available since home chemotherapy has become more common in the community as well as the acute care setting. Again professional journals, books, and drug- and medical-product companies have developed a variety of excellent resources for those needing information about the administration of chemotherapy. For home care nurses who have no experience in the area, continuing education programs with hands-on opportunities or supervision by an experienced nurse are as essential as the knowledge underlying this aspect of care. Many agencies have chemotherapy certification courses. Although home chemotherapy can be safe and effective in the hands of a knowledgeable team, it is not an area into which the novice should tread without preparation and assistance.

Support in Dealing with Responses to Cancer and Treatment

As cancer care in the home becomes increasingly high tech, there is the accompanying risk for home care nurses that preoccupation with the demands of complex care and equipment may at least temporarily override the need to be aware of and responsive to the human aspects of the cancer experience. Care directed toward the psychosocial needs of clients and families is an absolutely integral part of cancer care. The trajectory of cancer is often a complex one, with periods of rapid and sometimes devastating change, followed on occasion by long periods of stability. Issues of bodily changes, mortality, recurrence, and alterations in important areas of functioning, in roles, and in relationships all need to be explored with clients and their families over time. Those experiencing cancer will perceive it in a variety of ways and will deal with it in a variety of ways as well. There are, however, common experiences and needs that should be considered in assessment, planning, and intervention.

The initial impact of cancer has been described as a period when clients often face existential considerations—thoughts about the meaning and purpose of life, their own lives, and uncertainty about the future (Weisman, Worden, 1976-77). Family members experience the initial impact of the diagnosis in their own ways—with worries about the client, with concerns about themselves and their futures, and with uncertainty about the future of the family as a unit (Germino, 1987). As cancer becomes a more chronic illness, it is helpful to think about possible intervention in terms of key problem areas for chronic illness in general, as well as those specific to living with cancer over time. Prevention and management of medical crises, control of symptoms, management of treatment and self-care regimens, and preparation for the future (Strauss, 1984) are all areas in which nurses can assist through teaching, direct care, use of community resources, and perhaps most of all, their continuing, caring presence, which is available when the need arises. As the client's condition changes and family needs change as well, a variety of people and resources in the community can be drawn on. The ACS, for instance, has been mentioned as a source of information. In addition to information, however, the organization provides support groups for clients and families; educational programs for clients, families, and professionals; client visitation services, such as Reach to Recovery for mastectomy clients; transportation to and from treatment; and other needed services. Many comprehensive cancer centers and community hospitals also have client and family support groups, and other types of services may be available in the community. Home care nurses have a great deal of expertise in finding and using community resources of all kinds. The home care of cancer clients and their families may provide a great challenge over time to find a variety of resources to meet those needs.

Symptom Management

Over the last 20 years, there has been a rapidly growing body of knowledge fundamental to the understanding of symptoms and symptom distress and to the management of symptoms as an area of nursing intervention. Again, journal articles and books on managing side effects of chemotherapy and radiation, as well as pamphlets, audiovisuals, and the internet, are easily available to assist the home care nurse in the management of pain, anorexia, nausea and vomiting, hypercalcemia, skin and mucous membrane problems, central nervous system changes, fatigue, and infection. Specific resources are included in the list at the end of this chapter.

In the area of cancer symptom management the following 10 general principles guide nursing intervention, which are crucial for effectiveness:

- To make symptom-management decisions, it is essential to assess not only client variables, such as the disease process, treatment, age, physical status, and other illnesses, but also other major areas. For the client, it is important to have information on symptom patterns and the distress these symptoms are causing. Client goals and cultural and religious values are also important considerations in symptom-management decisions. Family variables, such as availability and willingness of family to participate in symptom management, ability of family members to be supportive of the client, other family member responsibilities, and family goals and values (especially where they may conflict with the client's), should be known to the nurse. Factors in the environment, its physical characteristics and limitations, and limitations of resources are other areas for consideration in decisions about managing symptoms.
- The goal is either care or cure, depending on the client's stage of illness and prognosis. Care is doing *with* people, not *to* them (Benoliel, 1976). Therefore clients have a right to the opportunity (if able) to participate in decisions affecting their lives.
- Contracting with clients and families to help them with symptom management is an important strategy. It implies a commitment to work with them until the goal has been accomplished or readjusted.
- Symptoms should be anticipated, whenever possible, based on disease processes, medications and treatments, age-related factors, and progression of illness.
- When a symptom is under control and the client is satisfied with symptom management, strategies should not be changed.
- In multisymptom management, only one strategy should be changed at a time, and the results are evaluated before making other changes. Otherwise, it will never be known which action was the effective one.

- The psychosocial component of physical symptoms, such as the anxiety component of pain, must be dealt with.
- As symptoms increase in number and complexity, there must be a balance of priorities in the symptom-management process. Symptom distress becomes more important.
- When someone is dying of cancer, certain therapeutic limits and contraindications become less relevant. For example, masking of certain symptoms by controlling others is irrelevant.
- Simple symptom-management strategies should be used before the complex. A preventive bowel regimen of adequate fluids, fiber, and prune juice, for example, can often be effective without need for laxatives and enemas.

Evaluation of Home Care

The effectiveness of any plan and set of interventions, of course, needs to be determined by monitoring both their implementation and outcomes. This includes not only objective indicators (such as relief of constipation), but also client and family satisfaction with the care. Use of a simple diary kept in the home for clients, family members, and professionals to note observations and comments about care and about the client's well-being can be an effective tool for the busy home care nurse in gathering maximal evaluative information to add to his or her own observation. Nursing research will continue to lead the way for improved outcomes for cancer clients. The practice for cancer nurses needs to be based on research.

CASE STUDY

Mr. M. was diagnosed with cancer of the head of the pancreas when he was 65 years of age. The cancer was advanced, and surgery and cure-oriented treatment were not realistic. The decision was made for him to return home and live out the last six months of his life in the comfort of his family. He was readmitted to a local hospital with the onset of esophageal bleeding. It was at this point that Mr. M. requested to go home to die. He wanted to be at his lake home with his wife, children, and grandchildren. Hospice was not available in the community, but Mr. M.'s daughter-in-law, who was a nurse, along with his local physician, was willing to honor Mr. M.'s last request. She contacted the home health nurse after formalizing the referral from Mr. M.'s physician, who agreed to visit once a week for the first month and then seek support for further visits as needed. She, herself, lived in a nearby lake cabin and would come and check on Mr. M. three times a day. The grandchildren would pick wild flowers and bring them for him to see. The grandchildren also would come and sing for their grandfather.

As the days passed, his wife of more than 40 years said one day to the home health nurse, "If he is going to be this sick, it's okay if he dies." His impending death was clear not only to his wife and children, but also to Mr. M.'s sister.

Mr. M.'s older sister had been very close to her brother and found his impending death very difficult. She thought having him at home was too difficult for the family. Mr. M. expressed frequently his joy at be-

ing home. When he could no longer swallow, he would chew beets, his favorite vegetable, and spit them out. He would smile. The nurse was very supportive, especially to Mr. M.'s daughter-in-law, and continued to encourage her that the care she was providing her father-in-law was good. Pain medications were obtained from the pharmacy with the physician cooperating with the necessary prescriptions.

After more than 2 weeks, Mr. M. went into a coma. The nurse encouraged the family to accept that death could take place very soon, within a day or two. Mr. M.'s daughter-in-law moved into the house to be available 24 hours a day. She checked her father-in-law every four hours at least. Very early one morning, Mr. M. was wide awake and able to talk; at the same time his legs and arms were ice cold. His daughter-in-law believed the end was near because of the coldness of his extremities and called all family members, including his sister, to come. As the family members surrounded his bed, each member spoke a few words to him, and he replied to each of them saying goodbye to them. His wife asked if he saw Jesus, and he replied, "yes." He stopped breathing and died. After a few moments at his bedside, the family members all moved into the living room, and for 3 hours talked about the life of Mr. M. The funeral home came and removed the body. Plans were made for his funeral, which became a joyous celebration for the family. His life had been exceptional, and his kindness had touched many.

Continued

CASE STUDY—cont'd

In the case study of this family, the immediate priorities had been taken care of. When Mr. M. requested home care, the priority was to bring him home. Back-up for both nursing and medical care was arranged.

The environment was most supportive of home care, despite inadequate plumbing (the house was a primitive lake cabin that did have running water). The social environment of the family was supportive despite a sister who was critical of the quality of care available in the home. Family resources were adequate, with Medicare covering the needed medical supplies. No treatment was necessary outside the home. Resources for providing care were available through Mr. M.'s daughter-in-law, daughter, and son, who were readily available 24 hours a day.

Family roles and relationships were maintained, and shifts in daily housework were easily accomplished. All members of the immediate family were committed to providing quality time for Mr. M.

Social support for the nurse daughter-in-law was the home health nurse. This was very helpful, since her nursing experience did not include having cared for a dying person at home. Her clinical experiences with death had been in the hospital setting. The home care nurse had the experience of helping with 3 to 4 clients dying at home each year.

Family goals and values were supportive of home care, especially since Mr. M. made it very clear that he wanted to be home. As his son carried him into the cabin from the hospital, Mr. M. remarked, "Home Sweet Home." Family devotions were held in the bedroom with Mr. M., who for years had been the leader of daily family devotions. His son took over that leadership when Mr. M. became too weak to continue.

The impact of the cancer on the family was the most difficult for Mr. M.'s wife, who had looked forward to retirement in a year. A trip around the world had been planned. However, the spouse appreciated the presence of all her children and grandchildren during this time. At the time of Mr. M.'s death, all his family were present except one son who had to return to work.

REFERENCES

Aranda S: Global perspectives on palliative care, *Cancer Nursing* 22(1):33-38, 1999.

Archbold PG et al: The PREP system of nursing interventions: A pilot test with families caring for older members, *Research in Nursing and Health* 18:3-16, 1995.

American Cancer Society (ACS): *Cancer Facts and Figures—2001,* New York, 2001, American Cancer Society.

Benoliel JQ: Overview: Care, cure, and the challenge of choice. In Earl A, Argonidizzo NT, Kutscher AH, eds: *The nurse as caregiver for the terminally ill patient and his family,* New York, 1976, Columbia University Press.

Braithwaite V: Caregiving burden, *Research on Aging* 14(1):3-27, 1992.

Brown JM: Home care models for infusion therapy, *Caring* 9(5):24-26, 1990.

Chekryn J: Cancer recurrence: Personal meaning, communication and marital adjustment, *Cancer Nursing* 7:491-498, 1984.

Corbin J, Strauss A: *Unending work and care: Managing chronic illness at home,* San Francisco, 1988, Jossey Bass.

Feeley N, Gottlieb LN: Nursing approaches for working with family strengths and resources, *Journal of Family Nursing* 6(1):9-24, 2000.

Feldman D: Chronic disabling illness: A holistic view, *Journal of Chronic Diseases* 27:287-291, 1974.

Germino B: Home health care. In Kozier B, Erb G: *Fundamentals of nursing,* Menlo Park, Calif, 1987, Addison-Wesley.

Germino B: Dying at home. In Corless I, Germino B, Pittman-Lindeman M, eds: *A challenge for living: Issues in death, dying, and bereavement,* Boston, 1995, Jones & Bartlett.

Germino B, Funk S: Cancer as a factor in parent-adult child relationships: Adult children's concerns after a parent's diagnosis, *Seminars on Oncology Nursing* 9(2):101-106, 1993.

Germino B, O'Rourke M: Cancer and the family. In Baird S, McCorkle R, Grant M, eds: *Cancer nursing,* ed 2, Philadelphia, 1996, WB Saunders.

Given B, Given CW: Patient and family caregiver reaction to new and recurrent breast cancer, *Journal of the American Medical Women's Association* 47:201-206, 1992.

Given BA et al: Determinants of family caregiver reaction, *Cancer Practice* 5(1):17-24, 1997.

Grace LA, Tomaselli BJ: Intravenous therapy in the home. In Terry J, Baronowski L, Lonsway RA, eds: *Intravenous therapy: Clinical principles and practices,* Philadelphia, 1995, WB Saunders.

Greenwald P: Role of dietary fat in the causation of breast cancer, *Cancer Epidemiology, Biomarkers & Prevention* 8(1):3-7, 1999.

Holland J: Fears and abnormal reactions to cancer in physically healthy individuals. In Holland JC, Rowland JH, eds: *Handbook of psychooncology: Psychological care of the patient with cancer,* New York, 1989, Oxford University Press.

Kearney N: New strategies in the management of cancer, *Cancer Nursing* 22(1):28-33, 1999.

Kurtz ME et al: Concordance of patient and caregiver reports of cancer patients' symptom distress, *Cancer Practice* 4:185-190, 1996.

Lewis FM: The impact of cancer on the family: A critical analysis of the research literature, *Patient Education and Counseling* 8:269-289, 1986.

Lewis FM: *Current issues and future directions for the family: Implications from the Family Impact and Family Functioning Studies.* Proceedings of the Sixth National Conference on Cancer Nursing, American Cancer Society, Atlanta, 1992.

Lewis FM: Psychosocial transitions and the family's work in adjusting to cancer, *Seminars in Oncology Nursing* 9(23):127-129, 1993.

Lewis FM: Behavioral research to enhance adjustment and quality of life among adults with cancer. II. *Preventive Medicine* 26(5):S19-S29, 1997.

Lowe JB et al: Psychologic distress in women with abnormal findings in mass mammography screening, *Cancer* 85(5):1114-1118, 1999.

Marino LB, Kooser JA: The psychosocial care of cancer clients and their families: Periods of high risk. In Marino LB: *Cancer nursing,* St Louis, 1981, Mosby.

McCorkle R: *Caring for the patient at home: Critical nursing behaviors in cancer care.* Proceedings of the Sixth National Conference on Cancer Nursing, American Cancer Society, Atlanta, 1992.

McCorkle R, Germino B: What nurses need to know about home care, *Oncology Nursing Forum* 11(6):63-69, 1984.

McCorkle R et al: A cancer experience: Relationship of patient psychosocial responses to caregiver burden over time, *Psycho-Oncology* 2:21-32, 1993.

McGuire E et al: Acute oral pain and mucositis in bone marrow transplant and leukemia patients: Data from a pilot study, *Cancer Nursing* 21(6):385-393, 1998.

McNally JC: Home care. In Baird S, McCorkle R, Grant M, eds: *Cancer nursing,* ed 2, Philadelphia, 1996, WB Saunders.

Mishel MH: Perceived uncertainty and stress in illness, *Research in Nursing and Health* 7(3):163-171,1984.

Mishel MH: Uncertainty in illness, *Image—The Journal of Nursing Scholarship* 20(4):225-232, 1988.

Morse SL, Fife B: Coping with a partner's cancer: Adjustment at four stages of the illness trajectory, *Oncology Nursing Forum* 25(4):751-760, 1998.

O'Connor A, Wicker C, Germino B: Understanding the cancer patient's search for meaning, *Cancer Nursing* 13(3):167-175, 1990.

O'Rourke M, Germino B: Spousal caregiving across the prostate cancer trajectory, *Quality of Life: A Nursing Challenge* 6(3):66-72, 1998.

Pasacreta J, McCorkle R: Psychosocial aspects of cancer. In McCorkle R et al, eds: *Cancer nursing,* Philadelphia, 1996, WB Saunders.

Penman DT et al: The impact of mastectomy on self-concept and social function: A combined cross-sectional and longitudinal study with comparison groups, *Women & Health* 11(3/4):101-130, 1986.

Penman DT et al: Predictors of strain in families of cancer patients: A review of the literature, *Journal of Psychosocial Oncology* 10(2):1-26, 1992.

Sales E, Schulz R, Biegel D: Predictors of strain in families of cancer patients: A review of the literature, *Journal of Psychosocial Oncology* 10(2):1-26, 1992.

Steinheiser MM: Vascular access device choices for home care patients, *Caring* 14(5):14-26, 1995.

Stoll B: Perimenopausal weight gain and progression of breast cancer precursors, *Cancer Detection and Prevention* 23(1):31-36, 1999.

Strauss AL: *Chronic illness and the quality of life,* St Louis, 1984, Mosby.

Tarzian A, Iwata P, Cohen M: Autologous bone marrow transplantation: The patient's perspective of information needs, *Cancer Nursing* 22(2):103-110, 1999.

Tornberg JM, McGrath BB, Benoliel JQ: Oncology transition services: Partnerships of nurses and families, *Cancer Nursing* 7(2):131-137, 1984.

Walker AJ, Pratt CC, Eddy L: Informal caregiving to aging family members: A critical review, *Family Relations* 44:402-411, 1995.

Weisman AD, Worden JW: The existential plight in cancer: Significance of the first 100 days, *International Journal of Psychiatry in Medicine* 7(1):1-15, 1976-1977.

Wynder E: The past, present, and future of the prevention of lung cancer, *Cancer Epidemiology, Biomarkers & Prevention* 7(9):735-748, 1998.

Zahlis EH, Lewis FM: Mothers' stories of the school-age child's experience with the mother's breast cancer, *Journal of Psychosocial Oncology* 16(2):25-43, 1998.

ADDITIONAL READINGS

American Cancer Society's *A Cancer Source Book for Nurses* is edited by Claudette Varricchio with Margaret Pierce, Carolyn Walker, and Terri Ades. This book is now in its seventh edition, and every nurse in home care working with cancer clients should obtain it.

American Cancer Society's *American Cancer Society Textbook of Clinical Oncology,* now in its second edition, is available from local offices of the American Cancer Society or by calling 1-800-ACS-2345.

CA: A Cancer Journal for Clinicians publishes every 2 months and is a journal of the American Cancer Society. This is an excellent journal and is free of charge from local offices of the American Cancer Society.

Cancer Practice, a multidisciplinary journal, contains articles of relevance to practitioners in all disciplines.

Cancer Nursing is an excellent clinical journal, and each home care office should have a subscription to it.

Journal of Pediatric Oncology Nursing is good if your agency is dealing with pediatric cancer clients.

Oncology Nursing Forum, the official journal of the Oncology Nursing Society, will assist home care nurses to keep up with the latest advances in cancer nursing care.

21 Stroke

Sandra MacKay

Stroke, the leading cause of long-term disability among adults in many industrialized countries, including the United States, is also one of the most challenging health care problems that nurses face. Each year, about 550,000 people in the United States have strokes, and about a third of them die. This means that a person has a stroke every minute, and a stroke kills someone every 3.7 minutes (American Heart Association [AHA], 1996). Although the United States has achieved one of the lowest mortality rates from cerebrovascular accidents (CVAs) in the world, stroke still ranks third as a cause of death—right after heart disease and cancer. This is comparable to stroke mortality rates in other industrialized nations. Despite long-term declines in stroke mortality in Japan (Tanaka et al, 1982), France (Alperovitch et al, 1986), Great Britain (Alfredsson, von Arbin, de Faire, 1986), Sweden (Terent, 1988) and several other nations (Thom, 1993; Feigin, Wiebers, Whisnant, 1994), cerebrovascular diseases (mainly stroke) are the third most common cause of death in most of the developed world (Bloom, Fineberg, 1997).

Both the economic and human costs of stroke are enormous. In 1993, the American Heart Association estimated the direct and indirect costs for stroke in the United States to be around $18 billion (AHA, 1993a). However, in May 1994, the National Stroke Association presented findings from the most comprehensive study ever undertaken on the economic burden of stroke indicating that it cost the nation $30 billion that year (Chaney, 1995; Matcher, 1997). These costs are over $40.9 billion now (Taylor et al, 1996; Wein, Hickenbottom, Alexandrov, 1998). Almost half of the total goes to direct medical costs, including hospitalization, physician fees, rehabilitation services, nursing home services, and equipment. The remainder is consumed by indirect costs, such as lost production (Chaney, 1995).

RISK FACTORS AND PREVENTION

Although strokes can occur in children and adolescents, as well as in adults (Savoiardo, 1986; Szmanda et al, 1994), there is a steep increase in the incidence of stroke with advancing age (Roper, 1982; Rosenwaike, Yaffe, Sagi, 1980). After the age of 55, stroke incidence rates double with every successive decade of life (AHA, 1996), and this trend is found in both men and women (Wolf, Kannel, McGee, 1986). The toll on blacks is great. Particularly, heavy blacks are twice as likely to have a stroke as whites, and they are twice as likely to die from strokes (National Stroke Association [NSA], 2000). Currently, there are more than 4 million Americans who have had one or more strokes (NSA, 2000), and many of them have long-term disabilities that make them dependent on assistance from their families and the health care system. Follow-up data from the Framingham Study indicates that 20% of stroke survivors require help walking, 31% need help caring for themselves, 70% still have impairment in their vocational abilities 7 years after the stroke, and 18% are institutionalized (AHA, 1996).

For years, the number of new cases of stroke and the stroke hospitalization rates did not fluctuate very much. However, the incidence of stroke seems to be increasing again, particularly

Acknowledgments: This chapter is based on randomized clinical trials of stroke rehabilitation conducted by the author in New Hampshire and Vermont as Principal Investigator for HSR&D Grants 596A and 016, awarded by the Research and Development Service of the Veterans Administration, Washington, DC.

in people who have underlying heart disease (Broderick et al, 1989; Whisnant et al, 1993; Wolf, D'Agostino, 1993). Atherosclerotic lesions (thickened and hardened lesions within the innermost layer of medium and large muscular and elastic arteries) are responsible for most cases of myocardial and cerebral infarction, since they can become so large they occlude the vascular supply to tissue in the area (Ross, 1996). Older people are not the only ones at risk.

The risk of developing heart disease in younger men and women is very high. According to the January 7, 1999, press release by the National Heart, Lung, and Blood Institute, one of every two men and one of every three women age 40 or younger will develop coronary heart disease unless they take immediate steps to reduce their risks. The major risks for stroke and heart disease are basically the same: e.g., diabetes, elevated cholesterol levels, hypertension, cigarette smoking, and lack of exercise (Easton, 1995). Nurses can address both of these diseases at the same time.

DEFINITION AND PHYSIOLOGICAL ASPECTS

The term *stroke* refers to the clinical symptoms that result from an infarction. To understand the mechanism of such an injury, the general characteristics of the affected area must be appreciated. A stroke damages the central nervous system, the main function of which is to integrate and respond to information from inside and outside the body. This system contains two parts: the brain and the spinal cord. Both are made up of soft, delicate tissue protected by cerebrospinal fluid and fibrous membranes. Externally, these structures are well protected by the bones of the skull and the vertebral column. The brain itself lies almost totally enclosed in the bony cavity of the skull and is connected to the spinal cord through a small opening in the base of the skull called the *foramen magnum*. Although these protective structures help prevent considerable trauma to the brain and spinal cord, they make the central nervous system extremely vulnerable to internal increases in volume and pressure. A stroke can occur anywhere in the central nervous system, although those involving the spinal cord are very rare; most strokes affect the brain (Buchan, Barnett, 1986).

Ischemia

Because the brain has no oxygen or glucose reserves of its own, it is highly sensitive to changes in its blood supply. Normally, regulatory mechanisms inside and outside the brain ensure that the brain receives a stable supply of oxygen and the other supplies it needs to maintain normal cerebral metabolism. However, if there is a disruption in blood flow and thus in the oxygen and blood glucose level in the central nervous system, such safety mechanisms cannot maintain a stable environment for very long (Mauro, 1996). Numerous studies indicate that each minute of ischemia is harmful to neurons at normal body temperatures. As Alberts (1997) notes in his review of the current state of knowledge regarding changes that occur after an ischemic stroke, such cerebral dysfunction may be reversible if the ischemia is of brief duration and is not very extensive. The brain can also withstand hours of insult if an adequate blood supply is maintained. However, if the blood flow is poor, the brain may not be able to withstand ischemia for more than a few minutes before infarction occurs. "Diminished cerebral blood flow triggers a cascade of events that includes defective protein synthesis, increased lactate production, glutamate release, depletion of adenosine triphosphate (ATP) stores, and calcium influx into cells" (Alberts, 1997).

Transient Ischemic Attack Versus Stroke

Both the duration and degree of cerebral ischemia are crucial in understanding the pathophysiology of a stroke. In some conditions, the cerebral ischemia is transient, whereas in others it is permanent. In a transient ischemic attack (TIA), the neurological deficit is often mild, and resolution of the focal ischemia occurs within 24 hours (Pulsinelli, 1996). In situations such as this, the client may have weakness or numbness in an arm that goes away in an hour. Or the client may experience numbness of one side of the face or one side of the body that resolves in a couple of hours. Such TIAs should always be medically evaluated to afford clients the best chance of preventing a full-blown stroke.

The National Stroke Association (NSA) Consensus Statement (1993) recommends that surgical intervention be considered if the cerebral ischemia resolves within the first 6 hours after the onset of symptoms. If there is carotid stenosis with arterial lumen blockage of more than 70%, an endarterectomy on the side causing the symptoms may reduce the risk of having a future stroke. In addition to TIAs, there are ischemic conditions that last longer than a day. A reversible ischemic neurological deficit (RIND) may last from 24 to 48 hours and then resolve in clients with lacunar or small-vessel strokes (Mauro, 1996). Lacunar strokes generally occur in the tiny vessels rather than perfuse areas deep within the brain. Microatheroma in these arteries are thought to cause stenosis and tiny holes in the brain, especially in the motor pathways and thalamus (Bronstein, Popovich, Stewart-Amidei, 1991).

When the ischemia persists for more than 24 hours and progresses to infarction with necrosis and permanent loss of brain tissue, the person is said to have had a stroke (Pulsinelli, 1996). Typically, such ischemic changes result in severe neurological dysfunction and extensive disability, if not death.

Major Causes of Stroke

Strokes are classified by how they develop. The two most important types result from occlusion or hemorrhage. Occlusive strokes can be caused by either thrombi or emboli. Hemorrhagic strokes are usually due either to an intracerebral hemorrhage or to a subarachnoid hemorrhage from an arterial aneurysm or an arteriovenous anomaly. Occlusive strokes account for 80% of all strokes (Mauro, 1996), but the 20% that are hemorrhagic (intracerebral and subarachnoid) are more life threatening. Hemorrhagic strokes usually begin without any warning while the person is active, then evolve over the course of a day. Astute clinical observations by nurses are vital in such cases, since there may be some question about when surgical intervention is needed (Sutin, 1986; Hornig, Dorndorf, Agnoli, 1986). According to Pulsinelli (1996), only 5% of strokes can be seen on computed tomographic (CT) scans that are done within the first 12 hours; 50% take 24 to 48 hours to become visible while 90% show up on CT scans in a week.

Completed Versus Progressive Strokes

A *completed stroke* is defined as one that is no longer evolving, as determined by both temporal and anatomical criteria. If there has been a stable neurological deficit of the carotid system for 24 hours or of the vertebrobasilar system for 72 hours, then the temporal criteria have been met (Green, 1986; Reeves, 1981). Any spontaneous return of neurological function is believed to be the result of decreased cerebral edema, the presence of collateral circulation to injured tissue, or the brain's use of alternative pathways in the same or the opposite hemisphere to compensate for its impaired function (Hier, 1986; Reeves, 1981). If the affected vascular territory has not been completely involved, additional brain cells are at risk of further ischemia unless treatment is started promptly (Pulsinelli, 1996).

The anatomical criteria for a completed stroke are met when the entire blood supply to a region is interrupted. Such lesions can occur deep within the brain, as well as on its surface (Zulch, 1981). Once cells have died, there is no effective way to reverse this process; subsequent treatment is aimed at reducing the cerebral edema and metabolic disturbances that follow the acute destructive lesion and compound its damage. A stroke is considered complete once neurological function has stabilized.

A *progressive stroke* refers to one that evolves over several hours to a week after the first symptoms. Such worsening of a stroke over time is fairly common, and progressive strokes are believed to occur in 20% to 35% of all hospitalized stroke clients (Bronstein, Popovich, Stewart-Amidei, 1991). The distinction between complete and incomplete strokes is seldom clear at the onset of a stroke, and Pulsinelli (1996) notes that clinicians often use the severity of functional loss (e.g., hemiplegia versus hemiparesis) as a basis for distinguishing this.

If there has been a gradual decrease in the blood supply to the affected area of the brain over a long enough period, there may have been time for collateral circulation to develop, which can protect neural cells in that area. Such collateral circulation increases the supply of oxygen to depressed neural tissues in marginal areas and often improves function over several days. However, this does not mean that no further damage will occur or that the stroke has been completed (Sutin, 1986).

Although strokes can affect any part of the brain, they often involve the cerebrum, which is the largest area. This area consists of a right and a left hemisphere connected by the corpus callosum.

Injury to one side of the brain generally produces defects on the opposite side of the body, owing to contralateral organization of the nervous system. Since each hemisphere is specialized, there are particular types of problems with left versus right hemispheric damage. For instance, impairment of the left cerebral hemisphere often produces weakness or paralysis on the right side of the body and can profoundly disrupt a person's ability to communicate with others. This occurs because 99% of right-handed people have most of their language control located in their left cerebral hemisphere, as do many left-handed people (Valenstein, 1981). For a more elaborate discussion of hemispheric function, the reader should refer to the research-based discussions provided by Bronstein, Popovich, and Stewart-Amidei (1991) and to the literature on split-brain research.

Consensus Statement on Stroke

In 1993, the NSA initiated a major effort to educate the public to respond to a stroke as an emergency and to support health care professionals in treating CVAs like other potentially life-threatening events. In line with this, NSA cosponsored a consensus statement by the American Academy of Neurology, American Association of Neurological Surgeons, American Society of Neuroimaging, Congress of Neurological Surgeons, International Stroke Society, and National Institute of Neurological Disorders to outline the evaluation and treatment of stroke within the first 6 hours (NSA, 1993). The panel focused on the first 6 hours because this was considered a feasible goal for clients to seek emergency treatment and yet was within the window of opportunity thought to be needed for successful therapy at that time (Alberts, 1997).

However, after publication of the National Institute of Neurological Disorders and Stroke rt-PA Stroke Study Group's findings (1995), many felt that 6 hours was too long. Intravenous tissue plasminogen activator (t-PA) was shown to reverse the effects of ischemic strokes in many clients, but it had to be administered within the first 2 to 3 hours after the onset of an acute ischemic stroke to work (Alberts, 1997). Unfortunately, by the time most clients were evaluated for stroke, this window of opportunity had closed. Since then, efforts have intensified to ed-

ucate health providers and the public that a stroke is a "brain attack," and treatment needs to be administered immediately in the nearest emergency department, just as it would be for someone with a heart attack. Although t-PA can be dangerous if it is given too late or to an inappropriate client, for the first time there is a drug to treat acute strokes in situations in which clinicians would otherwise be helpless (Grotta, 1997). When this drug is effective, it reduces the physical and cognitive deficits resulting from untreated strokes by about 30%.

When clients with symptoms of neurological dysfunction arrive in the emergency department, brain imaging can help to identify strokes, as opposed to subdural hematomas, neoplasms, and other conditions. A CT scan without contrast is needed to determine whether the stroke is hemorrhagic or ischemic. If the stroke is ischemic, the client should be kept in bed with the head of the bed flat to promote greater blood flow to the brain. By contrast, if the client has had a hemorrhagic stroke, the head of the bed should be raised 30 degrees and the client's head kept elevated to decrease congestion of the cerebral vessels and promote effective venous drainage (Bronstein, Popovich, Stewart-Amidei, 1991).

Time from Symptom Onset to Treatment

Jorgensen et al (1996) found that the milder the initial symptoms of a stroke were, the longer people delayed seeking treatment. Data from the Duke University/Durham Veterans Hospital Stroke Center registry indicate that less than half of all clients suffering from acute strokes (42%) come for treatment during the first 24 hours after the onset of symptoms; 25% arrive within 48 hours, and the rest do not come until after 48 hours (Alberts, Bertels, Dawson, 1990). A review of the recent literature on the time lapse between the first symptoms of a stroke and evaluation by a neurologist indicates that such delays are frequent in other medical centers as well (Alberts, 1997). Moreover, even clients who are already hospitalized in major medical centers, such as Yale and Duke, have been found to have delays averaging 2.5 hours between the onset of their symptoms and the time that they were evaluated. Such delays were much longer on some medical-center services than others. For instance, the median delay was only 30 minutes for clients hospitalized on the neurology service, but it was 20.5 hours for clients hospitalized on the surgical service at the same medical center (Alberts, 1997).

Until recently, delays such as these did not make any real difference in clinical outcomes because so little could be done for clients who had ischemic strokes. However, this is no longer the case. Early intervention and evaluation by a neurologist greatly increase stroke clients' chances for survival and decrease their length of hospitalization. CT scans, magnetic resonance imaging (MRI), arteriography, and ultrasonography all help pinpoint the extent and location of lesions, whereas neuroprotective agents, administered at the most efficacious time, reduce the insult to the brain. Placement of intravascular stents in stenosed carotid arteries is also increasingly used to prevent strokes from happening (Alberts, 1997; Iyer et al, 1996). Thus it is very important for nurses to respond to strokes as emergencies and to take steps to ensure prompt treatment of all strokes.

Focus on Prevention

According to a recent Gallop poll, 85% of Americans cannot identify the warning signs of a stroke, 80% are unaware of the risk factors for developing a stroke, and 76% do not even know what a stroke is (Alberts, 1997). This lack of information about stroke was even greater among African-Americans in this sample; 90% were unaware of the early symptoms of stroke, and 85% did not know the risk factors for developing a stroke, even though the incidence and mortality rates for stroke are particularly high in the black population.

In 1992 the mortality rate was 98% higher for black men who had had strokes than for white men, and it was 77% higher for black women than for white women (AHA, 1996). Information about such risk factors is of the utmost importance in stroke prevention and treatment for all clients, but especially those at high risk. This is a public health problem in which nurses can play major roles in reaching out to groups at risk and teaching them to take active steps to control their weight, avoid smoking, be physically active, eat heart-healthy meals, and keep their cholesterol, blood glucose, and blood pressure within normal limits. People who have diabetes are 2 times more likely to die from a stroke as those without diabetes. Being older and overweight and using too much salt are known to increase the risk of developing high blood pressure, and people with uncontrolled hypertension are 7 times more likely to have a stroke than those with normal blood pressure (Hernandez, Gazzaniga, 1996).

Primary and secondary prevention of stroke is far more effective than treatment and is also less costly. The average cost is $15,000 per person, just during the first 90 days after stroke; and for 10% of these people, costs exceed $35,000 (NSA, 2000). The chances of having a stroke can be reduced by making relatively modest changes in lifestyle (Wolf et al, 1988). Smoking increases the risk of having a stroke in men by 40% and in women by 60% (Hernandez, Gazzaniga, 1996), so nurses should educate clients on effective ways to quit smoking. Engaging in regular physical activity, on the other hand, not only decreases the likelihood of having a stroke, but it also beneficially modifies other risks associated with stroke, including hypertension, obesity, high lipid levels, and insulin resistance (Szmanda et al, 1994), so this should be encouraged. Unfortunately, American men, women, and children are becoming more sedentary. If all Americans remained at the appropriate weight for their age, height, and frame, it is estimated that there would be 35% fewer strokes a year (Hernandez, Gazzaniga, 1996).

Box 21-1 lists risk factors that have been associated with the development of stroke documented by the Hypertension Detection and Follow-up Program Cooperative Group (1982), the National Stroke Association Consensus Statement (1993b), Szmanda et al (1994), Petitti et al (1996), Hernandez and Gazzaniga (1996), and Kernan et al (2000). However, nurses should be aware that even those who make changes in their life styles can still have strokes (American Heart Association, 1993b), as can those who have no known risk factors (American Heart Association, 1996). The more risk factors a client has, the more likely he or she is to have a stroke. To improve outcomes, nurses should make every effort to educate the public about stroke symptoms and encourage people to seek care in the nearest emergency department immediately if they suddenly experience any of the early warning signs of a stroke (Box 21-2).

Box 21-1 Major Risk Factors for a Stroke

Heart disease
Hypertension
Diabetes
Acquired immunodeficiency syndrome (AIDS)
Sickle cell disease
Previous ischemic stroke
TIAs
Carotid stenosis
Cigarette smoking
Migraine headaches
Use of high-estrogen oral contraceptives
Use of diet, cough, and cold pills containing
  phenylpropanolamine
Serum cholesterol level greater than 200 mg/l
Recent drug abuse, particularly heroin and crack
  cocaine
Low socioeconomic status
Advanced age
African-American ethnic background
Family history of ischemic stroke

Box 21-2 Warning Signs of a Stroke

- Sudden weakness or numbness of the face, arm, or leg, especially on one side of the body
- Sudden difficulty seeing in one or both eyes or trouble seeing all parts of the visual fields
- Sudden confusion or trouble speaking or understanding
- Sudden severe headache, which may cause vomiting
- Sudden difficulty walking, standing, or maintaining normal coordination and balance
- Sudden decrease in ability or loss of ability to read, write, or use numbers
- Sudden difficulty pronouncing words clearly, using the tongue, or swallowing

---

Seeking treatment while a client is alert and oriented is vital. Higher levels of consciousness are associated with much better chances for survival in all stroke clients, but particularly in those with hemorrhages. If the client is on aspirin or other anticoagulants at home and there are signs of increased drowsiness, the nurse should withhold these medications and have the client evaluated in the emergency department. Home care

nurses also need to recognize that secondary hemorrhages can occur any time during the first few weeks of recovery from a stroke caused by an infarction and that this can be a life-threatening event at home.

HEALTH HISTORY AND PHYSICAL ASSESSMENT

Nurses are usually the ones who triage clients in an emergency department. While doing a nursing assessment of a stroke client, it is important to take a careful history from those who accompanied the client to the emergency department and inquire about the time of onset of any neurological deficits that have been observed, their anatomical location, and the course of these symptoms. Evidence of a headache, seizure, or change in the client's level of consciousness, as well as any concurrent problems and history of recent trauma, infection, and substance abuse, should be documented. Clients with hypertension, diabetes, cardiac disease, sickle cell disease, and acquired immunodeficiency syndrome (AIDS) should be assessed for symptoms of a stroke. Likewise, nurses should inquire about medications taken and the use of illicit drugs, such as heroin or cocaine, within the previous 24 hours, since the use of such drugs places clients at greater risk for ischemic and hemorrhagic strokes. The age, ethnicity, and gender of the client also have important implications. Women take 46% longer to seek care than men, and once in the emergency department, wait 49% longer to be seen. Black women have the highest rate of stroke in populations including whites and Hispanics (NSA, 2000).

Discharge Planning

While it is beyond the scope of this chapter to discuss the acute care of stroke clients in detail, the nurse's role in the hospital setting has been recently reviewed by Mower (1997). Clearly, hospital staff are under increasing pressure from managed-care organizations to discharge clients very early in the course of their illness, so it is important to begin discharge planning as soon as the client is stable. This means that stroke clients may be very ill when they are evaluated for discharge. However, whether the client is assessed by a nurse who has been providing daily care at the bedside or by a nurse who has been assigned discharge planning responsibilities for clients throughout the hospital, a comprehensive evaluation of the stroke client's nursing needs must be done before the client leaves the hospital. This should follow the general discharge planning principles outlined elsewhere in this text.

In planning services, nurses need to work with physical therapists, occupational therapists, nutritionists, social workers, neurologists, pharmacists, and family members so that all of the therapy can be continued at home and any needed supplies and equipment are available when the client is discharged. Many stroke survivors who need home care services may not be capable of returning to their previous occupations or will need to take on less-demanding work if they are able to return to work at all. If a client wants to return to work, a vocational counselor should be involved early in the rehabilitation process and made a member of the home care team. If the client is not going directly home from the hospital, but is being discharged to a stroke-rehabilitation facility or nursing home, the discharge plans should accompany the client to this facility.

Assessment before discharge Since no two strokes are exactly alike, the clinical assessment of the individual at the bedside is especially pertinent in making realistic discharge plans for stroke clients. In some hospitals clients have been referred for discharge home while they still have problems swallowing and handling their secretions without choking, still need tube feedings and frequent suctioning, and still have to master a walker or wheelchair. It would be a rare family who could take a stroke client home in this condition and safely manage his or her care without the assistance of a home care nurse, speech therapist, physical therapist, and home health aide.

Discharge planners will need to gather information about the client's neurological problems, as well as data about the degree of progress that is being made in physical therapy and other types of therapy. The bedside nurse and dietitian can provide valuable insight into the client's adjustment to daily routines, including any problems in eating, cutting up food, maintaining good oral hygiene, and doing other self-care activities. The speech therapist can provide suggestions for clients who are having difficulty swallowing, as well as understanding and using language. In some medical settings, the client's neurological

findings will be readily available in the client's chart. In other situations, these may be elsewhere, and the nurse will need to know how to take a history and conduct a brief neurological assessment to plan comprehensive follow-up care at home. The appendix contains a brief neurological evaluation developed by the author and her colleagues to assess aphasic stroke clients who were living in community settings. Findings from this and the other tests that were administered (MacKay et al, 1988) revealed that many elderly stoke clients who were living at home or in nursing homes were socially isolated and very severely impaired 2 years after their strokes. The burden of their care fell to caregivers who had not received adequate training to handle problems of this magnitude. Most of these caregivers were women, as is true for 72% of stroke survivors (NSA, 2000). Further instructions for conducting a neurological examination and taking a history after stroke can be found in Mauro (1996) and in neurology textbooks.

Mental status, insight, and judgment The neurological assessment in the appendix begins with a test of the client's mental status. Clients who have had strokes may fluctuate in their level of consciousness. To evaluate the mental status of a stroke client, the nurse should check to make sure that the client is not sleeping and then attempt to greet the client by name. While the nurse is attempting to make contact with the client, he or she should note whether the client is alert, lethargic, stuporous, or even comatose.

Alert clients will be aware of the nurse's presence and will be responsive to it. If clients cannot talk because of aphasia, they may still understand some of what is said. This may be revealed by the fact that their eyes focus on what the nurse says or does. Lethargic clients can be aroused to an alert state but will soon seem drowsy. Stuporous clients will be much more difficult to arouse and will seem very dull and sluggish even when responding. Comatose clients cannot be awakened, and their level of consciousness may be so depressed that there is no response to even deep pressure, pin pricks, or other painful stimuli.

Alert clients may be able to be cared for at home; however, this will depend on many other factors. If clients are able to talk, the nurse can learn a great deal about their ability to recall past events, their level of understanding, and their capacity for concentrated effort by taking brief family or work histories. Clues to their insight and judgment can be obtained by asking about their ability to perform a variety of routine chores and the implications of any difficulties they may experience in particular areas.

The amount of supervision needed at home will depend on clients' abilities to perform self-care activities in a safe manner. Clients with right-hemispheric lesions may have very poor judgment and a great deal of difficulty planning and carrying out activities. Hence, they may act in impulsive ways and be unable to modify their behavior even when they know that it is wrong.

Communication problems If there is damage to the left hemisphere, clients may have problems speaking, reading, writing, using numbers, following directions, and understanding what is said. To evaluate such clients, the nurse will need to listen very carefully to how clients talk. This is not easy to do with aphasic clients and requires considerable practice, since the early manifestations of certain types of aphasia can be so odd they are mistaken for dementia or psychosis. Home care nurses may find it helpful in their work with adults with speech and language disorders to incorporate some of the exercises that have been developed by visiting nurses into their evaluation process (Kilpatrick, Jones, 1977).

If a client who is not hard of hearing appears to have difficulty with normal conversational speech, it will be necessary to adjust speech to a much slower pace and to use short and simple sentences when talking with him or her. If there has not yet been a referral to a speech pathologist for a formal evaluation of the client's speech and language function, such a referral should be initiated through the proper medical and nursing channels.

Before the nurse can assess vision, hearing, speech, and other functions in a client whose stroke has affected the language system, the nurse will need to be sure that the client can indicate "yes" and "no" when asked, either verbally or nonverbally by nodding. If the client's nonverbal responses are reliable, they can be used in carrying out other parts of the neurological evaluation. The next sections (see appendix) cover assessing the client's orientation to time, place, and person, ability to name and use objects, and ability to comprehend both written and verbal instructions.

Although a detailed account of aphasia is beyond the scope of this chapter, the nurse should be familiar with the major syndromes that interfere with language use in stroke clients. In Broca's aphasia, which is the most common type of aphasia resulting from stroke, the lesion is in the anterior part of the language area of the brain, and the client's speech is very terse and impoverished. Clients who suffer from this type of aphasia may be able to say only a few words or make only a limited number of sounds. For example, the client may say "da, da, da" in answer to all of the nurse's questions. The ability to read, write, and use numbers may also be impaired. Nevertheless, the client may still be able to understand simple conversations about familiar subjects (Tonkonogy, 1986).

If the lesion is in the posterior area of the language zone of the brain, the impairment will be quite different. In Wernicke's aphasia, the client may produce meaningless words and phrases without being able to comprehend that he or she cannot be understood by others. There may also be unintelligible sounds pronounced as if they were words, difficulties naming objects, and an inability to understand simple questions or respond to simple commands. For many of these clients, reading, writing, drawing, and calculating are quite limited, if they are possible at all (Tonkonogy, 1986).

In global aphasia, the lesions involve both the anterior and posterior parts of the language area; consequently such clients are greatly impaired in their speech and communication abilities. This can result in an almost complete loss of speech, in addition to severe disturbances in comprehending, reading, writing, and using numbers (Tonkonogy, 1986).

Motor and sensory problems Independent performance of self-care activities is greatly facilitated by good muscle tone in both flexor and extensor muscle groups. Muscle strength in both arms and legs can be evaluated by the nurse while the client is in bed. By having the client initiate complete range of motion against the nurse's attempt to provide resistance, any weakness or loss of function in an arm or leg will be easy to detect. A physical therapist should be able to provide further information about the client's ability to use his or her affected limbs and any spasticity that may interfere with his or her ability to maintain balance, walk, and climb stairs.

Nurses are likely to be aware of the client's degree of bowel and bladder control and any feeding, bathing, and grooming difficulties. The nurses will also know how well the client turns in bed and whether or not he or she can transfer from a bed to a chair without assistance. This information needs to be conveyed to the social worker well in advance of discharge if the family members will need any special equipment or devices to care for the client at home. If the client does not have good visuomotor coordination or the manual dexterity needed for eating and dressing, an occupational therapist should be involved in rehabilitation as well.

Evaluation of the sensory system will require the nurse to enlist the client's cooperation in the assessment of deficits. Clients with impaired sensation tend to do better when they receive equal stimulation on both sides of the body at once, since this helps them detect any loss of feeling or numbness on one side. To assess sensation in the face, the nurse can gently stroke both of the client's cheeks and ask the client to indicate whenever he or she detects any change in sensation or feeling on one side. If the client can indicate awareness of touch on the face, the nurse can proceed to assess sensory changes in the trunk and the extremities in the same manner. Any abnormalities in sensation, perception, or pain awareness should be noted and can include burning, tingling, and the inability to discriminate between hot and cold, as well as a diminished response to touch.

Visuospatial problems Injury to the right hemisphere of the brain is often associated with difficulties in visuospatial tasks. Commonly such clients have difficulties perceiving visual patterns in the environment, in identifying objects by touching and holding them, and in perceiving themselves as whole people. To illustrate, the client may not be able to find multicolored clothes that are left on a patterned bedspread, or he or she may forget to brush the teeth on the left side or ignore the left hand if it becomes caught in the spokes of the wheelchair. If asked to draw a picture of a man, the client may fail to complete the left side of the figure in the drawing. Or, if asked to draw the face of a clock, he or she may be able to get the sequence of numbers right but spatially organize them so poorly that they only go half or three fourths of the way around the clock. To plan for the safe care of a client like this at home, the discharge planner needs to be sure that caregivers have been taught how to cope with visuospatial deficits and know how to supervise the client during shaving, bathing, food preparation, and other activities in which injury is possible.

Family and community resources Just as clients vary in their abilities to cope with a stroke at home, so do families and community agencies. In general, the fewer the client's cognitive disabilities and the more independent he or she is in performing self-care activities, the easier it will be to help manage his or her care at home, although even so-called minor strokes can be major to the people who are involved. In line with this, not every new stroke client can or should be cared for at home.

Nurses may find it ethically unacceptable to participate in discharging a client to a home situation that they consider unsafe. For instance, the nurses may learn that a cognitively impaired client would be left alone during most of the day while the family works or that an older caregiver has a serious health problem that limits the amount of physical care that can be given to a paralyzed spouse.

When the family members want to take the client home and seem able to provide safe and adequate care, the discharge planner should be sure that family members have been taught how to provide all of the nursing care that will be needed. In addition to teaching clients what they need to know, such education should prepare family members to give any medications the client cannot take himself or herself, as well as inform them how to contact the agency when needed and who to call in an emergency. Family members also need to be taught what types of exercises are needed and how frequently they should be done to improve client function and how to set up a plan that enables them to provide daily care at home. Teaching provided to clients and family members needs to be reinforced soon after the client leaves the hospital to prevent them from feeling overwhelmed with all of the new demands that are being made on them.

Community referrals The community health care agency should be provided with a referral that includes information about the client's diagnosis, treatment, nursing care, and functional abilities (see appendix). This referral should contain information about the client's medications, diet, abilities to perform self-care activities, and any teaching that the client and his family have received. If special assistive devices or medical equipment have been ordered for the client, they should be listed on the referral form, along with the arrangements made for their delivery. It may also be necessary to have the social worker teach a spouse or another caregiver how to handle bills and insurance forms if these were formerly handled by the client. Such support can serve a very important role in helping many elderly caregivers adjust to their new roles and decrease the anxiety produced by the necessity of dealing with complex medical insurance forms.

CARE OF THE CLIENT WITH SPECIAL NEEDS

A comprehensive home care program for stroke clients should include provision of all levels of nursing care, as well as various services provided by physical therapists, social workers, occupational therapists, nutritionists, and home health aides. Physicians who are involved in the clinical care of the stroke client need to be kept informed of changes in the client's health status, and a good working relationship needs to be maintained among all of the health care providers. Use of a tool, such as that in the appendix, can be provided to the home health nurse to help monitor progress in the community.

Bed-Fast Client

Home care of the client who has had a recent CVA will differ depending on whether the client is confined to bed, is able to use a wheelchair, or is ambulatory. When the client is confined to bed, much of the nursing care needs to be aimed at managing conditions associated with paralysis and loss of neurological control, as well as at preventing any further functional impairment and increased dependence on others.

Stroke clients with diabetes and circulatory problems are particularly vulnerable to decubitus ulcers when they are confined to bed. However, all stroke clients are at risk for developing pressure sores if they are limited in their mobility because of any muscular weakness or paralysis. If they also have impaired sensation, they may not know when their skin has been subjected to excessive pressure and may lie on an elbow or a hip for so many hours that the circulation to the area is reduced. Some clients also lose the ability to perceive pain and to locate body parts in space and can sustain serious injuries by lying on sharp objects or by dangling their extremities over the edge of the bed for a long time.

If a client cannot roll over, the visiting nurse should teach a family member how to turn him or her from side to side and how to lift him or her in bed without dislocating the shoulders or causing any trauma to the skin. It is possible to maintain the integrity of the skin in even a paralyzed client by teaching the family to turn him or her every 2 hours, to use a water bed or an alternating pressure mattress, and to ensure that he or she receives excellent hygiene and nutrition every day.

Caregivers should learn how to check the client's skin while they are assisting with the bath so that any early signs of a pressure sore can be immediately treated. The onset of a pressure sore usually begins with redness at the affected site, before the skin is actually broken. If the skin has been exposed to too much pressure, it will blanch to white when it is pressed, then turn red when the pressure is released.

If nursing measures are taken to alleviate pressure immediately, there will be no further damage to the tissue. Otherwise, pressure sores can progress rapidly from injury to the superficial tissue, as evidenced by abrasion or blistering, to injury that extends through the full thickness of the skin and penetrates muscle and bone. These latter wounds take a long time to heal and often require surgical intervention to close.

Whenever the nurse shows a family member how to care for a client in bed, it is important to do so in a way that will foster future rehabilitation goals. For instance, if a hemiplegic client is ever to walk normally, family members must be shown how to position him or her in bed so that external rotation of the hips and foot drop are prevented. To promote greater flexibility in hip, knee, and ankle joints, they also need to do passive range-of-motion exercises every day.

Bowel and bladder care If the client is incontinent, special attention needs to be directed to bowel and bladder care. Feces and urine are very irritating to the skin, and meticulous care must be taken to cleanse the client after each episode of incontinence to prevent any skin breakdown. Preventing urinary retention and infection requires that urinary output be monitored and an adequate intake of fluid be encouraged. If the client's temperature is elevated or the urine is cloudy and foul smelling, a culture is indicated (Shpritz, 1996). If incontinence is a recurrent problem, a formal bowel and bladder retraining program should be initiated, because such a program can prevent further damage to the client's self-esteem and reduce the demands placed on caregivers.

Alterations in bowel habits are seldom due to the stroke (Geibel, Kubalanza-Sipp, 1986) and often result from changes in a client's level of physical activity, difficulties in making toileting needs known to others, and changes in diet. The most frequent change in bowel habits after a stroke is constipation (O'Brien, Pallet, 1978; Lal, 1986). This is seldom difficult to correct if the client can establish regular times for toileting. To instill new patterns of behavior, family members should be instructed to establish a convenient time for bowel training and to adhere to the same routine every day. After a meal, when the gastrocolic reflex has just been stimulated, may be a good time to help the client go to the toilet. If the client needs a great deal of assistance getting onto the bedpan, it may be advisable to use a fracture pan and trapeze. Additional fluid and fiber in the diet help establish more regular bowel habits. If the client was dependent on laxatives before the stroke, stool softeners or glycerine suppositories may be needed afterward as well (Lal, 1986). A further discussion of nursing research-based interventions that are useful in bowel training can be found in Bronstein, Popovich and Stewart-Amidei (1991). If the client is sent home with a catheter to control urinary incontinence, the nurse should review procedures for its care and insertion with both the client and family members. By placing the client on a schedule for fluid intake throughout the day, it will be easier to help him or her establish regular times for voiding once the catheter is removed. To prevent accidents while the client is being retrained, toileting opportunities must be offered at frequent intervals with a gradual extension of the length of time between them. These intervals should be based on the client's previous pattern of voiding and the quantity of urine voided. If there are

problems with incontinence at night, liquids may need to be restricted after the evening meal and more extensive training procedures adopted (Pallet, O'Brien, 1985; Geibel, Kubalanza-Sipp, 1986; Bronstein, Popovich, Stewart-Amidei, 1991).

Such bowel and bladder retraining programs are of the utmost importance in rehabilitation. If a client can overcome incontinence, he or she will be more motivated to resume contacts with people outside the family and to continue working toward greater independence in other aspects of life. Continued incontinence, despite such retraining programs, is not a good prognostic sign (Kaplan 1986; Owen, Getz, Bulla, 1995; Gross, 1998) and often means that caregivers will need to assume most of the responsibility for these tasks.

Nutrition To help the client maintain good nutrition, the home care nurse should review the diet and identify any problems encountered in eating. Elderly homebound clients, who are deprived of sunlight and are poorly nourished, are susceptible to vitamin D deficiency, which further increases their risks of fractures of the hip and other sites (Gloth, 1995). Although the ability to swallow usually improves with the passage of time, some clients continue to choke on water and regular food for several weeks or longer after a stroke. During this time, thick soups, puddings, and fruit juices will be easier to swallow than clear liquids.

Family members should be instructed in how to prevent clients from choking during their meals by having the clients lean forward and toward the unaffected side when swallowing. If a client cannot handle regular food because of problems using the tongue or other neurological deficits, the nurse can teach the family to blend the food to a consistency that will be easier to manage. If there are any doubts about a client's ability to eat enough to stay well nourished, the nurse should have him or her evaluated by a speech therapist and nutritionist before resorting to a feeding tube. If there are problems with eye-hand coordination, the nurse can help the client do more by encouraging the family to buy special utensils that will make feeding easier. Assistive devices such as a plastic plate with a curved side aids in getting food onto the fork. A special spoon with a large plastic handle that is easy to grip is inexpensive and can make eating much less frustrating for a client who is regaining fine motor skills.

If the client tends to neglect food that is on the left side of the plate, the visiting nurse can teach him or her simple procedures to follow during meals to compensate for various perceptual deficits. To illustrate, the nurse can teach a client with a visual-field loss to turn his or her head and scan the whole plate before beginning to eat and to repeat this movement before finishing each meal. Another aid is to have the caregiver put the most nutritious food on the right side of the client's plate.

Often a client with facial droop and loss of sensation on the affected cheek does not actually swallow all of the food that is taken into the mouth. Partially chewed food then collects along the inner aspect of the cheek without the client's knowledge. To prevent aspiration of this food, the nurse should teach the client to use the index finger to check for any food that may still remain in the mouth and to rinse the mouth thoroughly after eating a meal. The client's family should also be taught to monitor the client's weight on a frequent basis and to keep a food diary so that meals can be varied over time.

Client in a Wheelchair

Being confined to bed for long periods is not healthy for any client, and every effort should be made to encourage early ambulation with a wheelchair. This requires that a client be able to sit up for a few hours without becoming too fatigued or light headed.

Nurses can use a number of neurophysiological programs while the client is still in bed to increase his or her strength and functional mobility (Mills, Wustenev, 1986). These generally include exercises in which the client progresses from lying, to rolling over, to sitting in bed, to sitting with both legs dangling over the edge of the bed, to eventually transferring from the bed to a wheelchair as weight bearing and balance improve. These exercises are especially important during the first few months after a stroke, when much spontaneous recovery usually occurs.

To ensure that correct body alignment is maintained while the client is in a wheelchair and prevent contractures of the trunk and neck, the client should be taught to sit so that the spine is correctly aligned, with the lower spine against the back of the wheelchair and the hips and knees at right angles. To prevent subluxation of the shoulder and contractures of the involved arm and hand, the affected extremity must be supported in a functional position and exercised on a regular basis (Pallet, O'Brien, 1985; Lal, 1986). To prevent falls when transferring, wheelchairs must also be safely locked and the foot rests swung out of the way before clients attempt to move in or out of them. If the nurse thinks that the client is likely to neglect either arm, a mobile arm support can be used in the wheelchair to help maintain function in the extremity and to protect it from injury (Pallet, O'Brien, 1985).

To help the client increase muscle strength in both legs, the nurse should teach the client to use the wheelchair without the foot support so that it is propelled with his or her feet. This exercise helps build the endurance and coordination that will be needed later for walking. The wheelchair chosen by the client should also be suitable for use wherever the client lives. For example, if the client lives in a rural area and will be wheeled outside over a large expanse of grass, a wheelchair with all-terrain tires, rather than thin tires, will be much easier to push. Likewise, it is exhausting for caregivers to have to lift a wheelchair into the trunk of a car several times a day to take the client to various appointments or to go shopping, so family members may want to purchase a chair-holding device that can be attached via a welded boat-pull to the rear of their car. Such devices can be purchased for about $125 and used to hold a folded wheelchair securely in place while driving.

Dressing and grooming   When a client first begins to use a wheelchair, it may be so taxing to transfer in and out of bed that other types of teaching have to be postponed. However, as the nurse observes the client gaining confidence in his or her ability to get in and out of bed, it is important to share these observations and to encourage resumption of self-care activities such as dressing, eating, and grooming in the rooms that are normally designated for these purposes.

Using the skills the client has already been taught (i.e., to roll over in bed and to raise the hips off the mattress), the visiting nurse can teach the client to begin dressing all or part of himself or herself before getting out of bed. This task will be simpler if the family members are taught to select clothing that is easy for the client to manage. Excellent choices might be sweat pants with elastic waist bands and cotton shirts with short sleeves and buttons up the front, rather than clothing with buckles, zippers, ties, and long sleeves, all of which are difficult for clients who have any weakness in their fingers.

Weak or hemiplegic clients should be taught to follow routines in which they always dress the affected leg first. After the client has dressed the lower part of the body, he or she should sit on the edge of the bed to put on the rest of his or her clothes.

When putting on a shirt, it is important to dress the affected arm first. The client can be instructed to start buttoning the shirt from the bottom up, to see what he or she is doing and button it evenly. If the client has difficulty managing buttons with one hand, he or she may need to use an assistive device, such as a button hook, or to wear shirts that have been modified with Velcro fasteners to minimize the amount of assistance that is required.

If there is any difficulty with right and left discrimination, it may be necessary to have a colored tag sewn inside the garment on the affected side to remind the client which side to dress first. A dressing technique that some clients use is to put the shirt in the lap with the buttons facing down, then reach inside the bottom of the shirt with both hands and pull it up over the head. This technique is particularly useful when range of motion in the client's shoulders is limited.

Shoes can be hard for any older person to put on and may be especially difficult for a stroke client who is limited to the use of one hand. These will be easier to put on if the client sits on the edge of the bed with both feet on the floor so that the unaffected leg can be used to help stabilize himself or herself. If a client cannot reach his or her feet, he or she may need to use a shoehorn with a long handle to get his or her shoes on properly. If the client requires the support of laced shoes, it may be necessary to use elastic laces that can be tied by someone else ahead of time.

In general, the use of small snaps, buttons, hooks, and more complicated fasteners on clothing should be avoided since they can be frustrating, if not impossible, for a client to use without assistance. If belts, buckles, and zippers are used on pants, the client should adjust them while standing up at the bedside, before transferring to a wheelchair.

Expanding self-care skills Clients who are already experiencing success using a wheelchair in the bedroom will be better motivated to venture into other rooms for self-care activities. To help them resume their normal routines, clients should be carefully supervised while they are learning to safely use the bathroom for toileting and bathing. In some cases, it may be necessary to modify the tub, toilet, or sink to meet the needs of a particular person. Grab bars attached to the wall beside the toilet and in the shower stall can be very useful to stroke clients. Clients who are too unsteady to safely shower standing up may be able to wash themselves quite well if they have a bench to sit on in the tub or shower stall and can spray themselves with a flexible, hand-held shower head. If the client has an altered body image, he or she should be encouraged to include bilateral activities in grooming routines and to compensate for any losses in perception and sensation by checking his or her grooming in a mirror (Geibel, Kubalanza-Sipp, 1986).

In supervising such clients, the nurse should ensure that clients always test the temperature of the water in the bath or shower with the unimpaired hand to prevent any possibility of getting burned. If a client is impulsive, lacks good judgment, or has any problems remembering instructions, it will be necessary for caregivers to adjust the temperature of the water themselves and to remain with the client in the bathroom so that he or she does not get injured. Temperature regulators may also have to be installed to ensure safety for such clients.

The concept of providing the client with only as much assistance as is needed is central to rehabilitation and can be extended to meal times and other activities. For example, if the family usually eats meals at a table that is too low to accommodate the client's wheelchair, the height of the table can be raised with small wooden blocks under its legs so that the client is able to eat with the rest of the family and does not need to be served by them. However, the client's neuropsychological, motor, and sensory deficits will need to be considered in determining whether he or she should be allowed to cook, use sharp knives, or engage in various other types of kitchen work.

As soon as the client can use a wheelchair to perform a variety of daily activities in the home, he or she should be encouraged to go outdoors and practice these activities in other settings. To take a client outside on a regular basis, it may be necessary to install a ramp at one of the exits to the house. Such a ramp should be extremely gradual in slope and wide enough to accommodate the wheelchair. Usually such ramps are constructed with a nonskid surface and have railings on both sides so the ramp is safe to use during all types of weather. Clients should be taught to use their wheelchairs on flat surfaces before navigating ramps. Some may not be able to safely manage their wheelchairs alone on an incline.

Prevention of pressure sores while using a wheelchair Pallett and O'Brien (1985) cite a number of potential sources of skin breakdown that nurses should be aware of as clients become more mobile. These include any clothing that constricts the client, irritates him or her, or concentrates pressure from buttons, heavy seams, zippers, and other types of fasteners. Breakdown can also occur from failure to protect the client's skin under braces, casts, splints, prostheses, and other types of assistive devices. Shearing pressure on the buttocks from using a sliding board improperly for transfers is also dangerous, as are wheelchairs that have been poorly designed or improperly adjusted or that are otherwise inadequate for a particular client. Sagging wheelchair seats can be a major problem for clients with impaired sensations, since they concentrate pressure on vertebral bodies and on the sacrum against the ischial tuberosities instead of on the thighs. Nursing attention to these matters and the use of a gel cushion in the seat of the wheelchair and exercises to increase circulation to the affected areas are excellent means for preventing the development of pressure sores at this stage of rehabilitation.

Social interaction As clients learn to use their wheelchairs for longer periods, the home care nurse should help them plan social outings that will build confidence and prevent them from becoming depressed and house-bound. Responses to the brief neurological evaluation in the appendix can help the nurse predict some of the difficulties that clients will encounter in public settings and can be used in designing trips and activities that are appropriate for each client. For example, the nurse might need to teach certain aphasic clients to use gestures when they interact with others to help them communicate more effectively. It might be necessary to demonstrate where a client with a visual-field deficit should place his menu so he or she can read it more easily in a restaurant. Other clients may avoid going out in public and may need to learn techniques that can help them handle uncomfortable social situations, such as having to ask for assistance when needed and learning how to refuse help when it is not needed. As clients gain experience using their wheelchairs for social events, they may find themselves being pushed beyond their limits. If clients show signs of becoming either fatigued or frustrated, they should be encouraged to conclude the activity as soon as possible so that they are not taxed beyond their present abilities. They may also require brief naps.

Interventions that are planned around a client's individual needs can have a direct impact on the quality of everyday life now and in the future. If a client's early interactions with others go well after a stroke, relationships with people outside the family are more likely to be maintained. This can help to prevent much of the social isolation that is commonly seen in stroke clients.

Ambulatory Client

Walking is an activity that most stroke clients look forward to. Though clients with weakness in the lower extremities can usually learn to walk with a walker or a quad cane once they regain sufficient balance and coordination, walking can be much more difficult for the hemiplegic client because the muscles in the affected leg may go into spasm and be very difficult to control. However, with proper physical therapy, many of these clients can eventually learn to walk with a normal gait. As they are learning to walk, it is important for caregivers to know how to assist them without injuring themselves or the client. It may also be necessary to use other safety measures, such as having railings installed throughout the house, removing any scatter rugs and furniture that could cause an unsteady client to trip and fall, using a bedside commode, and ensuring that clients always turn on a light before attempting to get out of bed at night.

Once the client becomes fully ambulatory, rehabilitation shifts mainly to the psychosocial aspects of care. By this time, many of the physical skills have been taught, and it is now up to the client to maintain them. This can be difficult for a person who finds it boring to do the exercises that are needed to keep a foot from dragging or hand from contracting, particularly when he or she cannot feel the hand or foot. Nevertheless, such daily exercises are necessary if the client is to maintain or improve his or her present level of functioning.

PSYCHOSOCIAL AND CULTURAL ASPECTS

A stroke can be very frightening. In fact, some people say that having a stroke is much more frightening to them than having a heart attack or being diagnosed with terminal cancer. As one man said after caring for his physically and cognitively impaired wife, "A stroke is much worse because it is a condition in which you are alive without having the mental and physical abilities that make life worth living." Other psychosocial stresses arise from a stroke survivor's fear of becoming a burden and being left by a spouse or partner.

The nurse should recognize that a stroke is a socially stigmatizing condition. Indeed, some clients and family members still believe that having a stroke is a punishment from God. The earliest descriptions of stroke were generally pejorative. Hippocrates (460-370 BC), used the Greek term *apoplexy,* which means "struck by violence," to refer to a stroke. This was in line with an early belief that the "hand of God" struck such clients for their wrongdoing (Bronstein, Popovich, Stewart-Amidei, 1991).

To a family member who has no training in anatomy and physiology, there is no reasonable explanation for the continuing neurological deficits that are seen long after the acute, life-threatening event has passed. Thus, if a stroke client cries uncontrollably or swears, a lay person may begin to question the client's sanity. Should the client drool, yell, and look disheveled, he or she is likely to be labeled "senile." And, if the client can no longer speak intelligibly, dress properly, eat without spilling, and use the toilet independently, the client may be treated as if he or she had reverted back to childhood or become "crazy." For those who still consider a stroke a punishment from God for past wrongdoing, a stroke has very clear moral implications as well. Contemporary use of the term *stroke* reflects this early history, as does the notion that a stroke is somehow the result of a "shock" or "accident" (Bronstein, Popovich, Stewart-Amidei, 1991).

Clients in an intensive care unit have been found to have an overwhelming psychosocial need to feel safe and well cared for by nurses (Hupcey, 2000). Nurses who care for stroke clients and their families should recognize how a loss of cognitive abilities can affect care providers. For example, since the brain is culturally regarded as the organ separating humans from animals and plants, in much of contemporary American society there can be a loss of personhood when a stroke causes severe brain damage. Health workers may begin to refer to such a client as "a vegetable" as they try to distance themselves from someone who is so upsetting to care for. Nurses can decrease the likelihood of this by making sure that their own language affirms the client's human dignity, rather than making such remarks.

Since 1968, prompted by the need for organ transplants (Cranston, 2001), the brain has had increasing importance in law as well. A person ceases to be alive from both a medical and a legal standpoint once the clerical criteria for brain death have been met. Decisions about giving or withholding intravenous fluids, antibiotics, tube feedings, and other forms of treatment before brain death will be more difficult to make if the client has not completed an advance directive, such as a "durable power of attorney for health care" (DPAHC), before he or she is too incapacitated to do so (MacKay, 1992). An advance directive states the client's wishes about these matters, and also cultural and religious practices for handling the body, clothes, and burial.

FACTORS AFFECTING RECOVERY

Fortunately, most people who have a stroke survive. Although good motor and physical skills are important in their rehabilitation progress, they alone are not sufficient for a good recovery (Bleiberg, 1986). Psychosocial adjustment problems are common in both clients and families, and the severity of the emotional distress that is experienced is not always related to the severity of the client's physical disabilities (Lal, 1986). Lal cites the sudden nature of a stroke, the fear of becoming a burden to loved ones, the reactions of family members and friends, financial worries, and the loss of social status as key factors contributing to the psychosocial problems observed after a stroke.

Bleiberg (1986) includes a person's premorbid personality as a factor in predicting the way that person will react to a stroke and notes that clients who rely on "vigilant focusing" mechanisms to protect themselves from feeling vulnerable before they become ill often create difficulties for therapists because they have a strong need to take charge of their rehabilitation. To prevent undue frustration in caring for such people, nursing care plans should specify exactly what routines are to be followed each day. These can be established with the client as a partner in a manner that allows more than one caregiver to be involved in his or her care. This permits clients to regain control over their situations.

Over the years, several researchers have explored the behavioral consequences of particular types of lesions (Kertesz, 1979; Naesser et al, 1981; Allen, 1983), and a few have identified which deficits seem to impose the greatest hardships on clients over time. Among the most incapacitating deficits are denial of illness, body image disturbances, neglect of hemiparesis, spatial disturbances, memory deficits, motor perseveration, and inattentiveness (Bleiberg, 1986). With creativity, it is possible to design nursing interventions that address each of these disturbances. For example, ambulatory clients with body image disturbances can be instructed to practice their exercises in front of a mirror, using audiotapes that remind them to exercise the neglected extremity.

If the client has motor perseveration problems, the nurse can teach a family member when to interrupt the client and help him or her switch to a new task. To increase the likelihood that a client will be attentive during conversations, the home care nurse may encourage visitors to bring up topics related to his or her former hobbies and interests. If a client has such a short attention span that he or she cannot focus on any task for longer than a few seconds, the nurse can show caregivers how to talk the client through an activity. In this way, the client may be able to sustain interest in a task for longer than he or she would otherwise and gradually increase his or her attention span (Halper, Mogil, 1986).

Since increased attentiveness is one of the best predictors of future improvement (Olson, 1986), it is one of the most important areas for a nurse to address very early in the client's rehabilitation.

Even clients with a poor prognosis may be able to make substantial gains in their rehabilitation if a program directed to problems such as these is started soon enough (Lieberman, 1986).

The psychosocial impact of a stroke can be devastating for both clients and their families. Feelings of anxiety, anger, and fear are very common, as are worries about having another stroke and suffering even greater disabilities in the future. These worries may begin in the hospital but be exacerbated when clients go home, as it gradually dawns on them that they will have continuing limitations in their physical, cognitive, and language abilities. For example, clients may realize that they can no longer work in their previous occupations or that they are unable to drive a car, balance a checkbook, or play golf with their buddies and become very depressed about such losses.

Psychological changes also relate to the site of the lesion in the brain. Depression has been reported in about 70% of clients with lesions involving the right hemisphere (Folstein, Mailberger, McHugh, 1977; Lal, 1986) and is seen after particular types of left hemispheric damage as well (Price, 1986). If the symptoms of depression are not recognized by professionals, it is unlikely that clients will receive adequate treatment for this condition, and their ability to cooperate in their rehabilitation may be seriously compromised.

Depression is a serious problem for stroke clients and more attention needs to be devoted to the recognition and treatment of this condition (Goodstein, 1983; Lofgren, Gustafson, Nyberg, 1999), since depression in any client who is not adequately treated is very apt to recur. After one depressive episode, the risk of a recurrence is 50%; after two episodes, it is 70%; and after three episodes, it is 90% (Depression Guideline Panel, 1993). Current guidelines for treating depression in healthy adults emphasize the importance of continuing antidepressive medications for at least 6 months after the onset of an initial depression to prevent such a recurrence and of continuing medication for longer than that if the client has had one or more depressions in the past. Depressed stroke clients should be assessed for the risk of suicide through direct questioning. Those who have made prior suicide attempts, feel hopeless, live alone, are elderly, are Caucasian, and are male are at increased risk, as are those with a history of psychosis, substance abuse, and medical illness. However, clients who are at highest risk are those who have made specific plans to kill themselves. Such suicidal clients should be immediately evaluated by mental health professionals and may have to be admitted to a hospital (Depression Guideline Panel, 1993).

Other abnormal behavior during stroke rehabilitation needs to be addressed as well, since this has been associated with greater disability at discharge and 12 months later (Clark, Smith, 1999).

Family Life

Rehabilitation outcomes have been shown to improve when there is a spouse in the home and the client's disabilities do not cause other family members to withdraw from him or her (Lieberman, 1986; Geibel, Kubalanza-Sipp, 1986). The more families know about stroke, the better they will be able to cope. Strokes that occur in clients who are married often place strain on a spouse, who may be an elderly caregiver with chronic health problems too (Williams, Freer, 1986). Besides the stress placed on caregivers when there is a stroke in the family, there are often marital difficulties. Not infrequently, a stroke disrupts the couple's sexual life, and there is an abrupt decrease in the client's sexual desire. Usually this has more to do with psychosocial changes than with changes of a physical nature. If the nurse encourages the client to discuss any fears about engaging in intercourse, this may be all that is required if the client has limited sexual activities out of fear of having another stroke. Other couples need information about how to handle the motor and sensory changes that have taken place (Geibel, Kubalanza-Sipp, 1986).

All caregivers of stroke clients are at greater risk of depression, poor health, and decreased social contacts than noncaregivers, and their life changes can be specifically assessed by nurses using the Bakas caregiving outcome scale (Bakas, Champion, 1999). If a couple needs more help than the nurse can provide, the nurse should refer them to a therapist who has expertise in counseling handicapped people and their significant others. Some couples need help with parent-child relationships. Children may resent their parents' disabilities and be embarrassed to be seen with them in public. If there are teenagers living at home, they may try to deny there are any problems, refuse to discuss what has happened to their family, and avoid bringing their friends home.

The nurse can encourage family members to discuss their feelings about the changes that have taken place by raising questions about how each of them is managing. This will give family members permission to talk further if they need to, without pressing them if they do not wish to pursue the subject at the time. The nurse can also inform them of support services that are available to stroke clients and their families in the area where they live. One of the most valuable resources for many families is a support group in which they can meet other people who have faced similar difficulties. Generally clients feel more comfortable sharing experiences with clients who have had strokes themselves and find it improves their self-esteem to be able to help others.

Nurses who work with stroke clients may discover that some of them come from cultural groups that are very different from their own. In the case study that follows, the client is a Native American who grew up on a reservation. The nurse must be aware of healing practices that the client and her daughters might be using in conjunction with or instead of those that were prescribed in the hospital. Although it is beyond the scope of this chapter to discuss complementary health practices in detail, such healing practices are widespread in contemporary American society (Eisenberg et al, 1993; Elder, Gillchrist, Minz, 1997) and may or may not be congruent with the dominant culture's biomedical paradigm. For example, Navajos believe in living in harmony with nature and consider illness an imbalance. They place great value on group consensus and equity in relationships. Navajo clients may consult medicine men; use smudging with smoke and eagle feathers; use tobacco with their morning prayers; and participate in sweat lodge ceremonies involving fire, water, smoke, rocks, and herbs to help restore balance (Kim, Kwok, 1998.)

In a recent study of 300 Navajo clients who were being seen in ambulatory care clinics, it was learned that 39% had been using native healers regularly, even though they considered themselves compliant with the advice received from their conventional medical providers. Those clients who consulted native healers for depression and anxiety were much less likely to consult Western medical providers for these conditions, and they never consulted medical personnel for sickness, family problems, or bad luck. On the other hand, those who consulted native healers for arthritis and diabetes were likely to consult medical providers as well (Kim, Kwok, 1998). The following case study involves a Native American client who has difficulty following medical advice and is referred to home health care services.

SUMMARY

Stroke is a global health problem that places enormous burdens on a society. This chapter has focused on increasing nurses' knowledge of both stroke prevention and treatment. Over 4 million Americans have had a stroke, and many of them have continuing cognitive and physical disabilities that require assistance from nurses. This requires a high level of clinical skill and judgment

---

CASE STUDY
NAVAJO WOMAN WITH A STROKE

Patricia is a 63-year-old Navajo woman who lives with her daughters in a San Francisco apartment. She is a newly diagnosed stroke client with a history of type 2 diabetes and hypertension. Recently she fell, broke a bone in her right foot, and was admitted to the municipal teaching hospital, where the diagnosis of a stroke causing mild visuospatial problems was made. After treatment of Patricia's broken foot, her blood glucose levels and blood pressure were difficult to maintain within the normal range. A referral was made for home care because of inconsistent progress and lack of retention of educational information by the client and her two daughters.

Orem's self-care deficit theory (1991) was used in teaching the client and family, and specific cultural information about the family's health practices was obtained. Patricia has limited English, so a Navajo interpreter was used during all visits, rather than relying on a particular daughter to interpret.

The nurse purposefully included Patricia in the instructions so that she could assume greater responsibility for controlling her diabetes and hypertension, both of which are risk factors for subsequent strokes. Key nursing diagnoses were self-care deficit: related to perceptual alterations, cognitive defects; immobility related to foot and other risk factors: family; technical procedure: impairment: family; and emotional stability: potential impairment: family. During the initial visits, the home care nurse focused on the technical procedures and emotional support, since this was the area in which the family needed help most of all, but in which they had been noncompliant in the hospital.

NURSING DIAGNOSIS: TECHNICAL PROCEDURE: IMPAIRMENT: FAMILY

Definition: A state in which the family lacks appropriate information or is having difficulty applying it to

their family member's medical regimen (diet, exercise, medication administration, and blood testing)

Data collection:

Assess for the following:
1. *Education and reading level of mother and adult daughters*
2. *Mother's and daughters' understanding of the interaction of medication, diet, and physical therapy exercises on stroke*
3. *Techniques used for blood testing that are accurate and prevent infection*
4. *Techniques used for monitoring blood pressure*
5. *Degree of participation of the mother in bathing, grooming, toileting, and other self-care activities*
6. *Strategies daughters are using to encourage adherence to medical regimen*

Outcome identification

The mother and daughters will be able to safely manage medications, exercises, and testing procedures by the end of the first 3 weeks of home visiting.
1. *Proper techniques for blood testing and blood pressure checks will be used by the mother and daughters.*
2. *The prescribed medications, diet, and exercises will be followed to help restore balance in life.*

Plan

Home care will focus on the evaluation and clarification of information necessary for proper diabetes and hypertension management and control.

Implementation (secondary and tertiary)

1. *Use the assessment information in planning instructional materials.*

on the part of the nurse to be effective, but it can result in much better outcomes for clients and their families. Stroke already costs the United States more than $40.9 billion annually, and most of this goes to rehabilitation and long-term care. However, the damage that strokes do can be prevented by clients modifying their lifestyles to decrease stroke risks and obtaining treatment during the first 3 hours of a CVA. Nurses who are knowledgeable about the importance of seeking early treatment can be pivotal in educating the public about the early warning signs of a stroke and the need to go to an emergency department for state-of-the-art therapy. They can also collaborate with other professionals to provide comprehensive rehabilitation services and effective discharge planning for stroke clients and their families in the community.

CASE STUDY
NAVAJO WOMAN WITH A STROKE—cont'd

2. Include the following as needed:
   a. Basic etiology and pathophysiology of diabetes, hypertension, and stroke
   b. Proper storage of medications and timely ordering of refills
      Use of one- and two-step commands and visual cues to develop medication routines
   c. Use of blood glucose monitor
      Use of alcohol when the finger is pricked to check glucose level each morning
      Review of the importance of more frequent blood testing if there is dizziness or change in mental functioning
   d. Signs of hypoglycemia and hyperglycemia
   e. Dietary instruction adapted to cultural beliefs
   f. Development of an individualized plan for daily physical therapy exercises
3. Include the daughters in teaching sessions, showing them how to make healthy, culturally appropriate selections of food from the exchange groups.
4. Include other family members (e.g., grandchildren) who care for the stroke client.

Evaluation

Review and monitor the family's progress in compliance with the therapeutic regimen. Maintain careful records of blood glucose values and blood pressure to assist in identifying additional educational needs.

NURSING DIAGNOSIS

Emotional stability: potential impairment: family. Definition: The state in which the family demonstrates a high risk for maladaptive behaviors in response to family stressors, such as Patricia's recent diagnosis of a stroke

Data collection

Observe for the following:
1. Family communication patterns regarding the diagnosis of stroke. Mother and daughters may be depressed, angry, or withdrawn. Sibling living elsewhere may feel excluded.
2. Any aggressive or acting-out behavior.
3. Available financial resources (including insurance).
4. Available social support from family members and friends.
5. Use of complementary health practices that are or are not compatible with medical regimen.

Outcome identification

Each daughter will identify personal stressors and discuss a plan to resolve tensions. Mother will be included in all discussions about adjusting family routines (e.g., meals, shopping, exercise)

Plan

Home care will provide guidance and support while assisting family members to use their strengths.

Implementation (primary)

1. Help daughters individually address their concerns about their mother's diagnoses and make plans for resolving conflicts. Decrease anxiety and confusion so that family can focus on these tasks.
2. Encourage mother to identify responsibilities that are congruent with her previous role and current limitations.
3. Provide information regarding community resources, such as Meals on Wheels, adult day care, and local stroke support group.

Continued

CASE STUDY
NAVAJO WOMAN WITH A STROKE—cont'd

4. Encourage the client and family to acknowledge any progress made in particular areas.
5. Encourage spiritual practices consistent with cultural values.

Evaluation

Review both the process and outcome of the journey that the home care nurse and family have taken together. Discuss areas where there has been growth and areas that may take more time to resolve. Make a joint decision about when to terminate the visits. Conduct periodic home visits to clarify the family's questions and concerns about managing the stroke and other health problems. If indicated, refer the client for counseling and assistance with financial matters.

REFERENCES

Alberts MJ: The need for early intervention in the treatment of stroke: Special report, *Postgraduate Medicine* 7-13, 1997.

Alberts MJ, Bertels C, Dawson DV: An analysis of time of presentation after stroke, *Journal of the American Medical Association* 263(1):65-68, 1990.

Alfredsson L, von Arbin M, de Faire U: Mortality from and incidence of stroke in Stockholm, *British Medical Journal* 292:1299-1303, 1986.

Allen M: Models of hemispheric specialization, *Psychopharmacology Bulletin* 93(1):73-104, 1983.

Alperovich A et al: Mortality from stroke in France, *Neuroepidemiology* 5:80-87, 1986.

American Heart Association: *Fact sheet on heart attack, stroke and risk factors,* AHA Pub No 51-1066, Dallas, 1993a, The Association.

American Heart Association: *Socioeconomic factors and cardiovascular disease: A review of the literature,* AHA Pub No 71-0035, Dallas, 1993b, The Association.

American Heart Association: *Heart and stroke facts: 1996 statistical supplement,* Dallas, 1996, The Association.

Bakas T, Champion V: Development of psychometric testing of the Bakas caregiving outcome scale, *Nursing Research* 48(5):250-259, 1999.

Bleiberg J: Psychological and neuropsychological factors in stroke management. In Kaplan PE, Cerullo LJ, eds: *Stroke rehabilitation,* Boston, 1986, Butterworth-Heinemann.

Bloom R, Fineberg HV: A healthy world view, *San Francisco Chronicle,* August 27, 1997.

Broderick JP et al: Incidence rates of stroke in the eighties: The end of the decline in stroke? *Stroke* 20(5):577-82, 1989.

Bronstein KS, Popovich JM, Stewart-Amidei C: *Promoting stroke recovery: A research-based approach for nurses,* St Louis, 1991, Mosby.

Buchan AM, Barnett HJ: Infarction of the spinal cord. In Barnett HJ et al, eds: *Stroke pathophysiology, diagnosis, and management,* New York, 1986, Churchill Livingstone.

Chaney EJ: Cost-effectiveness of antiplatelet therapy for stroke prevention. In *Reducing the odds of stroke: A special report,* Minneapolis, 1995, McGraw-Hill.

Cranston RE: The diagnosis of brain death, *New England Journal of Medicine* 345(8):616, 2001.

Depression Guideline Panel: *Depression in primary care: Detection, diagnosis, and treatment. Quick reference guide for clinicians,* No 5, AHCPR Pub No 93-05552, Rockville, Md, 1993, US Department of Health and Human Services, Public Health Service, Agency for Health Care Policy and Research.

Easton D: Preventing stroke, In *Reducing the odds of stroke: A special report,* Minneapolis, 1995, McGraw-Hill.

Eisenberg D et al: Unconventional medicine in the United States, *New England Journal of Medicine* 328(4):246-252, 1993.

Elder NC, Gillchrist A, Minz R: Use of alternative health care by family practice patients, *Archives of Family Medicine* 6(2):181-184, 1997.

Feigin VL, Wiebers DO, Whisnant JP: Update on stroke risk factors, *Journal of Stroke and Cerebrovascular Disease* 4(4):207-215, 1994.

Folstein MF, Mailberger R, McHugh PR: Mood disorder as a specific complication of stroke, *Journal of Neurology, Neurosurgery and Psychiatry* 40(10):1018-1020, 1977.

Geibel CA, Kubalanza-Sipp D: Nursing therapy and stroke rehabilitation. In Kaplan PE, Cerullo LJ, eds: *Stroke rehabilitation,* Boston, 1986, Butterworth-Heinemann.

Gloth FM et al: Vitamin D deficiency in homebound elderly persons, *Journal of the American Medical Association* 274(21):1683-1686, 1995.

Goodstein RK: Overview: Cerebrovascular accident and the hospitalized elderly—A multidimensional clinical problem, *American Journal of Psychiatry* 140(2):141-147, 1983.

Green D: Management of homeostatic factors. In Kaplan PE, Cerullo LJ, eds: *Stroke rehabilitation,* Boston, 1986, Butterworth-Heinemann.

Gross J: A comparison of the characteristics of incontinent and continent stroke patients in a rehabilitation program, *Rehabilitation Nursing* 23(3):132-140, 1998.

Grotta J: Should thrombolytic therapy be the first-line treatment for acute ischemic stroke? t-PA—the best current options for most patients, *The New England Journal of Medicine* 337(18):1310-1312, 1997.

Halper AS, Mogil SI: Communication disorders: Diagnosis and treatment, In Kaplan PE, Cerullo LJ, eds: *Stroke rehabilitation,* Boston, 1986, Butterworth-Heinemann.

Hernandez M, Gazzaniga JM, eds: *Heart disease and stroke fact finder,* Sacramento, 1996, California Department of Health Services and University of California, San Francisco, Cardiovascular Disease Outreach, Resources and Epidemiology (CORE) Program.

Hier D: Recovery from behavioral deficits after stroke, In Kaplan PK, Cerullo LJ, eds: *Stroke rehabilitation,* Boston, 1986, Butterworth-Heinemann.

Hornig CR, Dorndorf W, Agnoli AL: Hemorrhagic cerebral infarction: A prospective study, *Stroke* 17(2):179-185, 1986.

Hupcey J: Feeling safe: The psychosocial needs of ICU patients, *Journal of Nursing Scholarship* 32(4):361-367, 2000.

Hypertension Detection and Follow-up Program Cooperative Group: Five-year findings of the Hypertension Detection and Follow-up Program, *Journal of the American Medical Association* 247(5):633-638, 1982.

Iyer SS et al: Angioplasty and stenting for extracranial carotid stenosis: Multicenter experience, *Circulation* 94(suppl 1):1-58, 1996.

Jorgensen HS et al: Factors delaying hospital admission in acute stroke: The Copenhagen Stroke Study, *Neurology* 47(2):383-387, 1996.

Kaplan PE: Hemiplegia: Rehabilitation of the lower extremity. In Kaplan PK, Cerullo LJ, eds: *Stroke rehabilitation,* Boston, 1986, Butterworth-Heinemann.

Kernan W et al: Phenylpropanolamine and the risk of hemorrhagic stroke, *New England Journal of Medicine* 343(25):1826-1832, 2000.

Kertesz A: Recovery and treatment. In Heilman KM, Valenstein E, eds: *Clinical neuropsychology,* New York, 1979, Oxford University Press.

Kilpatrick K, Jones C: *Therapy guide for the adult with language and speech disorders,* vol 1, Akron, Ohio, 1977, Visiting Nurse Service.

Kim C, Kwok YS: Navajo use of native healers, *Archives of Internal Medicine* 158(20):2245-2249, 1998.

Lal S: Physiatric complications in stroke syndromes. In Kaplan PK, Cerullo LJ, eds: *Stroke rehabilitation,* Boston, 1986, Butterworth-Heinemann.

Lieberman J: Hemiplegia: Rehabilitation of the upper extremity. In Kaplan PK, Cerullo LJ, eds: *Stroke rehabilitation,* Boston, 1986, Butterworth-Heinemann.

Lofgren B, Gustafson Y, Nyberg L: Psychological well-being 3 years after severe stroke, *Stroke* 30(3):567-572, 1999.

MacKay S: Durable power of attorney for health care, *Geriatric Nursing* 13(2):99-108, 1992.

MacKay S et al: Expanding rehabilitation services for elderly stroke patients: A nursing research approach, *Geriatric Nursing* 9:177-179, 1988.

Matchar DB: Patient and caregiver quality-of-life considerations in the management of stroke: Special report, *Postgraduate Medicine,* March 7-13, 1997.

Mauro JA: *Instant nursing assessment: Neurologic,* Albany, NY, 1996, Delmar/International Thompson.

Mills V, Wustenev E: Physical therapy and the rehabilitation of patients with cerebrovascular accidents. In Kaplan PK, Cerullo LJ, eds: *Stroke rehabilitation,* Boston, 1986, Butterworth-Heinemann.

Mower DM: Brain attack: Treating acute ischemic CVA, *Nursing* 27(3):34-39, 47, 1997.

Naesser MA et al: Quantitative CT scan studies in aphasia, I, *Brain and Language* 12(1):140-190, 1981.

National Institute of Neurological Disorders and Stroke rt-PA Stroke Study Group: Tissue plasminogen activator for acute ischemic stroke, *New England Journal of Medicine* 333(24):76-81, 1995.

National Stroke Association (NSA) Consensus Statement: Stroke: The first six hours emergency evaluation and treatment, *Stroke Clinical Updates Special Edition* IV(1):3-12, 1993.

O'Brien MT, Pallet PJ: *Total care of the stroke patient,* Boston, 1978, Little, Brown.

Olson D: Management of non-language behavior in the stroke patient. In Kaplan PE, Cerullo LJ, eds: *Stroke rehabilitation,* Boston, 1986, Butterworth-Heinemann.

Orem DE: *Nursing: Concepts of practice,* ed 6, St Louis, 2001, Mosby.

Owen D, Getz P, Bulla S: A comparison of characteristics of patients with completed stroke: Those who achieve continence and those who do not, *Rehabilitation Nursing* 20(4):197-203, 1995.

Pallet PJ, O'Brien MT: *Textbook of neurological nursing,* Boston, 1985, Little, Brown.

Petitti DB et al: Stroke in users of low-dose oral contraceptives, *New England Journal of Medicine* 335(1):8-15, 1996.

Price TR: Progressing ischemic stroke. In Barnett HJ et al: *Stroke pathophysiology, diagnosis, and management,* vol 2, New York, 1986, Churchill Livingstone.

Pulsinelli WA: Cerebrovascular disease. In Bennett JC, Plum F, eds: *Cecil textbook of medicine,* Philadelphia, 1996, WB Saunders.

Reeves A, ed: *Disorders of the nervous system,* St Louis, 1981, Mosby.

Roper BA: Rehabilitation after stroke, *Journal of Bone and Joint Surgery, British Volume* 64(2):156-163, 1982.

Rosenwaike I, Yaffe N, Sagi PC: The recent decline in mortality of the extreme aged: An analysis of statistical data, *American Journal of Public Health* 70(10):1074-1080, 1980.

Ross R: Atherosclerosis. In Bennett JC, Plum F, eds: *Cecil textbook of medicine,* Philadelphia, 1996, WB Saunders.

Savoiardo M: CT Scanning. In Barnettt HJ et al, eds: *Stroke pathophysiology, diagnosis, and management,* vol 1, New York, 1986, Churchill Livingstone.

Shpritz DK: *Rapid nursing intervention: Neurologic,* Albany, 1996, Delmar/International Thomson.

Sutin JA: Clinical presentation of stroke. In Kaplan PE, Cerullo LJ, eds: *Stroke rehabilitation,* Boston, 1986, Butterworth-Heinemann.

Szmanda MT et al: Ischemic stroke in young adults: Results from the University of Wisconsin Stroke Registry, *Journal of Stroke and Cerebrovascular Disease* 4:188-193, 1994.

Tanaka H et al: Secular trends in mortality for cerebrovascular diseases in Japan, 1960-1979, *Stroke* 13(5):574-581, 1982.

Taylor TN et al: Lifetime cost of stroke in the United States, *Stroke* 27:1459-1466, 1996.

Terent A: Increasing incidence of stroke among Swedish women, *Stroke* 19(5):598-603, 1988.

Thom TJ: Stroke mortality trends: An international perspective, *Annals of Epidemiology* 3(5):509-518, 1993.

Tonkonogy JM: *Vascular aphasia,* Cambridge, Mass, 1986, MIT Press.

Valenstein E: Hemispheric function. In Reeves A, ed: *Disorders of the nervous system,* St Louis, 1981, Mosby.

Wein T, Hickenbottom S, Alexandrov A: Thrombolysis, stroke units and other strategies for reducing acute stroke costs, *Pharmacoeconomics* 14(6):603-611, 1998.

Whisnant JP et al: Stroke incidence with hypertension and ischemic heart disease in Rochester, Minnesota, *Annals of Epidemiology* 3(5):480-482, 1993.

Williams SE, Freer CA: Aphasia: Its effect on marital relationships, *Archives of Physical Medicine and Rehabilitation* 67(4):250-252, 1986.

Wolf PA, D'Agostini RB: Secular trends in stroke in the Framingham Study, *Annals of Epidemiology* 3(5):471-475, 1993.

Wolf PA, Kannel WB, McGee DL: Epidemiology of strokes in North America. In Barnett HJ et al, eds: *Stroke pathophysiology, diagnosis, and management,* vol 1, New York, 1986, Churchill Livingstone.

Wolf PA et al: Cigarette smoking as a risk factor for stroke, *Journal of the American Medical Association* 259(7):1025-1029, 1988.

Zulch K: *The cerebral infarct,* Berlin, 1981, Springer-Verlag.

Appendix

**Brief Neurological Evaluation of Clients
in the Community Stroke Study**

NAME _____   DATE TESTED _____

ADDRESS _____   BIRTH DATE _____

OCCUPATION BEFORE STROKE _____

Introduce self to client. If client is untestable for any item because too sick, withdrawn, etc., please write "untestable" and the reason by that item. Please check only one answer for each item.

I. MENTAL STATUS

    A. State of consciousness at examination
- ☐ Alert and responsive
- ☐ Lethargic
- ☐ Stuporous
- ☐ Comatose

    B. Verbal response indicator
- 1. Tester says to client, "Say 'yes' for me." (judge on actual verbal response only)
  - ☐ Clear verbal response of "yes"
  - ☐ Unclear verbal response but interpreted as "yes"
  - ☐ Unclear verbal response; unintelligible or inappropriate
  - ☐ No verbal response

- 2. Tester says to client, "Say 'no' for me." (judge on actual verbal response only)
  - ☐ Clear verbal response of "no"
  - ☐ Unclear verbal response but interpreted as "no"
  - ☐ Unclear verbal response; unintelligible or inappropriate
  - ☐ No verbal response

- 3. Tester says to client, "Shake your head 'yes'."
  - ☐ Clear nonverbal response of "yes"
  - ☐ Unclear nonverbal response but interpreted as "yes"
  - ☐ Unclear nonverbal response; unintelligible or inappropriate
  - ☐ No nonverbal response

    4. Tester says to client, "Shake your head 'no'. "
- ☐ Clear nonverbal response of "no"
- ☐ Unclear nonverbal response but interpreted as "no"
- ☐ Unclear nonverbal response; unintelligible or inappropriate
- ☐ No nonverbal response

C. Orientation to place
    1. Tester asks client, "Where are you?"
- ☐ Correct response (hospital, V.A., own home, etc.) (go to D.1.)
- ☐ Other response: _____ (write in)
- ☐ No response

    2. If response to C.1. is inappropriate or absent, tester gives clue. Tester asks, "Are you (where the client is, e.g., hospital, home, nursing home, etc.)?"
- ☐ "Yes" response (verbal or nonverbal)
- ☐ Other response: _____ (write in)
- ☐ Not sure or unclear response
- ☐ No response

D. Orientation to date
    1. Tester asks client, "What year is this?"
- ☐ Correct response (go to D.3.)
- ☐ Other response: _____ (write in)
- ☐ No response

    2. If response to D.1. is inappropriate or absent, tester gives clue. Tester asks client, "Is this (proper year inserted in sequence of 3 years, e.g., 1996, 1999, or 2002)?"
- ☐ "Yes" response (verbal or nonverbal)
- ☐ Other response: _____ (write in)
- ☐ Not sure or unclear response
- ☐ No response

    3. Tester asks client, "What month is this?"
- ☐ Correct response (go to E.1.)
- ☐ Other response: _____ (write in)
- ☐ No response

    4. If response to D.3. is inappropriate or absent, tester gives clue. Tester asks client, "Is this (proper month inserted in sequence of 3 months, e.g., January, April, or July)?"
- ☐ "Yes" response (verbal or nonverbal)
- ☐ Other response: _____ (write in)
- ☐ Not sure or unclear response
- ☐ No response

E. Orientation to person
    1. Tester asks client, "Who am I?"
- ☐ Appropriate verbal response (client says "Dr. Hunter" or "doctor")
- ☐ Appropriate nonverbal response (client selects correct physician from other names)
- ☐ Other response: _____ (write in)
- ☐ No response

II. PERCEPTUAL DEFICITS

A. Hearing, right ear

    1. Hearing, right ear
- ☐ Normal hearing (can hear fingers rubbed at ear)
- ☐ Slight impairment (can hear fingers snapped at ear)
- ☐ Moderate impairment (can hear hands clapped at ear)
- ☐ Severe impairment

    2. Tested right ear with hearing aid?
- ☐ Yes
- ☐ No

B. Hearing, left ear

    1. Hearing, left ear
- ☐ Normal hearing (can hear fingers rubbed at ear)
- ☐ Slight impairment (can hear fingers snapped at ear)
- ☐ Moderate impairment (can hear hands clapped at ear)
- ☐ Severe impairment

    2. Tested left ear with hearing aid?
- ☐ Yes
- ☐ No

C. Vision, right eye

    1. Vision, right eye
- ☐ Normal vision (can see numbers or letters of newsprint)
- ☐ Slight impairment (can see number or letters in headings of newsprint)
- ☐ Moderate impairment (can see finger move up and down at arm's length)
- ☐ Severe impairment or blindness

    2. Tested right eye with glasses?
- ☐ Yes
- ☐ No

D. Vision, left eye

    1. Vision, left eye
- ☐ Normal vision (can see numbers or letters of newsprint)
- ☐ Slight impairment (can see number or letters in headings of newsprint)
- ☐ Moderate impairment (can see finger move up and down at arm's length)
- ☐ Severe impairment or blindness

    2. Tested left eye with glasses?
- ☐ Yes
- ☐ No

    E. Right homonymous hemianopsia
        1. Tester says to client, "Look at my nose and point to the hand that moves." (Check all 4 quadrants of field of vision using 2 hands for each position)
            ☐ No field loss
            ☐ Mild field loss
            ☐ Moderate to severe field loss
            ☐ No response

    F. Left homonymous hemianopsia
        1. Tester says to client, "Look at my nose and point to the hand that moves." (Check all 4 quadrants of field of vision using 2 hands for each position)
            ☐ No field loss
            ☐ Mild field loss
            ☐ Moderate to severe field loss
            ☐ No response

    G. Eye paralysis
        1. Tester asks client, "Do you see double?"
            ☐ "Yes"
            ☐ "No"
            ☐ Not sure or unclear response
            ☐ No response

    H. Double vision
        1. Tester holds up one finger and asks, "How many fingers do you see?"
            ☐ "One"
            ☐ "Two"
            ☐ Not sure or unclear response
            ☐ No response

    I. Weakness or limitation of gaze (coordinated movement of both eyes)
        ☐ No weakness
        ☐ Slight weakness
        ☐ Moderate weakness
        ☐ Severe weakness

    J. Weakness, right eye
        1. Deviation
            ☐ Yes
            ☐ No (go to K.1.)

        2. Direction of weakness, right eye
            ☐ Inward deviation
            ☐ Outward deviation
            ☐ Alternating deviation

    K. Weakness, left eye
        1. Deviation
            ☐ Yes
            ☐ No (go to III.A.1.)

2. Direction of weakness, left eye
   ☐ Inward deviation
   ☐ Outward deviation
   ☐ Alternating deviation

III. LANGUAGE

A. Speech production
   1. Tester says, "Repeat after me: Round the rugged rocks the rascal ran."
      ☐ No dysarthria/clear pronunciation
      ☐ Slight dysarthria
      ☐ Moderate dysarthria
      ☐ Severe dysarthria
      ☐ No response

   2. Tester says, "Repeat after me: Methodist: episcopal."
      ☐ No dysarthria/clear pronunciation
      ☐ Slight dysarthria
      ☐ Moderate dysarthria
      ☐ Severe dysarthria
      ☐ No response

   3. Tester says, "Repeat after me: Billy Button."
      ☐ No dysarthria/clear pronunciation
      ☐ Slight dysarthria
      ☐ Moderate dysarthria
      ☐ Severe dysarthria
      ☐ No response

   4. Amount or quantity of sounds or words produced
      ☐ Normal (go to B.1.)
      ☐ Abnormal

   5. Abnormal quantity of sounds
      ☐ Decreased/terse
      ☐ Increased/verbose

B. Aphasic characteristics
   1. Naming of objects
      a. Tester shows client a pen and asks, "What is this?"
         ☐ Correct response (client says "pen")
         ☐ Other response: _____
                                          (write in)
         ☐ No response

      b. Tester shows client a safety pin and asks, "What is this?"
         ☐ Correct response (client says "safety pin" or "pin")
         ☐ Other response: _____
                                          (write in)
         ☐ No response

   c. Tester shows client a comb and asks, "What is this?"
- ☐ Correct response (client says "comb")
- ☐ Other response: _____
(write in)
- ☐ No response

2. Demonstration of use
   a. Tester shows client a pen and asks, "What do you do with this?"
- ☐ Correct response (demonstrates use of pen)
- ☐ Other response: _____
(write in)
- ☐ No response

   b. Tester shows client a safety pin and asks, "What do you do with this?"
- ☐ Correct response (demonstrates use of safety pin)
- ☐ Other response: _____
(write in)
- ☐ No response

   c. Tester shows client a comb and asks, "What do you do with this?"
- ☐ Correct response (demonstrates use of comb)
- ☐ Other response: _____
(write in)
- ☐ No response

3. Watch part identification
   a. Tester shows client a large wristwatch and asks, "What is this?"
- ☐ Correct response (client says "watch" or "wristwatch")
- ☐ Other response: _____
(write in)
- ☐ No response

   b. Tester points to hands of watch and asks, "What are these?"
- ☐ Correct response (client says "hands")
- ☐ Other response: _____
(write in)
- ☐ No response

   c. Tester points to the stem and asks, "What is this?"
- ☐ Correct response (client says "stem" or "winder")
- ☐ Other response: _____
(write in)
- ☐ No response

   d. Tester points to the watchband and asks, "What is this?"
- ☐ Correct response (client says "watchband", "band", "strap", or "bracelet")
- ☐ Other response: _____
(write in)
- ☐ No response

4. Responses to verbal requests
   a. Tester says to client, "Close your eyes."
- ☐ Correct response (client closes eyes)
- ☐ Other response: _____
(write in)
- ☐ No response

b. Tester says to client, "Stick out your tongue."
   □ Correct response (client sticks out tongue)
   □ Other response: _____
   (write in)
   □ No response

c. Tester says to client, "Raise your left (or right) hand."
   □ Correct response (client raises correct hand)
   □ Other response: _____
   (write in)
   □ No response

d. Tester says to client, "Touch your nose with your finger."
   □ Correct response (client touches nose with finger)
   □ Other response: _____
   (write in)
   □ No response

e. Tester says to client, "Touch your right (or left) eyebrow with your right (or left) middle finger."
   □ Correct response (client touches correct eyebrow with correct finger)
   □ Other response: _____
   (write in)
   □ No response

5. Responses to written requests
   a. Tester presents card that says, "Close your eyes."
      □ Correct response (client closes eyes)
      □ Other response: _____
      (write in)
      □ No response

   b. Tester presents card that says, "Stick out your tongue."
      □ Correct response (client sticks out tongue)
      □ Other response: _____
      (write in)
      □ No response

   c. Tester presents card that says, "Raise your right (or left) hand."
      □ Correct response (client raises correct hand)
      □ Other response: _____
      (write in)
      □ No response

   d. Tester presents card that says, "Touch your nose with your finger."
      □ Correct response (client touches nose with finger)
      □ Other response: _____
      (write in)
      □ No response

   e. Tester presents card that says, "Touch your right (or left) eyebrow with your right (or left) middle finger."
      □ Correct response (client touches correct eyebrow with correct finger)
      □ Other response: _____
      (write in)
      □ No response

6. Mimicking of behavior
   a. Tester says to client, "Watch me and copy what I do." Tester closes eyes.
      ☐ Correct response (client closes eyes)
      ☐ Other response: _____
        (write in)
      ☐ No response

   b. Tester says to client, "Watch me and copy what I do." Tester sticks out tongue.
      ☐ Correct response (client sticks out tongue)
      ☐ Other response: _____
        (write in)
      ☐ No response

   c. Tester says to client, "Watch me and copy what I do." Tester raises hand.
      ☐ Correct response (client raises either hand)
      ☐ Other response: _____
        (write in)
      ☐ No response

   d. Tester says to client, "Watch me and copy what I do." Tester touches nose with finger.
      ☐ Correct response (client touches nose with finger)
      ☐ Other response: _____
        (write in)
      ☐ No response

   e. Tester says to client, "Watch me and copy what I do." Tester touches right (or left) eyebrow with right (or left) middle finger.
      ☐ Correct response (client touches either eyebrow with either middle finger; credit not given for use of other than middle finger)
      ☐ Other response: _____
        (write in)
      ☐ No response

7. Aphasic defects

	YES	NO
a. Blocking	☐	☐
b. Perseveration	☐	☐
c. Mutism	☐	☐
d. Circumlocution	☐	☐
e. Wrong words	☐	☐
f. Word salad (mixed nouns)	☐	☐
g. Expletives	☐	☐

IV. OTHER NEUROLOGICAL FINDINGS

A. Motor defects, right arm (tester evaluates arm strength against moderate resistance)
   ☐ No weakness
   ☐ Slight weakness
   ☐ Moderate weakness
   ☐ Severe weakness or paralysis

B. Motor defects, left arm (tester evaluates arm strength against moderate resistance)
☐ No weakness
☐ Slight weakness
☐ Moderate weakness
☐ Severe weakness or paralysis

C. Motor defects, right leg (tester evaluates leg strength against moderate resistance)
☐ No weakness
☐ Slight weakness
☐ Moderate weakness
☐ Severe weakness or paralysis

D. Motor defects, left leg (tester evaluates leg strength against moderate resistance)
☐ No weakness
☐ Slight weakness
☐ Moderate weakness
☐ Severe weakness or paralysis

E. Touch sensation, face (tester strokes both sides of face at once using fingers)
☐ Intact (client feels both sides equally well)
☐ Mild loss
☐ Moderate loss
☐ Severe loss

F. Touch sensation, hands (tester strokes both hands at once)
☐ Intact (client feels both hands equally well)
☐ Mild loss
☐ Moderate loss
☐ Severe loss

G. Touch sensation, legs (tester strokes both legs at once)
☐ Intact (client feels both legs equally well)
☐ Mild loss
☐ Moderate loss
☐ Severe loss

H. Pain sensation, right hand (tester applies pressure with sharp and dull sides of safety pin)
☐ Intact (client feels dull and sharp equally well)
☐ Mild loss
☐ Moderate loss
☐ Severe loss

I. Pain sensation, left hand (test applies pressure with sharp and dull sides of safety pin)
☐ Intact (client feels dull and sharp equally well)
☐ Mild loss
☐ Moderate loss
☐ Severe loss

J. Pain sensation, right leg (tester applies pressure with sharp and dull sides of safety pin)
   ☐ Intact (client feels dull and sharp equally well)
   ☐ Mild loss
   ☐ Moderate loss
   ☐ Severe loss

K. Pain sensation, left leg (tester applies pressure with sharp and dull sides of safety pin)
   ☐ Intact (client feels dull and sharp equally well)
   ☐ Mild loss
   ☐ Moderate loss
   ☐ Severe loss

L. Position sense, right hand (tester asks client to touch a finger on the right hand to the tester's finger and then to the client's nose)
   ☐ Intact (client feels dull and sharp equally well)
   ☐ Mild loss
   ☐ Moderate loss
   ☐ Severe loss

M. Position sense, left hand (tester asks client to touch a finger on the left hand to the tester's finger and then to the client's nose)
   ☐ Intact (client feels dull and sharp equally well)
   ☐ Mild loss
   ☐ Moderate loss
   ☐ Severe loss

N. Coordination, right arm
   ☐ Intact (client feels dull and sharp equally well)
   ☐ Mild loss
   ☐ Moderate loss
   ☐ Severe loss

O. Coordination, left arm
   ☐ Intact (client feels dull and sharp equally well)
   ☐ Mild loss
   ☐ Moderate loss
   ☐ Severe loss

P. Handedness before stroke
   ☐ Right handed
   ☐ Left handed
   ☐ Ambidextrous
   ☐ No information available

22 Care of Clients with Alzheimer's Disease and Related Disorders

Ellen D'Errico, Betty Winslow, and Patricia Jones

Although identified in the twentieth century, dementia of the Alzheimer's type is certainly not new, since ancient Greek and Roman writers described similar symptoms. In 1906, a German physician named Alois Alzheimer described pathological changes in brain cells found in the autopsy of a client who had died after a progressive form of dementia. Thus *Alzheimer's disease (AD)* is the name for a debilitating condition that is increasingly prevalent in our globally aging society. Today, Alzheimer's disease and related disorders (ADRD) afflict more than 4 million people in the United States (National Institute on Aging, 1998). AD is the most common cause of dementia among people age 65 and older, and the prevalence doubles every 5 years after age 65 (National Institute on Aging [NIA], 1998). If current population trends continue and no cure is found, the number of people with the disease in the United States could double every 20 years. The burden of providing and financing care for this growing population produces strain on families and society and on a health care system that is already struggling to meet the chronic- and acute-care needs of its citizens.

As a result of the restructuring of health care systems in the United States, the home health care industry is experiencing a renaissance in the way care is being delivered and reimbursed. In the past, home health care agencies were reimbursed on a fee-for-service basis governed by specific criteria qualifying someone for services. The more visits a home care agency made, the more revenue it earned. This system of reimbursement is disappearing and is being rapidly replaced by prospective-payment and full-risk capitation contracts. Under these payment systems, a home care agency will be paid a predetermined amount of money for a particular skilled

need or diagnostic condition, and the agency will be held accountable for the outcomes of care. Survival in this arena is shifting from generating numbers of visits to appropriate care management. The philosophy behind this thinking is that the more directed, goal-oriented, and efficient health care is, the fewer visits the client will need, thereby preserving prepaid capital. Reimbursement would remain the same whether an agency made 2 visits or 20. An agency may contract for a population of clients that are an "assigned risk." These clients would be followed throughout the care continuum in a contracted health care system consisting of various provider partners (hospitals, medical groups, home health care agencies, rehabilitation facilities, and subacute care centers). Therefore home health care nurses will need to be adept at managing clients at the lowest-level cost in the least number of visits that is appropriate to meet the client's needs. Home health nurses will need to increase networking activities with other providers and community resources so that client and family equanimity can be maintained. There will be a greater emphasis on prevention strategies, anticipatory guidance, client and family caregiver education, and outcomes of care. It is with this in mind that AD management in home care will be approached. The client plan of care will vary depending on the stage of the disease.

PATHOLOGY OF ALZHEIMER'S DISEASE

AD is an irreversible, progressive brain disorder that develops gradually, resulting in memory loss, unusual behavior, personality changes, and a decline in thinking abilities (NIA, 1998). Hallmarks of the disease, documented on autopsy, include structural changes both inside and outside of neurons. Twisted strands of fiber called *neuro-fibrillary tangles* develop inside the neurons, and dense protein deposits called *neuritic plaques* develop outside the neurons. In the regions affected, neurons lose their connections with other neurons and later die.

To remain healthy and function normally, nerve cells depend on several processes, including intercellular communication, cellular metabolism, and cell and tissue repair. Communication between the billions of neurons in the human body is facilitated by chemical messengers, including neurotransmitters, hormones, and growth factors. Neurotransmitters are released from tiny sacs at the end of the axon and cross a very small space called a *synapse* to connect with the next neuron. Transmitters bind to receptor sites in the adjacent neuron and activate the cell to receive a message. The level of acetylcholine, a neurotransmitter used extensively in the hippocampus and cerebral cortex, naturally decreases some with aging but is markedly decreased in these areas in people affected by AD.

ETIOLOGY

There are two main types of AD: familial AD (FAD) and sporadic AD. FAD most often occurs before age 65, sometimes as early as age 30, whereas sporadic AD is more likely to occur after age 65. Development of AD has been found to be closely related to genetic factors. Mutated genes or 4 different chromosomes are known to be associated with AD; chromosomes 1, 14, and 21 are associated with early onset of the disease, and chromosome 19 with late onset. Chromosome 21 is also the gene implicated in Down syndrome. People with Down syndrome who survive into adulthood are known to develop plaques and tangles like those found in the brains of clients who die with AD.

Researchers expect to find that other chromosomes are also involved in AD and that other factors also contribute to development of the pathological manifestations. Glucose metabolism, for example, declines dramatically as neurons degenerate, but it is not known if metabolical changes lead to neuron degeneration or if neuron degeneration causes glucose metabolism to decline. In either case, neurons having a problem with glucose metabolism react abnormally to a neurotransmitter called *glutamate* and allow abnormal amounts of calcium to enter the cell. Too much calcium can kill a cell, and some researchers suspect that a rise in calcium may be what is killing neurons in AD (McNeil, 1995).

Estrogen is also considered a factor in the etiology and treatment of AD. Increasing evidence supports the possibility that estrogen protects neurons from degenerating and that estrogen therapy may delay the onset or slow the course of AD, particularly in cases of FAD, the early onset AD associated with a gene mutation on chromosome 14 (Mattson, Robinson, Guo, 1997). Laboratory studies show that estrogen suppresses oxidation and reduces the amount of cell death even when cells are exposed to oxidating substances. Oxidative processes produce free radicals that are thought to damage cells in the normal process of aging, as well as play a role in the development of AD. The body produces free radicals to help cells fight infection, among other things.

The presence of brain infarcts may be indicative in the development of AD, as proposed by the Nun Study. The postmortem brain tissue of 102 nuns 76 to 100 years of age from convents in the United States was studied. The brains containing brain infarcts were correlated with the subjects' premorbid degree of cognition and level of dementia. The more prevalent the number of brain infarcts, the higher the level of dementia. It was concluded that cerebrovascular disease may enhance the severity of the clinical symptoms of AD (Snowdon et al, 1997).

The search for risk factors is another important piece of AD research. It is believed there is no single cause of AD and that genetic mutations alone do not trigger onset of the disease. Other risk factors combine with a person's genetic makeup to increase the chances of developing AD. One breakthrough in the study of AD genetics and risk factors has been the development of the transgenic mouse. In 1996, University of Minnesota researchers developed a genetically engineered mouse by inserting human genes that are linked with AD (Holcomb et al, 1998). Other researchers continue to develop new transgenic mice with various combinations of genes that allow for studies to uncover the role of genes and risk factors and to document progress of the disease and outcomes of therapeutic interventions.

DIAGNOSIS

AD is characterized by progressive loss of memory, skills, time and space orientation, language, and abstract reasoning. AD attacks nerve cells primarily in certain regions of the brain: the basal forebrain, the hippocampus, and the cerebral cortex, usually in that order. As the disease process progresses from the forebrain to the hippocampus, memory loss, agitation, and wandering occur. Finally, when it reaches the cerebral cortex, language and reason are seriously affected. In the final stages, the person has difficulty recognizing family members and is totally dependent on others for care.

At present, clinical diagnosis is the primary method of diagnosing AD while the person is still alive. However, researchers aim to assist clinicians in this process. For example, genetic testing might be done after a clinical diagnosis to confirm the clinician's analysis and to reduce the small number of people who might be falsely diagnosed. Various other approaches to diagnosis are also being studied, including the measurement of structures in the brain through the use of magnetic resonance imaging (MRI) and single photon emission computed tomography (SPECT). The hippocampus often shrinks with AD. A number of research teams have found that by measuring the volume of the hippocampus, they can discriminate between people with mild cognitive impairment associated with AD and people without AD (Johnson et al, 1998; Convit et al, 1997).

Although an autopsy is still the only way to conclusively diagnose AD, advances are being made toward diagnosing AD while clients are still alive. Ultimately, it is hoped that AD can be diagnosed before the client has behavioral symptoms so that when drugs are available, they can be used early to slow the onset of symptoms. This will not only assist physicians in diagnosing and instituting treatments early, but also assist the client to maintain function and quality of life for a longer period.

SIGNS AND SYMPTOMS

Three general stages of AD have been identified. In the early stage, the disease begins insidiously, with small recent memory deficits and slight personality changes. As individuals begin to realize that something is wrong, depression becomes common. This stage of gradual symptom development usually lasts 2 to 4 years. In the middle stage, the progressive memory loss and lack of judgment become obvious. Clients have difficulty finding words, finishing thoughts, and recognizing sensory impressions. They may become lost in familiar places, have difficulty with basic skills such as dressing, forget socially acceptable behaviors, and become disoriented and restless. Feelings of frustration are evident and manifested in agitated behavior. Perseveration, a continuous repetitive motion, and hyperorality, the need to taste and chew continuously, are also manifested in stage two. The late stage is the terminal stage. During this time, clients lose most purposeful motor ability. Perseveration and hyperorality disappear, the appetite diminishes, and communication also diminishes. Clients become totally dependent on their families for care.

Depression, Delirium, and Dementia

When a person begins to experience memory loss, decreased psychomotor function, and loss of interest in surroundings, it is important to remember that these symptoms are not a normal part of the aging process. Clients suffering from depression, vision and hearing impairments, and substance abuse may also have these symptoms. It is understandable that when clients are informed that they are suffering from AD, they experience intense grief and sadness. However, when clients manifest symptoms such as feelings of extreme sadness, loss of energy, prolonged feelings of hopelessness, withdrawal, loss of appetite, sleeplessness, crying, despair, self-depreciation, poor hygiene, lack of initiative, and thoughts of suicide, they should be assessed for clinical depression.

Depression can be difficult to isolate because physical disorders, such as pain and the sufferings of chronic illness, can overshadow and mask symptoms of depression (Lundquist, Bernens, Olsen, 1997). Some depression may result from side effects of medications the client is taking. Clients with a history of depression are at greater risk of developing a major depression early in the course of AD (Teuth, 1995).

Dementia can be either primary, which is caused by pathophysiological changes in the brain and is irreversible, or secondary (delirium), resulting from acute, reversible conditions. Examples of acute reversible conditions resulting in delirium are medication side effects, exacerbation of chronic illness (e.g., acute pneumonia in a client with lung disease), and temporary physiological alterations (e.g., sepsis from a urinary tract infection). Once these conditions are resolved, a normal mental state should resume.

Depression can be superimposed with the symptoms of both primary and secondary dementia. Primary dementia usually develops gradually over several months or years. Delirium develops quickly, over several hours or days.

With proper medical intervention, depression is amenable to treatment and can improve considerably. Psychosocial intervention and antidepressant drug therapy can yield satisfactory outcomes. To effectively manage AD, the home care nurse needs to understand the differences between dementia, delirium, and depression, as well as know the ways sensory impairments can impact the client's mental presentation.

The home care nurse also needs to be aware that older adults may be abusing alcohol or prescription drugs as a dysfunctional response to major life changes, such as loss of a spouse or retirement, or in an effort to deal with poorly managed pain from a chronic illness. Symptoms manifested in these individuals may be incorrectly attributed to AD.

The clinical picture of the older substance abuser is quite different than that of younger people. Elderly people may live alone, do little driving, and have minimal social contact. Their drinking behaviors may be cleverly hidden (Hazelden, n.d.).

TREATMENT

The duration of AD averages from 4 to 8 years, but can be as long as 20 years. Once AD has been diagnosed, the use of drugs to control symptoms is essential. Scientists are looking for treatments that control a broad range of symptoms, that improve clients' activities of daily living (ADLs) and cognitive function, and that have no serious side effects. When behaviors such as aggression, agitation, wandering, and sleep disturbances can be

controlled, families will be able to manage health care in the home for much longer periods. There are new drugs that have been developed that look promising in decelerating the speed of progressive dementia.

The first drug to be approved by the FDA for use with AD clients was tacrine (Cognex), which became available in 1993. The second was donepezil hydrochloride (Aricept). Both of these act by inhibiting acetylcholinesterase, the enzyme that normally breaks down acetylcholine. Although both have a beneficial impact on symptom management, undesirable side effects limit their usefulness, and new cholinesterase inhibitors are being studied. However, even the new and potentially more effective of these will still not prevent the disease process from destroying the acetylcholine-producing nerve cells. Drugs are needed to help these cells survive to slow or prevent the development of AD.

Estrogen replacement after menopause has been shown to decrease the incidence of AD in women. In one study of menopausal women, a history of estrogen-replacement therapy was associated with reduced incidence of AD by about 50% and in another by 80% (NIA, 1998). Other clinical trial studies that examine the impact of estrogen in preventing AD are needed. Antiinflammatory drugs also appear to be associated with a reduced incidence of AD. There appears to be a link between inflammation and changes in the brains of AD clients. An interesting observation is that clients who had regularly used antiinflammatory drugs had a lower risk of developing AD than those who did not. However, until clinical trials are implemented, the actual relationship between these drugs and AD will not be known.

Antioxidants, such as vitamin E and selegiline, have been studied in regard to their impact in slowing the progression of the disease. In one study, taking vitamin E and selegiline extended the time it took for moderately impaired AD clients to lose their ability to do ADLs and need total care. The use of ginkgo biloba extract is also being examined for its antioxidant, antiinflammatory and anticoagulant properties. Not enough studies have yet been done to examine the impact of this product on AD or its side effects. In summary, lengthy clinical trial studies are needed to examine the impact of estrogen, vitamin E, antiinflammatory drugs, and natural substances such as ginkgo biloba on the development and progression of AD.

Palliative Care

Although new drug development is promising, most of the care and intervention related to the AD client is palliative in nature. To *palliate* means "to reduce the intensity of the symptoms of an illness or disorder" (Mish, 1985). Palliative treatment focuses on amelioration of the symptoms of an illness rather than cure of the disease.

The importance of proper nutrition, vitamin therapy, and exercise cannot be underestimated (Miziniak, 1994) in controlling symptom severity and progression of AD. However, the practical reality is that pharmacological intervention is usually indicated somewhere along the care continuum. Clients who develop psychotic syndromes, extreme paranoia, uncontrollable agitation, sleep disorders, and violent behaviors require drug therapy.

Advances are being made in using medications that do not excessively sedate, such as buspirone (BuSpar), trazodone (Desyrel), fluoxetine (Prozac), carbamazepine, valproic acid, propranolol, and clonidine (Hawkins, 1992). Traditional psychotropic medications (diazepam, sedative hypnotics, haloperidol [Haldol], thioridazine [Mellaril], lithium) in doses that have been carefully individualized can also lead to a successful decrease of disturbing behaviors.

Palliation of behavioral problems in clients with AD is best handled by clinicians who specialize in the care of the elderly or palliative medicine. Achievement of excellent symptom control is a process of trial and error until just the right combination of therapeutic agents in carefully tailored doses can be designed. Careful monitoring and much patience are needed on the part of the client's family to persevere through this process. The clinician must also be committed to reaching optimal outcomes and taking an individualized approach.

Assessment of Mental Status

The most reliable indicator of early AD is delayed recall (Welsh et al, 1992). This involves an inability to remember information recently presented after a short time span. Clients often try to preserve self-esteem and perpetuate denial that something may be wrong with them by covering up and concealing memory loss. They may blame others for not having informed them of a missed appointment or other responsibilities. At this stage, affected persons do not look ill, and their protestations can be taken at face value. Clients with likable personalities may be perceived as merely absent minded. What separates normal forgetfulness from pathological early AD is the increased frequency and persistence of memory loss.

A thoughtful, complete, and thorough assessment of the client's mental status is critical to avoid making inaccurate judgments about a client's cognition. Nurses who rely solely on measures of orientation to time, person, and place to determine cognition may risk an incomplete assessment, resulting in gaps in the client's plan of care (Dellasega, Cutezo, 1994). An impaired memory will impede the client's ability to remember information presented by the nurse or therapist. Strategies to improve recall are required to effect improvements in function.

For a more complete picture of a client's cognitive status, assessment and diagnostic tools using questions to assess computation skills, ability to do abstract thinking, language, recall, concentration, and judgment can be used (Box 22-1).

Mini-mental status examination The mini-mental status examination (Folstein, Folstein, McHugh, 1975) consists of orientation questions (client states day, date, month, year, season, and location); test of immediate recall (client repeats three unrelated words in order at different time intervals); attention and calculation exercises (client subtracts 7 from 100 five times or spells a word backward); and language exercises (client names objects, repeats a phrase, performs a three-step command, draws an object, or writes a sentence).

Clinical dementia rating scale The clinical dementia rating scale (Hughes et al, 1982) was originally designed as a research tool in a study of mildly demented individuals. It assesses not only memory, orientation, and problem solving, but also functional abilities related to community affairs, home, hobbies, and personal care.

Clock-drawing test The clock-drawing test (Boston Parietal Lobe Battery) is a visuospatial

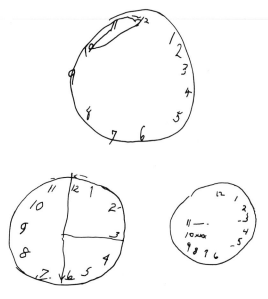

Box 22-1	Six-Item Blessed Orientation-Memory-Concentration Test

1. Say, "What year is it now?"
   Client's response:_____
   Actual year: _____
2. "What month is it now?"
   Client's response: _____
   Actual month: _____
3. Memory phrase: Say, "Repeat this phrase after me: John Brown, 42 Market Street, Chicago."
4. Say, "What time is it now?" (Within one hour)
   Client's response—hour _____ minutes _____
   □ AM   □ PM
   Actual time—hour_____ minutes _____
   □ AM   □ PM
5. Say, "Count backwards from 20 to 1."
   (If the client stops counting before completing the task, note # of their last response) _____
   If the client performed the count correctly, but only by **self correction** check this box □
6. Say, "Say the months in reverse order."
   (If the client stops before completing the task, note their last response)
   _____
   If the client performed the task correctly, but only by **self correction** check this box □
7. Say, "Repeat the memory phrase."
   Client's response in order—if the response is incorrect or there is no response, check this box □
   John □   Brown □   42 □   Market St. □
   Chicago □

From Katzman R et al: *The American Journal of Psychiatry* 140(6):734-739, 1983.

Fig. 22-1 Three spontaneous clock drawings from clients with SDAT. The time setting should be 10 minutes past 11 o'clock. *(From Goodglass H, Kaplan E: Assesment of aphasia and related disorders, Philadelphia, 1972, Lea & Febiger.)*

construction task evaluating the client's ability to plan and organize the spatial elements of a familiar object. It includes drawing from memory, copying, and setting a sequence (Fig. 22-1).

The Allen cognitive levels This tool using Allen's cognitive levels (1988) is a six-level categorization of cognitive impairment, with level six being most functional (normal) and level one being least functional (vegetative state). Functional ability needs to be accurately assessed to understand the full scope of the client's deficits. Individuals who score poorly on cognition tests may still be able to perform ADLs and other essential tasks. The nurse must examine the client from

both a cognitive and a functional perspective for a complete assessment (Dellasega, Cutezo, 1994).
Other tests There are many other tests that can be administered to the client by a gerontologist, psychologist, or psychiatrist to formulate a more definitive diagnosis. Diagnostic tests, such as computed axial tomography (CAT) scan, electroencephalogram, chest x-ray examination, and blood and spinal fluid studies are used to rule out other possible physiological causes of the client's impaired mental status.

Functional assessment includes assessment of both ADLs and instrumental ADLs (IADLs); ADLs are basic self-care activities such as bathing, dressing, toileting, eating, and transferring; IADLs are activities associated with independent living needed to support ADLs, such as shopping, cleaning, and paying bills. The latter are slightly more complex tasks that usually require cognitive and physical ability. In the AD client, functional assessment will uncover deficits in IADLs before those in ADLs. The person's ability to function is an indicator not only of whether independent living is still an option, but also of what specific kinds of assistance are needed.

Assessment of functional ability is best done through direct observation. Watching the client dress, toilet, wash, ambulate, or transfer provides valuable information regarding self-care abilities. Asking the person to demonstrate locks on doors, pour a glass of water, or make a cup of tea will indicate capabilities. Along with these requests, the nurse must build rapport with the client to provide a sense of security and to minimize the perceived threat of the performance part of the assessment.

Although assessment of IADLs is critical for the AD client living alone, it is still relevant for the AD client who is sometimes left alone by the caregiver for periods of time. In addition to questions regarding shopping, paying bills, and washing clothes, a demonstration by the client of actually unlocking the doors, dialing an emergency telephone number, and exiting the house is essential.

The home care nurse needs to ask the following questions on initial assessment:

1. When did the change in mentation begin?
2. Is the client taking any new medications or increased or decreased dosages of current medications?
3. Does the client use alcohol? If yes, how often and how much?
4. Are there possible food or drug interactions with the medications (including over-the-counter medications) that the client is taking?
5. Have there been any recent family or personal crises?
6. Has the client experienced a decline in physical status or exacerbation of illness?
7. Has the client had changes in hearing, vision, or sensory perception?
8. Has the client experienced a decline in his or her ability to perform ADLs?
9. How often does the client bathe? Does he or she need assistance? What kind?
10. Can the client dress independently? Does he or she need assistance? What kind?
11. Can the client still safely drive? Shop? Write a check? Count correct change?
12. Can the client fix a meal? Use appliances safely?

CAREGIVING FAMILY

Care for an individual with AD or related dementia should be understood within the context of the family. These diseases affect not only clients, but also those who most closely share their lives. In fact, family members are the ones who provide most of the care to people with AD. More than 70% of people with AD live at home, with almost 75% of their care provided by family and friends (Alzheimer's Association [AA], 1998). A recent survey indicated that, compared with other caregivers, Alzheimer's caregivers are twice as likely to provide more than 40 hours of care each week and that almost 40% of Alzheimer's caregivers have been providing care for more than 5 years (AA, National Alliance for Caregiving, 1999). In addition, the survey results report that 75% of these caregivers are women, many of whom have children or grandchildren under the age of 18 for whom they also care.

Impact on the Family

Caring for a relative with AD has been shown to produce stress-related physical- and emotional-health outcomes in the caregiver (Aneshensel et al, 1995; Baumgarten et al, 1992; Schulz, Visintainer, Williamson, 1990). As caregivers, women have been found to often have higher levels of burden than men who assume the caregiving role (Miller, Cafasso, 1992). The topic of caregiver stress and burden has been the focus of significant research efforts as scholars have sought to understand the predictors of caregiver burden and the effects of long-term caregiving on family members (Aneshensel et al, 1995; Gold et al, 1995; Leiberman, Fisher, 1995; Schulz et al, 1995; Whitlatch, Feinberg, Sebesta, 1997). Decreases in the client's cognitive ability, management of the client's problem behaviors, increases in caregiving tasks, amount and quality of social support for the caregiver, being a caregiving spouse, and severity of illness are some of the predictors associated with negative caregiver outcomes. Research has shown that the effects on caregivers of providing care for the person with AD have resulted in depression, anxiety, physical morbidity, and inability to sustain the caregiving role. Recently, the impact of interventions such as case management, support and educational groups, use of respite, and counseling services has been evaluated to see if they might ameliorate the negative outcomes of caregiving (Bedard et al, 1997; Mittleman et al, 1996; Winslow, 1997). Some of these studies have found that interventions assist family caregivers, but others have had limited or even negative effects.

Not all caregivers experience negative outcomes from caregiving. Some caregivers find that providing care gives meaning, purpose, and structure to their lives. Another focus in the study of family caregiving has begun to explore the gains that are experienced by family members as they care for loved ones (Kramer, 1997; Miller, Lawton, 1997). Positive outcomes have been found for adolescents when the family is engaged in caregiving (Beach, 1997). Husbands have also been found to express positive appraisal of their caregiving experience (Kramer, 1997). Recognizing that not all families will evaluate or experience their caregiving responsibilities as negative is an important insight for home health care nurses.

Family Caregiving Models

The experience of caring for a relative with AD has been described as a caregiving career (Aneshensel et al, 1995; Lindgren, 1993), as a stress process (Aneshensel et al, 1995; Pearlin et al, 1990), as coping with negative choices (Wilson, 1989), and as stages of bereavement (Jones, Martinson, 1992). Each of these conceptualizations of caregiving is briefly described to provide a framework for understanding the caregiving experience.

The progression of caregiving careers model includes stages described as role acquisition, role enactment, role disengagement, and the transition points of illness onset, nursing home admission, and client death (Fig. 22-2). During role acquisition, the caregiver recognizes the need for care and assumes the responsibility for care. The decision to become a caregiver is dependent on personal reasons that are related to the caregiver's history and composition of relationships. The enactment of the caregiving role is the time when role-related tasks are performed either in the home or in the formal setting of long-term care. Finally, role disengagement is the time when caregiving ceases and the caregiver experiences grief and readjustment, returning to other roles of life after the death of the impaired relative. It is likely that interventions from the home care nurse would be beneficial in each of these career stages.

Experiences associated with family caregiving can also be understood within the conceptual framework of the stress process (Aneshensel et al, 1995; Pearlin et al, 1990) Four domains make up the stress process: background and context, stressors, mediators, and outcomes. The background and context of the stress process include characteristics of the caregiver, aspects of the caregiving history, duration of caregiving, and health problems of the client. Stressors are the conditions, experiences, and activities that are problematic for the caregiver, which lead to other problems and hardships referred to as *secondary role strains* and

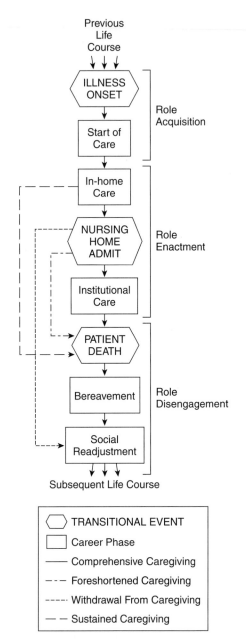

Fig. 22-2 The caregiving career model. *(From Aneshensel C et al: Profiles in caregiving: The unexpected career, San Diego, 1995, Academic Press.)*

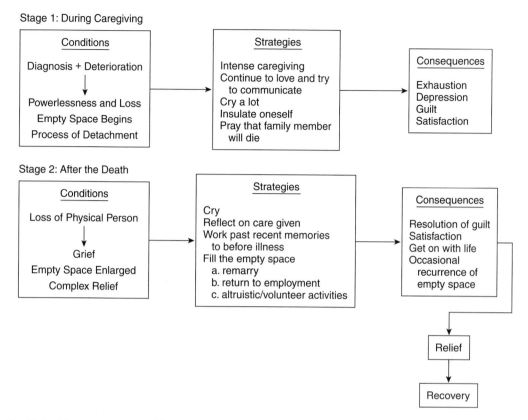

Stage 1: During Caregiving

Stage 2: After the Death

Fig. 22-3 Two-stage pattern of bereavement in family caregivers of an AD client. *(From Jones P, Martinson I: The experience of bereavement in cargivers of family members with Alzheimer's disease,* Image, *24:172-176, 1992.)*

intrapsychic strains. Mediators, such as social support and coping, are though to buffer the outcomes or effects of caregiving. Outcomes include whether or not the caregiver continues in the caregiving role or experiences a decline in physical or emotional health. Within the stress-process model, it may be possible for home health care services to reduce the negative outcomes of caregiving through mediating the stressors.

Coping with negative choices is another conceptualization of the caregiving experience based on a grounded-theory study conducted by nurse-researcher Wilson (1989). In her study, caregivers were described as attempting to cope with choices through a three-stage process, which she labeled "surviving on the brink." The stages that she described were "taking it on," "going through it," and "turning it over." The context of taking on the caregiving role is one of uncertainty, unpredictability, and lack of resources and understanding. Caregivers attempt to cope by talking to themselves, seeking spiritual solace, and talking out their problems with others who are ac-

cepting and nonjudgmental. The second stage is characterized by a long list of problems that include illness ambiguity, breakdown of shared meanings, disruptive household patterns, family conflicts, financial strain, and maintenance of the usual ADLs. Caregivers in this state of taking it on cope by taking care of business, using resources, and caring for themselves through protective governing. The final stage, turning it over, is a gradual process that involves the ultimate negative choice of entrusting the family member's care to an institutional facility. However, even when institutional placement occurs, many caregivers continue to be involved in their family member's care. For home health care nurses, this model suggests that family members experience inadequacy in health care services and could benefit from extended home care support services and survival strategies.

Based on a grounded-theory study of 13 family caregivers, a two-stage pattern of bereavement has been described in family caregivers of AD clients (Fig. 22-3). In stage one, the diagnosis of

AD can initiate a grief response. As the family experiences deterioration of the loved one's dignity, intellect, and personhood, feelings of loss and powerlessness ensue. This prolonged series of agonizing losses is accompanied by intense grief and is characterized by a process of detachment. Caregivers attempt to cope during this stage in varying ways and experience feelings of exhaustion, depression, satisfaction, and for some, even guilt. The second stage of grief follows the physical death of the client. This is a period of acute grief, which is accompanied by complex feelings of relief that require reflection and resolution on the part of the caregiver. Caregivers in this stage work out their painful memories, try to resolve any remaining guilt, and move on with their lives. The combination of experiencing bereavement while providing care can take a toll on the caregivers' physical and emotional health. Early recognition of the bereavement process and appropriate interventions by home care nurses are essential in maintaining the health of family caregivers and supporting them in their caregiving role.

Home Health Care and the Caregiving Family

Each of these descriptions of the family caregiving experience indicates a process of gradual decline of the client with changing responsibilities of the family caregiver. Opportunities for the home care professional to intervene at each stage of the caregiving experience are abundant. Understanding the caregiving experience is the first step in providing appropriate assessment and interventions. In addition to understanding the caregiver's experience, it is also important to understand that the caregiver possesses a unique knowledge of the client that can be used in developing appropriate plans of care for both the client and the caregiver (Harvath et al, 1994). Developing a partnership with the family is a strategy that supports development of individualized nursing care that will blend the personal knowledge of the family caregivers with the generalized knowledge of the home care nurse. Although the amount of knowledge a family has of a loved one can vary, many families possess a great deal of insight and understanding. Home health care nurses who work with families can initially acknowledge the families' personal knowledge, develop and enhance the families' knowledge when it is inadequate, and support the families' abili-

ties to problem solve when they are unable to do so on their own (Harvath et al, 1994). This development of a caregiving partnership, important in all home care endeavors, becomes especially important with families involved in dementia caregiving. Forming an alliance with the family caregiver will assist in delivery of care to the client and will also assist in providing the needed assessment and interventions of support, information, and referrals necessary to sustain the family caregiver.

STAGING APPROACH TO HOME HEALTH CARE MANAGEMENT
Early Stage

Client issues Home care clients with early stage dementia are usually seen for an unrelated primary condition. This is because clients in this stage may still be capable of a great deal of independence. However, any other condition that is medically necessary; requires the skilled care of a nurse, physical therapist, or speech pathologist; and causes the client to be homebound will qualify a client for home health care services (e.g., postsurgical hip-fracture client requiring gait training and incision dressing change). Dementia should be listed as an "other pertinent diagnosis" (Fig. 22-4).

Early stage dementia is traumatic. The client who was once active and independent must now learn to cope with memory lapse and a redefining or abandoning of expected roles. There can be grief, anger, and denial over the loss of cognitive function, role, and self as previously known.

Delayed recall and anomalies in communication are some of the early symptoms of AD. Circumlocution (talking around a topic), use of semantic jargon (nonsense words), difficulty finding the right words, repetition of the same words or phrases, irrelevant language, and reduced vocabulary are typical of the type of verbal processing problems that AD clients begin to experience (Roberto, 1998).

Clients are frustrated at trying to interpret complex information and are unable to process abstract ideas. Judgment, the ability to solve problems, and the ability to plan and organize things become impaired. For a client who had no past problems constructing a shopping list, driving to the supermarket, and obtaining and paying for groceries, these now become daunting, complicated tasks. Inability to handle finances,

Department of Health and Human Services
Health Care Financing Administration

Form Approved
OMB No. 0938-0357

HOME HEALTH CERTIFICATION AND PLAN OF CARE

1. Patient's HI Claim No. 000-00-0000	2. Start of Care Date 010599	3. Certification Period From: 010599 To: 030599		4. Medical Record No. 00-00-00	5. Provider No. 0000

6. Patient's Name and Address	7. Provider's Name, Address and Telephone Number
Ima Patient Elm Street Anytown, USA 00000-0000	Home Health Care Agency Main Street Anytown, USA 00000-0000 (000) 555-1234

8. Date of Birth 072420		9. Sex ☐ M ☒ F	10. Medications: Dose/Frequency/Route (N)ew (C)hanged

11. ICD-9-CM 820.8	Principal Diagnosis Fractured right hip	Date 123198	Donepezil Hydrocholoride 10 mg. PO qd @ HS Buspirone 15 mg. PO BID (N) Haloperidol 1 mg. PO TID (N) Docusate Sodium 100 mg. PO q AM & PM (N) Acetaminophen with codeine 30 mg. 1 PO q 4 hr. PRN pain Choral Hydrate 500 mg. PO @ HS PRN sleep
12. ICD-9-CM 79.35	Surgical Procedure ORIF right hip	Date 010299	
13. ICD-9-CM 331.0	Other Pertinent Diagnoses Alzheimers disease	Date 060497	

14. DME and Supplies Bedside commode, dressing supplies	15. Safety Measures: Fall precautions (See addendem)
16. Nutritional Req. Regular diet	17. Allergies: Penicillin

18.A. Functional Limitations				18.B. Activities Permitted					
1 ☐ Amputation	5 ☐ Paralysis	9 ☐ Legally blind		1 ☐ Complete bedrest	6 ☐ Partial weight bearing	A ☐ Wheelchair			
2 ☐ Bowel/bladder (incontinence)	6 ☐ Endurance	A ☐ Dyspnea with minimal exertion		2 ☐ Bedrest BRP	7 ☐ Independent at home	B ☐ Walker			
3 ☐ Contracture	7 ☒ Ambulation	B ☐ Other (specify)		3 ☐ Up as tolerated	8 ☐ Crutches	C ☐ No restrictions			
4 ☐ Hearing	8 ☒ Speech			4 ☐ Transfer bed/chair	9 ☐ Cane	D ☐ Other (specify)			
				5 ☐ Exercises prescribed					

19. Mental Status:	1 ☐ Oriented	3 ☒ Forgetful	5 ☒ Disoriented	7 ☒ Agitated
	2 ☐ Comatose	4 ☐ Depressed	6 ☐ Lethargic	8 ☐ Other

20. Prognosis	1 ☐ Poor	2 ☒ Guarded	3 ☐ Fair	4 ☐ Good	5 ☐ Excellent

21. Orders for Discipline and Treatments (Specify Amount/Frequency/Duration)

Skilled nursing 1 x week x 9 weeks
Assess & evaluate status of surgical incision for signs and symptoms of infection. Remove staples in one week if no infection is present.
Assess & evaluate nutritional status and amount of daily food/fluid intake.
If intake is <1,000 calories of food per day, <48 ounces of fluid per day, consult with dietician to increase food intake to 1800 calories, >48 ounces of fluid per day.
Assess & evaluate mental status/cognition. Teach caregiver strategies to cope with difficult behavior.
Assess & evaluate elimination patterns. Devise plan to manage incontinence. Instruct caregiver.
Develop and initiate bowel program. Evaluate effectiveness. Instruct caregiver.
Review all medications. Verify caregiver knowledge as to the purpose, doseage, administration, and potential side effects of all drugs. Teach and instruct caregiver as needed about medication management.
Assess & evaluate home environment for actual/potential safety hazards. Teach and instruct on home safety issues.

(See addendum)

22. Goals/Rehabilitation Potential/Discharge Plans
Surgical incision will heal without complication in one week. Staples will be removed without difficulty by 1/12/99
Patient will eat a nutritious, well-balanced diet of at least 1800 KCAL/day and at least 48 oz. Fluid per day by 3/5/99
Patient will be toileted every 2-3 hours while awake, use incontinence pad in panties, and move bowels every 2 days by 3/5/99
Caregiver will understand the purpose, dosage, administration schedule, and side effects of all drugs by 3/5/99 (See addendum)

23. Nurse's Signature and Date of Verbal SOC Where Applicable: Nancy Nurse RN 010599	25. Date HHA Received Signed POT

24. Physician's Name and Address Your Doctor Medical Office Building Ste. A Anytown, USA 00000-0000	26. I certify/recertify that this patient is confined to his/her home and needs intermittent skilled nursing care, physical therapy and/or speech therapy or continues to need occupational therapy. The patient is under my care, and I have authorized the services on this plan of care and will periodically review the plan.
27. Attending Physician's Signature and Date Signed	28. Anyone who misrepresents, falsifies, or conceals essential information required for payment of Federal funds may be subject to fine, imprisonment, or civil penalty under applicable Federal laws.

Form HCFA-485 (C-3) (02-94) (Print Aligned)

Fig. 22-4   Home health certification and plan of care.

Continued

ADDENDUM TO: ☐ PLAN OF TREATMENT			☐ MEDICAL UPDATE[69]	
1. Patient's HI Claim No. 000-00-0000	**2. SOC Date** 010599	**3. Certification Period** From: 010599 To: 030599	**4. Medical Record No.** 00-00-00	**5. Provider No.** 0000
6. Patient's Name Ima Patient		**7. Provider's Name** Home Health Agency		

8. Item No.

15. Fire/disaster evacuation plan, patient supervision at all times, non-skid rubber mat for tub/shower.

21. Assess & evaluate home environment for actual/potential safety hazards.

Teach and instruct caregiver on issues of home safety.

Home health aide: 2 X week X 9 weeks
Assist with bathing and personal care. Perform complete bed bath, oral care, skin care (apply moisturizing lotion following bath), comb hair, shampoo once a week, change bed linen, range of motion exercises as instructed by the physical therapist.

Physical therapist: 2 X week X 9 weeks
Assess and evaluate ambulation, gait, strength, level of conditioning.
Perform progressive ambulation and gait training.
Assess level of pain/discomfort with movement, report to MD if pain level is moderate to severe.
Develop home exercise plan and instruct caregiver in home exercise program for the patient.

Occupational therapist: 2 X week X 4 weeks
Assess and evaluate need for adaptive equipment option to aid in mealtime, dressing, bathing, and toileting safety.

Speech therapist: 1 X week X 4 weeks
Perform swallowing evaluation and report to MD.
Devise system for more effective communication with the patient and instruct caregiver in it's use.

Medical social worker: 1 X month X 2 months
Assist family with long range planning for patient care needs.
Evaluate caregiver/family stressors, refer to appropriate community resources.

22. Patient will be safe and free from injury by 030599
Patient will be able to ambulate 20 feet with one person assisting by 030599
Patient will exhibit no verbal or non-verbal signs of pain when moving by 030599
Patient will participate in home exercise program by 030599
Patient will use prescribed adaptive equipment correctly by 030599
Caregiver will be knowledgeable and demonstrate competency in use of communication tools by 030599
Caregiver and family agree on options for long range plan for patient by 030599
Caregiver and family access all available, appropriate community resources by 030599

9. Signature of Physician	**10. Date**
11. Optional Name/Signature of Nurse/Therapist Nancy Nurse RN	**12. Date** 010599

Fig. 22-4, cont'd   Home health certification and plan of care.

such as balancing a checkbook, and poor insight into how their behavior affects others emerge. Simpler, over-learned tasks, such as dressing, grooming, and bathing and orientation to time, place, and person, are usually still intact. However, clients begin to have periods of confusion and increased anxiety in unfamiliar situations.

Preservation of autonomy   It should not be automatically assumed that clients are incapable of making decisions about their health care just because they have cognitive impairments in early AD (Caralis, 1994). It is important to talk and listen to clients concerning issues of future care while they still have the ability to state preferences. Clients have the right to voice their desires about the following:

1. Handling of their property
2. Management of their financial affairs
3. Choice of help when they cannot function independently
4. Placement in a care facility
5. Preferences for future medical treatment (aggressive or palliative)
6. Initiation of do-not-resuscitate orders and use of artificial feeding and hydration
7. Advance directives and conservatorship or guardianship (Goldstein et al, 1991).

In one study of client preferences, only 7.5% of 332 clients studied had completed living wills. In this same group, only 15.1% had executed a durable power of attorney for health care. The remaining clients and their families in the sample group had not considered either option. This was true even though caregiving families had been confronted by the client's deterioration for extended lengths of time and had stated that they were generally very concerned for the client's uncertain future (Brechling, Schneider, 1993).

Although this is challenging, discussion of these matters needs to begin early in the course of the disease. Some days the client may be performing better cognitively than others; many AD clients function better in the morning (Brechling, Schneider, 1993). It is during these good moments that discussion of these issues should be initiated. If delayed, the window of opportunity will eventually close, and the client's wishes may never be known. This can complicate the execution of appropriate medical, legal, and economic decisions on the client's behalf and can be a source of discord, doubt, and guilt for the caregiving family.

Readiness of discussion of autonomy issues must be carefully predicted as such topics can be emotionally charged. The home care nurse needs to be sensitive to the delicate nature of introducing these topics at the right time and should not be intimidated when strong emotions are elicited from this activity. Consultation and referral to the home care medical-social worker are often required.

Caregiver and Nurse Interventions

1. Suggest use of memory aids (lists, calendars, written schedules, pill dispensers, or notes on a bulletin board or refrigerator door).
2. Establish set routines.
3. Keep distractions to a minimum.
4. Do not overload the client with too much information at once.
5. Do not expect the client to function well in new and unfamiliar situations for long periods of time.
6. Break down instructions into small manageable steps.
7. Provide feedback on communication patterns between caregiver and client. Suggest more effective strategies if needed (e.g., modify rate of speech, word choice, topic selections, and amount of information given at one time) (Roberto et al, 1998).
8. Allow ample time for client responses.
9. Avoid use of indefinite pronouns (he, she, and they), ambiguous words, and too many questions (Roberto et al, 1998).
10. Use repetition.
11. Avoid explanations using abstract concepts.
12. Explain the pros, cons, and long-term consequences to the resistive client as simply and directly as possible.
13. Initiate discussion of advance directives and other issues related to the preservation of client autonomy.

Measurable Expected Outcomes

1. Client will verbalize or demonstrate decreased level of frustration by (date).
2. Client's forgetfulness will be minimized by _____% through use of memory aids by (date).
3. Client's medications will be administered on schedule with no missed doses by (date).
4. Client's communication difficulties will be reduced by _____% by (date).
5. Client will state preferences regarding issues of autonomy and execute advance directive by (date).

Family issues As has already been noted, in the early stage of dementia, home care clients are usually seen for other unrelated primary conditions. However, the secondary diagnosis of dementia may already be having an impact on the caregiving family.

Assessment and implications During this early stage, family members may be aware of the memory lapses, errors in judgment, and communication difficulties, but have not yet taken the client for an evaluation. The family caregiver may need validation that these symptoms are not part of the normal process of aging and need to be encouraged to seek appropriate medical evaluation of the client. If the diagnosis has already been made, caregivers and clients may be unclear as to the usual progress of the disease and may request information about the disease and future expectations. This is also a time when caregivers may be searching for a quick cure and be susceptible to alternative therapies that may be harmless or, in some instances, detrimental to the client. Assessment by the home care nurse should include whether medical evaluation for dementia has been obtained and what information is needed by the family to understand the medical diagnosis. Assessment should also include what remedies are being used or considered by the client and family.

In the early stage, caregivers may already be feeling frustrated with responding to the client's repeated communication and apparent obstinate behavior. These clients are at risk of caregiver abuse and neglect, since they may possess several factors associated with the mistreatment of elderly individuals, including dependency, isolation, and stressed caregivers (Abraham et al, 1994). As the burden of providing care for the client increases, the risk of neglect also builds. The home care nurse should assess the high-risk situation and intervene with the family in a proactive manner (Fulmer, Burkenhauer, 1992).

Families may also be concerned with financial and legal arrangements for the client. The home care nurse can facilitate discussion of their concerns and guide them to appropriate community resources for financial and legal assistance.

CAREGIVER INTERVENTIONS   Early stage interventions for some clients and families may involve referral for a medical evaluation. Information regarding the disease process and practical answers to family questions are also needed in this early period. Caregivers can be given literature and referred to books such as *The 36-Hour Day* (Mace, Rabins, 1990) as sources of information regarding AD. Caregivers may also be referred to the Alzheimer's Disease Education and Referral (ADEAR) Center and the National Alzheimer's Association for current information regarding the disease, resources available, and caregiving tips. Both of these agencies have internet sites that may be accessed by the caregiver (see Appendix A). Another excellent resource for family members may be a local AD support group, where they can receive education regarding the disease, as well as support from others who are experiencing a similar situation. Families considered at risk for abuse or neglect may need referral to the appropriate community social service agency. Referral to financial and legal services may also be appropriate at this time. The office of the local Area Agency on Aging (AAA) may have information on low-cost legal services for elders and on information regarding financing of long-term care (see Appendix A for additional resources).

MEASURABLE EXPECTED OUTCOMES

1. Caregivers will assist client in receiving a medical evaluation by (date).
2. Caregivers will be able to describe the usual symptoms and progress of AD by (date).
3. Caregivers will have established some form of personal support through either formal or informal sources by (date).
4. Caregivers will have discussed financial and legal arrangements with client and significant family members and begun to make appropriate arrangements by (date).

Middle-Stage

Client issues   As the disease progresses to the middle stage, mild symptoms worsen and become more pronounced. New symptoms that require ever-increasing adjustment and coping for both the client and caregiving family emerge. Seemingly endless amounts of time, strength, energy, patience, and resourcefulness are necessary for the client to be maintained at home. Stress skyrockets. Without thoughtful, careful home management, clients may be prematurely institutionalized.

At this stage of AD, clients are only able to do concrete thinking. The client relies on verbal cues to know how to behave. Clients are unable to dress and groom themselves in a precise manner and need supervision, assistance, or both, to complete these tasks satisfactorily; therefore clients cannot safely be left alone for long. They have little understanding of what constitutes a dangerous situation. They can be impulsive and exhibit poor judgment as a result of an increasingly limited capacity for analysis, problem solving, and critical thinking. Eventually, the client will exhibit some or all of the problems described in this section: agitation, catastrophic reactions, wandering, feeding problems, toileting problems, sleep and rest pattern disturbances, and inappropriate sexual behavior.

Agitation, anxiety, and resistance Agitation, anxiety, and resistance behaviors surface as AD clients try to cope with an increasingly stressful environment that is difficult for them to interpret— one that seems threatening and dangerous to them. Once familiar places, people, and processes now seem alien. Feeling "lost" is disconcerting at best and overwhelming at its worst. This stimulates a primitive fight-or-flight reaction as a way of adapting and trying to reclaim security, equilibrium, and control.

In an examination of the cognitive and behavioral problems of this disease, Kolanowski (1996) recommends that the client's preillness personality be explored for evidence of past abusive and controlling behaviors toward others, inflexibility, aggressiveness, alcoholism, and substance abuse. Also, questions should be asked about the client's exposure to life-threatening and stressful events in the past and ways the client coped with such events. Research suggests that persons with histories of these kinds of behaviors are at greater risk of exhibiting more rapid cognitive decline and have higher levels of agitation, anxiety, stubbornness, wandering, shadowing, and catastrophic reactions.

CLIENT INTERVENTIONS In the book, *The 36-Hour Day* (Mace, Rabins, 1999), the authors recommend using the "6 Rs" approach to client management: restrict, reassess, reconsider, rechannel, reassure, and review.

1. Restrict. Through the use of gentle firmness, tact, cajoling, and distraction, the goal is to get the client to stop unwanted behavior. A more direct approach will be needed if the client is engaged in harmful or unsafe actions toward the self or others. A possible outcome of this strategy may be increased agitation. However, that must be weighed against the degree of harm the client or others may sustain if the behavior is continued.

2. Reassess. All behavior has meaning. Clients with AD have a hard time expressing their needs in a conventional manner. What may be interpreted as senseless, annoying behavior may be an attempt to communicate a problem or discomfort the client cannot put into words. For example, the client who is agitated and tries to undress himself or herself may be trying to communicate the need to void. Perhaps the client is becoming physically ill or has pain. Caregivers should assess beyond the obvious to a more subtle representation of what the client may be trying to communicate and reduce and eliminate stressors from the client's environment.

3. Reconsider. Caregivers should imagine themselves in the client's situation. Considering the client's impairment, how might they be interpreting the environment? A tall marble plant stand may look like a urinal to a male client. A female client may think someone is trying to break into her home to attack her when in reality it is only a noisy television program. Caregivers should reduce unnecessary noise and commotion from the client's environment.

4. Rechannel. Becoming adept at using distraction techniques is particularly useful. Caregivers should engage the client in safe, pleasant activities to replace objectionable ones and be realistic about what is expected of the client. Just because clients could easily perform activities or tasks in the past does not mean they can do them now. Things should be kept simple.

5. Reassure. A calm, patient, confident, nonconfrontational approach will help foster interpersonal relationships in clients with AD. Caregivers should be open, loving, and reassuring. The world of the dementia client is a confusing, puzzling, and frightening place. A positive attitude toward an acceptance of the client is needed to reduce fear and alleviate accompanying acting-out behaviors. Caregivers should develop and follow a set routine for the client.

6. Review. Caregivers should think about what, when, and why situations trigger problems; assess which strategies do and do not work; and learn from trial and error. Sharing that knowledge with others via caregiver support groups and Alzheimer's internet chat sites can be helpful and therapeutic for the caregivers and others.

ACTIVITIES It is important to determine purposeful and enjoyable activities with which to engage the client. Nurses can explore with the client (if possible) and caregivers what those activities may be. This will be based on inquiries into the life-long interests and lifestyle preferences of the client. The "pleasant events schedule" is a tool devised by researchers in dementia care that can help the nurse identify and design an individualized activity program for the client (Teri, Logsdon, 1991) (Fig. 22-5).

Pleasant Events Schedule - Alzheimer's Disease

This schedule contains a list of events or activities that people sometimes enjoy. It is designed to find out about things the patient has enjoyed during the past month. Please rate each item *three times*. The first time, rate each item on how many times it happened in the past month (frequency); the second time, rate how available it has been (availability); and the third time, rate each event on how pleasant it has been (enjoyability), either now or in the past.

Because this list contains events or activities that might happen to a wide variety of people, you may find that many of the items have not happened to the patient in the past month. It is not expected that anyone will have done all of these things in one month. There are no right or wrong answers.

Frequency directions:
How often have these events happened in the patient's life in the past month? Please answer each item by putting an X in the appropriate column according to how often the item has occurred.
    Not at all - This has *not happened* for the patient in the past month.
    A few times- This has *happened a few times* (1 to 6 times) in the past month.
    Often- This has *happened often* (7 or more times) in the past month.

Availability directions:
How available are these events to the patient? Please answer each item by putting an X in the appropriate column according to how available the item is.
    Not at all- This item has *not been available* during the past month.
    A few times- This item has been *available a few times* (1 to 6 times during the past month.
    Often- This item has been *available often* (7 or more times) during the past month.

Enjoyability directions:
How enjoyable are these events to the patient? Please rate each item by putting an X in the appropriate columns (one or both if they both apply) according to how enjoyable the item is.
    Now enjoys- The patient has enjoyed doing this item *in the last month.*
    Enjoyed in the past- The patient has enjoyed doing this item in the *past* (in the last 5 years).

Example:
Item #1 is "Being outside." If the patient has been outside three times during the past month, place an X in the box marked "a few times" under *frequency.* If the patient has had an opportunity to be outside seven or more times during the past month, place an X in the box marked "Often" in the *availability* column. Finally, if the patient has enjoyed being outside in the past, but did not enjoy it during the last month, place an X in the "Enjoyed in the past" column. Even if the patient hasn't experienced something on the list in the past month, it is still necessary to rate its enjoyability.

Important: Some items will list more than one event; for these items, check how often the patient has done any of the listed events. For example, item #3 is "Planning trips or vacations, looking at travel brochures, traveling." You should rate item #3 on how often the patient has done *any* of these activities in the past month.

Fig. 22-5   Pleasant events schedule—Alzheimer's disease. *(From Logsdon RG, Teri L: The Gerontologist 31[1], 1997.)*

	Frequency			Availability			Enjoyability	
	Not at all	A few times	Often	Not at all	A few times	Often	Now enjoys	Enjoyed in the past
1. Being outside (sitting outside, being in the country)								
2. Meeting someone new or making new friends								
3. Planning trips or vacations, looking at travel brochures, traveling								
4. Shopping, buying things (for self or others)								
5. Being at the beach								
6. Reading or listening to stories, novels, plays, or poems								
7. Listening to music (radio, stereo)								
8. Watching T.V.								
9. Camping								
10.. Thinking about something good in the future								
11. Completing a difficult task								
12. Laughing								
13. Doing jigsaw puzzles, crosswords, and word games								
14. Having meals with friends or family (at home or out, special occasions)								
15. Taking a shower or bath								
16. Being with animals or pets								
17. Listening to nonmusic radio programs (talk shows)								
18. Making or eating snacks								
19. Helping others, helping around the house, dusting, cleaning, setting the table, cooking								
20. Combing or brushing my hair								
21. Taking a nap								
22. Being with my family (children, grandchildren, siblings, others)								
23. Watching animals or birds (in a zoo or in the yard)								
24. Wearing certain clothes (such as new, informal, formal, or favorite clothes)								
25. Listening to the sounds of nature (birdsong, wind, surf)								
26. Having friends come to visit								
27. Getting/sending letters, cards, notes								
28. Watching the clouds, sky, or a storm								
29. Going on outings (to the park, a picnic, a barbeque, etc.)								
30. Reading, watching, or listening to the news								
31. Watching people								
32. Having coffee, tea, a soda, etc. with friends								
33. Being complimented or told I have done something well								
34. Being told I am loved								

Fig. 22-5, cont'd For legend see opposite page.

Continued

MEASURABLE EXPECTED OUTCOMES

1. Control of fear and anxiety will be consistently demonstrated by fewer than _____ resistant episodes per week by (date).
2. Agitation will be successfully controlled through distraction techniques and simple repetitive-task performance by (date).
3. Client will be able to be taken on short outings for needed services, such as barber, doctor, podiatrist, and shoe store by (date).
4. Client will adhere to and cooperate within an established daily routine by (date).
5. Client will participate in _____ pleasant activities _____ times per week by (date).

35. Having family members or friends tell me something that makes me proud of them											
36. Seeing or speaking with old friends (in person or on the telephone)											
37. Looking at the stars or moon											
38. Playing cards or games											
39. Doing handwork (crocheting, woodworking, crafts, knitting, painting, drawing, ceramics, clay work, other)											
40. Exercising (walking, aerobics, swimming, dancing, other)											
41. Indoor gardening or related activities (tending plants)											
42. Outdoor gardening or related activities (mowing lawn, raking leaves, watering plants, doing yard work)											
43. Going to museums, art exhibits, or related cultural activities											
44. Looking at photo albums and photos											
45. Stamp collecting, or other collections											
46. Sorting out drawers or closets											
47. Going for a ride in the car											
48. Going to church, attending religious ceremonies											
49. Singing											
50. Grooming self (wearing makeup, having hair done)											
51. Going to the movies											
52. Recalling and discussing past events											
53. Participating or watching sports (golf, baseball, football, etc.)											

Fig. 22-5, cont'd   For legend see p. 394.

Catastrophic reactions   High amounts of sensory stimuli and unfamiliar people, places, and routines can trigger an outburst of such proportion that the client becomes completely overwhelmed and acts out in an extreme manner. The client's temper becomes explosive and produces a temper tantrum of hostility, anger, aggression, and screaming. These outbursts can happen anywhere and anytime. They are particularly disturbing when they occur in public places.

CAREGIVER AND NURSE INTERVENTIONS

1. Determine circumstances that trigger catastrophic reactions in the client.
2. Avoid circumstances that trigger adverse reactions.
3. Identify and eliminate client's perceived stressors.
4. Reduce stimuli during a catastrophic episode. Simplify the environment. Create a quiet and calm atmosphere.
5. Do not shout at, argue with, or laugh at the client.

MEASURABLE EXPECTED OUTCOMES

1. The client will maintain self control _____% of the time by (date).
2. Factors contributing to catastrophic reactions will be identified and avoided by (date).
3. The client will refrain from verbal outbursts and antisocial behaviors by (date).

Wandering   Wandering is one of the most common and potentially dangerous behaviors in clients with AD. It is a major safety concern. Once thought to be purposeless, aimless motor activity, wandering behaviors have meaning to the client and can actually have some benefits if carefully supervised. Wandering can be an outlet with which the client can cope with stress, find security, and fill a need unable to be articulated. Two primary types of wandering have been identified: continuous and sporadic. Each requires a different management approach (Thomas, 1995).

CONTINUOUS WANDERING   The continuously wandering client is constantly on the move and can expend enormous amounts of energy with hour upon hour of movement. The client does not have the judgment to associate fatigue with the need to sit or rest. These clients can have a difficult time maintaining proper weight and will not be still long enough to sit and eat a meal. Continuous wanderers have a greater degree of cognitive impairment and generally are in the more advanced states of dementia (Lucero et al, 1993). Their single purpose is movement. They are not successfully lured to distraction by guidance to a chair or diversional activity. These wanderers are less communicative and interactive. Continuous wanderers are cued by objects in the environment. For example, if the client is wandering and comes upon a door, he or she will open the door to go out. They will pick objects up and carry them off when encountering objects on tables or furniture. Attempts to physically restrain clients are usually met with great agitation, thereby increasing the client's stress level and potential for a catastrophic episode.

SPORADIC WANDERING Clients who engage in sporadic wandering are in motion about half of the time. Their reasons for wandering are more goal oriented, such as wanting to go home, go to work, or search for someone or something. These clients have better cognitive ability and are generally more verbal and interactive with others. It may also be more difficult to deter these individuals because they can be very focused on wanting to achieve their goal. Sporadic wanderers are occasionally able to be distracted from their desire to leave by engaging them in games, meals, or other activities, since once successfully distracted, they may forget (for a while) their original mission.

SAFETY CONCERNS FOR THE WANDERER First, it is important to assess for a safe environment in and around the client's home and community. Evaluate inside the home for potential and actual safety hazards, such as location of exits and staircases, placement of furniture and rugs, hallway obstructions, pets underfoot, fire evacuation routes, presence of smoke alarms, location of bedroom in relationship to exits, and existence of nonedibles the client may mistake for food. Other important safety considerations are the availability and storage of sharp objects, tools, chemicals, and firearms; condition and access of electrical appliances; and the presence of smokers in the home.

Second, it is important to assess the area outside of the home for proximity to traffic and busy intersections, availability of sidewalks, numbers of pedestrians on the streets, environmental hazards

and barriers (businesses or industry near the home, swimming pools, bus stops, open stairwells, tunnels, and accessibility of trash containers), and the type of neighborhood. Is the client well known to the neighbors? Do neighbors look out for one another? Are they aware of the client's impairment? Would they intervene if they observed the client outside the home without supervision?

CAREGIVER AND NURSE INTERVENTIONS

1. Place alarm devices on windows and doors.
2. Replace doorknobs with specially designed ones that are difficult for a client with dementia to manipulate.
3. Never allow the client to smoke unsupervised.
4. Lock up all matches, lighters, and other smoking materials and firearms.
5. Create, if feasible, a securely fenced continuous circuitous pathway in the backyard, free of distracting objects and barriers, for the continuous wanderer to walk.
6. Camouflage doorways and other potential exits so that the client is not cued to leave.
7. Install window locks and staircase gates as needed.
8. Remove knobs, dials, and switches from stoves and appliances.
9. Use methods of distraction and stalling when possible.
10. Eliminate the client's access to vehicle keys.
11. Register the client for the Safe Return program (nationwide 24-hour program that keeps client information and photos to alert local police and others if the client becomes lost; sponsored by the Alzheimer's Association).

MEASURABLE EXPECTED OUTCOMES

1. Environmental risks and hazards will be identified and either removed or minimized by (date).
2. Client will live and function in a safe, secure environment by (date).
3. Appropriate barriers to prevent falls and unwanted exit from home will be in place by (date).
4. Alarm systems will be in place and in good working order by (date).
5. Hazardous materials and objects will be securely stored and inaccessible to the client by (date).

6. Fire evacuation route and disaster plan will be formulated by _(date)._

Sexually aggressive behavior Most people experience a great deal of discomfort when faced with a client engaging in inappropriate sexual behavior. Disrobing in public; masturbating compulsively; touching, grabbing, or pinching inappropriately; exposing genitals; expressing desire for intercourse; and shouting obscenities are all acts associated with shame and embarrassment.

The sex drive is fundamental in human beings and basic to the psyche. Problem behavior can be triggered by deficits in the following five areas: (1) disturbance in memory and judgment; (2) unmet affection needs; (3) age-related changes with decreased impulse control; (4) death anxiety; and (5) underlying physical problems, such as urinary tract infections, urinary retention, colorectal pain, vaginitis, and fecal impaction (Philo, Richie, Kaas, 1996).

CAREGIVER OR NURSE INTERVENTIONS

1. Assess for physiological reasons that may be contributing to behavior.
2. Provide opportunities for the client to go to the bathroom every 2 to 3 hours while awake.
3. Post pictures near room entrances that illustrate the purpose of the room.
4. Provide tactile stimulation, such as a rag doll, stuffed animal, differing textures of cloth, or a pet.
5. Stop inappropriate public exhibitions quickly; provide clothing; or remove client to a private area.
6. Use modified clothing that is not easily removable by the client (overalls, shirts or blouses that button up the back, turtle-neck sweaters, pull-over tops, or elasticized-waist sweat pants with a cinch that can be tied).
7. Spend quality time with client; reward positive behavior with appropriate rewards.
8. Use therapeutic touch, such as hand massage (Snyder, Egan, Burns, 1995) (Box 22-2).
9. Reassure client of self-worth.
10. Use pharmacological agents as ordered by physician to deal with unmanageable behaviors and to decrease anxiety and agitation.
11. Teach purpose, preparation, dosage, administration, and side effects of prescribed medications; verify caregiver's knowledge and competency in medication management.

Box 22-2   Protocol for Hand Massage

1. BACK OF HAND MASSAGE
   A. Short/medium length straight strokes from wrist to fingertips using moderate pressure (effleurage)
   B. Large half-circular stretching strokes from center to side of hand using moderate pressure
   C. Small circular strokes over entire back of hand using light pressure (making little O's with thumb)
   D. Featherlike straight strokes from wrist to fingertips using very light pressure
2. PALM OF HAND MASSAGE
   A. Short/medium length straight strokes from wrist to fingertips using moderate pressure (effleurage)
   B. Gentle milking/lifting of tissue of entire palm of hand using moderate pressure
   C. Small circular strokes over entire palm of hand using moderate pressure (making little O's)
   D. Large half-circular stretching strokes from center of palm to sides using moderate pressure
3. FINGER MASSAGE
   A. Gentle squeezing of fingers from base to tip on sides and top/bottom using light pressure
   B. Gentle circular range of motion of each finger followed by a gentle squeeze of the nail bed
4. COMPLETION OF HAND MASSAGE
   Lay client's hand on yours and cover it with your other hand. Gently draw your top hand toward you several times. Turn client's hand over and gently draw the other hand toward you several times.

From Snyder M, Egan EC, Burns KR: *Geriatric Nursing* 16(2):60-63, 1995.
NOTE: Do not massage any injured, reddened, or swollen portion of the hand.

MEASURABLE EXPECTED OUTCOMES

1. Inappropriate displays of sexually demonstrative behaviors will cease by _(date)._
2. Anxiety and mood will be controlled by _(date)._
3. Need for affection, reassurance, and self-worth will be met by _(date)._
4. Any side effects of prescribed medications will be recognized and immediately reported.

5. Caregiver will demonstrate competency in medication management by (date).

Sleep and rest pattern disturbances   Many clients with AD sleep more during the day and become restless at night, depriving the caregiver of much-needed sleep. Once again, rather than attributing this process solely to the disease itself, the nurse must investigate other factors that may be implicated. Because of a decline in functional capabilities and an inability to initiate activities, the AD client may spend too much time during the day sitting and dozing. Daytime inactivity can lead to sleeplessness at night. It can be helpful to keep the client occupied during the day with tasks such as washing dishes, raking leaves, folding laundry, watering the lawn, sorting coins, and other simple repetitive tasks.

Obvious reasons for nighttime waking, such as caffeine intake, an overstimulating environment in the evening, physical discomfort, and the need to void or have a bowel movement, should be explored. Fewer visual and auditory cues at night to compensate for declining mental abilities may be responsible for the client losing his or her orientation completely, resulting in increased anxiety, agitation, and panic. This phenomenon is commonly referred to as *sundown syndrome.* Clients can be upset all night long. As soon as the sun rises and familiar routines, sights, and sounds return, they feel more secure and fall asleep. If this pattern is not broken, it will reinforce disrupted sleep and rest patterns.

CAREGIVER AND NURSE INTERVENTIONS

1. Make a list of appropriate daytime diversional activities within the client's capabilities.
2. Initiate tasks periodically throughout the day.
3. Assess for depression and refer if necessary for appropriate treatment.
4. Avoid caffeine several hours before bedtime.
5. Provide an opportunity for the client to go to the bathroom before going to bed for the night.
6. Install and turn on night lights.
7. Restrict extended napping during daytime hours.

MEASURABLE EXPECTED OUTCOMES

1. Client will establish sleep and rest pattern by (date).
2. Client will retire for the night at _____ PM and wake at _____ AM by (date).

3. Client will awaken no more than _____ times per night by (date).
4. Client will return to sleep within _____ minutes by (date).

Nutrition and feeding problems   Decreased food intake in clients with AD can result from depression, difficulty making selections when presented with multiple food choices, and an inability to remember how to swallow or use a fork, knife, or spoon. Wanderers may not be able to be lured to sit at the dinner table long enough to ingest a proper meal. Continuous wanderers expend so much effort that it may be difficult for them to keep up with their energy needs. Clients who are paranoid may believe the food has been poisoned and refuse to eat. Some AD clients prefer high-sugar foods and empty calories and can develop vitamin and protein deficiencies. Eating in restaurants increases stress because of change of routine, too many menu choices, and the commotion in the restaurant.

Clients still living at home alone need to be monitored for safe food-handling techniques. Clients living alone may be eating rotten, rancid food because they no longer understand the concept of fresh versus spoiled. They have been known to mix all foodstuffs into a single pot or pan making an inedible concoction because they cannot remember the steps for food preparation (Hall, 1994).

CAREGIVER AND NURSE INTERVENTIONS

1. Avoid overstimulating activities, such as exercise or bathing, just before mealtime.
2. Prepare small frequent feedings cut into bite-size pieces, finger foods, and snacks that the client can eat "on the run."
3. Avoid the use of caffeine.
4. Use supplemental formulas or fortified milkshakes for clients who are losing weight.
5. Feed clients who no longer know how to use utensils. Cue verbally to chew and swallow if needed.
6. Prepare blended foods when swallowing difficulties increase.
7. Leave ample time for feeding. Maintain an unhurried, relaxed atmosphere. Turn off the radio and TV.
8. Consider the client's past food preferences, eating patterns, and cultural norms surrounding food when meal planning. Use the

feeding behavior inventory tool to identify client-specific patterns (Box 22-3).

9. Monitor dentition and oral status. Provide referral for routine dental care. Have dentist adjust ill-fitting dentures.

MEASURABLE EXPECTED OUTCOMES

1. Minimum caloric intake will be _____ Kcal/day by (date)
2. Protein intake will be at least _____ g/day by (date).
3. Fluid intake will be at least _____ ml/day by (date).
4. Client will achieve body weight of _____ lb by (date).

5. Food and meal activities will not trigger increased anxiety or catastrophic reactions by (date).
6. Client will have pain-free dentition for chewing (or well-fitting dentures) by (date).
7. Client will receive routine dental check-up on (date).

Elimination and toileting   Before urinary or fecal incontinence is attributed to the inevitable decline in functioning inherent in AD, many factors must be considered. Common physical causes, such as urinary tract infection and drug effects, should be ruled out. Although some causes of urinary or fecal incontinence can be determined and treated by the nurse, others will require further

---

Box 22-3   Feeding Behavior Inventory

Code appropriate response:
X   Behavior is seen
O   Behavior is not seen
N/A   Behavior could not be assessed at this time
Non-food items: trays, cups, bibs, napkins, covers, etc.
Impatient behaviors: banging, yelling, demanding food
Condiments: salt, pepper, catsup, mustard, jelly, sauces, etc.

RESISTIVE/DISRUPTIVE BEHAVIORS

1. Attempts to leave table before finishing ☐
2. Distracted from eating ☐
3. Sets food or plate aside before finished eating ☐
4. Plays with food or non-food items ☐
5. Hoards, hides or throws food ☐
6. Stares without eating ☐
7. Impatient behaviors demonstrated during or prior to meal time ☐
8. Verbally refuses to eat or states, "No more," "Not hungry," or "I'm finished" ☐
9. States, "I can't afford to eat," etc. ☐
10. Searches for food at non-meal times ☐
11. Demands food at non-meal times ☐
12. Refuses to go to dining room or eating place ☐

ORAL BEHAVIORS

1. Holds food in mouth (stuffs food/pockets) ☐
2. Does not chew food prior to swallowing ☐

3. Refuses to open mouth ☐
4. Spits food out ☐
5. Prolonged chewing without swallowing ☐

PATTERN OF INTAKE

1. Eats others' food ☐
2. Eats dessert or sweets and neglects other foods ☐
3. Eats paper goods, condiments or other non-food items ☐
4. Eats only certain food groups or only liquids ☐
5. Eats everything and anything (food and non-food) ☐
6. Eats pieces too big for safe intake ☐
7. Eats too fast for safe intake ☐

STYLE OF EATING

1. Uses straw incorrectly ☐
2. Uses knife incorrectly ☐
3. Uses spoon incorrectly ☐
4. Uses fork incorrectly ☐
5. Uses cup or glass incorrectly ☐
6. Eats non-finger food with hands ☐
7. Mixes inappropriate foods together ☐
8. Uses condiments incorrectly ☐

Total % of foods consumed _____
Total % of protein consumed _____

Total time available to eat _____

From Durnbaugh T, Haley B, Roberts S: *Geriatric Nursing* 17(2):63-67, 1996.

medical work-up. Physiological incontinence may be caused by neurological malfunction, infection, spasms, and fistulas affecting the urinary and gastrointestinal tract.

A study done by Hutchinson, Leger-Krall, and Wilson (1996) identified the act of toileting to be a 21-step sequence of events from start to finish. As the client's cognition deteriorates, the ability to perform the toileting process in the correct order becomes lost. Clients may feel the urge to urinate or defecate but forget where the bathroom is. Once in the bathroom, the client may not remember that the next step is to unfasten their clothing and pull down their underwear. The client can become baffled at any one of the numerous steps in the toileting process. This ultimately leads to nonphysiologically induced incontinence.

Self-care in elimination is a necessity done in private by normal adults. It may seem unnatural and embarrassing to the client to need assistance with this most personal task. The client's poor insight into his or her inability to completely carry out the toileting procedure can contribute to problems with resistance when attempting to assist.

Constipation can become a recurring problem if not monitored regularly. Clients with AD will not remember when they last had a bowel movement, nor will they be able to determine whether the bowel movement was of sufficient quantity. Clients who are not physically active and have poor fluid intake are at greater risk for constipation and fecal impaction. The home care nurse needs to assess bowel function and emphasize to caregivers the importance of monitoring the frequency and amount of the client's stools. Procedures such as enemas and manual disimpaction of stool are traumatic for these clients and can initiate a catastrophic reaction. It is far better to plan and implement a successful bowel program so that the client's bowels move on a regular basis.

CAREGIVER AND NURSE INTERVENTIONS (HUTCHINSON, LEGER-KRALL, WILSON, 1996)

1. Follow routine toileting schedule to fit with individual client routines; adhere to schedule.
2. Preserve client dignity by speaking about toilet issues with them in private and being discreet in front of others.

3. Use signs and pictures to indicate location of bathroom.
4. Provide cognitive assistance when needed (verbal cues as to the appropriate next step in toileting process).
5. Provide physical assistance in a gentle, matter-of-fact, nonthreatening, dignified manner.
6. Use panty liners or incontinence products for the occasional "accident."
7. Keep tract of the frequency and amount of the client's bowel movements.
8. Determine sufficient bowel frequency.
9. Devise actions to be taken when the client does not meet normal bowel frequency pattern

MEASURABLE EXPECTED OUTCOMES

1. Urinary incontinence will be managed by (date).
2. Client will have a bowel movement every day(s) by (date).
3. Client's verbal and nonverbal cues indicating the need to eliminate will be recognized and responded to promptly by (date).
4. Action plan will be initiated when bowel frequency does not meet threshold by (date).

Family issues As the disease progresses, caregivers often find themselves overwhelmed with the many tasks of caregiving. In addition to the physical tasks of assisting the client with ADLs, the caregiver is also required to handle most of the IADLs, such as providing transportation, cooking, doing laundry, and paying bills. As described earlier in this chapter, caregivers may experience feelings of burden, overload, depression, anxiety, and decreased personal health. Caregivers may also experience feelings of grief and loss as they care for a loved one who is in the process of becoming a stranger (Jones, Martinson, 1992; Wuest, Ericson, Stern, 1994). Much of the assessment and many of the interventions for the client at this stage involve the family caregiver and the process of teaching the caregiver to provide care when the professional is not available.

Caregivers should be assessed as to the level of knowledge related to the care they are required to give. "Knowing how to provide care to someone with dementia is not an innate skill . . . acquired solely through the motivation to care; [but] . . . it is learned and acquired through guidance, experiences, and support from knowledgeable providers of caregiver education and support" (Kelley, Buckwalter, Maas, 1999). The preparedness, enrichment, and predictability (PREP) program is a home health care nursing intervention designed to increase caregiver preparedness for caregiving, enrich the caregiving experience, and increase predictability and control in caregiving. This intervention has shown positive outcomes for the caregiver and has decreased hospital costs (Archbold et al, 1995). This preliminary study of a specific nursing intervention with caregivers lends support to the notion that home care services directed to the family caregiver can produce positive outcomes. Other studies have also shown that caregivers who participate in interventions that support the development of caregiving-specific skills and knowledge and that enhance social support, problem solving skills, and the use of community-based services are more satisfied in their caregiving (Collins, Given, 1994). In general, the role of the home care nurse during this stage becomes one of providing support, education, and referral.

Assessment Caregiver stress and burden should be evaluated during the home visit. Several burden assessment instruments are available in the research literature. (See Vitaliano, Young, Russo [1991] for a comprehensive review of 10 of these measures.) Given the array of these tools, it may be useful for the home health care agency to adopt or modify an existing instrument that matches the characteristics of its client-patient population (Winslow, Carter, 1999). Another tool for measuring caregiver overload that has been found to be valid and reliable is in Appendix B. It may be useful in evaluating the caregivers' subjective experience of caregiving (Pearlin et al, 1990). Assessment of caregiver depression and perceived physical health should also be evaluated.

NURSE INTERVENTIONS FOR CAREGIVERS Caregivers at this stage need specific caregiving instruction on how to deal with client behaviors described in the client section. They also need instruction on how to provide safe physical care. As discussed earlier, caregivers may also need assistance in knowing how to effectively communicate with clients.

Interventions at this stage will likely include referrals to other community services. Caregivers continue to need support and may benefit from ongoing involvement in a support or educational

group or in counseling. They may also need some in-home assistance with chores or with respite to get some time away from their caregiving responsibilities. Out-of-home respite may also be an alternative for the caregiver. Social or Alzheimer's day care or day health care are potential resources for caregivers. Caregivers may also be interested in placing the client into some type of short-term, out-of-home respite such as board and care, to have a few days off from the rigors of caregiving. Referrals to the local Alzheimer's Association, AAA, or Eldercare Locator will provide caregivers with information regarding respite, day care, and in-home supportive services available in their areas (see Appendix A).

Finally, caregivers need to be encouraged to care for themselves. Several strategies have been suggested by Mace and Rabins (1999) in *The 36-Hour Day.* Those strategies include taking time, giving themselves a present, staying connected with friends, avoiding isolation, and accepting additional help if it is needed. For some caregivers, the acceptance of help is not an easy step. For those wives who care for their husbands, the role of providing care sometimes makes it nearly impossible to accept help, especially in the home (Winslow, 1998). These caregivers need to be listened to and supported as they make decisions that are profoundly difficult in light of what they perceive as their responsibility.

MEASURABLE EXPECTED OUTCOMES

1. Caregivers will be able to demonstrate appropriate caregiving strategies for providing physical and instrumental assistance with ADLs by (date).
2. Caregivers will be able to demonstrate satisfying communication strategies that they have developed with the client by (date).
3. Caregivers will be able to identify and access community resources that are needed in the particular caregiving situation by (date).
4. Caregivers will describe _____ strategies that they will use to care for themselves by (date).
5. Caregivers will identify _____ sources of support for themselves by (date).

Late Stage

Client issues Late-stage AD is the terminal phase of the illness. It is characterized by the progressive, relentless disintegration of all physical and mental capabilities. The personality traits and characteristics that make an individual unique are destroyed by the entropy taking place in the brain. This unraveling of all learning is the inverse of normal growth and development. The client with AD becomes infantile, requiring care like a baby. The client regresses to the extent that only the most basic reflexes are left intact. Advanced AD is the turnabout of normal skill acquisition (Reisberg, 1983).

Researchers at New York University's Aging and Dementia Center developed a staging scale known as the functional assessment staging (FAST) scale. This scale consists of 16 functional stages. When applied periodically throughout the course of the disease, this scale can help document the rate of decline in the AD client. The client who is at or beyond stage seven of the FAST scale is reaching the terminal stage of AD.

In some respects, it is easier to care for a client in the late stage of AD than in the middle stage. Caregivers no longer have to contend with wandering, catastrophic reactions, misplaced items, or being constantly shadowed by the client. Clients eventually become bedbound and essentially contained. Excellent care of the bedbound, immobile, minimally responsive client is now the focus of care. The client needs to be turned every 2 hours when in bed, have incontinence managed, be hand fed and lifted to sit in a chair, and receive meticulous skin and oral care. Prevention of decubitus ulcers and sufficient food and fluid intake are also areas of concern.

Even though the physical care in the late stage of AD becomes more predictable and routine, this stage often presents with excruciatingly difficult psychosocial and ethical dilemmas. These are spawned by differing viewpoints among family members as to the appropriate end-of-life care the client should receive in the absence of advance directives. This debate generally commences with the question of whether or not to insert a feeding tube for artificial nutrition and hydration when the client loses the ability to swallow. There can also be disagreement about if, when, and where to institutionalize the client. Conflicts arise between the factions of the family who provide the actual physical care of the client with other family members who do not provide care, but compel others to either continue efforts to keep the client alive or to cease life-prolonging measures.

Differences in values, beliefs, religious perspectives, and culture can affect the nature of the debate on terminal care. Unresolved guilt and other relationship issues that have been unsatisfactorily dealt with can come to light and rekindle family turmoil. There is no one correct answer as to what constitutes appropriate care for every client. What one family deems as right and proper may be totally inappropriate for another. The home care nurse needs to identify and clarify what is essential to the core values of the family system and support the family's decision regarding care for the client once consensus has been reached.

CAREGIVER AND NURSE INTERVENTIONS

1. Provide optimal care of the immobile client including skin care, oral care, turning and positioning, range-of-motion exercises, use of pressure-reducing devices, adequate hydration and nutrition (usually requires hand feeding), adequate oxygenation, and prevention of constipation and infections.
2. Evaluate for hospice appropriateness (Box 22-4).

MEASURABLE EXPECTED OUTCOMES

1. Client will receive oral care _____ times per day by (date).
2. Client will be turned and positioned in bed every 2 to 3 hours by (date).
3. Client will not develop decubitus ulcers or contractures.
4. Client will have a fluid intake of _____ ml per day by (date).
5. Client will have an intake of calories per day by (date).
6. Client will not become constipated.
7. Client will be referred to hospice care when appropriate.

Family issues   The late stages of caregiving are often marked with transitions to institutional care. Even if institutionalization does occur, caregiving does not cease (Winslow, 1998; Zarit, Whitlatch, 1992). Most caregivers continue to assist their loved ones with physical care, such as feeding and grooming while assuming the role of client advocate if the client moves to institutional care. For other families, caregiving is continued in the home environment often with the support of home health care or hospice services.

Box 22-4   Worksheet for Determining Prognosis Dementia

The purpose of this worksheet is to guide initial and recertification assessment. It must be accompanied by narrative documentation. These are guidelines only; clinical judgment is required in each case. Construct a narrative from the information on this worksheet and information from the patient's physician and record on back. The patient should be re-evaluated at specific intervals set by the interdisciplinary team and within 60 days of clinical stabilization. This form may be used for initial and subsequent re-evaluation.

Pt. Name: _____ ID# _____
Date: _____

Both 1 and 2 must be present as evidence of hospice appropriateness.

1. Is patient severely demented?   ☐ YES ☐ NO
   Patient should be at or beyond Stage 7 of the Functional Assessment Staging Scale. Check level:
   ☐ 7A Ability to speak is limited to approximately 6 intelligible words or fewer, in the course of an average day or in the course of an intensive interview.
   ☐ 7B Speech ability is limited to the use of a single intelligible word in an average day or in the course of an intensive interview (the person may repeat the word over and over).
   ☐ 7C Ambulatory ability is lost (cannot walk without personal assistance).
   ☐ 7D Cannot sit up without assistance (e.g., patient will fall over if there are not lateral rests (arms) on the chair).
   ☐ 7E Loss of ability to smile.
   ☐ 7F Loss of ability to hold up head independently.

Patient should show **all** of the following characteristics. Check all that apply:
   ☐ inability to ambulate independently (cannot walk without personal assistance)
   ☐ unable to dress without assistance
   ☐ unable to bathe properly
   ☐ incontinence of urine and stool (occasionally or more frequently, over the past weeks as reported by a knowledgeable informant or caregiver)
   ☐ unable to speak or communicate meaningfully (see 7A above)

2. Has the patient had one or more of the following medical complications related to dementia during the past year?   ☐ YES ☐ NO
   (Conditions should have been severe enough for hospitalization whether or not hospitalization occurred) Check all that are appropriate:
   ☐ aspiration pneumonia
   ☐ upper urinary tract infection
   ☐ septicemia
   ☐ decubitus ulcers, multiple, stage 3-4
   ☐ fever recurrent after antibiotics
   ☐ inability or unwillingness to take food or fluids sufficient to sustain life; not a candidate for feeding tube or parenteral nutrition
   Patients who are receiving tube feedings must have documented impaired nutritional status as indicated by either:
   ☐ unintentional, progressive weight loss of greater than 10% over prior 6 months, or
   ☐ serum albumin less than 2.5 gm/dl (may be helpful prognostic indicator but should not be used by itself)

From Stuart B et al: *Medical guidelines for determining prognosis in non-cancer diseases,* ed 2, Washington, DC, 1996, National Hospice Organization.

Assessment   As the client's condition deteriorates, the family may find that it no longer is able to provide the level of care required. Stress and burden may be very high in these families. Along with the feelings of stress, there may also be feelings of guilt, especially if there has been a high expectation to always provide care. Deterioration of the caregivers' own health may be a precursor to the sense that caregiving can no longer be carried out. Continuing assessment of the care-givers' stress and emotional and physical health is important at this stage. Assessment of the caregivers' knowledge and use of community resources, as well as connection to personal support systems, is also important. Spiritual support is an important facet of caregiving and should be included in the assessment of the personal support system. Assessment of the caregivers' ability to provide more complex levels of physical care, when provided with adequate instruction, should also be completed. Attention should also be given to the caregivers' concerns regarding their ability to continue providing care. CAREGIVER AND NURSE INTERVENTIONS   At this stage, the home care nurse's role continues to be one of direct care provider to the client, educator of the family caregiver, provider of appropriate referrals, and counselor for the family caregiver. Specific interventions will likely include instruction in increasingly complex physical care of the client. Interventions may also include careful listening to the caregivers' concerns regarding continuation of home care. Caregiving families may need support and information as they are faced with the option to continue home care or place the relative in institutional care (Winslow, 1998). The option of home hospice care can also be explored with the caregiving family. Hospice care is also available in selected skilled nursing facilities that work with local community-based hospice organizations. Families will likely benefit from continuing involvement in a caregiver support group and spiritual support systems as they explore their options at this stage of caregiving.

MEASURABLE EXPECTED OUTCOMES

1. Caregivers will be able to demonstrate appropriate caregiving skills that satisfy the increasing complexity of the client's needs by (date).
2. Caregivers and family will be able to describe the caregiving options of in-home and out-of-home care available to them by (date)
3. Caregivers and family will decide on the type of care (home, institutional, or hospice) that fits within their values, needs, and desires by (date).
4. Caregivers will describe personal sources of support that they can use by (date).
5. Caregivers will describe strategies that they can use to care for themselves by (date).

ROLE OF THE INTERDISCIPLINARY TEAM
Physical Therapist

The role of the physical therapist is to preserve clients' physical function, mobility, and safety for as long as possible. The physical therapist specializes in large muscle groups and can design a plan of care that focuses on keeping the client mobile through safe ambulating. The physical therapist can perform home-safety evaluations, devise home-exercise programs to improve and maintain range of motion for all joints, recommend equipment that aids walking, and suggest strategies to keep wanderers in a secure, obstacle-free environment.

Occupational Therapist

The occupational therapist specializes in the preservation and maintenance of the fine muscle coordination necessary for independence in performance of ADLs. The occupational therapist's skills range from activity analysis and task equivalents to recommending modifications so that tasks can be executed in a simple, efficient manner. This may involve the use of various types of adaptive equipment, such as special eating utensils and dressing aids. The occupational therapist helps the client and family focus on assets rather than deficits and helps clients use their remaining abilities for as long as possible (Maddox, Burns, 1997).

Speech Therapist

The speech therapist can help in the development of communication aids for AD clients. Because of their extensive knowledge of the physiology and function of the parts of the brain, they can assess what part of the brain is impaired by an examination of speech and cognitive deficits. As the disease progresses, the speech therapist can perform swallowing analysis tests and make recommendations for more effective feeding techniques.

Medical-Social Worker

The medical-social worker is an invaluable team member who can assist in referring families to community resources and mediate when a family has unresolved issues regarding long-range plans for the client's care. If there is suspected or actual abuse and neglect occurring because of high levels of stress and fatigue on the part of the caregivers, the medical-social worker can recommend support groups and respite options. For the client who lives alone and has no available friends or family and is no longer safe living independently, the medical-social worker can help arrange for conservatorship and facility placement.

Dietitian

Dementia alone causes a host of feeding problems and issues that have been addressed earlier in this chapter. In addition, many AD clients may be suffering from other (sometimes several) chronic illnesses that require dietary modifications. This type of scenario needs the input of registered dietitians. They can suggest interventions based on the client's food preferences, dietary restrictions, height, weight, energy use, activity level, and cultural considerations. When the home care nurse assesses that the client is at nutritional risk, there should be documented evidence that the registered dietitian was consulted.

Advanced-Practice Nurses

Home care nurses will be collaborating with colleagues such as family, adult, and geriatric nurse practitioners or clinical nurse specialists. Increasingly, public agencies, private care facilities, and managed care groups are recognizing the beneficial role that advanced-practice nurses play in terms of client and family satisfaction, effective use of resources, and improved quality of life for AD clients.

These nurses are often a source of referrals to home health care agencies when clients develop skilled needs and are going home. Important information can be shared between the home care nurse and advanced-practice nurses to maintain optimal continuity of care as clients transition between home and other care settings.

SUMMARY

As the overall population ages, there will be increased numbers of individuals with AD who will need care. Since many of these clients will be living in the community, the home care nurse will play an important role in helping families manage these clients throughout the stages of this debilitating, incurable illness. The nurse must be knowledgeable and proficient in assessing mental status and cognition, as well as have a working knowledge of management strategies that can help reduce the symptoms and behavioral manifestations of the disease. The home care nurse must be able to recognize signs of stress, overload, and fatigue in clients and their caregivers and have a caring concern for the caregivers who are undertaking the burden of care for their loved one. The home care nurse will need to collaborate and coordinate the client's plan of care with the other members of the interdisciplinary team. This will help reduce the incidence of dis-

comfort and disability and will promote quality of life for both the client and caregiving family.

REFERENCES

Abraham I et al: Care environments for patients with Alzheimer's disease, *Nursing Clinics of North America* 29(1):157-172, 1994.

Allen CK: Occupational therapy: Functional assessment of the severity of mental disorders, *Hospital Community Psychiatry* 39(2):140-142, 1988.

Alzheimer's Association [AA]: Statistics/prevalence (On-line) 1998, http://www.alz.org/testweb/facts/rtstats.htm.

Alzheimer's Association [AA], National Alliance for Caregiving: *Who cares? Families caring for persons with Alzheimer's disease*, Washington, DC, 1999, The Association.

Aneshensel C et al: *Profiles in caregiving: The unexpected career*, San Diego, 1995, Academic Press.

Archbold P et al: The PREP system of nursing interventions: A pilot test with families caring for older members, *Research in Nursing Health* 18(1):3-16, 1995.

Baumgarten M et al: The psychological and physical health of family members caring for an elderly person with dementia, *Journal of Clinical Epidemiology* 45(1):61-70, 1992.

Beach D: Family caregiving: The positive impact on adolescent relationships, *The Gerontologist* 37:233-238, 1997.

Bedard M et al: Associations between dysfunctional behaviors, gender, and burden in spousal caregivers of cognitively impaired older adults, *International Psychogeriatrics* 9:277-290, 1997.

Brechling BG, Schneider CA: Preserving autonomy in early stage dementia, *Journal of Gerontological Social Work* 20(1-2):17-33, 1993.

Caralis PV: Ethical and legal issues in the care of Alzheimer's patients, *Medical Clinics of North America* 78(4):877-893, 1994.

Collins C, Given B, Given C: Interventions with family caregivers of persons with Alzheimer's disease, *Nursing Clinics of North America* 29:195-207, 1994.

Convit A et al: Specific hippocampal volume reductions in individuals at risk for Alzheimer's disease, *Neurobiology of Aging* 18(2):131-138, 1997.

Dellasega C, Cutezo E: Strategies used by home health nurses to assess the mental status of homebound elders, *Journal of Community Health Nursing* 11(3):129-138, 1994.

Durnbaugh T, Haley B, Roberts S: Assessing problem feeding behaviors in mid-stage Alzheimer's disease, *Geriatric Nursing* 17(2):63-67, 1996.

Folstein M, Folstein S, McHugh P: Mini-mental state examination: A practical method for grading the cognitive state of patients for the clinician, *Journal of Psychiatric Research* 12:189-198, 1975.

Fulmer T, Birkenhauer D: Elder mistreatment assessment as a part of everyday practice, *Journal of Gerontological Nursing* 18(3):42-45, 1992.

Gold D et al: Caregiving and dementia: Predicting negative and positive outcomes for caregivers, *International Journal of Aging and Human Development* 41(3):183-201, 1995.

Goldstein MK et al: Managing early Alzheimer's disease, *Patient Care* 25(18):44-73, 1991.

Goodglass H, Kaplan E: *Assessment of aphasia and related disorders,* Philadelphia, 1972, Lea & Febiger.

Hall GR: Chronic dementia: Challenges in feeding the patient, *Journal of Gerontological Nursing* 20(4):21-30, 1994.

Harvath T et al: Establishing partnerships with family caregivers: Local and cosmopolitan knowledge, *Journal of Gerontological Nursing* 20(2):29-35, 42-43, 1994.

Hawkins JW: Nonsedating treatments for Alzheimer's patients with behavioral problems, *Journal of Clinical Psychiatry* 53(3):1992.

Hazelden: *How to talk to an older person who has a problem with alcohol or medications,* Center City, Minn, Author.

Holcomb L et al: Accelerated Alzheimer-type phenotype in transgenic mice carrying both mutant amyloid precursor protein and presenilin I transgenes, *Nature Medicine* 4(1):97-100, 1998.

Hughes CP et al: A new clinical scale for the staging of dementia, *British Journal of Psychiatry* 140:559-572, 1982.

Hutchinson S, Leger-Krall S, Wilson HS: Toileting: A biobehavioral challenge in Alzheimer's dementia care, *Journal of Gerontological Nursing* 22(10):18-27, 1996.

Johnson-Wood K et al: Amyloid precursor protein processing and Abeta 42 deposition in a transgenic mouse model of Alzheimer disease, *Proceedings of the National Academy of Sciences USA* 94(4):1550-1555, 1997.

Jones P, Martinson I: The experience of bereavement in caregivers of family members with Alzheimer's disease, *Image: Journal of Nursing Scholarship* 24:172-176, 1992.

Katzman R et al: Validation of a short orientation-memory-concentration test of cognitive impairment, *American Journal of Psychiatry* 140(6):734-739, 1983.

Kelley L, Buckwalter K, Maas M: Access to health care resources for family caregivers of elderly persons with dementia, *Nursing Outlook* 47(1):8-14, 1999.

Kolanowski A: Everyday functioning in Alzheimer's disease: Contribution of neuropsychological testing, *Clinical Nurse Specialist* 10(1):11-19, 56, 1996.

Kramer B: Gain in the caregiving experience: Where are we? What next? *The Gerontologist* 37:218-231, 1997.

Lieberman M, Fisher L: The impact of chronic illness on the health and well-being of family members, *The Gerontologist* 35:94-102, 1995.

Lindgren C: The caregiver career, *Image: Journal of Nursing Scholarship* 5:214-219, 1993.

Lucero M et al: Wandering in Alzheimer's dementia patients, *Clinical Nursing Research* 2:160-175, 1993.

Lundquist RS, Bernens A, Olsen CG: Comorbid disease in geriatric patients: Dementia and depression, *American Family Physician* 55(8):2687-2694, 2703-2704, 1997.

Mace N, Rabins P: *The 36-hour day,* ed 3, Baltimore and London, 1999, Johns Hopkins University Press.

Maddox MK, Burns T: Positive approaches to dementia care in the home, *Geriatrics* 52(suppl 2):S54-58, 1997.

Mattson MP, Robinson N, Guo Q: Estrogens stabilize mitochondrial function and protect neural cells against the pro-apoptotic action of mutant presenilin-1, *NeuroReport* 8(17):3817-3821, 1997.

McNeil C, Public Information Office, National Institute on Aging: *Alzheimer's disease: Unraveling the mystery,* 1995, The Institute and National Institutes of Health.

Miller B, Cafasso L: Gender differences in caregiving: Fact or artifact? *The Gerontologist* 32:498-507, 1992.

Miller B, Lawton M: Introduction: Finding balance in caregiver research, *The Gerontologist* 37:216-217, 1997.

Mish FC, ed: *Webster's ninth new collegiate dictionary,* Springfield, Mass, 1985, Merriam-Webster.

Mittleman M et al: A family intervention to delay nursing home placement of patients with Alzheimer's disease, *Journal of the American Medical Association* 276:1725-1731, 1996.

Miziniak H: Persons with Alzheimer's: Effects of nutrition and exercise, *Journal of Gerontological Nursing* 20(4):21-30, 1994.

National Institute on Aging, National Institutes of Health: *Progress Report on Alzheimer's Disease,* 1998, The Institutes.

Pearlin L et al: Caregiving and the stress process: An overview of concepts and their measures, *The Gerontologist* 30:583-591, 1990.

Philo S, Richie MF, Kaas MJ: Inappropriate sexual be-havior, *Journal of Gerontological Nursing* 22(11):17-22, 1996.

Reisberg B, ed: *Alzheimer's disease,* New York, 1983, Free Press.

Roberto KA et al: Communication patterns between caregivers and their spouses with Alzheimer's dis-ease: A case study, *Archives of Psychiatric Nursing* 12(4):202-208, 1998.

Schulz R et al: Psychiatric and physical morbidity ef-fects of dementia caregiving: Prevalence, corre-lates, and causes, *The Gerontologist* 35:771-791, 1995.

Schulz R, Visintainer P, Williamson G: Psychiatric and physical morbidity effects of caregiving, *Jour-nal of Gerontology* 45(5):181-191, 1990.

Snowdon D et al: Brain infarction and the clinical ex-pression of Alzheimer disease: The Nun Study, *Journal of the American Medical Association* 277(10):813-817, 1997.

Snyder M, Egan EC, Burns KR: Efficacy of hand mas-sage in decreasing agitation behaviors associated with care activities in persons with dementia, *Geriatric Nursing* 16(2):60-63, 1995.

Stuart B et al: *Medical guidelines for determining prog-nosis in non-cancer diseases,* ed 2, Washington, DC, 1996, National Hospice Organization.

Teri L, Logsdon RG: Identifying pleasant activities for Alzheimer's patients: The pleasant events sched-ule, *The Gerontologist* 31(1):124-127, 1991.

Thomas D: Wandering: A proposed definition, *Jour-nal of Gerontological Nursing* 21(9):35-41, 1995.

Tueth MJ: How to manage depression and psychosis in Alzheimer's disease, *Geriatrics* 50(1):43-46, 49, 1995.

Vitaliano P, Young H, Russo J: A review of measures used among caregivers of individuals with de-mentia, *The Gerontologist* 31:67-75, 1991.

Welsh KA et al: Detection and staging of dementia in Alzheimer's disease: Use of the psychological measures developed for the Consortium to Estab-lish a Registry for Alzheimer's Disease, *Archives of Neurology* 49(5):448-452, 1992.

Whitlatch C, Feinberg L, Sebesta D: Depression and health in family caregivers: Adaption over time, *Journal of Aging and Health* 9:222-243, 1997.

Wilson H: Family caregiving for a relative with Alzheimer's dementia: Coping with negative choices, *Nursing Research* 38(2):94-98, 1989.

Winslow B: Effects of formal supports on stress out-comes in family caregivers of Alzheimer's pa-tients, *Research in Nursing and Health* 20:27-37, 1997.

Winslow B: Family caregiving and the use of formal community support services: A qualitative case study, *Issues in Mental Health Nursing* 19:11-27, 1998.

Winslow B, Carter P: Patterns of burden in wives car-ing for husbands with dementia, *Nursing Clinics of North America* 34(2):275-287, 1999.

Wuest J, Ericson P, Stern P: Becoming strangers: The changing family caregiving relationship in Alzheimer's disease, *Journal of Advanced Nursing* 20:437-443, 1994.

Zarit S, Whitlatch C: Institutional placement: Phases of the transition, *The Gerontologist* 32:665-672, 1992.

Sources of Information and Referral for Caregiving Families

Alzheimer's Association
1-800-272-3900
The Alzheimer's Association provides education and information for caregivers and referrals to local Alzheimer's Associations.

Elder Care Locator
1-800-677-1116
The Elder Care Locator provides community support for older persons, including referral to local Area Agency on Aging (AAA).

International Parish Nurse Resource Center
1-800-556-5368

Safe Return
1-800-272-3900
Safe Return provides an identification bracelet and centralized identification program for elders. Safe Return is sponsored by the Alzheimer's Association.

Alzheimer's Disease Education & Resource (ADEAR) Center
1-800-438-4380
ADEAR provides information on Alzheimer's disease and family caregiving.

Hospice Link
1-800-331-1620
Hospice Link provides information and referral to local hospice providers within the United States.

National Family Caregivers' Association
1-800-896-3650
http://www.nfcacares.org
National Family Caregivers Association provides education and information for family caregivers on ways to improve caregivers' quality of life.

APPENDIX
B
Measurement of Caregiver Overload

Here are some statements about your energy level and the time it takes to do the things you have to do.

How much does each statement describe you?

	Completely	Quite a Bit	Somewhat	Not at All
You are exhausted when you go to bed at night.	4	3	2	1
You have more things to do than you can handle.	4	3	2	1
You don't have time just for yourself.	4	3	2	1
You work hard as a caregiver but never seem to make any progress.	4	3	2	1

NOTE: A higher score indicates a higher level of overload.
From Pearlin L et al: *The Gerontologist* 30:583-594, 1990.

23 Heart Failure and Home Care

Bonnie Huiskes

The prevalence of congestive heart failure, a condition once known as *dropsy* and now more commonly referred to as *chronic heart failure,* or simply *heart failure,* has increased significantly in adults since the mid 1970s (Fig. 23-1) as an estimated 400,000 new cases are diagnosed each year (Konstam et al, 1994). The number of people in the United States with the diagnosis of heart failure is currently estimated at 4.8 million, 70% of whom are 60 years of age or older (Thom, Kannel, 1997). The growing prevalence of this condition has been attributed to the overall aging of the population and advances in the management of coronary artery disease, valvular lesions, and hypertension (Starling, 1998), thus creating a group of persons with predisposing factors who live long enough to develop heart failure.

Hospitalization rates have also grown significantly. The number of hospitalized heart failure clients increased between 1985 and 1995 from 577,000 to 871,000 per year (Haldeman et al, 1999). For clients 65 years of age and older, congestive heart failure (CHF) is the most common reason for hospital admission. After an initial hospitalization for heart failure, readmission is common, ranging from 26% to 47% within 3 to 6 months after discharge (Foote, 1997).

Although the mortality rate from cardiovascular disease in general has seen declines in the past 2 decades (Rich, 1999b), heart failure has until very recently been estimated at a 50% mortality rate 5 years after diagnosis (National Heart, Lung and Blood Institute [NHLBI], 1996). However, in a study reported in 1998, the Centers for Disease Control and Prevention (CDC) found that the heart failure mortality rate for people 65 years of age and older declined between 1988 and 1995 at an average annual rate of 1.1%. The average annual decline was greatest in black men (3.0% per year) and black women (2.2% per year), followed by white men (1.7% per year) and white women (0.5% per year). The decline in the mortality rate may reflect improved detection and treatment of hypertension, myocardial infarction, and heart failure (CDC, 1998).

Heart failure is considered a major public health burden because of the increasing prevalence, frequent hospital admissions, associated costs, and resultant disability. An estimated $17.8 billion was spent caring for heart-failure clients in hospitals, physician offices, home care, and nursing homes in 1993 (NHLBI, 1996). The bulk of that expenditure is for inpatient stays, many of which are considered preventable with improved outpatient care (Konstam et al, 1994).

CHANGING PARADIGMS IN HEART FAILURE

The past 2 decades have witnessed a considerable increase in the scientific understanding of the pathophysiological mechanisms leading to heart failure. Beginning in the early 1980s, the application of those findings to clinical research in medical treatment has resulted in the current evidence-based approach to managing heart failure. Pathophysiology and treatment approach are two of the heart-failure paradigms that have changed significantly (Table 23-1). Other contrasts between current heart-failure management and that of 2 decades ago, which will be addressed in this chapter, include the focus of the physical examination in determining fluid status, the active role of clients, the emphasis on exercise and rehabilitation rather than rest, and the location of care for the heart-failure client.

DEFINITIONS

Heart failure may be said to exist when there is an abnormality of cardiac function. Systolic heart failure occurs when the heart fails to contract

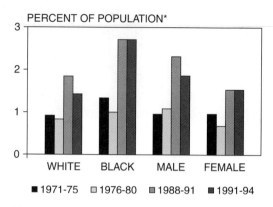

PERCENT OF POPULATION*

Fig. 23-1 Prevalence of congestive heart failure by race and sex, age 25-74, United States, 1971-1975 to 1991-1994. *(From National Institutes of Health, National Heart, Lung, and Blood Institute:* Morbidity and mortality: 1998 chartbook on cardiovascular, lung and blood diseases, *Bethesda, Md, 1998, The Institutes.)*

■ 1971-75   ▢ 1976-80   ▩ 1988-91   ▪ 1991-94

*Age-adjusted to the 2000 standard.

Table 23-1   Changing Paradigms in the Management of Heart Failure

Paradigm Aspects	Old	New
Definition	Pump	Pressure
Physical examination focus	Rales	Jugular venous pressure (JVP)
	Peripheral edema	Abdominojugular reflux
Client role	Compliance	Self-management
Fluid restriction	Usual	Serum sodium level <130 mEq/L
Daily weight	Optional	Essential
Medications	Digoxin	Angiotensin-converting enzyme (ACE) inhibitors
	Diuretics	Angiotensin II blockers
		Diuretics
		Digoxin
		Beta-blockers
		Second-generation calcium channel blockers
		Spironolactone
Use of beta-blockers	Contraindicated	Recommended
Prognosis	Dismal	Improving
Activity	Rest	Exercise and rehabilitation
Timing of care	Episodic	Continuum based
Location of care	Inpatient	Outpatient or home

normally, and diastolic heart failure occurs when the contraction is normal but the relaxation is abnormal. The most common syndrome of heart failure is caused by left ventricular systolic dysfunction, and it is said to exist when the ejection fraction (EF),* which normally ranges from 55% to 70%, is less than 40% (Heywood, 1999).

When there is evidence of fluid overload, such as elevated neck veins or pulmonary edema, and the heart is contracting normally (as evidenced by a normal EF), diastolic heart failure (diastolic dysfunction) may be diagnosed (Heywood, 1999). Diastolic heart failure occurs in approximately one third of CHF cases, more commonly in elderly individuals than in those under 60 years of age (Zile, 1998). Diastolic dysfunction most frequently results from coronary artery disease or hypertension (Konstam et al, 1994).

---

*Ejection fraction is the percentage of blood pumped out of the heart with each beat and is most commonly measured by echocardiogram (ultrasound of the heart).

Table 23-2 Selected Components of Neuroendocrine Activation in Heart Failure

Chemical Mediator	Source	Effects
Norepinephrine Epinephrine	Adrenergic nerve fibers	Increases heart rate Increases contractility Causes vasoconstriction Stimulates secretion of renin
Renin*	Kidney	Combines with angiotensinogen and ACE to form angiotensin II
Angiotensin II*	Angiotensin (from the liver) + renin + ACE = angiotensin II	Causes vasoconstriction Stimulates norepinephrine release Stimulates secretion of aldosterone
Aldosterone*	Adrenal cortex	Causes sodium retention Causes water retention Causes potassium excretion
Arginine vasopressin (antidiuretic hormone)	Pituitary gland	Causes water retention Causes vasoconstriction
Endothelin	Endothelial cells lining blood vessels	Causes vasoconstriction Stimulates growth of myocytes

*Collectively known as *RAAS (renin-angiotensin-aldosterone system)*.

Currently, the term *heart failure* is often used rather than the term *congestive heart failure* because many clients do not manifest pulmonary or systemic congestion (Konstam et al, 1994). These clients may have mild ventricular dysfunction, or they may have more severe dysfunction that has been treated adequately with recommended therapies such as ACE inhibitors and beta-blockers.

Another term, *chronic heart failure,* also removes the "congestive" from CHF (Starling, 1998) and rightly describes the long-term nature, rather than the acute or episodic nature, of the condition. This terminology revision is significant, since an understanding of the nature of chronic illness in general, and of chronic heart failure in particular, is essential for successful management in inpatient, outpatient, and home care settings.

In some instances, the term *cardiomyopathy* is used interchangeably with *heart failure.* However, *cardiomyopathy* is used most frequently to describe primary myocardial disease, either of specific or unknown etiology (Hosenpud, 1994). Many clinicians prefer the term *cardiomyopathy* for all types of myocardial dysfunction because it does not convey the ominous tone to clients of heart *failure.*

PATHOPHYSIOLOGY

Left ventricular systolic dysfunction (diastolic dysfunction is addressed in Appendix A) begins with an initial injury or insult to the heart muscle, which impairs contractile function and causes decreased ventricular emptying. Volume or pressure overload in the poorly emptying ventricle leads to ventricular dilatation (more common acutely) or hypertrophy of the left ventricle, which is seen in long-standing hypertension. The high ventricular filling pressures resulting from decreased emptying and the widespread compensatory response of neurohormonal activation (Table 23-2) are responsible for the congestive symptoms (dyspnea on exertion, orthopnea, ascites, hepatomegaly, and peripheral edema), which characterize the syndrome known as *CHF.* Angiotensin II (one of the neurohormones) production, for instance, results in vasoconstriction, thus increasing the workload of the failing heart, which must pump against higher resistance. Angiotensin II also stimulates the secretion of aldosterone, which promotes sodium reabsorption in the kidney and thus fluid retention (Goran, Johantgen, 1998). The production of angiotensin II and other neurohormones is initially compensatory but eventually causes not

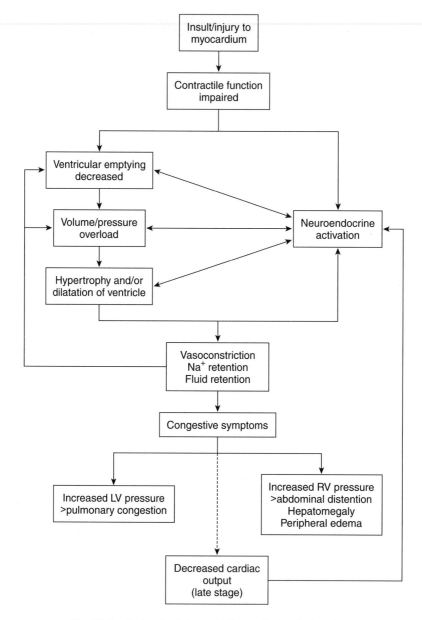

Fig. 23-2 Pathophysiology of left ventricular dysfunction.

only the congestive symptoms, but also further injury as the neurohormones exert a direct toxic effect on myocardial cells (Eichhorn, Bristow, 1996). Eventually, in end-stage heart failure, cardiac output falls and results in decreased renal blood flow and hypoperfusion of the skin and skeletal muscle. The pathophysiological processes of heart failure and their interrelationships are summarized and illustrated in Fig. 23-2.

ETIOLOGY

Coronary artery disease and hypertension are the most common causes of heart failure. Other causes of myocardial damage resulting in heart failure include toxins, such as alcohol, amphetamines, cocaine, or doxorubicin (Adriamycin), which exert a direct effect on the myocardium. Cardiomyopathy may also result from viral disease or aortic or mitral valvular disease or may

Box 23-1	New York Heart Association Functional Classification

FUNCTIONAL CLASS I

Clients with cardiac disease but without resulting limitations of physical activity. Normal daily activity does not result in symptoms.

FUNCTIONAL CLASS II

Clients with cardiac disease resulting in slight limitations of physical activity. Normal daily activity results in symptoms, but symptoms subside with rest.

FUNCTIONAL CLASS III

Clients with cardiac disease resulting in marked limitation of physical activity. Minimal activity results in symptoms; clients are usually comfortable at rest.

FUNCTIONAL CLASS IV

Clients with cardiac disease resulting in inability to carry on any physical activity without symptoms. Symptoms also present at rest.

Box 23-2	Symptoms Suggestive of Heart Failure

Paroxysmal nocturnal dyspnea (PND)
Orthopnea
Dyspnea on exertion
Lower-extremity edema
Decreased exercise tolerance
Unexplained confusion, altered mental status, or fatigue in an elderly patient
Abdominal symptoms, such as nausea or pain, that are associated with ascites

Modified from Konstam MA et al: *Heart failure: Evaluation and care of patients with left ventricular systolic dysfunction. Clinical Practice Guideline No 10,* AHCPR Pub No 94-0612, Rockville, Md, 1994, Agency for Health Care Policy and Research, Public Health Service, US Department of Health and Human Services.

be considered idiopathic when no known cause can be found. Additional primary or contributory causes of heart failure include tachycardia, hyperthyroidism, and anemia. The insult to the myocardium may have a relatively rapid onset, as in the case of viral cardiomyopathy, or be gradual, as in the long-standing pathological processes that damage the cardiac muscle.

Diastolic dysfunction (see Appendix A) typically occurs when the myocardial wall is hypertrophied and stiff from hypertension. The condition may also result from other causes, such as myocardial ischemia or infiltrative processes, such as amyloidosis. Some cases of heart failure are a combination of both systolic and diastolic dysfunction.

NEW YORK HEART ASSOCIATION CLASSIFICATION

The New York Heart Association (NYHA) classification (Box 23-1) is the subjective scale most commonly used in clinical practice to describe the severity of symptoms of heart disease. This rough measure of functional status, first introduced by the NYHA, assigns clients to one of four functional classes, based on the degree of effort needed to elicit symptoms (Packer, Cohn, 1999). The classification is useful in describing the impact of the disease on a client's life and serves as a means to track improvement (or decline) over time. Functional class does not correlate well with degree of left ventricular systolic dysfunction, however. Clients with mild reduction of cardiac function may have NYHA Class IV symptoms, and others with severe disease may experience little impact on their functional status. Most heart-failure clients followed by home care are NYHA Class III or IV.

SYMPTOMS

Symptoms that suggest a diagnosis of heart failure are found in Box 23-2. The presence of these symptoms does not necessarily mean that the client has heart failure. Dyspnea, for instance, may be the result of pulmonary disease, deconditioning, volume overload from nephrotic syndrome or renal failure, intermittent cardiac ischemia, anxiety, or acute lower respiratory infection. Other symptoms, such as lower-extremity edema, also may be found to have a noncardiac cause (Konstam et al, 1994).

DIAGNOSIS

The first step in evaluating heart-failure symptoms is to obtain a complete medical history,

Table 23-3 Recommended Tests for Clients with Signs and Symptoms of Heart Failure		
Test	Finding	Suspected Diagnoses
Chest x-ray study	Cardiomegaly	Heart failure
	Pulmonary venous congestion	
Electrocardiogram	Acute ST-T wave changes	Myocardial ischemia
	Atrial fibrillation or another tachyarrhythmia	Thyroid disease or heart failure caused by rapid ventricular rate
	Bradyarrhythmias	Heart failure caused by low heart rate
	Previous myocardial infarction (MI) (e.g., Q waves)	Heart failure caused by reduced left ventricular performance
	Low voltage	Pericardial effusion
	Left ventricular hypertrophy	Diastolic dysfunction
Complete blood count (CBC)	Anemia	Heart failure caused by or aggravated by decreased oxygen-carrying capacity
Urinalysis	Proteinuria	Nephrotic syndrome
	Red blood cells (RBCs) or cellular casts	Glomerulonephritis
Serum creatinine level	Elevated	Volume overload caused by renal failure
Serum albumin level	Decreased	Increased extravascular volume caused by hypoalbuminemia
Thyroxine (T_4) and thyroid-stimulating hormone (TSH) levels (if atrial fibrillation, evidence of thyroid disease or age >65)	Abnormal T_4 or TSH levels	Heart failure caused by or aggravated by hypothyroidism or hyperthyroidism

Modified from Konstam MA et al: *Heart failure: Evaluation and care of patients with left ventricular systolic dysfunction. Clinical Practice Guideline No 11,* AHCPR Pub No 94-0612, Rockville, Md, 1994, Agency for Health Care Policy and Research, Public Health Service, US Department of Health and Human Services.

including information regarding previous myocardial infarction; angina; other heart disease or surgery; hypertension; diabetes; renal, pulmonary, thyroid, or gastrointestinal disease; substance abuse (including alcohol); family history; and medications. The initial physical examination may reveal the following findings, which tend to support a diagnosis of heart failure (Konstam et al, 1994):

- elevated JVP or positive hepatojugular reflux
- third heart sound (S3)
- laterally displaced apical impulse
- pulmonary rales that do not clear with cough
- peripheral edema

The echocardiogram is an essential diagnostic test, which should be performed whenever symptoms and physical examination support the probable diagnosis of heart failure. Information gained from this noninvasive test includes atrial and ventricular size, wall motion, valvular structure and function, and estimation of the left ventricular EF and pulmonary artery pressure. Ventricular diastolic function can also be assessed by echocardiogram. Additional recommended diagnostic testing, findings, and suspected diagnoses can be found in Table 23-3.

TREATMENT

Treatment of heart failure begins with a search for a modifiable or treatable underlying cause or causes. Clients with ongoing ischemia may require percutaneous transluminal coronary angioplasty (PTCA) or coronary artery bypass graft (CABG) surgery to restore blood flow to the hypoperfused myocardium. Surgical correction of valvular lesions must be considered if the valve's pathology is the etiology of the heart failure. Untreated hypertension should be managed aggressively, with a target systolic blood pressure as low as 90 mm Hg, plus the EF in cases of markedly reduced (<20% EF) left ventricular function (Heywood, 1999). Control of tachycardia will improve the function of the failing left ventricle. If sinus rhythm can be restored in cases of atrial fibrillation, the normal "atrial kick" will augment ventricular function. Anemia should be corrected so that myocardial workload is decreased. If alcohol or amphetamines are implicated as causes of heart failure, they must be avoided, since abstinence is likely to result in improved heart function. Derangements of thyroid function should also be treated.

Medications

Medications shown in clinical research trials to improve survival and quality of life for heart-failure clients should be used in recommended doses. Titrating medications to optimal levels while monitoring clinical response is one of the most important components of heart-failure management. ACE inhibitors, angiotensin II blockers, diuretics, beta-blockers, and digoxin are currently accepted first-line therapeutic agents. Other medications that may be added to the regimen include spironolactone, second-generation calcium channel blockers, anticoagulants, amiodarone, nitrates and positive inotropic agents such as dobutamine and milrinone. Medications that should be avoided in heart failure are first-generation calcium channel blockers, most antiarrhythmics, and nonsteroidal antiinflammatory drugs.

ACE inhibitors and angiotensin II blockers

ACE inhibitors have become the cornerstone of effective management of heart failure (Levine, Hall, 1998), opposing the activation of the renin-angiotensin system, which results in vasoconstriction and sodium and water retention. Benefits of ACE inhibitors include reduction in mortality, improvement in functional class, and fewer hospitalizations for heart failure. The Agency for Health Care Policy and Research (AHCPR) guidelines recommend that all clients with heart failure from left ventricular dysfunction be given ACE inhibitors unless the following contraindications exist: (1) history of intolerance (intractable cough not a result of fluid overload) or adverse reactions (angioedema of the oropharyngeal region), (2) serum potassium >5.5 mEq/L that cannot be reduced, or (3) symptomatic hypotension (Konstam et al, 1994). Because ACE inhibitors are titrated to recommended dosages, diuretics may require simultaneous reduction, discontinuation, or use on an as-needed basis only when target ACE inhibitor dose levels are reached. Failure to reduce diuretics concurrently may result in the hypotension commonly thought to represent ACE inhibitor intolerance. Angiotensin II blockers such as losartan (Cozaar) and irbesartan (Avapro) are used to block the renin-angiotensin system when ACE inhibitor intolerance is responsible for cough.

Diuretics

Diuretics are used in heart-failure clients who have signs and symptoms of volume overload. Options include thiazide diuretics for mild heart failure; loop diuretics, such as furosemide (Lasix) or bumetanide (Bumex), for maintenance in cases of persistent volume overload; or intravenous furosemide for severe fluid overload (Konstam et al, 1994). Another option for severe fluid overload is the addition of a second oral diuretic, such as metolazone (Zaroxolyn), a potent thiazide-related diuretic. Outpatients treated with metolazone must be monitored closely for signs of hypovolemia and hypokalemia (Levine, Hall, 1998). It is important to remember that in advanced, severe heart failure, the "good" weight figure may need to be adjusted downward as clients lose body weight. Conversely, when clients improve, they may gain body weight as their appetites return, and the dry or "good" weight figure must be adjusted upward.

Beta-adrenergic blockers

Heart-failure clients have high levels of plasma norepinephrine, evidence of increased sympathetic activity (Michael, Parnell, 1998). As is the case with the renin-angiotensin system, activation of the autonomic nervous system (resulting in the high levels of norepinephrine) is linked to the progression of myocardial dysfunction after an initial insult to the heart's function (Smith, Levine, 1999). A clinical trial using carvedilol (Coreg), a nonselective beta-blocker with alpha-adrenergic blockade and antioxidant properties in clients with mild to moderate heart failure because of left ventricular dysfunction showed a 65% reduction in the mortality rate (Packer et al, 1996). In a recent clinical trial of another beta-blocker, metoprolol, in NYHA classes II and III, there was a 35% reduction in the mortality rate for those clients treated with the drug (MERIT-HF Study Group, 1999.) These agents must be started at very small doses and titrated slowly to higher levels while clients are carefully monitored for evidence of worsening heart failure or symptomatic bradycardia.

Digoxin The AHCPR guidelines recommend that digoxin be used routinely in clients with severe heart failure and added to the medical regimen for clients with mild or moderate heart failure who remain symptomatic after optimal management with ACE inhibitors and diuretics (Konstam et al, 1994). More recently, the Heart Failure Society of America (HFSA) guidelines recommend that digoxin, in addition to standard therapy, be considered for clients who have symptoms of heart failure caused by left ventricular systolic dysfunction (Adams et al, 2000). Digoxin has a narrow therapeutic margin of safety and should be used with caution in clients with renal failure, advanced chronic pulmonary disease, hypothyroidism, or electrolyte abnormalities or in elderly clients (Smith, Levine, 1999). The nurse should be aware of digoxin's toxic effects: arrhythmias, disorientation, nausea, anorexia, and visual disturbances (Guthery, Schumann, 1998).

Other medications The following additional medications may also be used in the management of chronic heart failure: second-generation calcium channel blockers (amlodipine and felodipine), anticoagulants (warfarin and aspirin), spironolactone (potassium-sparing diuretic that blocks aldosterone), nitrates (in oral short- or long-acting forms and transdermal patches), and amiodarone (the only antiarrhythmic considered safe in clients with reduced left ventricular function). Positive inotropic agents may be used in selected clients whose conditions remain severely symptomatic despite maximal doses of standard medications for heart failure.

HOME CARE

More than 65,000 heart failure clients receive home care each year (NHLBI, 1996). According to one study, CHF clients were older than most home care clients and had chronic health problems. More than half of the clients studied would not have been able to remain in their own homes

Box 23-3	Home Care Client Referral Criteria

Clients with a diagnosis of heart failure who:
   Have more than 2 readmissions for heart failure per year
   Require additional training in self-management of:
      Medications
      Dietary sodium intake
      Self-monitoring (weight, symptoms, and blood pressure [BP])
   Have unstable comorbidities (diabetes, hypertension, chronic obstructive pulmonary disease [COPD])
   Have caregiver issues that impact adherence to the heart-failure regimen
   Are elderly or fragile

without a caregiver. The fragility of the population is evidenced by the study finding that less than half of the study group were discharged from the home health care agency in improved conditions, and many were discharged to other health care facilities (Anderson, Pena, Helms, 1998).

A hospital discharge planner, insurance case manager, cardiologist, or primary care physician may refer heart-failure clients to home care. Referral criteria are listed in Box 23-3. Home care has a pivotal role in shifting care for heart-failure clients from an inpatient to outpatient location (Sherman, 1995). With same-day or next-day home care visits, for instance, clients can be discharged earlier from the acute care setting than would have otherwise been advisable. Adjustment of diuretics or administration of intravenous diuretics for fluid overload, based on the assessment of the home care nurse, may prevent an emergency department visit or hospitalization. In addition, the home care nurse provides education about heart failure and training in self-management, which supplements and reinforces the often-abbreviated educational opportunities in the hospital.

Background and Training of Heart-Failure Home Care Nurses

Experience in the care of cardiac clients and a critical care background are important requirements for home care heart-failure nurses (Hohenleitner, Minniti, 1998). Certainly, advanced physical-assessment skills (including estimating JVP and recognizing an S3) provide the nurse with the needed tools to evaluate the heart-failure client in the home. Excellent clinical judgment skills are also important in caring for these clients outside the hospital environment, since they may be very ill or only marginally stable. Home care nurses should be knowledgeable regarding the pathophysiology and treatment of heart failure and should be comfortable with training clients to be illness self-managers. Ideally, home care nurses should spend time working with clinicians in a heart-failure clinic to gain expertise in assessment and familiarity with the clinical management issues this client population presents. Ongoing continuing education in heart-failure management is also important because the treatment of this complex condition continues to evolve as new information from clinical research trials becomes available and guidelines are updated.

Home Care Interventions

The following list summarizes the range of home care nursing interventions for heart-failure clients.

1. Perform assessments (Box 23-4)
2. Train illness self-managers: client and family or caregiver
3. Perform venipuncture for laboratory tests and track results
4. Maintain close communication with primary medical doctor (PMD), nurse practitioner (NP), and cardiologist
5. Administer IV diuretics
6. Administer IV inotropes

The first step in the examination is to weigh the client on his or her own scale and to review his or her weight record. Physical assessment should be carried out in relative privacy so that the chest can be observed as well as auscultated. The cardiac examination requires a good stethoscope and a quiet environment whenever possible (the television and phone should be turned off). The examination should include orthostatic blood pressure measurements; these data are of particular importance if the client has been lightheaded or if fluid volume depletion is suspected. Since pulmonary rales and peripheral edema are relatively nonspecific indicators of fluid status (Levine, Hall, 1998), the nurse should

---

Box 23-4   Assessment of the Heart Failure Client

Subjective report
  Level of dyspnea
  Level of fatigue
  Orthopnea
  PND
  Chest pain or pressure
  Abdominal distention
  Appetite
  Swelling of legs and ankles
Physical examination
  Weight
  Blood pressure, seated and standing
  Apical heart rate and regularity
  Respiratory rate and effort
  Temperature
  JVP
  Abdominojugular reflux (AJR)
  Heart
      Location of the point of maximal impulse
        (PMI)
    Murmurs
    Presence of an S3
  Abdomen
  Extremities
    Edema
    Temperature
Functional status
Psychosocial issues
Environmental assessment
Self-monitoring and treatment plan adherence
  Weight record
  Medications
  Low-sodium diet
  Exercise

---

be comfortable assessing JVP and the presence or absence of the AJR. Pillows can be arranged on the bed or sofa to elevate the head and chest for the assessment of neck veins.

Physical assessment findings, along with current medication dosages and pertinent laboratory values, can be tracked using a flow sheet format that provides an overview of client trends. (See Appendix B for a sample flow sheet.) The in-depth assessment and trending will alert the nurse to early indicators of decompensation or other factors that might precipitate hospitalization for an acute exacerbation of heart failure.

These factors include an acute febrile illness, anemia, onset of atrial fibrillation, dietary sodium restriction or medication-plan nonadherence, and psychosocial crises. Ideally, assigning the same nurse to follow the client consistently results in the recognition of subtle changes, which may be missed by providers unfamiliar with the client.

Home Care and Treatment Plan Adherence

Clients fail to adhere to the medical regimen because "(1) they do not understand what they are supposed to do; (2) they forget to follow the advised regimen; (3) they have not been convinced that the treatment is beneficial; or (4) they cannot follow the regimen because of financial or other constraints" (Dracup et al, 1994). Identifying the barriers to adherence and planning interventions to address them are key roles for the home care nurse. Home visits may uncover problems that would otherwise have gone undetected (Stewart, Pearson, Horowitz, 1998). Often it is the home care nurse who discovers that the heart-failure client is unaware of the sodium content of various condiments regularly added to food, that the client is unable to read, that the medication expenses are beyond the individual's financial resources, that cognitive or functional impairment is greater than what was evident in the outpatient clinic, or that the constraint of incontinence is the real reason for nonadherence to a diuretic regimen. The home care nurse may assist in setting up reminders, such as medication boxes and instruction sheets, to help ensure regular adherence to the complex regimens. The next step beyond considering adherence or nonadherence to a treatment regimen is that of training clients to become self-managers of their treatment for heart failure.

Client Education: Training Self-Managers

The treatment of chronic conditions requires significant client involvement and ownership, since clients bear responsibility for the day-to-day care of a condition that has become a permanent part of their lives. The concept of client self-management of chronic illness provides a striking contrast to that of compliance, which implies a passive role and unquestioning fulfill-

ment of health care–provider instructions (Coates, Boore, 1995). Although the concept of adherence positions the client in a collaborative role with the health care provider, it lacks the empowerment and self-efficacy training focus included in the notion of self-management. To support the evolving role of client as self-manager, the role of the health care provider changes to one of coaching and mentoring newly empowered clients, rather than simply dispensing information or instructions.

As hospital length of stay for heart failure continues to shorten, the location for the self-management education and training moves more and more into the home setting. An important aspect of the home care nurse's role is to assess self-management potential to identify clients and caregivers with inherent management talent and those with strong management potential (given adequate training and coaching). These clients and caregivers will benefit from disease self-management training. However, not all clients are able or willing to undertake self-management. Those who have limitations that preclude self-management or who display a lack of interest or motivation will require closer ongoing follow-up by the home care nurse and medical provider to ensure that treatment-regimen adherence is maintained and that readmissions are prevented. When client limitations are significant, heart-failure management training may be directed to the caregiver.

As would be appropriate for any management training, the scope of the work to be undertaken is first described (Box 23-5). It may be useful for clients to think of the management of their heart failure as work, since the notion of *work* validates the occupied time, frustrations, and even exhaustion associated with adherence to a complex regimen. The home care nurse should define the coach or mentor role and the self-manager role, outline mutual expectations for the training, and describe the interactive nature of the process. The home care nurse then assesses the strengths and limitations of the knowledge and skill base and develops a self-management training contract with the client and caregiver. Each home care visit becomes an opportunity for providing information, teaching skills, reinforcing prior learning, and affirming growing management expertise. For instance, the home care nurse may

Box 23-5   Training Client Self-Managers at Home: Summary of the Process

1. Describe or define the work to be done
2. Describe roles of health care provider, client, and family
3. Communicate expectations of each role
4. Identify strengths, support systems, and resources
5. Identify areas for knowledge and skill development
6. Negotiate an education contract outlining roles and expectations
7. Provide focused mentoring or coaching
8. Titrate supervision as competence in self-management emerges

note an increased level of dyspnea with activity, a change that the client did not realize was significant. This teachable moment permits the nurse to review the basic pathophysiology of heart failure, review other self-monitoring parameters such as weight, and have an interactive discussion with the client regarding possible responses to changes in status. Going beyond the traditional approach to client education is needed to achieve a more solid relationship between client learning and effective health behaviors (Dunbar, Jacobson, Deaton, 1998).

Educational content and materials   The self-management approach requires solid educational resources for clients. Brochures, books, diagrams, audiotapes, videotapes, the internet, and computer-assisted learning modules are available for use in education. Much of the material available for heart-failure clients, however, provides fairly general information that does not prepare them to become self-managers of their illness. Although these materials may address the medical and pharmacological aspects of management, they do not describe well the patient's role in on-going care (Harrison, Toman, 1998). This limitation has led some programs to develop their own comprehensive teaching manuals (Foote, 1997; Harrison, Toman, 1998), which serve as self-contained client resources and provide consis-

tency in teaching materials. One such interactive manual is organized in topical sections, with questions clients must answer before moving on to the next section of information. The content is also available on disk for clients with computers (Foote, 1997). Client manuals may also contain sections for weight-monitoring records, medication records, specific instructions, and appointment reminders.

The AHCPR clinical practice guideline for heart failure recommends that clients and families be counseled on the following topics: the nature of heart failure, drug regimens, dietary modifications, activity and exercise, self-monitoring, symptoms of worsening heart failure, response to worsening symptoms, and prognosis (including advance directives). An expanded content outline suitable for individual client and family or group education can be found in Box 23-6.

The self-monitoring of daily weights deserves special attention, not only because it has a pivotal role in determining fluid status, but also because of the surprising complexity of the subject. Many clients resist the notion of daily weights, either dismissing the scale as an insignificant adjunct in the age of medical miracles and high-tech equipment or feeling sensitive about the very personal (and possibly negative) subject of how heavy they are. Once the psychological barriers have been addressed and the role of weight in monitoring fluid status explained, a number of issues must be addressed (Box 23-7). For instance, one misconception many clients hold is that the home scale is not accurate if it does not give the same weight as the hospital or clinic scale. Others may believe they should weigh themselves repeatedly during the day to detect the first sign of fluid overload. Occasionally, clients with limited vision will need a caregiver to read the dial for them. Some heart-failure programs have provided scales to clients who are unable to afford them, believing the cost to be a small investment in readmission prevention (Lasater, 1996).

Documenting client education   Ideally, documenting the education of client and caregiver begins in the inpatient setting and continues on the same record in the outpatient clinic or in the home. The hospital CHF program, for instance, can send a copy of the teaching checklist (and the discharge medication list) to home care and fax a

Box 23-6   Core Content for Heart-Failure Client Education

Explanation of how the heart works (basic anatomy and physiology)

Explanation of what happens in heart failure (basic pathophysiology)

Causes and symptoms of heart failure

Treatment of heart failure

Medications—clients should know the following about each medication:

   Trade and generic names

   Dosage and time of administration (with or without food)

   Purpose and expected benefit

   Common side effects

   Significant adverse reactions

   Drug and food interactions

   Medication management

   Methods to enhance regular dosing

   Refills and new prescriptions

   Financial issues and available support

   Over-the-counter medications

Nutrition and fluids

   Basics of healthy eating

   Low-sodium diets (see Appendix C for low-sodium guidelines)

      Rationale for sodium restriction

      Foods to avoid

      Seasoning substitutes

   Fluid restriction (advised for serum sodium levels <130 mEq/L only)

Self-management of heart failure

   Self-monitoring

      Weight

      Blood pressure and pulse

      Symptoms

      Activity tolerance

Health care–provider roles

Circumstances under which to call the physician or home care nurse

Exercise and activity

   Deconditioning in heart failure and the role of exercise

   Initiation of a walking (or stationary cycle) program

   Monitoring of the level of exertion

   Sexual activity

Coping with heart failure

   Coping challenge of a chronic illness

   Personal and family impact of a chronic condition

   Coping styles and methods

   Support groups and information sources

Advance directives

   Definition

   Advance directive completion

   Home do-not-resuscitate (DNR) directives (appropriate for advanced, end-stage heart failure)

Box 23-7   Obtaining an Accurate Daily Weight in the Home

Questions to ask:
1. Does the client have a scale?
2. Does the scale have a readable dial? (Digital readout is preferable.)
3. Is the scale on a solid surface?
4. Is the scale kept in one place, or is it moved around?
5. Is good lighting available in the vicinity of the scale?
6. If the scale requires a battery, is a spare available?

Instructions to give:
1. Weigh every morning at approximately the same time.
2. Weigh after urinating and before eating breakfast.
3. Weigh in the same amount of clothing (or no clothing) every day.
4. Wear your glasses if you need them to see the dial or digital display.
5. Write your weight down every day.
6. When your weight is up _____ pounds in 24 hours, you should _____.
7. If your weight is the same or has increased the next day after taking extra water pills, you should _____.
8. Make a note of any change in diuretic dose in your weight record.
9. Take your weight record with you when you see your doctor.

Tom was a 44-year-old man with an idiopathic cardiomyopathy who had had two to three ED visits a month for dyspnea and two hospitalizations for CHF in the past 6 months. After the most recent hospitalization, he was referred to home care. Tom did not understand what was wrong with his heart, took his medications irregularly, and did not own a scale. He lived alone and frequently ate take-out food or canned soup "because it was easy." Tom was eager to learn how to break the hospitalization and ED-visit cycles, and was open to learning how to self-manage his heart failure.

The home care nurse began assessing his heart-failure knowledge and skill base at the first visit and developed an educational contract outlining the roles and expectations for each of them. When Tom understood why the medications were prescribed and how they benefited his heart, he began to take them more regularly. He was surprised at the sodium content in much of what he ate but struggled with shopping for and preparing palatable low-sodium meals. The home care dietitian suggested meal plans and seasoning alternatives, some of which he explored. After a few weeks of coaching, Tom began to consistently monitor and record his daily weight. When he understood the significance of 2- to 3-lb overnight weight gain and its relationship to his sodium intake, the home care nurse affirmed this as major progress in his transition to self-management. Working with his physician, the nurse developed a diuretic-adjustment plan for a 24-hour weight gain. Tom required ongoing coaching in person and over the phone but eventually became independent in the management of his medications, weight, and low-sodium diet. In the following 6 months, he had no hospitalizations and no ED visits for heart failure.

copy to the physician's office, ensuring that all providers are aware of content that has been covered and content that has not been communicated. Transmission of these records must include a cover sheet that addresses the privileged and confidential nature of the client records and provides direction for handling communications sent in error to other than the intended office.

Using the same record and format (or an on-line documentation system) will also promote consistency in the information provided and in the self-management emphasis, which is vital for all health care providers, whether in the home, clinic, or hospital (Dunbar, Jacobson, Deaton, 1998). If, for instance, the hospital instructs the client to adopt a strict fluid limit that has not previously been part of the treatment plan, the maintenance diuretic dose may be too high and the client may become volume depleted. Likewise, a client who is instructed to begin a walking plan for exercise and who encounters another provider with the old paradigm of rest prescriptions for heart failure will be confused and stalled in self-management growth. An example of an educational map for heart failure clients that includes documentation is found in Appendix D.

Client education: Summary and case study
Clients benefit greatly from information about their chronic illness along with training in self-management so that they can integrate the approaches into their chosen lifestyle (Coates, Boore, 1995). Many clients are relieved to learn that heart failure does not mean their hearts are about to stop and that treatment advances translate into greatly improved quality of life in most cases and an improved prognosis, as well. Breaking the cycle of acute dyspnea and emergency department (ED) visits and hospitalization and feeling that they have some control returned to their lives are tremendous rewards for the work of self-management. The case study above illustrates the role of the home care nurse in educating and mentoring a heart-failure client as he moved into the role of self-manager of his condition.

COMMUNICATION WITH MEDICAL TEAM

Optimal chronic-illness management requires collaboration among all providers to ensure an even flow of information about the current status and treatment plan for a particular client. Faxing the flow sheet to the physician or nurse practitioner after a visit will provide him or her with important information about client trends. With prompt home care intervention for early signs of decompensation, many heart-failure admissions can be avoided. In some instances, team conferences regarding the management of challenging client situations may be warranted.

INTRAVENOUS DIURETICS AT HOME

Clients with severe fluid volume overload may require intermittent administration of intravenous furosemide, since the intestinal edema associated with excess fluid impairs absorption of oral medications (Levine, Hall, 1998). In one study, the administration of intravenous (IV) diuretics for symptomatic clients at home prevented hospital admission (Vinson et al, 1990). Clients treated with intravenous diuretics require careful follow-up to ensure adequate potassium supplementation and to monitor renal function. Daily weights provide evidence of diuresis or the absence of response to intravenous diuretics. If fluid overload persists despite this therapy, hospital admission is warranted.

INOTROPE ADMINISTRATION

IV inotropes are indicated for advanced heart-failure clients (NYHA class III or IV) who are unresponsive to conventional oral therapy with diuretics, ACE inhibitors, and beta-blockers or are intolerant of these agents. When clients are fluid overloaded, inotropes may improve the action of diuretics by improving renal perfusion (Levine, Hall, 1998). Hospitalized end-stage clients who are not weanable from inotropic therapy may be discharged with inotrope administration in the home (Feldman, 1999). Improvement in client functional status may be seen with home inotrope therapy, and hospital admissions, length of stay, and cost of care are reduced (Berkland, 1995; Harjai et al, 1997).

Intravenous Inotropic Agents

Two inotropic agents are currently administered intravenously to advanced heart-failure clients: dobutamine (a beta-adrenergic agonist) and milrinone (a phosphodiesterase inhibitor). Both dobutamine and milrinone enhance cardiac contractility by increasing myocardial cellular levels of cyclic adenosine monophosphate, thus increasing the intracellular concentration of calcium (Mehra et al, 1997).

The usual dosage range for dobutamine infusions in an outpatient setting is 2 to 5 mcg/kg/minute (Levine, Hall, 1998). After intermittent administration of dobutamine, symptomatic improvement of heart failure symptoms may persist for a week or more, a phenomenon that is not well understood (Mehra et al, 1997).

Important side effects of dobutamine are myocardial ischemia and ventricular arrhythmias. Continuous infusion may result in the development of tolerance to the drug, which may be prevented by intermittent infusions if the client is not inotrope dependent. Intermittent infusion allows down-regulated beta-receptors to be up-regulated during drug-free periods (Mehra et al, 1997).

Milrinone is not only a positive inotropic agent, but also a direct-acting vasodilator; unlike dobutamine, milrinone does not increase myocardial oxygen consumption. Another difference is that unlike dobutamine, hemodynamic tolerance to milrinone has not been observed (Katz et al, 1997). Milrinone, because of its vasodilatory properties, is more likely than dobutamine to cause hypotension, particularly in the setting of renal insufficiency (Mehra et al, 1997). The dosage range for milrinone is 0.25 mcg/kg/minute to 0.75 mcg/kg/minute.

For both dobutamine and milrinone, clinical indicators of a beneficial response include an increase in arterial blood pressure, increase in urine output, and subjective improvement in fatigue level and dyspnea (Katz et al, 1997). Weight, functional status, renal function (blood urea nitrogen [BUN] and creatinine levels), and potassium levels should also be monitored regularly. Dosage, frequency, and length of the inotrope infusion can be titrated based on the client's clinical response.

Intravenous Access

Reliable venous access is essential for home infusion therapy and should be established in the hospital setting before discharge. Three types of long-term central venous access devices are used in the home: peripherally inserted central catheters (PICC lines), tunneled central catheters, and implanted ports. PICC lines are inserted through the basilic or cephalic vein in the antecubital fossa and advanced to the superior vena cava (Konick-McMahan, 1997).

Tunneled catheters (Hickman, Broviac, and Groshong) are surgically inserted into the subclavian vein; the catheter is then tunneled under the chest-wall skin to an exit site, usually located on the anterior chest midway between the nipple and sternum. Implanted ports are also surgically inserted under the skin near the clavicle, providing direct access to the subclavian vein without external catheters (Camp-Sorrell, 1995). Discussion of the advantages and disadvantages of each type of catheter, complications, and the care of central venous access devices can be found in the previously referenced article by Konick-McMahan (1997) and the chapter authored by Camp-Sorrell (1995).

Infusion pumps for home use are generally portable and more user friendly than those found in the hospital. Both fixed-rate and programmable pumps are available. Some fixed-rate pumps are disposable. The portable pumps allow clients to move about freely, to shower, and to pursue activities outside the home, thus contributing to an improved quality of life (Konick-McMahan, 1997).

Home Care Role

The home care nurse needs to be knowledgeable regarding inotropic medications, their role in the management of advanced heart failure, home infusion protocols, and trouble-shooting of central venous access devices and infusion pumps. Since inpatient stays are brief, the nurse will also be responsible for the majority of client and caregiver education. Training the client and caregiver will require frequent visits initially, since the management of access site and infusion pump is a more complex issue than those routinely encountered by heart-failure clients. Eventually, the nurse will shift responsibility for ongoing care to the client and family and plan less-frequent visits to monitor heart-failure status, perform venipuncture, provide ongoing mentoring in self-management, and assess client and caregiver burden and coping. An on-call home care nurse must be available on a 24-hour basis for trouble-shooting for clients receiving home infusion therapy.

Client and Family Education

Home infusion therapy requires knowledgeable, committed caregivers and clients to ensure success. Education should begin in the hospital when the medical management of heart failure in the home includes the administration of an IV inotrope. Since the therapy has been associated with an increased mortality rate and since appropriate candidates for inotropes are those with severe, advanced heart failure, education in the hospital or home should address advance directives and cardiopulmonary resuscitation (CPR).

A suggested content checklist for training clients and caregivers can be found in Box 23-8. Education and training activities and client and

---

Box 23-8   Home Inotrope Client and Family Self-Management Training Checklist

MEDICATION
- ☐ Trade name
- ☐ Generic name
- ☐ Beneficial action
- ☐ Dosage
- ☐ Side effects
- ☐ Adverse effects
- ☐ Expiration date
- ☐ Storage

ACCESS
- ☐ Type of access
- ☐ Site inspection
- ☐ Dressing changes
- ☐ Disposal of supplies

INFUSION PUMP
- ☐ Type of device
- ☐ Infusion set-up

INFUSION PUMP—cont'd
- ☐ Current settings
- ☐ Alarms and trouble-shooting
- ☐ Battery change

OTHER INFORMATION
- ☐ Electrical safety
- ☐ Signs and symptoms to report
- ☐ Numbers to call for questions or problems
  Pharmacy
  Durable medical equipment supplier
  Home health agency
  Physician or nurse practitioner
- ☐ Advance directive
- ☐ Prehospital DNR form

Modified from Konick-McMahan J: *RN* 60(4):25-28, 1997.

HOME INOTROPE THERAPY

Harold was a 73-year-old client with an ischemic cardiomyopathy who had been followed in a heart-failure clinic for 5 years. He was significantly limited in his functional status when he entered the clinic, but after optimization of medical therapy and education in self-management skills, he enjoyed nearly 4½ years of relative stability, traveling, pursuing his gardening hobby, and enjoying his grandchildren. His cardiac function began to deteriorate 4 months before his death, and balancing aggressive diuresis with the maintenance of adequate blood pressure and renal function became a major challenge. Within a few weeks of the onset of his decline, intermittent dobutamine infusions were scheduled in the outpatient unit. Harold managed to travel to the hospital for two of those appointments, but as his heart-failure symptoms continued to worsen, three outpatient visits per week became untenable. A PICC line was inserted while he was in the outpatient unit, and daily home dobutamine infusions were initiated. Harold's wife was a capable and committed woman who learned the technical aspects of site and pump care readily, although she described herself as not mechanically adept. The home care nurse titrated her visits from daily to weekly as Harold and his wife became more

independent in the management of his infusions. At the next clinic visit, the cardiologist and advanced-practice nurse initiated a discussion with Harold and his wife about Harold's current medical status, his prognosis, and issues related to advance directives and end-of-life care. They reassured the couple that they would be available to support them in their desire to remain at home (they did not wish hospice referral) and would work along with the home care team to ensure his comfort. Harold completed an advance directive stating his wishes for comfort care only, and a DNR form for use in the home was completed. Over the next 2½ months, the home care nurse, the client and his wife, and the advanced-practice nurse collaborated on a daily basis to manage Harold's symptoms at home. The dobutamine infusion maintained his blood pressure so that IV diuretics could be used on an intermittent basis as his cardiac function worsened. Nausea became Harold's most distressing symptom, and guidance regarding medications to control the nausea was obtained from the hospice team. As his cardiac and renal function deteriorated further, Harold slept more of the time. He died quietly in his sleep approximately 3 months after the home dobutamine infusion was started.

caregiver levels of mastery evidenced in return demonstrations should be documented and communicated to those involved in the care of the client.

Current Issues in Home Inotrope Therapy

Home inotrope therapy for advanced heart failure appears to reduce hospital admissions and improve quality of life, but it is associated with an increased mortality rate. Current research does not show a clear benefit from the administration of inotropes in heart failure. Questions that remain to be answered include (1) which clients are appropriate for the therapy, (2) which agents should be used, (3) what doses of inotropes are to be used, and (4) what effects might be expected (Packer, Cohn, 1999). Another unanswered question concerns the role of hemodynamic monitoring, either to establish a recom-

mended inotrope dose level or to monitor hemodynamic status concurrently with an inotrope infusion (Feldman, 1999).

Where should these infusions take place? The number of nurse-managed outpatient CHF-treatment centers, in which clients receive intermittent IV inotropes on individually adjusted schedules, has grown in recent years (Feldman, 1999). For most clients with severe, advanced heart failure and a class IV functional status, however, inotrope administration in the home setting is preferable to intermittent trips to an outpatient center.

CASE FOR COMORBIDITIES

The home care nurse should identify the heart-failure client's other medical conditions and take them into consideration when developing a plan of care, since unstable comorbid conditions are frequently responsible for hospital admissions and readmissions in clients with heart failure (Buckle, 1999). These other illnesses include COPD, diabetes mellitus, renal disorders, and hematological problems. The fragility of many heart-failure clients with multiple comorbidities (and multiple medications for each comorbidity) is not well understood by many health care providers. Many times, issues related to the pathophysiology or treatment of one condition will have a negative impact on the other. For example, consider the case of a 47-year-old woman with a long-standing history of insulin-dependent diabetes mellitus who was unable to keep her heart-failure medications down because of intractable vomiting and was admitted with severe shortness of breath. She was diagnosed during that admission with gastroparesis, a complication of her diabetes. The diabetic neuropathy of the autonomic nervous system causes a marked delay in the emptying time of the stomach and can result in severe vomiting. Treatment of this complication of her comorbidity had a profound impact on the treatment of her heart failure.

EXERCISE AND ACTIVITY LEVELS

Rest was once a key element of heart-failure treatment. Cardiac enlargement and heart failure were considered relative or absolute contraindications to exercise training in the early years of cardiac rehabilitation. Several studies have shown, however, that exercise training in heart-failure clients results in improvement in functional capacity and psychosocial status (Kavanagh et al, 1996; McKelvie et al, 1995; Stevenson et al, 1995). The improvement in exercise tolerance appears to be a result of skeletal muscle adaptations (Wegner et al, 1995). For clients with stable heart failure, a regular exercise program, such as walking, is recommended. In conjunction with the physician's treatment plan, the home care nurse should instruct clients to gradually increase walking distance over several months while monitoring their symptoms. If clients feel tired the day after exercising, they have overexerted themselves and should adjust their program accordingly (Dracup et al, 1994). See Appendix E for home exercise guidelines for heart-failure patients.

Referral to a supervised rehabilitation program should be considered for clients who are anxious about exercising or dyspneic at a low work level, who have angina, or who have had a recent MI or recent CABG surgery (Konstam et al, 1994). A program with experience in exercising heart-failure clients should be selected, since the severe deconditioning that is often associated with the condition makes these clients poor candidates for a traditional cardiac-rehabilitation program.

MULTIDISCIPLINARY TEAM APPROACH

Heart-failure clients benefit from a multidisciplinary approach to home care. Physical therapy is indicated for clients who are severely deconditioned or who require specific training to maintain or resume functional status. Occupational therapists can assess the home environment for safety and make recommendations for energy conservation. When clients require extensive education for dietary modifications related to heart failure or other comorbid conditions, the dietitian should participate in the client's care. For many clients, the social, financial, psychological, or spiritual issues they face are the major barriers to treatment plan adherence, and involvement of the home care social worker, psychiatric clinical nurse specialist, or chaplain may be a key element of the continuing care plan.

REDUCING READMISSION RATES: HOME CARE ROLE

Heart-failure clients are frequently readmitted to the acute care hospital, increasing not only the cost of care for this population, but impacting the quality of life for both the client and caregiver. Many of these readmissions are avoidable, since a number of the factors implicated in precipitating readmissions appear to be modifiable (Rich et al, 1995). Both medical and social factors are associated with readmission of clients to the hospital, including a prolonged previous admission, comorbidities, hypoalbuminuria, nonadherence to a low-sodium diet, nonadherence to a medication regimen, social isolation, and inadequate client and caregiver education about heart-failure management (Chin, Goldman, 1997; Shah et al, 1998; Vinson et al, 1990).

Health care providers in various settings have designed interventions to address the frequent readmission rates of heart-failure clients. The approaches have included hospital-based discharge planning by geriatric-trained advanced-practice nurses (Naylor et al, 1999), collaborative-practice hospital-based CHF clinics (Smith et al, 1997), home care–directed disease management (Hohenleitner, Minniti, 1998), and mailings of client educational materials, data gathering, and notification by an independent monitoring service (Shah et al, 1998). One research study intervention provided a single visit by a nurse and pharmacist to newly discharged heart-failure clients (Stewart-Pearson, Horowitz, 1998).

Virtually any intervention that provides education and close follow-up for heart-failure clients will result in fewer hospital admissions. Hospital days, number of admissions, and number of ED visits were decreased, in some cases dramatically, by these interventions. The implication for home care is that addressing both medical and social factors will have a significant impact on ED and hospital use for the heart-failure client. Indeed, two studies using retrospective chart review found that the frequency and intensity of home care correlated inversely with hospital readmissions in clients with heart failure (Dennis et al, 1996; Martens, Mellor, 1997).

Moreover, home care reduces readmissions by connecting the continuum of care, which easily develops "cracks" where chronic illness is concerned. Situational "cracks" include the following:

1. The client who runs out of his ACE inhibitor medication and cannot get it refilled because it is no longer covered by his insurance plan and cannot get through to his physician's office because the phone lines are always backed up, then wakes short of breath at 2:00 AM 3 days later and calls 911
2. The fragile client with both IDDM and heart failure who is discharged after a diabetes-related hospitalization by providers unfamiliar with her heart-failure management (who reduced her cardiac medications drastically) who is readmitted within a week for an exacerbation of heart failure
3. The client who continually visits the ED with an 8- to 10-lb weight gain and severe dyspnea but whose diet recall never includes the canned sardines the home care nurse finds in her cupboard ("they're just a snack")

4. The client who is experiencing increasing shortness of breath but cannot get an appointment with the physician for 2 weeks

In the first two scenarios, home care involvement will address and remedy the situations that precipitate the readmissions. In the third instance, the value of the home care intervention of "pantry and refrigerator assessment" for sodium sources is obvious and is likely to prevent further readmissions precipitated by excessive sodium intake. For clients in distress, as in the fourth example, the home care nurse navigates the health care system and ensures access to a provider and to needed care in a timely fashion.

CARE MAPS

Home care clinical pathways or care maps for heart failure should be based on current practice and clinical guidelines. Assessment, educational interventions, and behavioral modifications can be integrated into a CHF pathway. The pathway should be individualized to each client and include relevant outcome measures (Barella, Monica, 1998; Hohenleitner, Minniti, 1998). Involving clients and caregivers in the care plan will promote their growth as heart-failure self-managers. Ideally, the care map or pathway is continuum-based, including the hospital, outpatient clinic, and home settings.

Care map planning should also consider all phases of the disease, including remissions and maintenance (see Appendix F for a status-based care map). Unlike acute-illness episodic care, a chronic illness such as heart failure may require varying levels of intervention over the course of the disease, depending on a number of factors that either support continued client stability or precipitate decompensation. For example, one previously fragile and frequently hospitalized elderly heart-failure client was trained and mentored in self-care by her home care nurse. She had completed nearly 6 months of stable self-management when she contracted herpes zoster and gained 8 lb in less than a week. She was no longer receiving home care visits because she had mastered self-monitoring skills but had been called by the home care nurse on a weekly basis. This regular home care phone contact provided early warning about a potential crisis that may have precipitated a hospital admission. She was seen in the heart-failure clinic and given intra-venous furosemide (Lasix) and then followed with home care visits until she had returned to her previous level of stability.

HOSPICE FOR END-STAGE HEART FAILURE

Hospice care for dying clients focuses on comfort and quality of life, rather than on interventions and cure. Hospice care is an alternative to lengthy hospitalization for end-stage heart-failure clients, since hospice services provide additional support for clients and caregivers that can be tailored to meet individual client or family needs. Clients who exhibit progressive symptoms despite max-imal medical therapy and have clinical evidence of end-stage disease are appropriate for referral to hospice (Head, 1997).

Several challenges exist in providing hospice care for heart-failure clients. Unlike cancer clients, who have a clear phase of decline, chronic illness clients tend to have a declining course that resists accurate prognosis. Thus chronic illness generally lacks an identifiable failing phase, when clients would most likely be referred to hospice care (Skolnick, 1998). The number of heart-failure clients who would potentially benefit from hos-pice care is further reduced by the sudden, unex-pected nature of a significant number of deaths.

Another challenge is that hospice providers are unaccustomed to cardiology clients, since ap-proximately 85% of hospice clients have a cancer diagnosis (Head, 1997). Hospice nurses and other care providers who are unfamiliar with heart-failure symptoms and treatment may be less com-fortable managing this client population. More-over, in end-stage heart failure, comfort care such as the administration of IV diuretics and in-otropes (and in some cases, thoracentesis for re-current pleural effusions) may appear to resem-ble treatment intervention and not palliation.

In addition, some heart-failure clients may be deterred from accepting hospice care if they fear the prohibition on ED use, particularly if they have been frequent users of emergency services for acute dyspnea. These clients may be unaware of the hospice commitment to symptom control and the round-the-clock availability of hospice nurses.

One solution is a joint approach to manage-ment. The interdisciplinary teams of a heart-

Box 23-9	Clinical Characteristics of End-Stage Clients

Maximal medical therapy
Systolic BP <80 mm Hg
Marked elevation of JVP
Serum sodium level <130 mEq/L
Rising BUN and creatinine levels
Cool extremities

failure program and a hospice program can work together to design an overall plan of care address-ing the needs of advanced and end-stage heart-failure clients and collaborate in the management of specific clients.

HEART-FAILURE PROGRAM ROLE IN HOSPICE REFERRAL

When end-stage clients are identified (see Box 23-9 for clinical characteristics of end-stage clients), frank discussions with the client and family concerning medical status provide a springboard for offering options, such as hospice referral, for care in the final phase of the disease. The discussion also provides an opportunity to reassure clients and family members that they will not be abandoned but that the focus of care will shift to maximizing comfort. Clients should be informed about advance directives far earlier in the course of the disease so that their health care choices can be known and so that a surro-gate decision-maker can be identified.

LEFT VENTRICULAR ASSIST DEVICE (also called *Left Ventricular Assist System*)

The most common reason for adult cardiac trans-plantation is left ventricular systolic dysfunction with the resulting heart-failure symptoms (Smith, Levine, 1999). Each year, approximately 2300 peo-ple receive a transplanted heart (Chillcott, Atkins, Adamson, 1998), but approximately 20% of cli-ents waiting for a transplant die before receiving a donated heart (Smith, Levine, 1999). One alter-native treatment for advanced heart failure is the implantation of a mechanical left ventricular as-sist device (LVAD) (Stevenson et al, 2001), cur-rently used as a "bridge" to cardiac transplant,

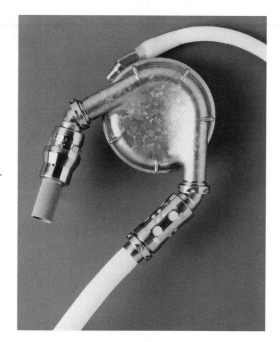

Fig. 23-3 HeartMate vented electric LVAS.

Box 23-10   Home Care Maintenance Phase—Follow-up Call Questions

1. How are you feeling?
2. What is your weight today?
3. Is there any change in how short of breath you become with activity?
4. How many pillows are you sleeping on?
5. Do you wake up short of breath during the night?
6. Do you have any swelling in your legs or ankles?
7. How is your appetite?
8. Has there been any change in the amount of sodium you are getting in your food?
9. Has there been any change in the way you take your medicines?
10. Do you need refills on any of your medicines?
11. Are there any major changes in your life?

Box 23-11   Heart-Failure Outcome Measures in Home Care

Hospitalizations
Hospital length of stay (LOS)
ED visits
Caregiver and family burden
Client satisfaction
Client quality of life (QOL)

Number of clients on ACE inhibitors at recommended doses
Number of clients on beta-blockers
NYHA class
Home care resource utilization

supporting the failing heart until a suitable donor heart is available. The implantation of newer, electric motor-driven pumps is being researched as a permanent option for clients who are not transplant candidates. These clients, as well as clients awaiting transplant, can be discharged home with the battery-powered pump after extensive client and caregiver education. Home care nurses, who also require specific training, become involved with the client before discharge to help ease the transition to home. Home care–visit frequency is determined by individual client needs (Chillcott, Atkins, Adamson, 1998). One such device, the HeartMate Vented Electric LVAS, is shown in Fig. 23-3.

TELEMANAGEMENT

The close follow-up many heart-failure clients (particularly those with advanced disease) require can be greatly expanded by using technology. Technological approaches range in complexity from the scripted telephone interview regarding weight and symptom status (Box 23-10) to the use of sophisticated monitoring equipment in the home, which transmits data via modem to a hospital central monitoring station (Schiller, Bondmass, Avitall, 1997), and video-conferencing capabilities (Laing, Behrendt, 1998). Internet applications may eventually provide heart-failure clients with information, communication, and decision assistance. These adjuncts to face-to-face encounters are useful for gathering serial client data, reinforcing self-management behaviors, and offering options for early intervention when required by changing client status. Research protocols currently in progress will provide more information regarding the cost-effectiveness and client satisfaction associated with technology-assisted client care in the home.

TRACKING OUTCOMES

Expected outcomes of home care intervention have not been well defined in the literature (Mitty, Mezey, 1998). Current reimbursement issues will encourage the use of outcome measures to justify disease-management approaches and to market agencies and programs to managed-care companies and other third-party payors. Internal review of outcome measures also provides the basis for program revision or development of other disease-management approaches. Suggested outcome measures for home care heart-failure clients include those found in Box 23-11.

One tool to measure quality of life is the Minnesota Living with Heart Failure Questionnaire, which consists of 21 questions assessing the client's perception of how heart failure has impacted physical, emotional, and social aspects of his or her life in the past month (Rector, Kubo, Cohn, 1987). The tool can be administered at admission to home care and then at serial intervals, such as 6 and 12 months, and then yearly. Another quality-of-life tool is the Medical Outcomes Trust SF-12 Health Survey standardized questionnaire, which monitors clients' perceptions about their illness, mental well-being, and ability to engage in activities (Hohenleitner, Minniti, 1998; Ware, Kosinski, Keller, 1996). The longer version, the Medical Outcomes Study 36-Item Short-Form Health Survey (SF-36), measures 8 health concepts: physical functioning, bodily pain, role limitations resulting from physical health problems, role limitations resulting from personal or emotional problems, general mental health, social functioning, energy and fatigue, and general health perceptions. This survey also includes a single item that provides an indication of perceived change in health (Ware, Sherbourne, 1992).

REIMBURSEMENT: CHALLENGE ON THE HOME FRONT

Changing home care reimbursement patterns both for Medicare and managed-care organizations provide further impetus for health care providers to organize care for chronic illnesses across a continuum. Home care agencies will work closely with hospital-based and payor-based case managers, cardiologists, primary-care physicians, and mid-level providers, such as nurse practitioners and physician assistants, to optimize resource utilization. Home care nurses will be challenged to use the most efficient and cost-effective methods to provide services that support self-management by clients and avoid inpatient stays whenever possible. Using innovative approaches to refine their home-based management and tracking the outcomes for a population, such as heart-failure clients, will position home care as a key element of a disease-management program for this costly chronic illness.

J.P., an 83-year-old Latina, was referred to the heart-failure program of a university-based hospital after the most recent of a series of hospitalizations for exacerbations of CHF. She had symptoms of dyspnea with minimal exertion (walk distance <20 feet), two-pillow orthopnea, and PND 2 to 3 times per night. An echocardiogram performed during the recent hospital stay showed an EF of 15% (normal 55% to 70%). Her medications included benazepril 2.5 mg daily, furosemide 20 mg three times daily, digoxin 0.125 mg daily, and isosorbide dinitrate 20 mg three times daily. Blood pressure was 94/50 mm Hg in clinic.

She was referred to home care for continued titration of the ACE inhibitor; diuresis as needed; follow-up laboratory work; and education in self-management, including daily weights, medications, symptom awareness, and a low-sodium diet. In collaboration with the heart-failure clinic advanced-

practice nurse via phone, the ACE inhibitor was carefully titrated to the recommended dosage of 10 mg twice daily. The process took several weeks of frequent visits (daily at first) as the diuretic was simultaneously down-titrated and weight, BP, and JVP monitored. The client's symptoms were markedly improved, with a decrease in her level of dyspnea and no episodes of PND. The home care nurse also provided extensive client and family education, and as the client and family assumed greater levels of self-management, the home care nurse visits were titrated down, and the client was eventually discharged from home care.

Over the next 2 years, the client was hospitalized only twice, once for pneumonia and once for heart-failure exacerbation. Home care referral for brief periods following the hospitalizations helped ensure a return to the client's usual stability.

REFERENCES

Adams KF et al: HFSA guidelines for the management of patients with heart failure due to left ventricular systolic dysfunction—Pharmacological approaches, *Congestive Heart Failure* 6(1):11-39, 2000.

Anderson MA, Pena RA, Helms, LB: Home care utilization by congestive heart failure patients: A pilot study, *Public Health Nursing* 15(2):146-162, 1998.

Barella P, Monica ED: Managing congestive heart failure at home, *AACN Clinical Issues* 9(3):377-388, 1998.

Berkland D: Creative solutions: Home dobutamine infusions, *AACN Clinical Issues* 6:443-451, 1995.

Buckle JM: Manage comorbidities in individuals with CHF for optimal outcomes, *Medical Management Network* 7(1):4, 1999.

Camp-Sorrell D: Advances in tunneled and non-tunneled catheters: Nursing management strategies. In Connors RB, Winters RW, eds: *Home infusion: Current status and future trends,* Chicago, 1995, American Hospital.

Centers for Disease Control and Prevention: Changes in mortality from heart failure—United States, 1980-1995, *Morbidity and Mortality Weekly Report* 47(30):633-637, 1994.

Chillcott SR, Atkins PJ, Adamson RM: Left ventricular assist as a viable alternative for cardiac transplantation, *Critical Care Nursing Quarterly* 20(4):64-79, 1998.

Chin MH, Goldman L: Correlates of early hospital readmission or death in patients with congestive heart failure, *American Journal of Cardiology* 79:1640-1644, 1997.

Coates VE, Boore JRP: Self-management of chronic illness: Implications for nursing, *International Journal of Nursing Studies* 32(6):628-640, 1995.

Croft JB et al: National trends in the initial hospitalization for heart failure, *Journal of the American Geriatrics Society* 45:270-275, 1997.

Dennis et al: The relationship between hospital readmissions of Medicare beneficiaries with chronic illness and home care nursing interventions, *Home Healthcare Nurse* 14:303-309, 1996.

Dracup K et al: Management of heart failure. II. Counseling, education, and lifestyle modifications, *Journal of the American Medical Association* 272:1442-1446, 1994.

Dunbar SB, Jacobson LH, Deaton C: Heart failure: Strategies to enhance patient self-management, *AACN Clinical Issues* 9(2):244-256, 1998.

Eichhorn EJ, Bristow MR: Medical therapy can improve the biological properties of the chronically failing heart: A new era in the treatment of heart failure, *Circulation* 94:2285-2296, 1996.

Feldman AM: The use of intermittent inotrope therapy in the management of end stage heart failure: A therapeutic and economic conundrum, *Congestive Heart Failure* 5(1):46-47, 1999.

Foote M: Innovations in the management of heart failure in the home health care environment, *Home Health Care Management and Practice* 9(4):35-42, 1997.

Goran SF, Johantgen M: Heart failure. In Kinney MR et al, eds: *AACN's clinical reference for critical care nursing,* St Louis, 1998, Mosby.

Guthery D, Schumann L: Congestive heart failure, *Journal of the American Academy of Nurse Practitioners* 10:3331-3339, 1998.

Haldeman GA et al: Hospitalization of patients with heart failure: National Hospital Discharge Survey, 1985 to 1995, *American Heart Journal* 137:352-360, 1999.

Harjai KJ et al: Home inotropic therapy in advanced heart failure: Cost analysis and clinical outcomes, *Chest* 112:1298-1303, 1997.

Harrison MB, Toman C: Hospital to home: Evidence-based education for CHF, *The Canadian Nurse* 94(2):36-42, 1998.

Head B: An overview of hospice home care. In Spratt JS, Hawley R, Hoye RE, eds: *Home health care: Principles and practices,* Delray Beach, Fla, 1997, GR/St Lucie Press.

Heywood JT: Personal communication, January 1999.

Hohenleitner SG, Minniti MJ: Developing effective disease state management programs, *Home Health Care Management and Practice* 10(4):11-19, 1998.

Hosenpud JD, Jarcho JA: The cardiomyopathies. In Hosenpud JD, Greenberg SA, eds: *Congestive heart failure: Pathophysiology, diagnosis and comprehensive approach to management,* ed 2, New York, 2000, Springer-Verlag.

Katz SD et al: Outpatient management of severe congestive heart failure. In Rothkopf MM, ed: *Standards and practice of homecare therapeutics,* ed 2, Baltimore, 1997, Williams & Wilkins.

Kavanagh T et al: Quality of life and cardiorespiratory function in chronic heart failure: Effects of 12 months' aerobic training, *Heart* 76:42-49, 1996.

Konick-McMahan J: Discharged with dobutamine, *RN* 60(4):25-28, 1997.

Konstam MA et al: *Heart failure: Evaluation and care of patients with left ventricular systolic dysfunction. Clinical Practice Guideline No 11,* AHCPR Pub No 94-0612, Rockville, Md, 1994, Agency for Health Care Policy and Research, Public Health Service, US Department of Health and Human Services.

Laing G, Behrendt D: A disease management program for home health care patients with congestive heart failure, *Home Health Care Management and Practice* 10(2):27-32, 1998.

Lasater M: The effect of a nurse-managed CHF clinic on patient readmission and length of stay, *Home Healthcare Nurse* 14(5):351-356, 1996.

Levine BS, Hall ML: Management of chronic heart failure in the outpatient, *AACN Clinical Issues* 9(2):257-267, 1998.

Martens KH, Mellor SD: A study of the relationship between home care services and hospital readmission of patients with congestive heart failure, *Home Healthcare Nurse* 15(2):123-129, 1997.

McKelvie RS et al: Effects of exercise training in patients with congestive heart failure: A critical review, *Journal of the American College of Cardiology* 25(3):789-796, 1995.

Mehra MR et al: The unique management of refractory advanced systolic heart failure, *Heart and Lung* 26:280-288, 1997.

MERIT-HF Study Group: Effect of metoprolol CR/XL in chronic heart failure: Metoprolol CR/XL randomized intervention trial in congestive heart failure (MERIT-HF), *Lancet* 353:2001-2007, 1999.

Michael KA, Parnell KJ: Innovations in the pharmacologic management of heart failure, *AACN Clinical Issues* 9(2):172-191, 1998.

Mitty E, Mezey M: Integrating advanced practice nurses in home care: Recommendations for a teaching home care program, *Nursing Health Care Perspectives* 19(6):264-270, 1998.

National Heart, Lung and Blood Institute: *Data fact sheet: Congestive heart failure,* Bethesda, Md, 1996, US Department of Health and Human Services.

Naylor MD et al: Comprehensive discharge planning and home follow-up of hospitalized elders: A randomized clinical trial, *Journal of the American Medical Association* 281:613-620, 1999.

Packer M, Cohn JN, eds: Consensus recommendations for the management of chronic heart failure, *The American Journal of Cardiology* 83(2A):1A-38A, 1999.

Packer M et al: The effect of carvedilol on morbidity and mortality in patients with chronic heart failure, *New England Journal of Medicine* 334:1349-1355, 1996.

Rector TS, Kubo SH, Cohn JN: Patient self-assessment of their congestive heart failure: Content, reliability and validity of a new measure, the Minnesota Living with Heart Failure questionnaire, *Heart Failure* 3:198-209, 1987.

Rich MW: Heart failure, *Cardiology Clinics* 17(1):123-135, 1999a.

Rich MW: Heart failure disease management: A critical review, *Journal of Cardiac Failure* 5(1):64-75, 1999b.

Rich MW et al: A multidisciplinary intervention to prevent the readmission of elderly patients with congestive heart failure, *New England Journal of Medicine* 330:1190-1195, 1995.

Schiller AE, Bondmass M, Avitall B: Technology-based home care for disease management, *Remington Report* 5(5):8, 10-12, 1997.

Shah NB et al: Prevention of hospitalizations for heart failure with an interactive home monitoring program, *American Heart Journal* 135:373-378, 1998.

Sherman A: Critical care management of the heart failure patient in the home, *Critical Care Nursing Quarterly* 18(1):77-87, 1995.

Skolnick AA: MediCaring project to demonstrate, evaluate innovative end-of-life program for chronically ill, *Journal of the American Medical Association* 279:1511-1512, 1998.

Smith JJ, Levine HJ: Systolic dysfunction of the ventricle in congestive heart failure: Pathophysiology, diagnosis, and therapy, *Congestive Heart Failure* 5:10-16, 19-26, 1999.

Smith LE et al: Symptomatic improvement and reduced hospitalization for patients attending a cardiomyopathy clinic, *Clinical Cardiology* 20:949-954, 1997.

Starling RC: The heart failure pandemic: Changing patterns, costs, and treatment strategies, *Cleveland Clinic Journal of Medicine* 65(7):351-358, 1998.

Stevenson LW et al: Improvement in exercise capacity of candidates awaiting heart transplantation, *Journal of the American College of Cardiology* 25:163-170, 1995.

Stevenson LW et al: Mechanical cardiac support 2000: Current applications and future trial design, *The Journal of Heart and Lung Transplantation* 20(1):1-38, 2001.

Stewart S, Pearson S, Horowitz JD: Effects of a home-based intervention among patients with congestive heart failure discharged from acute hospital care, *Archives of Internal Medicine* 158:1067-1072, 1998.

Thom TJ, Kannel WB: Congestive heart failure: Epidemiology and cost of illness, *Disease Management and Health Outcomes* 1(2):75-83, 1997.

Vinson JM et al: Early readmission of elderly patients with congestive heart failure, *Journal of the American Geriatrics Society* 38:1290-1295, 1990.

Ware J, Kosinski M, Keller SD: A 12-item short-form health survey: Construction of scales and preliminary tests of reliability and validity, *Medical Care* 34(3):220-233, 1996.

Ware JE, Sherbourne CD: The MOS 36-item short-form health survey (SF-36): I. Conceptual framework and item selection, *Medical Care* 30:473-483, 1992.

Wegner NK et al: *Cardiac rehabilitation. Clinical Practice Guideline No 17,* AHCPR Pub No 96-0672, Rockville, Md, 1995, US Department of Health and Human Services, Agency for Health Care Policy and Research, National Heart, Lung and Blood Institute.

Weinberger HD: Diagnosis and treatment of diastolic heart failure, *Hospital Practice* 34(3):115-118, 121-122, 125-126, 1999.

Zile MR: Diastolic dysfunction and heart failure in hypertrophied hearts, *Congestive Heart Failure* 4(6):32-42, 1998.

Diastolic Dysfunction

DEFINITION

Diastolic dysfunction of the ventricle occurs when myocardial relaxation and filling are impaired and the ventricle is unable to accept an adequate volume of blood from the venous system, fill at low pressure, and maintain normal stroke volume. When heart failure is caused by diastolic dysfunction alone, the heart size and EF will be normal (Zile, 1998).

PREVALENCE

In nearly 40% of cases of heart failure, systolic function is normal and diastolic function is abnormal. Diastolic dysfunction appears to be strongly age related, since the average incidence for people with heart failure who are younger than 65 is 8% but increases to 32% for those older than 65 (Weinberger, 1999).

ETIOLOGY AND PATHOPHYSIOLOGY

The leading causes of diastolic dysfunction are coronary artery disease, hypertension, diabetes, obesity, and aortic stenosis (Weinberger, 1999). Other causes include genetic hypertrophy, infiltrative cardiomyopathies, and constrictive pericarditis (Zile, 1998). The increased interstitial collagen deposition in the myocardium, which is associated with aging, also contributes to decreasing ventricular compliance. Ischemia decreases relaxation of the ventricle because it reduces the availability of the high-energy phosphates required to rapidly remove calcium from the cell; hypertrophy slows the rate of myosin-actin dissociation and also decreases left ventricular compliance (Weinberger, 1999). The processes that reduce compliance, and thus filling of the left ventricle, result in an increase in left-ventricular filling pressures and ultimately the symptoms of CHF.

DIAGNOSIS

The congestive symptoms of heart failure (such as exertional dyspnea) caused by diastolic dysfunction may be very similar to those of systolic dysfunction. Diastolic heart failure is diagnosed when there are classic signs and symptoms of CHF with an EF greater than 40% in the absence of significant valvular or pericardial disease (Heywood, 1999). Thus the diagnosis of diastolic dysfunction requires an evaluation of the size and thickness of the left ventricle and of the systolic (pumping) function (Zile, 1998) to exclude the diagnosis of systolic dysfunction. An echocardiogram is most commonly used to assess cardiac structure and function, but some of the information can also be obtained from radionuclide ventriculography (gated blood-pool scanning, sometimes called a *MUGA scan*) or during a cardiac catheterization, using contrast ventriculography (Weinberger, 1999; Zile, 1998).

TREATMENT

The treatment of diastolic dysfunction, unlike that of systolic dysfunction, has not been evaluated in large-scale randomized clinical trials. Currently, the medications most frequently used are beta-blockers, calcium channel blockers, and ACE inhibitors. Beta-blockers slow the heart rate so that filling time is lengthened. Calcium channel blockers improve diastolic function to a small degree and reduce ischemia and ventricular hypertrophy. ACE inhibitors are believed to improve left ventricular compliance and reduce hypertrophy (Rich, 1999a). Diuretics are also used but in smaller doses than would be used for systolic dysfunction (Zile, 1998). In diastolic dysfunction, it is important to avoid overdiuresis because the less-compliant left ventricle relies on adequate filling to maintain stroke volume and cardiac output (Rich, 1999a). Treatment also includes modifying etiological factors, such as myocardial ischemia and hypertension, to the greatest extent possible.

SELECTED NURSING CONSIDERATIONS

Clients with diastolic dysfunction tend to have more difficulty with exercise. They also tolerate smaller changes in weight status and should be monitored more closely for increases or decreases in their weight. Diastolic dysfunction clients should be assessed for signs and symptoms of overdiuresis, such as hypotension, cognitive impairment, or prerenal azotemia (Rich, 1999a). Increases in heart rate should be reported, since a rapid rate will reduce left ventricular diastolic filling time and thus worsen heart-failure symptoms.

B Home Care Flow Sheet: Heart Failure

Client Name _____ DOB _____ ID# _____

DATE								
Weight								
BP								
Heart Rate								
NYHA Func Class								
JVP/AJR								
Lungs								
Edema								
MEDS								
ACEI								
AII blocker								
Diuretic								
Second diuretic								
Digoxin								
Beta-blocker								
Warfarin								
LABS								
Na								
K								
BUN								
Creat								
Dig level								
TSH/T4								
PT/INR								
Hgb/Hct								

Adapted with permission from the flow sheet developed by Sharon Fabbri, RNP, for use in the Cardiomyopathy Program at Loma Linda University Medical Center in Loma Linda, Calif.

C Client Guidelines for Low-Sodium Eating

*T*he reason for decreasing the sodium in what you eat is that when the heart is having difficulty with pumping, the kidneys believe they should hold onto sodium. This causes the body to hold onto water as well. The extra fluid causes the swelling in your abdomen, ankles, and legs and the shortness of breath you have most likely experienced. Lowering your sodium intake will help decrease the swelling and shortness of breath.

LOW-SODIUM DIET PRINCIPLES

1. Aim for a total of 2000 mg of sodium per day.
2. Become a label reader. You will be surprised at the number of "hidden" sources of sodium in processed foods. Foods do not have to taste salty to contain large amounts of sodium.
3. Remember to look for the number of servings on a food label. If the package or can contains more than one serving, you will have to multiply the number of servings by the amount of sodium listed on the label to get the total amount of sodium.
4. Prepare more of your food at home, using fresh ingredients, which are naturally low in sodium and taste better, as well.
5. Banish the salt shaker from your table. Use other ingredients to flavor your food (e.g., herbs, spices, onion, garlic, lemon juice, or vinegars). Avoid onion or garlic salt.
6. Before using a salt substitute, check with your doctor. Most salt substitutes contain potassium, which may raise your blood potassium level.
7. Keep a supply of low-sodium snacks in your kitchen—raw vegetables, fresh fruit, unsalted rice or popcorn cakes, low-fat or nonfat yogurt, popcorn kernels to prepare without salt, or frozen juice bars.

8. Look for sodium on the labels of over-the-counter medications (e.g., sodium bicarbonate, sodium citrate, sodium phosphates, sodium saccharin, and sodium biphosphate).
9. While the initial adjustment to eating food with less salt may make the taste buds complain, within a month or two, many people actually prefer lower-sodium foods.
10. *If you have not been following a low-sodium diet and decide to begin reducing your intake, be sure to contact your physician or nurse practitioner. He or she may reduce your water pill dose (you may not need as much water pill if you are not retaining as much water!).*

FOODS TO AVOID OR CHOOSE LESS OFTEN

1. Cured or processed meats—bacon, ham, salt pork, corned beef, sausage, hot dogs, luncheon meats, canned meat or fish, frozen fish in salt solution, and smoked fish.
2. Sauces and seasonings—barbecue sauce, gravy and other sauce mixes, bouillon, canned broth, marinades, prepared salad dressings, prepared mustard, catsup, monosodium glutamate (MSG), soy sauce, teriyaki sauce, cooking wine, and tomato sauce.
3. Vegetables—canned vegetables with sodium, sauerkraut, pork and beans, tomato juice, vegetable juice, pickled vegetables, and frozen vegetables with sauce or breading.
4. Other canned or packaged products—stews, pot pies, frozen TV dinners and entrees, baking mixes, instant pudding, and packaged potato, rice, or pasta mixes.
5. Dairy products—buttermilk, most cheeses (especially processed cheese), and regular cottage cheese.

6. Snacks and condiments—salted popcorn, pretzels, salted nuts, chips and dips, salted crackers, pickles, olives, and salad peppers.
7. Desserts—pastries, cheesecake, and some cookies and cakes (read the labels).
8. Fast food—nearly all fast food (hamburgers, hot dogs, burritos, tacos, fried chicken, and pizza) is very high in sodium.

FOODS TO CHOOSE

1. Fresh meat and fish
2. Dried beans and peas
3. Unsalted tofu (soybean curd)
4. Fresh eggs
5. Pasta and rice, cooked without salt
6. Hot cereals (regular, not instant types)
7. Dry cereals (read the labels, since they vary greatly in sodium content)
8. Breads (read the labels)
9. Fresh fruits and vegetables
10. Fruit juices and fruit drinks
11. Dried fruits, such as raisins and prunes
12. Unsalted crackers, pretzels, chips, and nuts
13. Fruit ices, sherbet, frozen fruit juice bars, or popsicles
14. Low-sodium cottage cheese; unsalted butter; low-sodium margarine; and low-sodium cheese, cream cheese, and milk
15. Anything you prepare yourself, using fresh and low-sodium ingredients

Educational Map
for Heart Failure Clients

LOEB RESEARCH INSTITUTE
Partners in Care Education Map:
Congestive Heart Failure©

Continuity
of
Care

PROFILE:
Patient's name:_____
Address: _____
_____
Phone number: _____

Instructions:
At the top of the column for each module: sign your name, status, and the date of teaching. If material needs to be re-taught, continue to add name(s) and date(s) appropriately. For each session, initial in the column as each component is completed. General content is in the patient education booklet, organized by modules.

Nursing:	Module #1	Module #2	Module #3
	Nurse's signature and date: _____ _____	Nurse's signature and date: _____ _____	Nurse's signature and date: _____ _____
Assessment	☐ level of prior learning ☐ patient perception/readiness ☐ learning challenges	☐ review of activity sheet #1 ☐ respond to questions arising ☐ level of understanding achieved	☐ review of activity sheet #2 ☐ respond to questions arising ☐ level of understanding achieved
Planning	☐ decision on readiness to learn ☐ strategies to meet learning challenges (identify these at top of page 2)	☐ decision to re-teach previous session ☐ decision to progress ☐ learning strategies in place	☐ decision to re-teach previous session ☐ decision to progress ☐ learning strategies in place
Interventions	**Teaching content:** ☐ overview of the teaching program ☐ the heart as a living pump (basic anatomy, physiology) ☐ personal responsibility ☐ controllable aspects of CHF ☐ present Activity sheet #1	**Teaching content:** ☐ principal components of CHF management ☐ specific signs/symptoms from patient's experience ☐ self-monitoring skills ☐ present Activity sheet #2	**Teaching content:** ☐ patient's medications for CHF management ☐ patient's related cardiac medications ☐ non-prescription medications used by the patient ☐ signs/symptoms of high and low potassium (if required) ☐ use of the medication record ☐ present Activity sheet #3
Evaluation (patient outcomes)	☐ verbalizes readiness to learn ☐ acknowledges personal involvement in managing CHF ☐ verbalizes controllable aspects of CHF	☐ identifies self-monitoring skills ☐ relates individualized signs and symptoms of CHF to basic heart function ☐ participates with learning activity sheet	☐ identifies personal medication management components: name, dose frequency, description, and side effects ☐ identifies self-monitoring aspects of own medications

Courtesy MB Harrison, C Toman, and J Logan.

Current Medications:

_____

_____

_____

_____

_____

_____

_____

_____

_____

Previous CHF status: _____

Present CHF status: _____

Learning challenges: _____

_____

Strategies for meeting challenges: _____

Designated learner(s): _____

(Client, family member, other caregiver) _____

Module #4	Module #5	Module #6	Module #7
Nurse's signature and date:	Nurse's signature and date:	Nurse's signature and date:	Nurse's signature and date:
_____	_____	_____	_____
_____	_____	_____	_____
☐ review of activity sheet #3 ☐ respond to questions arising ☐ level of understanding achieved	☐ review of activity sheet #4 ☐ respond to questions arising ☐ level of understanding achieved	☐ review of activity sheet #5 ☐ respond to questions arising ☐ level of understanding achieved	☐ review of activity sheet #6 ☐ respond to questions arising ☐ level of understanding achieved
☐ decision to re-teach previous session ☐ decision to progress ☐ learning strategies in place	☐ decision to re-teach previous session ☐ decision to progress ☐ learning strategies in place	☐ decision to re-teach previous session ☐ decision to progress ☐ learning strategies in place	☐ decision to re-teach previous session ☐ decision to progress ☐ learning strategies in place
Teaching content: ☐ diet in the management of CHF: components of weight control, salt and sodium, fat and cholesterol, fluids, use of alcohol ☐ food preparation ☐ planning for special occasions ☐ changes in appetite ☐ present Activity sheet #4	**Teaching content:** ☐ role of exercise, rest and energy conservation in CHF ☐ reflection on present levels ☐ benefits ☐ techniques for use ☐ related self-monitoring skills ☐ present Activity sheet #5	**Teaching content:** ☐ Stress management, relaxation and environmental influences ☐ related self-monitoring skills ☐ techniques for use ☐ present Activity sheet #6	**Teaching content:** ☐ resources and support systems for CHF ☐ patient role ☐ professional's role ☐ community resources ☐ present wall chart guide for daily self-care activities
☐ identifies main CHF dietary components ☐ recognizes relation of diet to own signs/symptoms ☐ recognizes importance of changed appetite ☐ evaluates current dietary practices	☐ identifies self-monitoring aspects ☐ identifies preferred techniques ☐ participates in self-monitoring skills	☐ identifies personal situations of stress ☐ identifies own preferred coping techniques	☐ identifies personal sources of support ☐ identifies community resources for continued learning about CHF ☐ review of draft forms for patient education related to CHF

1. Check with the physician for client-specific guidelines for an exercise program. The physician may wish to order an exercise test before recommending exercise.
2. Delay (or suspend) an exercise program if the client has any of the following:
   a. Recent MI or CABG surgery
   b. Symptomatic fluid overload
   c. Angina
   d. Severe lightheadedness
   e. Symptomatic dysrhythmias
3. Advise client to do the following to develop and maintain a walking regimen:
   a. Choose good walking shoes and comfortable clothing
   b. Choose a time of day when the client's energy level is highest
   c. Avoid extremes of temperature (very hot or humid or very cold weather)
   d. Select a level area to walk whenever possible
   e. Begin with the client's current level of activity (e.g., 1 minute down an indoor hallway, 100 feet to the mailbox, or 1 block in front of the house) once or twice a day
   f. Gradually increase distance or frequency as the client tolerates
   g. Alternate periods of rest and activity
   h. Keep record of daily exercise
4. Instruct clients to avoid activities such as weightlifting (or swimming underwater) that require holding the breath or bearing down during the activity.
5. Time exercise at least 1 hour after a meal.
6. Instruct clients to stop exercise and call their physician if they experience palpitations, lightheadedness, a change in the pattern of their chest pain, or a marked increase in shortness of breath (mild shortness of breath is expected with exercise).
7. If clients experience unusual fatigue on the day after any increase in exercise duration or intensity, they should rest that day and reduce their level of activity when they resume exercise.

Status-Based Care Map for Management of Heart Failure

	Initial Visit	Follow-up Visits	Maintenance Phase	Crisis Visits	Posthospital
Assessment	Complete assessment guidelines for the heart-failure client in the home (Box 23-4). Assess current activity level (e.g., walk distance). Administer QOL tool.	Perform cardiovascular (CV) assessment. Assess knowledge about heart failure. Evaluate self-management skills. Assess functional status. Assess psychosocial status. Assess stability of comorbid conditions. Assess caregiver burden.	Per phone contact, using scripted questions (Box 23-10). Per home visits at intervals based on client stability and mastery of self-management.	Phone assessment to triage need for immediate intervention. Home visit: CV Assessment Assessment of nature and severity of condition	Discharge weight Medication changes CV assessment Functional status Stability of comorbid conditions Caregiver and support system function
Nursing Action	Develop individualized care plan for client based on assessment. Communicate with other disciplines involved in care. Communicate plan to medical provider.	Modify plan of care and determine frequency of visits based on client stability and progress in self-management. Involve other disciplines as indicated. Communicate modifications in plan of care to medical provider. Perform venipuncture for ordered laboratory tests. Collaborate in titration of medications (ACE inhibitor, beta-blocker) as ordered by medical provider.	Modify plan of care and determine frequency of visits based on client stability and continued self-management. Address preventive health measures: influenza and pneumonia vaccines, ongoing medical care, and self-management of comorbid conditions. Consider discharge from home care for clients who are: 1. Medically stable 2. NYHA Class I or II 3. Independent in self-management	Respond to call with visit within 1 to 2 hours. Call physician or NP as indicated. Administer IV diuretic if ordered. Adjust oral medications if ordered. Perform venipuncture for ordered laboratory tests. Call emergency medical services (EMS) system if transport to hospital is required.	Identify and address precipitating factors for hospitalization. Modify plan of care and determine frequency of visits based on client status. Communicate with medical provider to clarify any changes in medication regimen or other aspects of treatment plan. Communicate with medical provider about changes in client status.

Continued

QOL, Quality of life.

	Initial Visit	Follow-up Visits	Maintenance Phase	Crisis Visits	Posthospital
Education	Assess knowledge base about heart failure. Assess level of self-management. Assess pantry and refrigerator for foods with high sodium content. Plan education for client and caregiver for suggested content (Box 23-6).	Continue education and training in self-management as per plan developed at initial visit.	Continue education related to new medications or treatments. Review relevant content in response to client and caregiver questions.	Validate appropriate calls from client or caregiver about new or worsening symptoms. Provide education about interventions as indicated. Identify and address precipitating factors for crisis.	Review aspects of education related to precipitating factors for hospitalization. Provide education about medication or other treatment plan changes.
Outcomes	Daily weight chart is initiated. Client and caregiver know medication schedule. Client and caregiver are able to access appropriate resource for questions or crises.	There is evidence of increased self-management: Daily weight record Medication adherence Low-sodium diet adherence Knowledge of symptoms to report Functional status is stable or improved. Walking distance is increased.	No hospitalizations or ED visits for CHF Influenza and pneumonia vaccines administered to all clients at recommended intervals Stable or improved functional status Stable or improved QOL score Completed advance directives	Precipitating factors for crisis are identified and addressed.	Precipitating factors for CHF hospitalization are identified, addressed, and tracked. Plan for prevention of future exacerbations is in place.

24 Renal and Genitourinary Disorders

Susan A. Pfettscher and Lowanna S. Binkley

Kidney disease affects a significant segment of the American population. Alteration in renal and lower urinary-tract function on an acute or chronic basis undoubtedly affects millions of people, although complete numbers are not available. Many of these problems are treated conservatively and may require only infrequent outpatient care and treatment. The most dramatic treatment for diseases of the renal and genitourinary (GU) systems is renal replacement therapy. In 1998, more than 200,000 clients were treated with hemodialysis, peritoneal dialysis, and renal transplantation (US Renal Data System, 1999). Clients with diseases involving their kidneys and urinary tracts may experience concern and fear about requiring these lifelong therapies. It should be emphasized, however, that many people with renal and urinary tract diseases do not require these replacement therapies.

As the American population has aged and is subjected to chronic disease states, more individuals may well have significant changes in renal function that require monitoring and treatment with or without the use of replacement therapy. The nurse providing home care should have a strong renal knowledge base and understanding of the current and potential renal and urinary problems that the client has or may develop. This will enable the nurse to appropriately and adequately assess the client, as well as to intervene with appropriate therapies and education in those situations that warrant it.

RENAL ANATOMY AND PHYSIOLOGY
Gross Anatomy of the Kidney and Urinary Tract

The healthy human is born with two separate kidneys, weighing approximately 150 g each and located retroperitoneally on either side of the vertebral column between the twelfth thoracic and third lumbar vertebrae. They are well protected by the rib cage (two thirds of the kidney tissues lie within the rib cage). Although both kidneys are approximately the same size, the right kidney rests slightly lower in the body because of the position of the liver above it (Fig. 24-1). These bean-shaped organs are enclosed in a smoother, collagenous renal capsule and are also covered by a thick layer of perirenal fat (Sherwood, 1997).

The structures of the ureter, bladder, and urethra complete the system that removes the urine formed in the kidneys. The ureter arises from the renal pelvis and is a smooth, muscle-walled tube connecting the kidney to the bladder. Fluid is propelled down the ureter by the muscular function of the ureter.

The urinary bladder serves as a reservoir for urine before urination. This hollow structure consists of highly distensible, contractile smooth muscles, thus allowing for the collection of large quantities of urine (sometimes exceeding 1 L). The urethra extends from the lower neck of the bladder and is made of smooth muscle, which can contract or relax as stimulated. When the urethra is relaxed, urine flows out of the bladder and thus out of the body. Although this activity is usually called *voiding* or *urinating,* many colloquial terms describe this function and may be used by clients. The sensations of distensibility in the bladder and the ability to constrict or relax the urethra are neurologically mediated and can be consciously controlled. Neurological damage and diseases of various types, however, can interfere with recognition and control of these functions (Guyton, Hall, 2000).

Vascular Structure

The structure and functions of the blood vessels are the most important features of the kidneys. The kidneys receive 25% of the cardiac output

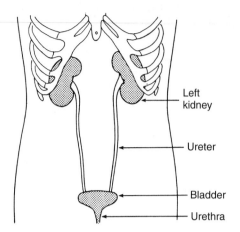

Fig. 24-1 The kidneys lie well protected within the rib cage. *(From Binkley L, Banton H:* Journal of Nephrology Nursing *3(4):139-158, 1986.)*

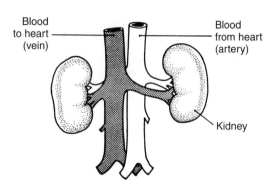

Fig. 24-2 Blood supply to the kidney. *(From Binkley L, Banton H:* Journal of Nephrology Nursing *3(4):139-158, 1986.)*

per minute, with nearly 90% of the body's total blood supply circulating through the kidneys every 5 minutes. This is achieved because the renal arteries arise from the abdominal aorta, thus providing high-volume, high-pressure blood flow to the kidneys. Venous return from the kidneys is directly from the renal vein into the inferior vena cava (Fig. 24-2). This high-pressure, high-flow system is not intended to maintain the kidney tissue oxygenation and viability, but rather to maintain the metabolic functions of the kidney.

To accommodate the high blood flow required to perform its functions, the circulation of the kidneys has to be extensive. Branching from the renal artery are several interlobar arteries, which divide into the arcuate arteries and then into the interlobular arteries. These smaller arteries continue to branch and become the afferent arterioles; an afferent arteriole is a blood vessel that leads into the glomerulus of each nephron; an efferent arteriole carries blood away from the glomerulus and forms the peritubular capillary network that nourishes the nephron. Blood flows from this capillary network into the venous system and enters the vena cava. Thus any condition that compromises blood flow to the kidneys or causes vascular changes compromises the ability of the kidneys to function normally (Guyton, Hall, 2000).

Microscopic Structure

Each kidney contains approximately a million nephrons, the functional units of the kidney. A nephron consists of a glomerulus, which acts as a filtering mechanism; Bowman's capsule, which serves as a collecting area for the filtrate; the tubular network, which achieves dynamic adjustments in fluid, electrolyte, and acid-base balance depending on systemic needs; and the collecting duct and tubule, which drain the urine into the pelvis of the kidney, and accomplishing final water balance as required (Fig. 24-3).

Physiology and Pathophysiology of the Kidneys

Several activities in the body are influenced by and influence renal function. The kidneys are the primary organs of excretion of end products of metabolism. Thus all end products of cellular function are excreted by the kidneys. In addition, the kidney is a regulatory organ for the following: (1) fluid balance, (2) electrolyte balance, (3) acid-base balance, (4) calcium-phosphorus balance, (5) blood-pressure control, (6) erythropoietin production, and (7) metabolism of other hormones. Thus kidneys should be seen as having both excretory and endocrine functions.

Many functions of the kidney can be measured by clinical laboratory (blood and serum) testing. Table 24-1 lists selected normal values for various kidney functions; because individual lab-

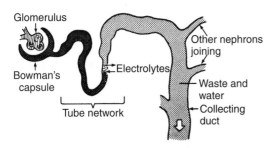

Fig. 24-3   The nephron is the functioning unit of the kidney. *(From Binkley L, Banton H:* Journal of Nephrology Nursing *3(4):139-158, 1986.)*

Table 24-1	Normal Laboratory Values
Test	Normal Values
BUN	9-15 mg/dl
Creatinine	0.9-1.4 mg/dl
Sodium	135-145 mEq/L
Potassium	3.4-5.0 mEq/L
Phosphorus	3.5-4.5 mg/dl
Calcium	8.5-10.5 mg/dl
Albumin	3.2-5.0 g/dl
Carbon dioxide	24-34 mEq/L

oratory ranges vary slightly, the nurse is advised to consult the laboratory values that are used in testing for the individual client. However, the nurse should be aware of the "generally normal" values for these laboratory studies.

End products of metabolism excreted by the kidneys are usually measured via the blood urea nitrogen (BUN) and serum creatinine (end product of muscle-mass metabolism). Nitrogenous waste products (urea nitrogen) are formed as end products of protein metabolism. Thus the amount produced depends on the amount of protein ingested (oral, enteral, or parenteral) and the state of protein metabolism experienced by the individual (anabolism [positive protein balance] or catabolism [negative protein balance in which the client's metabolic needs are not met with adequate protein intake]).

Other metabolic end products and organic salts are also excreted but may not be measured by blood studies, The products are often referred to

by physicians (along with urea nitrogen and creatinine) as *toxins* or *poisons*, but all are normally occurring products of metabolism. When these end products of metabolism are retained in the blood because they cannot be excreted by malfunctioning or nonfunctioning kidneys, the condition was historically known as *uremic poisoning;* its more modern term is *uremia.* The effects of uremia are systemic and result in death if untreated (Bullock, Henze, 2000; Sherwood, 1997).

Single values of urea nitrogen and creatinine provide information about the immediate function of the kidneys in excreting the end products of metabolism. However, serial measurements provide much better information about the client's state of renal function, In addition, these values cannot be adequately interpreted without knowing the general medical status (acute and chronic) of the client.

Fluid balance (excretion and reabsorption) is regulated within the tubular network of the nephron. Fluid is freely filtered at the glomerulus and enters the tubular system. Urinary concentration (reabsorption of water) takes place in the loop of Henle, with final concentration occurring in the distal tubule and in the collecting duct; antidiuretic hormone (secreted from the posterior pituitary gland) influences the final volume of urine to be excreted. Although 180 L of fluid are filtered through the glomeruli in a 24-hour period, only about 1500 ml (1 to 2 L) are excreted as urine. Nighttime concentration of urine is a normal function, which is regulated by various systemic functions; the loss of this function is called *nocturia* and is one of the very early symptoms of renal dysfunction or disease. Fluid excretion and reabsorption are manipulated and altered by many human functions (e.g., volume of fluid intake and activity states) that may not identify renal disease; in addition, many therapeutic interventions (many drugs including diuretics, hormones, and antihypertensives), as well as other diseases, influence fluid balance. Thus an accurate history must be obtained before interpreting the client's urination pattern and volume excreted. Renal function in the excretion and reabsorption of fluid is a major component in the fluid-volume status of an individual client. If excretion is diminished, the client will develop fluid overload in the vascular and interstitial compartments. All of the signs, symptoms, and complications of fluid-volume excess will be present. Conversely, the kidneys will maximally reabsorb water in a state of acute fluid loss or dehydration to the point that the client will exhibit oliguria or anuria. This is not a measure of renal dysfunction or disease; rather, it measures maximal renal function in the acute situation and is a powerful sign of fluid imbalance (Bullock, Henze, 2000).

In addition to control of fluid volume in the vascular compartment, the kidneys control blood pressure in two other ways: through elimination of sodium and through production of renin. These functions set into motion the responses that are shown in Fig. 24-4.

The renin-angiotensin system is a powerful controller of systemic blood pressure and fluid volume. In response to a perceived decrease in renal perfusion (usually because of decreased circulating volume or because of an obstruction in the renal blood vessels [a stenosis that causes decreased blood flow into the kidneys]), renin is secreted from the juxtaglomerular apparatus located in the nephron. Renin stimulates the release of angiotensinogen, which is synthesized to an-

giotensin I by the liver. An enzyme then converts angiotensin I to angiotensin II in the lungs; this enzyme is referred to as the *angiotensin-converting enzyme (ACE)*. Angiotensin II is a powerful vasoconstrictor that directly increases systemic blood pressure. In addition, angiotensin II stimulates the release of aldosterone from the adrenal glands; aldosterone increases sodium and water reabsorption within the kidney (distal convoluted tubule), resulting in expanded extracellular fluid volume and increased blood pressure (Fig. 24-5). In an effort to control this response causing hypertension in many individuals (who are not experiencing fluid volume deficits), the group of antihypertensive medications known as *ACE inhibitors* (e.g., captopril [Capoten], enalapril [Vasotec]) have

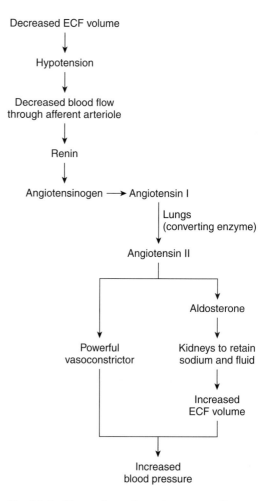

Fig. 24-4 Juxtamedullary nephron is the source of renin production in the macula densa.

Fig. 24-5 The renin-angiotensin system. *Courtesy Phoenix Educational Systems, Inc.*

been developed; these medications directly block the conversion of angiotensin I to angiotensin II in the lungs. In addition, a medication (losartan [Cozaar]) to block angiotensin II at its receptor site has also been developed for use as an antihypertensive (Guyton, Hall, 2000; McKenry, Salerno, 1998).

Excretion of excess water and sodium not excreted in situations of compromised or decreased renal function can also be improved with the use of diuretics. Multiple classes of drugs and various preparations are available to stimulate renal excretion of excess water and are used in clients with or without kidney dysfunction to maintain water balance, prevent fluid overload, or treat hypertension by enhancing the excretion of sodium, as well as water (Lilly, Aucker, 1999; McKenry, Salerno, 1998).

Electrolyte and acid-base balance are critical functions of the tubules. Selective reabsorption of sodium, chloride, potassium, magnesium, and phosphate occurs throughout the entire length of the tubular system to precisely regulate electrolyte excretion. When renal function is decreased significantly, electrolyte imbalances are clinically measurable. Sodium will be retained and enhance water retention. Of most critical significance is the retention of potassium because of its effects on cardiac muscle leading to fatal arrhythmias. Hydrogen ions are produced as a by-product of normal metabolism, including the digestion of food. An accumulation of hydrogen ions can alter body pH and cause metabolic acidosis. The role of the kidneys in acid-base balance is to ultimately correct changes in pH that may arise from any metabolic or respiratory alteration. This is done by regulating bicarbonate production in the kidney tubules and neutralizing (buffering) and excreting acids. Thus medications that alter acid-base balance can alter the pH of the urine and may create complications, such as the formation of calculi (stones), or contribute to the development of urinary tract infections.

Calcium and phosphorus are often considered minor electrolytes but are critically important in the assessment and treatment of clients with renal dysfunction or failure. Serum calcium levels are controlled by renal excretion in conjunction with parathyroid function. Thus the kidneys excrete excess serum calcium and retain amounts needed in response to complex hormonal functions. In their role in the calcium-phosphorus balance, the kidneys are responsible for the conversion of vitamin D (ingested through the gastrointestinal [GI] tract or absorbed from sunlight) to its metabolically active form, which then allows calcium to be absorbed from the GI tract during digestion; thus renal dysfunction results in a decreased serum calcium level even when adequate amounts of calcium are ingested. Calcium and phosphorus (another product absorbed from the GI tract during digestion) maintain a reciprocal relationship in the blood compartment—as one decreases, the other increases. This reciprocal relationship is exacerbated when the kidney is unable to excrete excess phosphorus; thus an even lower serum calcium level is produced. In clients with renal disease or failure, a low serum calcium level and a high phosphorus (phosphate) level usually occur. In addition, the hypocalcemic state triggers the release of parathormone from the parathyroid glands. Increased parathormone levels cause calcium to be resorbed (taken out) of bones to raise the serum calcium level. This response results in a complication known as *renal osteodystrophy* that can lead to significant morbidity. In addition, if the serum phosphorus level remains elevated, the calcium and phosphorus ions will precipitate and form crystals; these often deposit in soft tissues and joints and cause significant vascular calcification. For clients with osteoporosis or bone disease from other causes, this complication is additive to the severity of their bone disease and increases morbidities (fractures, vertebral collapse, and bone pain) (Brunier, 1996; Guyton, Hall, 2000; Pfettscher, 1999).

Erythropoietin is a glycoprotein produced in the peritubular capillaries in the cortex of the kidney. It is generally referred to as a hormone because its receptor site is the bone marrow, where it stimulates the conversion of stem cells to red blood cells. Secretion of erythropoietin is increased in response to hypoxic states (anemia), although low levels are secreted continually. When a person with normal renal function experiences anemia, erythropoietin secretion is increased. In states of acute blood loss, this response is useful in the endogenous response to the loss of and the increased production of red blood cells. In a person with renal disease or failure, this substance is no longer produced and a normochromic, normocytic anemia develops.

Modern biotechnological processes have allowed for the synthesis of this glycoprotein. It is manufactured as epoetin alfa (Epogen or Procrit) and is prescribed for people with the anemia of renal disease (Levin, 1992; Lundin, 1990).

The kidneys' role in the production of various growth and sex hormones is not clearly understood. It is clear that children with kidney disease do not grow at the same rates as other children and that adults with kidney disease do not produce adequate amounts of epidermal growth hormone. It is also known that men and women with kidney disease produce inappropriate amounts of luteinizing and follicle-stimulating hormones; there may be decreases in testosterone in male clients and in progesterone and estrogen in female clients.

Because the kidneys are the primary organs for the excretion of end products of metabolism, alterations in renal function also alter the rate of metabolism and excretion of drugs. Because so many drugs are both metabolized and excreted by the kidney, measurement of drug levels and use of certain drugs must be considered carefully for the person with renal dysfunction. The nurse should carefully assess clients for signs and symptoms of drug toxicity.

Finally, the functioning kidney also metabolizes and excretes insulin (endogenous and exogenous). For the client with diabetes mellitus (DM), decreased renal function can result in episodes of hypoglycemia, even though the client is eating correctly and following the prescribed regimen. Some clients with type 2 DM who have been taking insulin may not need to take any injections because their endogenous insulin is more available as they develop renal failure; they may mistakenly think or report that their diabetes is cured or gone. Persons with type 1 DM may also experience increased and more profound episodes of hypoglycemia on their prescribed regimen. The home care nurse can identify these episodes and report them appropriately. In addition, education of clients is critically important to ensure their understanding and acceptance of changes in their therapeutic regimen.

IMPAIRED RENAL FUNCTION AND FAILURE

The kidneys are remarkably able to respond to changes in homeostasis and to continue functioning maximally in the face of major physiolog-

ical alterations. There are two distinct phenomena that cause renal dysfunction and failure. In one, renal function can be restored, but in the other, significant disease processes cause irreversible damage. The two distinct processes have been labeled as *acute* and *chronic*. At the outset, it may not be clear which of these the client has developed. However, the diagnostic interventions performed along with the client's history will assist in determining which process is occurring. The signs and symptoms of renal failure (uremia) are the same in both acute and chronic renal failure. Therefore clinical laboratory studies (BUN, creatinine, and electrolyte levels and creatinine clearance) will not reveal or assist in the diagnosis of an acute or chronic problem. Greater attention may be paid to the BUN/creatine ratio in acute situations. Increases in urea that exceed increases in creatinine elevations are usually associated with GI bleeding, catabolic drugs, and decreased urine flow (prerenal). In acute tubular necrosis (ATN), the ratio may be maintained at 10:1, indicating parenchymal (intrarenal) damage (or chronic disease). In addition, for clients with minimal muscle mass (cachectic individuals or elderly persons), serum creatinine will remain at lower values than for an individual with large muscle mass with the same level of renal failure. Finally, the client's prior medical history and the circumstances bringing the client to the acute care setting may be very useful in determining whether the condition is likely to be acute or chronic. The following explanations should be useful to the nurse caring for individuals with renal problems (Vaughn, 1999).

Acute Renal Failure

Acute renal failure is a sudden, rapid deterioration of renal function that is usually (but not always) characterized by the onset of oliguria (less than 400 ml per day of urine output), azotemia (BUN level greater than 30 mg/dl), or uremia (clinical findings of renal failure). Acute renal failure is also potentially reversible; after the acute event, normal renal function can be restored as measured by various laboratory studies if clients had normal renal function previously. The cellular damage that occurs in the nephron (the tubule) causing renal dysfunction or failure is repaired during the recovery process. It remains unclear why repair occurs in this situation.

Acute renal failure is also further categorized as prerenal, intrarenal, or postrenal and assists in understanding the physiological and pathophysiological processes that have occurred. Understanding these processes also allows for more specific interventions and treatments to assist in the restoration of renal function (Bullock, Henze, 2000; Stark, Melander, 1999).

Prerenal failure   Prerenal azotemia and uremia imply that the acute renal failure has occurred as a result of decreased blood flow to the kidneys. Causes for this condition include the following:

1. Hypovolemia from hemorrhage, burns with fluid shifts or loss, or excessive fluid loss from any cause (e.g., GI losses, perspiration, vomiting, or excessive diuretic use)
2. Peripheral vascular changes (dilatation) from antihypertensives, sepsis, antiarrhythmics, drug overdose, neurogenic shock, and anaphylaxis
3. Cardiac disorders, such as myocardial infarction (MI), congestive heart failure, arrhythmias, or cardiac tamponade causing decreased cardiac output resulting in decreased renal perfusion
4. Renal artery lesions, such as occlusion, stenosis, thrombus, embolus, trauma with tears or occlusion, or aneurysm (including abdominal aortic aneurysms)

In these situations, there is inadequate blood flow into the vasculature of the kidneys to maintain renal functions associated with homeostasis (excretion and reabsorption of substances). If adequate renal perfusion is restored, the uremic state will not develop. In acute situations (e.g., traumas, burns, MIs, or hemorrhage), great attention is paid to the prevention of decreased renal perfusion to prevent the complication of acute renal failure.

Intrarenal failure   Intrarenal azotemia or uremia occurs as a result of insult or injury to the renal tissue (nephrons) and their surrounding tissue. ATN is the most common cause of intrarenal failure and of acute renal failure. When a prerenal condition cannot be reversed in a short time, tubular damage or necrosis develops, and the client progresses to ATN. Other causes of ATN include the following:

1. Acute renal diseases, such as interstitial nephritis, acute medullary necrosis, and acute cortical necrosis
2. Nephrotoxic agents, such as aminoglycosides; diuretics; iodinated or hyperosmolar contrast media; heroin; other antibiotics; salicylates; pesticides; organic solvents; heavy metals; heme pigments; and plant and animal substances, such as poisonous mushrooms and snake venom
3. Inflammatory processes, including autoimmune and hypersensitivity diseases
4. Radiation nephritis
5. Obstruction secondary to stones, scar tissue, or neoplasms
6. Intravascular hemolysis, such as transfusion reactions or disseminated intravascular coagulation (DIC)
7. Systemic and vascular disorders, such as renal vein thrombosis, nephritic syndrome, multiple myeloma, sickle-cell disease, malignant hypertension, DM, and systemic lupus erythematosus

Note that this list is varied and sometimes also includes conditions listed under the prerenal heading because of their progressive nature. In ATN, the client usually develops significant uremia and requires replacement therapy until tubular regeneration takes place.

Postrenal failure   Postrenal failure (azotemia or uremia) occurs when urine flow from the kidneys into the bladder or the emptying of the bladder through the urethra is obstructed. Urine continues to be produced and increases in volume either in the kidneys (ureteral obstruction) or from the bladder into the ureters and kidneys (urethral obstruction). Causes of these obstructions include the following:

1. Enlargement of the prostate (benign or malignant) with urethral obstruction
2. Congenital anomalies of the urinary tract, usually diagnosed in infancy or early childhood
3. Pregnancy with mechanical obstruction of one or both ureters by the enlarged uterus
4. Tumors in the abdominal or pelvic cavity that mechanically obstruct one or both ureters by direct pressure
5. Stone formation in the ureters (usually must occur in both, which is very rare); large stone formations in renal pelvis (both kidneys)
6. Postradiation fibrosis (rare because of improved radiation techniques)

Although the client may be uremic at the time of acute presentation, relief of the obstructive lesion usually provides a relatively immediate resolution of the signs and symptoms of acute renal failure. When the obstruction is removed, diuresis may begin immediately. Nephron damage by urine stasis takes an extended time to develop. Most clients seek more urgent medical assistance when they cannot void or are already receiving treatment for one of the causative problems.

Clinical course Most individuals with acute renal failure will be hospitalized when this complication develops or will be hospitalized because of the acute nature of the symptoms. Whereas acute renal failure is a loss of kidney function, the effect is a systemic one in which all organ systems can be involved. Some clients may experience only fluid and electrolyte imbalances (azotemia) that may last for a few hours or days. Other clients may experience complex problems that persist for weeks to months, requiring dialysis for life support (uremia). However, acute renal failure is an acute episode; the client with previously normal renal function who survives may expect return of normal or near-normal renal function. If the client has experienced other major trauma or illness, death may occur secondary to the primary problems or to other medical complications.

It is thought that approximately 10% to 20% of adults and 50% of children who develop ATN are found to have preexisting chronic renal disease (often undiagnosed). Thus, while they may be acutely ill, they do not meet the most stringent definition of acute renal failure (having previous normal renal function). Their acute presentation may indicate irreversible progression of their disease states or development of another acute condition that further and irreversibly compromises their remaining renal function.

An individual who is recovering from an episode of acute renal failure will be justifiably concerned about future kidney problems. The home health nurse who is caring for the client after discharge can provide support and information to the client and family about current kidney function through review of laboratory studies (Are values returning to normal?) and the client's therapeutic regimens (Is the client still receiving dialysis or other renal-specific therapies?).

Chronic Renal Failure

Progressive deterioration in kidney function over a considerable length of time moves through several phases. During this period, the person may not be aware of the presence of altered renal function. Only in the later stages of renal failure do significant signs and symptoms develop. People who see health care providers on a regular basis may be diagnosed with renal abnormalities based on laboratory studies; however, even slight elevations occur only after the disease has developed (not when it first begins). The stages of renal disease may be described as follows.

Renal insufficiency is a reduction in renal function characterized by few or no physical symptoms, serum creatinine generally between 2 and 5 mg/dl for a healthy adult, azotemia with the BUN level elevated between 20 and 40 mg/dl, few or no electrolyte abnormalities, and few other blood chemistry abnormalities (no anemia or calcium-phosphorus derangements). The person feels well and may not be diagnosed if no routine laboratory tests are performed. People may be diagnosed if they seek medical assistance for acute symptoms (unrelated) or if they have other diseases, such as hypertension, cardiac disease, or diabetes (type 1 or 2).

Chronic renal disease is characterized by a serum creatinine level >5 mg/dl; BUN level >40 mg/dl; increasing inability to maintain fluid, electrolyte, and acid-base balance; hypertension; anemia; and beginning symptoms of general malaise.

Chronic renal failure and end-stage renal disease (ESRD) are characterized by elevations of BUN >80 mg/dl; serum creatinine elevations to >8 mg/dl; and creatinine clearance of <15 cc/minute. The person may be experiencing nausea with vomiting, loss of appetite, edema, oliguria, hypertension, and fatigue secondary to significant anemia. People who have not been seeing a physician may seek medical care for these symptoms and report that they have had the "flu" for a longer time than expected.

If untreated, the client with ESRD (uremia) will die. Uncontrolled vomiting, hypertension, generalized edema (anasarca), seizures, and coma (uremic encephalopathy) will develop; death will occur secondary to cerebral edema with brainstem herniation. Such cases are rarely, if ever, seen in the United States today. Renal replacement therapies are initiated to prevent or reverse these problems. If a client chooses not to undergo treatment, conservative management of fluid intake and other symptoms, such as vomiting, make death much easier. Clients will usually die of hyperkalemia and its resulting cardiac arrest if treatment is supportive in the hospital or home (Albee, Beckman, Shell, 1996; Bullock, Henze, 2000; Lancaster, 1995; Pfettscher, 1999).

Special populations at risk   Elderly individuals experience a decline in renal function secondary to the normal aging process. Loss of nephrons occurs with aging. Creatinine clearance is diminished even though serum creatinine levels are minimally increased. Decreased intake of protein may prevent a substantial rise in BUN, even in the face of diminished renal function. If the elderly person has other illnesses, such as hypertension, cardiac disease, or DM (and many elders have all three of these diseases), the risk of renal disease or renal failure increases.

If the client experiences events leading to hypotension or hypoperfusion (episodes of dehydration), the risk increases more dramatically. In addition, the administration of radiographic contrast agents can cause a nephrotoxic event that may not be reversible. If the elderly client has renal dysfunction, he or she may experience alterations in drug metabolism and even further renal dysfunction. The home care nurse seeing such clients who are exposed to any of these risks may be able to prevent or minimize further insults to the renal system through careful monitoring of medication administration, tests being performed, and health status of the client.

Types 1 and 2 DM are associated with high rates of chronic renal disease and failure. Both the glomerular and vascular structures suffer damage secondary to diabetes, resulting in loss of renal function. A very early sign of renal involvement is the development of microalbuminuria. The Diabetes Complications and Control Trial (DCCT) (1993) and other studies being undertaken in type 2 DM clients have shown that early and intensive control of blood glucose can significantly delay or possibly even prevent the development of renal failure. Because almost half of clients receiving ESRD treatment have diabetes, such prevention can have a significant impact. The home health nurse may be seeing a client with DM either for monitoring or other illnesses or problems and may be able to identify early signs and symptoms of renal involvement. The nurse may also play a significant role in support and education of the client in preventing progression of renal disease (DCCT Research Group, 1993; Keane, Eknoyan, 1999).

End-Stage Renal Disease

ESRD is generally determined to be the state in which the individual's kidney function has deteriorated to the point that death is imminent unless renal replacement therapy is begun. The uremic state has been previously described. If clients have been receiving care by a health care provider, they may begin replacement therapy before they experience the actual state of uremia, thus avoiding this episode of illness.

Other clients may come to the health care provider (even to the emergency department) in obvious uremia without any prior knowledge or diagnosis of renal disease. Because they may not understand the insidious nature of chronic renal failure, such clients may consider that their illness is sudden and that they will recover. These clients may need extensive support and education as they begin life-long treatment (Albee, Beckman, Shell, 1996; Dunn, 1993; Sosa-Guerro, Gomez, 1997; Lancaster, 1995; Pfettscher, 1999).

Treatment of end-stage renal disease   Generally, two forms of dialytic therapy and renal transplantation are the available treatments for ESRD in the United States. Variations in the way dialytic therapy is accomplished may vary for the individual client. The principles underlying these therapies remain unchanged. Dialysis is a treatment for ESRD that cleanses the blood of accumulated waste products. The two types of dialysis currently used are hemodialysis and peritoneal dialysis (Lancaster, 1995; Pfettscher, 1999).

Hemodialysis   Hemodialysis is sometimes called *the blood type of dialysis* and uses blood that is withdrawn from a specially constructed blood vessel (vascular access) and circulates it through an artificial kidney, where the metabolic waste products and excess water are removed by principles of diffusion, filtration, osmosis, and pressure gradients. This extracorporeal circuitry allows the blood to be efficiently returned to the client through the vascular access. Because blood is flowing through an extracorporeal circuit, the client undergoing hemodialysis usually receives heparin at the initiation of treatment to prevent clotting in this circuit. The heparin dose is administered at the initiation of dialysis; clients may receive additional doses during the treatment period. Dosage and administration are calculated for return to a near-normal clotting time by the end of the dialysis treatment (Daugirda, Ing, 1994; Lancaster, 1995; Pfettscher, 1999).

Vascular access for hemodialysis remains a primary problem in the delivery of this treatment. The surgical creation of an arteriovenous (A-V) fistula or an A-V graft is generally required to access the volume and rate of blood required for efficient hemodialysis treatment. Fistulae using the client's own artery and vein may work well for some clients, but may not be able to be created for the client with significant vascular disease or who requires immediate dialysis. A-V grafts are created using an artificial vascular graft material (usually expanded polyfluorotetraethylene) to create a conduit from an artery to a vein. One problem associated with vascular accesses is clotting of blood in the vessel lumen (generally does not extend into more distant vessels). Stenotic lesions may also develop at the surgical anastomoses, causing flow problems or aiding in the clotting process. Procedures to "declot" these accesses or to replace them may be required on multiple occasions for some clients, although other clients will rarely experience access problems. To perform hemodialysis, two needles must be placed in the vascular access. Because of their large gauge and the high-pressure, high-flow nature of the access, bleeding at the end of treatment is similar to that from arterial punctures. Some clients experience episodes of bleeding after they leave the dialysis unit and may require emergency interventions. Hemodialysis clients are at increased risk of local or systemic infections because of these multiple needle sticks. Rigorous aseptic care is taken when needles are placed and removed during the hemodialysis treatment. Clients are instructed how to care for their accesses, including monitoring of patency, cleanliness, and general inspection of sites for redness or infection. Because clients are seen in the dialysis unit so frequently, this assessment is also performed by staff at the time of each treatment (Beathard, 1994; Brunier, 1996; Hartigan, 1993, 1994; Kaufman, 1997).

An alternative short- or long-term vascular access may be created with placement of a multiple-lumen (dual or triple) central venous catheter. Manufactured primarily for hemodialysis access, these catheters may be left in place for weeks to months to provide access routes for hemodialysis. The usual procedures for the care of central venous catheters apply to lines. They may be inserted in either the subclavian vein or the internal or external jugular vein and threaded into the superior vena cava. Between dialysis treatments, these catheters have heparin instilled into the lumens (ports) and are appropriately clamped, capped, and bandaged. Some dialysis programs may use home care nurses to provide catheter care, including changing of the heparin locks or cleaning and redressing the catheter site. Procedures specific to that facility should be obtained to ensure consistent care and to avoid heparin administration errors (Ouwendyk, Helferty, 1996; Northsea, 1996).

Hemodialysis clients usually need to take medications as an adjunct to their dialysis treatment. Many require antihypertensive therapy to control the effects of fluid overload between treatments or to treat underlying hypertensive disease. Phosphorus binders are taken with meals since phosphate is poorly dialyzed out; current therapy usually uses a form of calcium carbonate or acetate (Tums or Phoslo) that binds phosphorus in the gut and excretes it through the GI tract. Multivitamin preparations that include folic acid are usually prescribed to replace the water-soluble vitamins that are removed with the dialysis treatment. Folic acid is required in the manufacture of red blood cells. In addition, oral iron may be taken to assist in the manufacture of red blood cells; iron studies are routinely performed to monitor for the need for iron therapy. Intravenous iron administration is preferred to minimize the side effects of oral iron agents.

Some medications are administered intravenously during the hemodialysis treatment, thus enhancing their complete absorption and ensuring their administration. Most commonly, epoietin alfa (Epogen) is administered intravenously or subcutaneously at the time of treatment. This drug has been most useful in the treatment of anemia associated with renal failure. Various drugs may also be given intravenously to treat the hyperparathyroidism associated with calcium-phosphorus imbalances in an attempt to prevent renal osteodystrophy. Iron replacement can also be administered intravenously during hemodialysis to enhance its absorption. If required, other medications (e.g., antibiotics, parenteral nutrition, or vaccinations for hepatitis, flu, or pneumonia) are administered in the hemodialysis unit to maintain the health of these clients.

Hemodialysis can be performed in the home by trained clients and a trained partner (often a family member). This allows the client to control the schedule of treatment rather than have to follow the schedule at the dialysis facility. Both the client and partner are trained with the knowledge and skills necessary to perform the dialysis treatment and to solve any problems that might arise with the equipment or the treatment (Fig. 24-6). The popularity of home dialysis has waxed and waned in the United States, primarily because of governmental policies related to payment (e.g., programs that paid partners to assist once existed). Currently, there are no financial incentives specifically directed to home dialysis performance. In addition, the geographic proximity to outpatient hemodialysis units in most communities may serve as a disincentive for clients to undertake home hemodialysis. There are currently some trials underway using new equipment that may allow hemodialysis clients to dialyze at home without a partner while they sleep (overnight) on a nightly basis. It is thought to provide better therapy than intermittent treatment. It is unclear at this time if nightly home hemodialysis will prove useful for a significant number of people.

Peritoneal dialysis Peritoneal dialysis is a form of dialysis that allows the client to provide his or her own treatment outside of a dialysis facility. Clients who choose peritoneal dialysis are trained independently by professional nursing staff to perform this procedure.

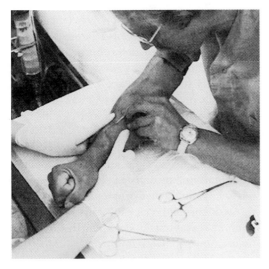

Fig. 24-6 Self-venipuncture performed by hemodialysis client, using a large-bore 15-gauge needle.

Peritoneal dialysis uses the semipermeable membrane and its rich vasculature in the peritoneal cavity to perform dialysis on a continuous basis. A soft catheter is implanted into the peritoneal cavity; dialysis solution flows by gravity through this catheter into the peritoneal cavity (Lancaster, 1995; Lewis et al, 1996). The fluid dwells there for approximately 4 hours before it is drained by gravity into a collection bag and then immediately replaced with another volume of fluid. The principles of diffusion and osmosis allow for the movement of metabolic waste products and water from the blood vessels into the dialysate solution (Daugirda, Ing, 1994; Lancaster, 1995; Pfettscher, 1999).

Continuous ambulatory peritoneal dialysis (CAPD) usually requires four exchanges of fluid in 24 hours. The first three exchanges are usually done during the waking hours, and the final instillation is done at bedtime. Technical improvements in the design of the dialysate bags and the tubing required for exchanges have decreased the number of connections and disconnections required in performing an exchange. Thus the risk of contamination and development of peritonitis through the introduction of organisms into the sterile peritoneal cavity has been decreased. In addition, these advances have made this procedure simpler for clients to perform.

Medications can be administered via the peritoneal cavity by adding them to the bag of dialysate solution. Local or systemic administration of antibiotics is achieved by injecting the antibiotics into the solution bag when peritonitis is suspected. In addition, many clients with DM who require insulin inject regular insulin into their exchange bags and thus receive insulin on an almost constant basis.

Continuous cyclic peritoneal dialysis (CCPD) uses the same principles of peritoneal dialysis but it is scheduled and delivered somewhat differently. The equipment used is a small machine that is programmed to deliver several exchanges of fluid during the night, cycling the fluid in and pumping it out when the dwell time has been completed. Fluid is usually instilled at the end of the night and remains in the peritoneal cavity during the day—the reverse schedule of CAPD for most clients. Dialysis is constant with this method but provides the client with freedom from exchanges during the day. For the client who works during the day, this technique allows for independence from the dialysis facility and freedom from need to perform exchanges during the workday.

Peritoneal dialysis use is minimal compared to the number of clients who continue to undergo hemodialysis; fewer than 20% of clients in the United States use peritoneal dialysis. However, special populations have found this therapy especially useful: clients who wish to control their therapy rather than having it provided, people with DM who find that their visual changes are stabilized (heparin use with hemodialysis has been implicated in the development of retinal hemorrhages), and people who are essentially homebound who have peritoneal dialysis provided by another person in the household. Clients who have had multiple vascular access problems with hemodialysis may be encouraged to use peritoneal dialysis to prevent this continuing problem. Finally, because peritoneal dialysis is continual, the diet restrictions (fluid, sodium, and potassium) usually required for hemodialysis are not as stringent. Indeed, some clients find that their diets are less restricted and near normal; most peritoneal dialysis clients are encouraged to eat larger quantities of protein, since some protein is lost through the peritoneal membrane.

In addition, peritoneal dialysis is administered by specially trained staff in nursing homes for their residents, thus decreasing the transportation difficulties that may arise with need for outpatient hemodialysis. Home care nurses may visit clients undergoing peritoneal dialysis for other problems and needs, so understanding the principles and schedules of this treatment modality can help in assessing the client's condition and well-being. Communication with the dialysis staff is useful to verify the schedule and prescription for dialysis, medications, and diet. It is also useful in preventing or resolving problems in the household or with treatment that could interfere with successful peritoneal dialysis therapy.

Clients undergoing peritoneal dialysis continue to see the peritoneal dialysis nursing staff on a regular basis for outpatient follow-up. All dialysis clients (hemodialysis and peritoneal dialysis) receive direct care from a nephrologist who may also serve as their primary physician. In addition, all ESRD facilities in the United States are required to have social workers and dietitians specializing in the care of renal clients on their staffs.

Renal Transplantation Renal transplantation can be performed for individuals with ESRD with the expectation of excellent outcomes. The primary limitation of renal transplantation is the availability of human donor kidneys. New immunosuppressive drugs are more specifically targeted to treat rejection episodes while decreasing the level of systemic immunosuppression that is required (Young, Koda-Kimble, 1995).

Renal transplantation requires the donation of a healthy kidney from another individual. Current procedures use family members who share genetic identity with the recipient. Outcomes of this transplantation procedure are generally excellent, since the kidney is genetically more compatible or nearly identical. Although the typical donor is a close family member, such as a sibling, parent, or adult child, more distant relatives have also served as donors with good outcomes (Hilton, Starzonski, 1994).

Cadaveric organ donation provides other clients with kidney transplants. A cadaveric donor is an individual from whom the kidneys are removed (often along with other organs and tissues) after brain death has occurred. A complex system of organ procurement agencies throughout this country arranges for cadaveric organ donation and is charged with ensuring that the most compatible recipient receives the donated kidney. From a cadaveric donor of two healthy kidneys, two recipients will receive transplants (Chabealewski, 1996).

With the advent of improved, more specific immunosuppressive medications, some renal transplant centers also use biologically unrelated donors; these are usually adults who have an emotional bond or relationship to the potential recipient. They may be spouses, close friends, or work colleagues. Although these transplants are reported to have a similar success rate to cadaveric transplants, the advantage is in their timeliness; the extended waiting period of 4 to 5 years for a cadaveric transplant is eliminated. In addition, the living donor is ensured of being in excellent health, in contrast to the cadaveric donor who may have suffered massive injuries or trauma resulting in brain death; the donated kidney has not been subjected to any hemodynamic or systemic insults.

All donors and recipients undergo a series of immunological tests to determine the degree of tissue compatibility. Blood type should also be compatible between donor and recipient. If a living donor donates the kidney, that individual's health status is subjected to complete examination to ensure that his or her health is not compromised by this surgical procedure and the loss of one kidney. Recent developments in the use of laparoscopic surgery to remove the donor's kidney have decreased the recuperative time that the donor faces and may make living donation more acceptable to people who are fearful of the traditional nephrectomy operation. Recipients remain hospitalized for less than 1 week if no postoperative problems or complications develop. Outpatient office visits with laboratory studies to monitor renal function and immunosuppressive therapy are frequently (at least weekly) performed in the early period after the transplantation. If the client experiences no problems after the early postoperative period, medical-visit frequency decreases. After the first year, the client may need to be seen on a monthly basis or even less frequently. The client may be seen by his or her local nephrologist (not the transplant team) for long-term care, especially if there are geographic barriers involved.

Immunosuppressive drug regimens are guided by the principles of balancing the therapeutic effects of these drugs while minimizing their side effects and complications. Immunosuppressive drug therapy may need to be discontinued for the client who develops major complications (e.g., infections or cancer). Current immunosuppressive drugs used for renal transplantation include the following:

- Cyclosporine (Sandimmune and Neoral) suppresses T-cell formation (preventing acute rejection) and may also suppress B-cell formation (preventing chronic rejection).
- Mycophenolate (CellCept) suppresses T- and B-cell proliferation. It is a new, more specific immunosuppressive agent.
- Tacrolimus is a potent immunosuppressive that can be used as a primary agent but may be reserved for treatment of an acute rejection episode.
- Corticosteroids (prednisone) have been one of the primary immunosuppressive drugs. It has both immunosuppressive and antiinflammatory actions. Its large number of side effects and complications (notably the Cushingoid appearance) makes it a less acceptable drug for transplant recipients.
- Azathioprine (Imuran) is a nonspecific immunosuppressive drug that may have effects on both acute and chronic rejection

because it suppresses white blood cell formation by the bone marrow.

Clients may be on various combinations of these drugs as stabilization of transplant function occurs. Increases in drug dose and frequency of administration may be ordered if there is possibility of rejection activity. If rejection does not occur, drug doses may be tapered to baseline amounts; if multiple drug therapy is used, some of the immunosuppressives may be discontinued if renal function remains normal. Other immunosuppressives (antithymocyte globulin and murine monoclonal antibody) may be administered intravenously at the time of a rejection episode in an attempt to suppress rejection (Payne, 1992; Young, Koda-Kimble, 1995).

Renal transplantation is not a cure for ESRD. The client may enjoy return of normal renal function and reversal of some of the other systems complications that have occurred with ESRD; however, clients must adhere to the medication regimen, must pay careful attention to their health status to avoid opportunistic infections, and may need to follow a sodium-restricted diet. In addition, the client lives with the possibility of other complications of drug therapy or rejection of the transplanted organ even years after the surgical implantation, Currently, the cost of drug therapy after renal transplantation provides a barrier for some clients; the average cost of maintenance immunosuppressive therapy can be greater than $10,000 per year.

The home care nurse who provides services for a renal transplant recipient needs to be sensitive to the socioeconomic burdens that ESRD and renal transplantation may place not only on the client, but also on his or her family. Renal transplantation provides the client with options to return to a more normal lifestyle unencumbered by the demands of dialysis treatment. For many, it provides an opportunity to return to the workplace or to engage in other life activities made difficult with dialysis schedules.

Discontinuation of ESRD treatment The ESRD client may determine that his or her illness is terminal and choose to discontinue dialysis therapy. Federal regulations governing the delivery of ESRD services support this decision. State regulations also generally uphold such client decision-making under various statutes and case law. When an ESRD client discontinues treatment, death may come very quickly or more slowly (usually a maximum of 2 weeks' survival). The client may be referred to hospice services in the community for support and care during the dying period; the family also needs support during this period. Death may come easily, with development of hyperkalemia leading to cardiac arrest; death from hyperkalemia may be relatively pain free unless the client experiences chest pain from hypoxia (oxygen can be administered as a comfort measure). There appears to be little reason to maintain the potassium-restricted diet when the client has chosen to discontinue dialysis; some clients choose to enjoy the foods that they had previously had to exclude from their diet. Excess sodium and fluid intake should be avoided because the development of congestive heart failure and pulmonary edema causes hypoxia, difficulty in breathing, and a sensation of suffocation and results in more suffering during the final stages of dying. The home care nurse caring for the client who has chosen to terminate treatment may find it challenging to provide care; referral to hospice or other agencies may assist the client, family, and nurse in continuing to provide excellent nursing care. Interaction with the dialysis staff may also be of support during this time (National Kidney Foundation, 1996; Pfettscher, 1999).

HOME CARE NURSING ASSESSMENT AND INTERVENTION

Successful nursing intervention for the client who has chronic renal failure is dependent on astute nursing assessment. Assessment of the client should be based both on what the client tells the nurse and on what the nurse observes in the home setting. Any signs or symptoms (nausea, vomiting, diarrhea, constipation, increasing fatigue, dyspnea, shortness of breath, and mental confusion) that indicate increasing renal deterioration in the client who has not yet initiated therapy or the development of these and other signs and symptoms (pruritus, numbness and tingling in extremities, sleeplessness, and increasing sleep) in the client undergoing dialysis should be noted and reported. Consultation with the dialysis unit staff—nurses, physicians, social workers, and dietitians—can allow for timely interventions and correction of problems and complications.

The nurse who can identify the cause of symptoms and who understands the principles of the ESRD treatment that the client is undergoing can contribute to his or her care and well-being. Communication with the health care staff ensures the client of coordinated care. Tables 24-2 and 24-3 summarize and provide additional

Text continued on p. 462

Table 24-2	Symptoms, Possible Causes, and Suggested Nursing Interventions in Clients with Chronic Renal Failure ○	
Symptoms	**Possible Causes**	**Nursing Interventions**
Dizziness	Medications Fluid deficit Orthostasis	Review medications for any that might cause dizziness and instruct client on their use. If dizziness is severe and intolerable, inform physician for possible drug change. If dizziness is mild and tolerable, determine if side effect is self-limiting or may become tolerable. Check multipositional blood pressure of client on antihypertensive medications. If orthostasis is present, instruct client about slow position changes. If client is hypotensive, assess for fluid loss (vomiting or diarrhea) and weight loss and assess skin turgor and mucous membranes.
	Cardiac output Cerebral blood flow	Auscultate for carotid bruit, mental confusion or alterations in memory or behavior, and previous episodes of syncope. Auscultate heart sounds. Assess for bradycardia, tachycardia, or other arrhythmia. Assess for evidence of congestive heart failure.

Symptoms	Possible Causes	Nursing Interventions
Shortness of breath	Fluid excess	Weigh client, if able, to do accurate comparison to previous weights.
		Assess edema in extremities, sacral area, and face.
		Assess lung fields for wheezes, rhonchi, and decreased breath sounds.
		Assess vital signs for evidence of CHF, hypertension, or hypotension with fluid volume excess.
Nausea with or without vomiting	Medications Ulcerations	Elicit history of nausea, use of OTC or prn medications, bowel function (diarrhea or constipation) with or without use of medications, blood in emesis or stool, use of NSAIDs (prescription or OTC), digitalis toxicity, hypercalcemia, and use of herbs.
	Acidosis (venous CO_2 level <19 mEq/L)	Treat with sodium bicarbonate or sodium citrate (Bicitra).
		Start dialysis or increase dialysis time.
	Uremia (BUN level >80 mg/dl)	Restrict protein intake in diet.
		Initiate dialysis therapy.
		If BUN level is >100 mg/dl in dialyzed client, increase treatment time or frequency.
Pruritus	Dry skin	If skin is dry and flaky, start intensive therapy with water-based lotions (Eucerin).
		Use tepid water for bathing.
		Soak client in tub with oils or oatmeal bath preparations added to water.
		Avoid harsh soaps.
		Apply liberal amounts of water- or lanolin-based creams or lotions several times per day.
	Serum phosphorus level >6 mg/dl	Administer phosphorous binding with meals or snacks.
		Assess diet for phosphorus.
		Reduce or eliminate dairy products and beans.
Diarrhea	Diabetic gastroenteropathy	Assess use of metoclopramide (Reglan) or ranitidine for control, use of diphenoxylate and atropine (Lomotil) for short periods, and intake of sorbitol in sugar-free foods.
	Hyperkalemia	Assess for other signs and symptoms of fatigue, muscle weakness, cardiac arrhythmias, bradycardia, dietary indiscretions or use of potassium-containing drugs, and use of herbs.
	Drugs	Assess for use of laxatives, cathartics, other stool softeners, over-the-counter agents, magnesium-containing laxatives, and sodium polystyrene sulfonate (Kayexalate) with sorbitol.
Fatigue	Anemia	Identify if client is receiving epoetin alfa.
		Assess for blood loss, vomiting, diarrhea, hemorrhoids, and menstrual period.
		Identify if client is taking or receiving folate or iron (oral or intravenous) supplements.
		Assess for increasing uremia requiring initiation of dialysis.
		Increase dialysis time.
	Depression	Assess sleep pattern, participation in normal activities, and reported feelings of sadness or depression.
		If client reports sleepiness, assess for use of sedatives, antidepressants, and other drugs that may cause sleepiness.
		Assess for signs and symptoms of sleep apnea.
Irritability, sadness, mental sluggishness	Uremia	Initiate dialysis or increase frequency or time.
	Vitamin B deficiency	Initiate vitamin B replacement.
	Grief over loss of renal function	Initiate counseling regarding normal response.
		Make referral regarding adaptation to chronic illness.

CHF, Congestive heart failure; *OTC,* over-the-counter; *prn,* as needed; *NSAIDS,* nonsteroidal antiinflammatory drugs; *CO₂,* carbon dioxide.

Table 24-3 Guidelines for Care of Client with Chronic Renal Failure

Dos	Don'ts
If blood needs to be drawn, use the limb without the vascular access.	Don't take blood pressures or use tourniquets or venipunctures in limb with vascular access.
For clients with diabetes (types 1 and 2), encourage use of blood glucose testing with greater frequency to prevent episodes of hypoglycemia.	Don't rely on client signs and symptoms of hypoglycemia since these may not be reliable.
Use concentrated glucose sources (sugar, glucose tablets, and hard candies) to treat hypoglycemia.	Don't use orange juice to treat hypoglycemia; potassium content is too high.
Encourage use of various spices for seasoning foods—garlic powder, onion powder, and Mrs. Dash—to replace salt.	Don't permit salt substitutes. They contain potassium chloride or other electrolytes.
Always measure blood pressure multipositionally—while client is lying, sitting, and standing.	Don't accept a supine (lying) elevated blood-pressure reading without obtaining a sitting and standing blood pressure. Blood pressure may change because of antihypertensive drugs.
Assess vascular access function by auscultating for the bruit; palpate the thrill to ensure patency of access.	Don't occlude the vascular access with constrictive clothing, blood pressure cuff, tourniquet, or name bracelet or other jewelry. Remind client not to place heavy objects against the access.
Encourage the client to assume as much responsibility for self-care as possible.	Don't encourage dependency and complacency, since these may contribute to decreased quality and quantity of life.
Teach and encourage client to follow prescribed regimen of diet, medications, and dialysis treatment.	
Educate and reinforce that complications and death can result from nonadherence.	

CASE STUDIES

MR. B.

Mr. B. is a 52-year-old man with type 1 DM. He has developed diabetic nephropathy and currently loses 4 g of protein every 24 hours in his urine. He is on an 1800-calorie American Dietetic Association (ADA) diet prescription, with 60 g of high-biologic-value protein and 20 g of low-biologic-value protein, 6 mEq/l potassium, and 2-g sodium restriction for his progressive renal failure. His insulin requirements are neutral protamine Hegedorn (NPH) 72 U in the morning and 45 U in the evening. Other medications include furosemide 80 mg twice daily (bid) and enalapril 5 mg bid, along with stool softeners and a multivitamin. The home health nurse has been asked to see Mr. B. because of a blister that has developed on his right great toe. The plan of care developed by the home care nurse for Mr. B. is as follows:

NURSING DIAGNOSES	NURSING INTERVENTIONS
Alteration in tissue perfusion	Assess circulation to toes, feet, and legs.
Impairment of skin integrity with potential for infection	Treat toe as ordered; ensure that client understands appropriate foot care and can perform required procedures.
Potential knowledge deficit	Reinforce knowledge of symptoms of hypoglycemia and appropriate measures to take; teach client that the ability to metabolize and excrete insulin decreases as renal function decreases and that insulin requirements may decrease; emphasize need for frequent glucose testing.
Alteration in fluid volume	Assess fluid balance by measuring weight changes, blood pressure, and presence of edema; review use of diuretics; teach client the importance of eating all the protein ordered to replace losses because these losses lead to an increase in edema.

MRS. L.

Mrs. L. is a 43-year-old mother of three who has systemic lupus erythematosus with accompanying lupus nephritis. She has been placed on hemodialysis and receives treatment three times a week at a local outpatient dialysis clinic. The home care nurse has been *asked to see this client because she recently underwent mitral valve replacement surgery and has just been discharged from the hospital. Among other things, the plan of care for Mrs. L. would include the following diagnoses and interventions:*

NURSING DIAGNOSES	NURSING INTERVENTIONS
Ineffective breathing pattern	*Assess and monitor respiratory rate and rhythm; assess for signs and symptoms of distress (chest pain, dyspnea, and decreased breath sounds); reinforce teaching for deep-breathing exercises provided in hospital; reinforce need to perform exercises frequently.*
Potential for alteration in cardiac output	*Assess heart sounds, rate, and rhythm; assess for evidence of edema and changes in fluid balance; reinforce need to maintain prescribed sodium and fluid restrictions.*
Impaired mobility	*Assess degree of limitation; encourage exercise regimen as prescribed before discharge; encourage range-of-motion exercises; encourage ambulation; use pain-relief medications before performing activity.*
Potential for ineffective coping	*Assess changes in mental status; ask client to identify benefits of surgery, complications she has experienced, or fears she has; identify assistance available from family and friends for chores and activities.*
Potential for vascular-access dysfunction	*Assess vascular access for patency; review assessment techniques of palpation and auscultation with client; teach proper action to take if access function changes or is absent.*

MS. J.

Ms. J. is a 45-year-old woman who has had a long history of bladder stones and bladder infections. She recently was hospitalized and underwent an ileal conduit *for urinary diversion secondary to ureteral scarring. Her home care nurse's plan of care includes the following:*

NURSING DIAGNOSES	NURSING INTERVENTIONS
Potential for alteration in tissue perfusion	*Assess stoma for color (should be bright red and moist); encourage client to perform leg exercises to prevent deep vein thrombosis (DVT); assess healing of incisions.*
Alteration in urinary elimination	*Evaluate stoma; ensure that client has been fitted with appropriate pouch system; teach client how to replace drainage pouch; teach client to test urine with pH paper every 3 to 5 days to ensure acidity; teach client to add vinegar (small amount) to pouch to neutralize urine odor.*
Impairment of skin integrity	*Remove appliance (bag) and inspect skin for rash, excoriation, or allergic response to face-plate; teach client to clean stoma and surrounding skin; teach client to place 4 × 4 gauze in stoma to prevent urine leakage when changing bag; teach client to use hair dryer on low setting to dry skin quickly.*
Disturbance in self-concept	*Provide opportunity for client to discuss implications of surgery; explore client's expectations of this surgery and changes in activities; discuss client's feelings of attractiveness, desirability, and worth.*

information that may assist the home care nurse in providing care for the client with renal disease.

CLIENT AND FAMILY TEACHING

An important component of nursing care of the renal client involves client and family teaching. Perhaps the simplest way to address this is to look at the various elements to be considered and some issues and information for teaching. Home care nurses may be able to reinforce teaching that

has been done elsewhere. If nurses are unsure of the information that should be taught or reinforced, they should speak with the physician, dialysis nurse, or social worker–dietitian. Dialysis units have many teaching materials—books, booklets, charts, and posters—that nurses may find useful in their own continuing education about this complex disease and its treatment. Table 24-4 reviews some of the information that is most commonly taught to clients with renal failure undergoing dialysis treatment.

Table 24-4 Teaching Guide for Clients and Families	
Element	Information and Hints
Anatomy and physiology of the kidney	Normal renal function
Kidney disease	Client's specific disease
	Symptoms of kidney malfunction
	Signs and symptoms to report to health care practitioner
Vital signs	Taking of own vital signs
	Acceptable limits for clients
	Appropriate action if vital signs are beyond established limits
	Convenience and reliability of automated equipment
Medications	Name, purpose, dose, frequency, side effects, and administration of drugs
	Appropriate action if adverse reaction occurs
	Written lists or charts for reinforcement or reference
Clinical manifestations of disease	Causes of various symptoms
	Control of symptoms
	Signs and symptoms to report to health care practitioner
Skin care	Physiological basis for interventions
	Use of creams and lotions
	Avoidance of creams and lotions (avoidance of alcohol-based creams because they are drying)
	Maintenance of good skin care
Nutrition	Proper diet as the most important medical treatment
	Potential harm of certain foods
	Use of labels to determine sodium and potassium content of foods
	Relationship between weight, fluid intake, blood pressure, and sodium intake
	Hyperglycemia and hypoglycemia
Dialysis	Goals of treament for the individual client (established collaboratively)
	Assessment of vascular access
	Care of peritoneal catheter
	Performance of dialysis procedures as appropriate
Chronicity	Importance of resuming activities of daily living if possible
	Maximal level of self-care possible
	Client's potential
	Long-term adjustments

GENITOURINARY DISORDERS

The lower urinary tract is subject to a variety of diseases and medical problems arising from urine formation, metabolic alterations, trauma, and changes in tissue integrity and function. Common problems or those requiring ongoing health care services by the home care nurse are discussed here. In addition, the home care nurse may be caring for clients who have histories of GU disorders that have been successfully treated. The client, however, may continue to experience sequelae of this treatment and require continuing treatment, education, and support.

Urinary Calculi

Stones formed in the urinary tract are known as *urinary calculi,* and they can pose considerable discomfort and severe pain. In addition, they can lead to altered function of the urinary tract (obstructions). Most stones are formed in the kidney and progress down the ureter to the bladder before they are expelled through the urethra.

Causes Causes of urinary calculi are not completely understood, but some factors are associated with their formation and incidence. For example, sedentary occupations may be associated with increased incidence. The southeastern and arid southwestern United States have a higher incidence than other areas. Abnormal metabolism of some products in foods, such as calcium (dairy products), oxalate (green, leafy vegetables), and purines (meat, fish, poultry, and organ meats), has been implicated as a causative factor in stone formation. Long-term use of calcium carbonates, vitamin D, antacids, megadoses of vitamin C, probenicid, acetazolamide, and triamterene can also lead to stone formation. Gout, resulting in the retention of uric acid (from purines), may also lead to the formation of urinary calculi in this systemic disease.

Individuals with long-term indwelling Foley catheters may tend to develop gravel or sludge that clogs the catheter, necessitating its replacement. These particles are not usually classified as stones.

Some stones form better in a certain urinary pH. Thus adjustment of the urinary pH through diet or drugs can decrease stone formation. The urine is usually acidic, with a pH of 3 to 5. Measurement of urine pH can be easily performed with dipstick testing (Fischbach, 2000; Guyton, Hall, 2000; Sherwood, 1997).

Treatment To determine the cause of stone formation, clients should save and strain all urine during an episode of passing a urinary stone. Pain during this time can be excruciating (often called *renal colic*) and may require hospitalization for pain control and for assessment of urinary tract patency. If a stone can be obtained, laboratory analysis will identify its content. If the substance (e.g., calcium or purine) can be eliminated through dietary control, the client should receive dietary instruction to prevent future stone formation. If urine pH is implicated as a cause, the diet may be altered and drugs may be administered to alter the pH appropriately; acidification is frequently accomplished through the intake of cranberry juice or administration of potassium and sodium phosphates (Neutra-Phos). If the client develops sludge from minimal urine formation and flow, increased fluid intake is indicated to flush out the urinary tract.

Stones that cannot be passed can cause urinary tract obstruction and result in altered renal function (flow of urine out of the kidney). Some stones are so large that they completely fill the renal pelvis and extend into the calyces of the kidney; traditionally, a nephrectomy was performed to remove this stone with the assumption that the kidney was no longer functional. The newer technology of lithotripsy has decreased the need for open surgical procedures for stone removal or nephrectomy. Lithotripsy uses high-intensity sound waves to shatter a large stone in the urinary tract (usually the kidney), breaking it into many very small pieces that can be expelled through the urinary tract. This noninvasive procedure has been highly successful in the treatment of kidney stones and is readily available in most communities (Tierney, McPhee, Papdakis, 1999).

Incontinence

Incontinence is the involuntary leakage of urine from the bladder through the urethra; it occurs after the age of toilet training. It occurs as a problem through the lifespan and is particularly prevalent in the elder population. There are several types of incontinence: stress, overflow, instability, urge, constant incontinence, and overactive bladder. In addition, some people may have signs and symptoms of more than one of these types of incontinence.

Stress incontinence When pressures within the bladder exceed the urethral closure pressure, urine is forced through the urethral sphincters in the absence of an appropriate detrusor-muscle contraction (as occurs in normal urination). Stress incontinence is more commonly seen in women. There are two primary causes of stress incontinence: pelvic muscle relaxation and bladder neck (internal sphincter) incompetence. Pelvic fracture, transurethral resection of the prostate in men, bladder-neck surgery in women, and multiple antiincontinence procedures are all associated with stress incontinence resulting from internal-sphincter incompetence. Obesity is also thought to play a role.

Stress incontinence is manifested by a leakage of urine with coughing, sneezing, laughing, or any maneuver that precipitates a rise in intraabdominal pressure. Urgency and nocturia usually accompany these signs. Urinary tract infection may also be a problem, especially if there is incomplete emptying of the bladder.

Nursing interventions include encouraging weight loss, teaching a series of exercises to strengthen pelvic-floor muscles (Kegel exercises), and assessing for other problems that may be repaired by surgical interventions (significant cystocele, rectocele, or uterine prolapse).

Instability incontinence Neurogenic bladder is the primary cause of instability incontinence. Cerebrovascular accidents, brain tumor, multiple sclerosis, or other neurological diseases may result in loss of normal neuronal function. Spontaneous micturition with normal sphincter responses occurs at a particular bladder volume. Cystitis can also cause instability incontinence, as can vaginitis or carcinoma of the bladder wall.

Overflow incontinence *Nurses' bladder* is so named because of the perceived inability to interrupt work for micturition. Overflow incontinence is the leakage of urine in the presence of a large residual. Many individuals with overflow incontinence are not aware of their inability to empty the bladder. Signs and symptoms associated with overflow incontinence include urgency, frequency, nocturia, and a dribbling, intermittent urine stream. Low back pain may result from bladder enlargement. Bladder outlet obstruction (a stricture in the bladder neck or urethra) may also be a cause of overflow incontinence.

Urge incontinence and overactive bladder The client feels a strong, uncontrollable urge to urinate. The bladder apparently is overly sensitive to volume, resulting in stimulation of the contractions opening the bladder neck and expelling urine if the external sphincter is weak. Overactive bladder is thought to occur in female clients after menopause as a result of weakening of the external sphincter from hormonal alterations.

Constant incontinence Constant incontinence can occur with a fistulous tract or from any mechanism in the urinary tract resulting in continuous urine leakage. Cystitis is a common occurrence. A fistula that has developed between the urethra and the vagina is an example of this problem; urine constantly flows from the vagina.

The management and treatment of incontinence are best accomplished if the client has had a complete evaluation of the urinary tract, particularly the bladder and urethral sphincter. Urologists and advanced-practice nurses have formed specialized practices for diagnosing and treating the problem of adult incontinence (particularly in women). Biofeedback and electrical stimulation may be used to stimulate pelvic floor and bladder muscle contractions and thus decrease incontinence. Surgical correction to support the bladder neck may also improve or eliminate incontinence in women. Collagen implants may be performed; collagen is placed around the urethra near the bladder neck and creates a seal that prevents urine leaking in stress incontinence.

Other industries have responded to this problem with the manufacture and sale of adult incontinence pads and underwear (adult diapers). Medications may also be prescribed to decrease overactivity of the bladder or to increase complete emptying. Bladder retraining may be successful in overcoming overactive bladder.*

Benign Prostatic Hypertrophy and Prostate Cancer

Prostate disease in men generally occurs in the second half of life. Benign prostatic hypertrophy (BPH) is the progressive enlargement of the prostate gland, causing narrowing of the urethra;

---

*AHCPR, 1992; Palmer et al, 1992; Skoner, 1994; Turner, Plymat, 1988; Wyman et al, 1993.

it is usually associated with aging and occurs in virtually all men over the age of 50. Signs of prostate enlargement include decreased force and caliber of the urinary stream, dribbling after urination, nocturia, a significant residual urine volume, and acute urinary retention leading to azotemia, and rarely, uremia.

Prostate cancer also occurs in older men (over age 50) and presents with the same signs and symptoms as BPH. The prostate-specific antigen (PSA) test is a blood test that may identify prostate cancer when there is an elevation of PSA; it is used as an initial screening test. Definitive diagnosis is made by biopsy of the prostate tissue.

BPH may be treated medically with the administration of alpha-1 blockers (e.g., terazosin [Hytrin]); these drugs, commonly used to treat hypertension, cause the prostate to contract, thus relieving the obstruction caused by the enlargement.

Both BPH and prostate cancer may be definitively treated with surgery. Transurethral resection of the prostate (TURP) is a commonly used surgical intervention for these conditions. Suprapubic or retropubic prostatectomy may also be used. These procedures may leave the client with incontinence; a suprapubic catheter may be left in place permanently after resection of the urethra. In addition, many men may have erectile dysfunction after prostatectomy as a result of nerve damage that occurs during the procedure (Bullock, Henze, 2000; Guyton, 2000; Tierney, McPhee, Papdakis, 1999).

Urinary Diversions

Several types of urinary diversions may be surgically created for the client who has obstructions in the urinary tract that cannot be resolved medically. Removing portions of the urinary tract (e.g., resecting the bladder for carcinoma) or bypassing a neurogenic bladder may require such permanent diversions.

Urinary catheterization   Foley-catheter placement may be considered as a diversion if the reason for its placement is urethral obstruction; the Foley catheter allows drainage of urine from the bladder when the urethra is obstructed or sphincter control is altered. Although it is preferable not to place a long-term Foley catheter, there are situations in which this cannot be avoided. The goals of urinary

drainage are to keep the bladder empty of urine, prevent urinary tract infection because of stagnant urine, and keep the client dry and comfortable. It is not uncommon for clients living at home to have a Foley catheter placed to meet these goals. For the male client, placement of an exdwelling (condom) catheter may meet these same goals. The client or family member requires instruction on caring for the client, the catheter, and the drainage bag. Changing an indwelling Foley catheter on a regular schedule is controversial; there are no clear data to determine if it should be done regularly or how frequently it should be done.

Intermittent self-catheterization   Intermittent self-catheterization is a clean procedure that the client performs three or four times a day. After the meatus is cleansed, a clean French catheter is inserted through the urethra into the bladder. After the bladder is emptied into the toilet or other reservoir, the catheter is removed, cleaned with soap and water, hung to dry, or placed in a small, clean container. The goals of this procedure are the same as those for a Foley catheter. Data have shown that this procedure does not increase the likelihood of urinary tract infection. It is used by many individuals with neurogenic bladders secondary to various conditions, such as spinal cord injury and spina bifida (Charbonneau-Smith, 1993; Moore et al, 1993).

Suprapubic catheters   Suprapubic catheters placed directly into the bladder also bypass the bladder neck and urethra; they are also placed as a diversion to urethral obstructions. Although these may be permanent routes, they require minimal or no surgery; reversal of their use if function is restored is through their simple removal.

Ileal conduit   An ileal conduit is constructed by taking a segment of the ileum (with intact mesentery and blood flow), suturing one end closed, and bringing the other end out through the abdominal wall to create a stoma. Both ureters are anastomosed into the ileal segment, and urine drains continuously through the stoma into an external pouch. A "continent" ileal conduit may be formed by creating a pouch that is deep enough to collect and hold urine until it is drained by a catheter placed through the stoma. This procedure may be more aesthetically pleasing and acceptable to the client who requires urinary diversion above the bladder.

Ureterostomy Occasionally a ureterostomy may be established in someone who cannot undergo an ileal conduit. This is a procedure that surgically brings the ureters to the skin surface in a stoma; the ureters drain into external pouches (urostomy bags). This procedure is less acceptable because it subjects the kidneys more directly to infection. In addition, there is a fairly high rate of stenosis in the ureters.

Nephrostomy tubes Small-gauge drainage tubes may be placed in the pelvis of the kidneys to drain urine above the level of the ureters. This procedure is used when there is bilateral involvement or constriction of the ureters. These are generally not permanent drainage systems. They may be attached to a small bag or drain onto padded dressings, which require frequent changes. These tubes place the client at high risk of infection directly into the kidney (pyelonephritis) (Turner, 1997).

SUMMARY

The urinary tract is a complex system that includes the kidneys, ureters, bladder, and urethra. Because of its life-sustaining functions, alterations in various components of this system can have a major impact on the client's well-being and on other systemic organ systems and their functions. The home care nurse who is knowledgeable about the functions, dysfunctions, and specific treatments used for the myriad diseases that may occur and the complications that may develop can provide excellent care, education, and support to the client and family in the home setting.

REFERENCES

Agency for Health Care Policy and Research (AHCPR): *Clinical practice guidelines for urinary incontinence in adults,* AHCPR Pub No 92-0038, Rockville, Md, 1992, US Department of Health and Human Services.

Albee B, Beckman NJ, Shell HM: Patients with end-stage renal disease. In Cloches JM et al, eds: *Critical Care Nursing,* ed 2, Philadelphia, 1996, WB Saunders.

Beathard GA: The treatment of vascular access dysfunction: A nephrologist's view and experience, *Advances in Renal Replacement Therapy* 1:131-147, 1994.

Brunier G: Care of the hemodialysis patient with a new permanent vascular access: Review of assessment and teaching, *ANNA Journal* 23:547-556, 1996.

Charbonneau-Smith R: No-touch catheterization and infection rates in selected spinal-cord injured population, *Rehabilitation Nursing* 18:296-299, 1993.

Daugirda JT, Ing TS, eds: *Handbook of dialysis,* ed 2, Boston, 1994, Little, Brown.

Diabetes Control and Complications Trial (DCCT) Research Group: The effect of intensive treatment of diabetes on the development and progress of long-term complications in insulin-dependent diabetes mellitus, *New England Journal of Medicine* 329(14):977-986, 1993.

Dunn SA: How to care for the dialysis patient, *American Journal of Nursing* 93(6):26-33, 1993.

Guyton AC: *Textbook of medical physiology,* ed 10, Philadelphia, 2000, WB Saunders.

Hartigan MF: Maintaining hemodialysis vascular patency, *Nephrology Nursing Today* 3:6, 1993.

Hartigan MF: Vascular access and nephrology nursing practice: Existing views and rationales for change, *Advances in Renal Replacement Therapy* 1:155-162, 1994.

Hilton B, Starzonski R: Family decision-making about living-related kidney donation, *ANNA Journal* 21:346-381, 1994.

Kaufman JL: What is the duty of the surgeon in dialysis vascular access? *Contemporary Dialysis and Nephrology* 18:18-21, 1997.

Keane WF, Eknoyan G: Proteinuria, albuminuria, risk, assessment, detection, elimination (PARADE): A position paper of the National Kidney Foundation, *American Journal of Kidney Diseases* 33:5, 1004-1010, 1999.

Lancaster L, ed: *ANNA core curriculum for nephrology nursing,* ed 3, Pitman, NJ, 1995, American Nephrology Nurses Association.

Levin NW: Session II: The impact of epoetin alfa—Quality of life and hematocrit level, *American Journal of Kidney Diseases* 20(suppl 1):16-20, 1992.

Lewis SL et al: Nursing practice related to peritoneal catheter exit site care and infections, *ANNA Journal* 23:609-617, 1996.

Lundin AP, Delano BG, Quinn-Cefaro R: Perspectives on the improvement of quality of life with epoetin alfa therapy, *Pharmacotherapy* 10:22S-26S, 1990.

Moore KM et al: Bacteria in intermittent catheterization users: The effects of sterile versus clean reused catheters, *Rehabilitation Nursing* 18:306-309, 1993.

National Kidney Foundation: *Initiation or withdrawal of dialysis in end-stage renal disease: Guidelines for the health care team,* New York, 1996, The Foundation.

Northsea CL: Continuous quality improvement: Improving catheter patency using urokinase, *ANNA Journal* 23:567-571, 1996.

Ouwendyk M, Helferty M: Central venous catheter management: How to prevent the complications, *ANNA Journal* 23:572-583, 1996.

Palmer MH et al: Detecting urinary incontinence in older adults during hospitalization, *Applied Nursing Research* 5:174-180, 1992.

Payne JL: Immune modification and complications of immunosuppression, *Critical Care Nursing Clinics of North America* 4:43-61, 1992.

Pfettscher SA: Chronic renal failure and renal transplantation. In Bucher L, Melander S, eds: *Critical Care Nursing,* Philadelphia, 1999, WB Saunders.

Sherwood L: *Human physiology: From cells to systems,* Belmont, Calif, 1997, Wadsworth.

Skoner M: Self-management of urinary incontinence among women 31-50 years of age, *Rehabilitation Nursing* 19:339-343, 1994.

Sosa-Guerro S, Gomez NJ: Dealing with end-stage renal disease, *American Journal of Nursing* 97(10):44-50, 1997.

Stark J, Melander S: Acute renal failure. In Bucher L, Melander S, eds: *Critical care nursing,* Philadelphia, 1999, WB Saunders.

Tierney LM, McPhee SJ, Papdakis MA: *Current medical diagnosis and treatment,* Stamford, Conn, 1999, Appleton & Lange.

Turner S, Plymat K: As women age: Perspectives on urinary incontinence, *Rehabilitation Nursing* 13:132-135, 1988.

Vaughn G: *Understanding and evaluating common laboratory tests,* Stamford, Conn, 1999, Appleton & Lange.

Wyman JF et al: Influence of functional, urological, and environmental characteristics on urinary incontinence in community-dwelling older adults, *Nursing Research* 42:270-275, 1993.

Young LY, Koda-Kimble MA, eds: *Applied therapeutics—The critical use of drugs,* Vancouver, Wash, 1995, Applied Therapeutics.

25 HIV/AIDS and the Home Care Client

Helen Miramontes and Brian K. Goodroad

In 1981, a southern California physician reported four cases of *Pneumocystis carinii* pneumonia (PCP) to the Centers for Disease Control (CDC) (now the Centers for Disease Control and Prevention) in four gay, white men with severely compromised immune systems. Soon the disease became known as acquired immunodeficiency syndrome (AIDS), manifested by severe infections with numerous opportunistic diseases, PCP being one of the major infections. The etiological agent, the human immunodeficiency virus (HIV), was finally identified in late 1983 in France and in early 1984 in the United States (Shilts, 1987).

Since that time, HIV has been identified throughout the world. In December 2001, the World Health Organization (WHO) and the United Nations AIDS (UNAIDS) Program announced that 40 million people were living with AIDS worldwide, that more than 20 million people had died from AIDS, and that 2.6 million deaths occurred in 1999 alone. Approximately 5 million people were newly infected in 2001 (13,699 per day); 8.2 million children had become AIDS orphans since the beginning of the epidemic; and in North America, 9,200,000 people were living with HIV or AIDS in 1999. About one third of those currently living with HIV and AIDS are between the ages of 15 and 24 (UNAIDS, 2001). Most of them do not know they carry the virus.

In the United States, new HIV infections continue to spread unchecked (Weiss, 1998), even though the progression to AIDS has slowed and the death rate from AIDS has dropped by 21% as a result of more intensive antiretroviral therapies (Palella et al, 1998). In spite of the media attention predicting a potential end to the epidemic, or at least control of the current epidemic, no one has yet been cured of AIDS. In addition, some people are experiencing failure of the complex HIV treatment regimens (Perlman, 1997; Schoofs, 1996). More recent data indicate that the rapid decline in AIDS deaths observed in the United States during 1997 and 1998 is beginning to level off. This leveling suggests that perhaps the peak benefit of the new HIV treatments has been reached (Centers for Disease Control and Prevention [CDC], 1999).

Given these facts, it remains clear that people will continue to need care and treatment, including home care for those individuals at later stages of HIV disease. Researchers, in a study cited in the Agency for Health Care Policy and Research (AHCPR) newsletter (1997), interviewed 1,727 HIV-infected adults over a 12-month period and found that 39% of persons with AIDS (PWAs) received formal home care and 38% received informal care from family and friends. The need for services was related to increased levels of physical impairment, levels of fatigue, and prior hospitalizations.

The care and treatment regimens needed by PWAs are often complex and frustrating. The complexity of medication regimens renders them especially difficult for many clients to manage and presents major challenges for the home care nurse. Strategies to enhance clients' adherence to a regimen must be designed to meet the needs of the individual client and are based on the skills and the expertise of the nurse to engage the client in a shared decision-making process. The purpose of this chapter is to provide a brief overview of HIV disease and its associated manifestations. The pathogenesis of HIV is reviewed, and disease effects on the immune system are presented. Common infections and malignancies affecting those with HIV are described and the treatments for these maladies are reviewed. A comprehensive assessment of clients in the home care setting is reviewed and care-planning suggestions are provided. The special focus of the chapter is meant to acquaint the professional home care nurse with the dimensions of adherence and the significant role of the nurse in facilitating clients' abilities to manage these complex regimens.

PATHOGENESIS OF HIV

To understand the complexity of HIV disease management, it is essential to comprehend the pathogenesis of HIV. Knowledge about the pathogenesis of HIV has significantly changed during the past several years. The assumption had been that viral replication latency paralleled clinical latency, but since the definitive research of David Ho, M.D. (1995), it is known that viral replication is continuous from the moment of infection, even though clinical manifestations of infection may not be apparent. In fact, even during early stages of infection, HIV is replicating at astronomical rates of 5 to 10 billion virions per day.

HIV is classified as a retrovirus. This means that instead of deoxyribonucleic acid (DNA) as the gene codes, HIV has ribonucleic acid (RNA) in its core. The method by which HIV enters the host immune cells and replicates uses a cellular enzyme called *reverse transcriptase (RT)*. This enzyme helps to synthesize HIV RNA into HIV DNA. The class of antiretroviral drugs known as *reverse transcriptase inhibitors* works by inhibiting this particular phase of viral replication. Once the viral RNA has been turned into DNA, another cellular enzyme known as *integrase* helps to integrate viral DNA into the host immune cells. Once infected, the host cells become viral factories that produce large amounts of new HIV. A final cellular protein called *protease* is used in the assembly and cleaving of these new virions. Protease inhibitors work by preventing successful assembly of new HIV (Flaskerud, Ungvarski, 1999).

The cells of the immune system most affected by HIV are the CD4 T-helper cells. These cells act as the "conductor" of the human immune system in that they direct all types of immune responses. Once infected, these cells can no longer carry out their conductor function and begin to replicate new HIV. The immune system mounts an aggressive response to HIV infection, producing millions of CD4 cells and antibodies to combat the viral infection. The immune system is often able to maintain this response, which is approximately equitable to the viral clearance rate, for long periods of time (Phair, Murphy, 1997). However, over time the immune system is typically overwhelmed by HIV, manifested by lower numbers of CD4 cells and higher measures of virus in the blood. No longer able to fight off infections, the person with HIV is vulnerable to illnesses that a competent immune system would normally keep at bay. These bacteria, fungi, viruses, and other infections take the opportunity of a dysfunctional immune system to cause acute illness in the person with HIV. As a result, to monitor a person with HIV, health care providers will order CD4 cell counts. This simple blood test is a measure of an individual's immune-system function. In addition, the amount of HIV circulating in the bloodstream will be measured through complex techniques called *polymerase chain reaction (PCR)* or *branched-chain DNA (bDNA)*. More commonly, these tests are just called *viral load measurements*. Together, the quantitative CD4 count and the viral load indicate how immunocompromised an HIV-infected person is and how actively the virus is replicating. Medications to fight HIV and its associated infections are initiated and changed based on careful assessment of these laboratory findings and the client's clinical signs and symptoms.

HIV infection is differentiated into three stages. The first stage is the primary acute infection stage, lasting 2 to 12 weeks. The second stage is the clinical latency period, lasting 1 to 20 years (usually about 10 years). The third stage is the clinical symptomatic period, usually referred to as *AIDS,* and lasting a few months to 5 years or longer (Phair, Murphy, 1997).

Primary infection typically occurs 2 to 4 weeks after exposure to HIV, although incubation periods of 6 days to 6 weeks are not uncommon (Carr, Cooper, 1999). During the initial or acute stage, viral replication is rapid, and viral load, if measured in the blood, is high. The virus infects CD4 cells of the central nervous system, bone marrow, and lymphoid tissue (Casey, Cohen, Hughes, 1996). The client may experience flulike symptoms, such as fever, malaise, and lymphadenopathy; some individuals may develop a rash. During this acute stage, cellular and humoral responses are mounted by the individual's immune system, and symptoms disappear and viral load drops (Casey, Cohen, Hughes,

1996; Phair, Murphy, 1997). Data suggest that a lower set-point of viral load after primary infection indicates a better prognosis and less chance for rapid disease progression (Carr, Cooper, 1999). During this stage, the screening test used for HIV testing, called the *enzyme linked immunosorbent assay (ELISA)*, would most likely be negative, even though the person is infected and can transmit the virus. The ELISA is a test for HIV antibodies, which in this stage have not yet been produced by the immune system. This period is often called the *window period.*

The next stage is the clinical latency stage, often referred to as an *asymptomatic period.* During this stage, rapid viral replication continues, primarily in lymphoid tissue, and stimulates the immune system's response, maintaining a steady-state of viral clearance while HIV continues to spread to susceptible cells. It is estimated that productively infected cells have an average life span of 2 days, but billions of virions are produced each day. Approximately 99% of the viral production is located in the active CD4 cells, with the remaining 1% located in the macrophages and inactive CD4 cells. Approximately 30% of the virions and 5% of the CD4 cells are replaced each day. Reverse transcriptase is an error-prone enzyme, and with rapid viral production, viral mutations occur quickly. These viral mutations are likely to confer resistance to HIV medications, which has significant implications for treatment (Phair, Murphy, 1997). Phenotypic and genotypic testing of viral mutations is now being used in care. These tests are measures of mutations in the viral genome, which may indicate the development of resistance to HIV medications. The predictive validity of these measures is not yet understood, and clinical outcomes related to viral mutations have not been established. However, as these tests become readily available, they will be powerful tools to assist with antiretroviral-medication management.

The third stage is the symptomatic stage with mild to severe symptomatology. This is the stage most likely to be seen in the home care setting. Manifestations of numerous opportunistic infections (OIs) occur during this phase and are related to the severely compromised immune system. OIs may occur as viral, bacterial, protozoal, and fungal infections; as neoplastic processes; as neuropsychiatric disorders; as hematological abnormalities;

and as wasting syndrome (Casey, Cohen, Hughes, 1996). An individual's CD4 count is a reliable indicator for assessing the risk for developing OIs. Typically, candidiasis and tuberculosis occur with CD4 count between 250 and 500/mm³; Kaposi's sarcoma, lymphoma, and cryptosporidiosis with CD4 count between 150 and 200/mm³; PCP, *Mycobacterium avium* complex (MAC), toxoplasmosis, cryptococcosis, and esophageal candidiasis with 75 to 125/mm³; and cytomegalovirus (CMV) retinitis with CD4 <50/mm³ (Kocurek, Hollander, 1999). These OIs are frequently intractable and difficult to treat; medications are usually prescribed prophylactically for many of the OIs. Death associated with AIDS usually occurs from one of the OIs.

MEDICATION TREATMENTS
Antiretroviral Medications

Zidovudine (ZDV, formerly AZT) was the first antiretroviral drug approved by the Food and Drug Administration (FDA) in 1987, for the treatment of HIV infection. ZDV is one of the nucleoside analogue reverse transcriptase inhibitors (NRTIs), a category of drugs in which the mode of action is inhibition of the synthesis of reverse transcriptase, an enzyme required by HIV to synthesize its DNA (Folks, Hart, 1997). Currently there are five approved drugs in this category, with seven used in some combination (Wolbach et al, 2001).

Another category of antiretrovirals is the non-nucleoside reverse transcriptase inhibitors (NNRTIs). These drugs differ from nucleoside reverse transcriptase inhibitors in that they do not require intracellular phosphorylation to an active metabolite. However, this class of drugs has an inhibitory effect on HIV that occurs in a very similar manner as NRTIs. There are currently three approved drugs in this category. A common side effect of this entire class is rash.

A third category of current antiretrovirals is the protease inhibitors (PIs). Protease is another enzyme essential to HTV replication (Phair, Murphy, 1997). Specifically, protease is necessary to assemble the new virions correctly. When this enzyme is inhibited, the infected CD4 cells assemble new virions, but they lack the ability to infect other cells. There are six approved drugs in this category. Besides the side-effect profile of each drug individually, drugs in this class have been associated with hyperglycemia.

Antiretroviral Drugs in Development

In addition to the development of new drugs in the aforementioned categories, clinical trials are underway on a class of antiretrovirals known as *integrase inhibitors*. This class of drug, if proven beneficial, will attack HIV replication in a portion of the replication cycle not yet affected by currently available treatments. Also, a number of medications called *fusion inhibitors* are being studied. These drugs inhibit the attachment of HIV to healthy CD4 cells. Together with current treatments, these new classes of antiretrovirals may offer significant improvement in the control or eventual elimination of HIV.

Antiretrovirals and the P-450 System

The cytochrome P-450 (CYP) monooxygenases are a system of 30 enzymes located in the hepatocytes (liver) that metabolize many drugs, as well as some food and hormones. Knowledge of the CYP enzymes is essential to the HIV clinician because this enzyme system can either be sped up (induced) or slowed down (inhibited) by exposure to antiretrovirals, many of the other medications used to treat HIV-related OIs, antibiotics, and certain chemicals in food. Drug-drug interactions may cause severe problems, including side effects or the rendering ineffective of antiretroviral therapy. It is essential that the home care nurse assess the client for use of any complementary therapies, nutritional supplements, recreational drugs, or medications provided by a prescriber other than the HIV care provider and relate this information to the prescribing provider.

Antiretrovirals, Diabetes, and Lipodystrophy

Since the advent of multiple–antiretroviral-drug cocktails, an interesting and difficult to manage syndrome has occurred for many people on multiple medications. This syndrome includes several metabolic complications, including effects on carbohydrate tolerance (high fasting glucose and insulin levels and onset or exacerbation of existing diabetes) and plasma lipid levels (increase in serum cholesterol and triglyceride levels). In addition, changes in distribution of body fat have been described. These fat distribution level changes include (1) increase in abdominal girth, (2) increase in breast size (in women), (3) accumulation of dorsocervical fat tissue (buffalo hump), and (4) loss of facial and limb fat tissue. The causes of these changes are not yet understood but are thought to be multisystem in nature. Treatment has included lipid-lowering agents, diet, exercise, and in some cases, surgery to remove fat or improve facial wasting symptoms (da Silva, Lowe, 1999). Some people with HIV have been so bothered by these symptoms that they have discontinued HIV treatment. In addition, early onset cardiac disease, including myocardial infarction, has been associated with these problems. Further understanding of the pathogenesis of this syndrome and potential treatments are urgently needed.

These categories of antiretrovirals, in various combinations, are prescribed to aggressively treat clients with HIV disease. These regimens are called *highly active antiretroviral therapy (HAART)*. The regimens are complex, difficult to take, have significant side effects, and require daily ingestion of many pills. Dosage varies; some require food to be taken with the pills, and some pills should not be taken with food. Considering that these clients are usually on prophylactic drugs to prevent the numerous OIs also, the number of pills that a client is required to take daily may vary from 20 to 40 or more pills per day. It is obvious that maintaining this complex regimen may prove very difficult for the client and require intensive nursing intervention to facilitate the process. (See Appendix A for the list of current antiretroviral medications.)

Medications for the Treatment and Prophylaxis of OIs

Some of the common OIs are PCP, CMV infections, toxoplasmosis, disseminated MAC, candidiasis, cryptococcosis, cryptosporidiosis, herpes, tuberculosis, skin infections, bacterial pneumonias, gastroenteritis infections, cognitive and organic disorders, and neoplasms. Some OIs are treated prophylactically, such as PCP, MAC, candidiasis, and herpes; others may be treated when diagnosed (Phair, Murphy, 1997). (See Appendix B for specific medications to treat some of the common OIs.)

Guidelines for Treatment

The *Guidelines for the Use of Antiretroviral Agents in HIV-Infected Adults and Adolescents* (Department of Health and Human Services [DHHS],

Kaiser, 2001) was released by the Department of Health and Human Services and the Henry J. Kaiser Family Foundation. These guidelines and principles of therapy were developed by 2 expert panels convened by the National Institutes of Health (NIH). These guidelines are now available on the web. Access information and a brief synopsis of the guidelines are provided in Appendix C.

HOME HEALTH CARE NURSING ASSESSMENT OF PEOPLE WITH HIV AND AIDS

With the advent of HAART, the severity of illness and frequency of end-stage infections have decreased. Thus a significant decrease in the number of people with AIDS seeking home care has also occurred. Some experts believe that this is a short-lived reprieve before wide-scale failure of HAART for many people (Deeks, 1999). Nonetheless, many people with HIV and AIDS still require home nursing skills. Home care for people with HIV and AIDS is most likely to be undertaken during later stages of the disease. Care may focus on the treatment of an OI and teaching of the client regarding infection prevention, activities of daily living, or medication regimen. Whatever the focus of care, a comprehensive assessment is the first necessary element of developing the home care plan. The collection of baseline data provides the framework on which the home care nurse structures the plan of care. Assessment should be an interaction with the client, significant other, family members, and service providers. This is a time to introduce the role of the home care nurse, establish relationships with all care providers, and develop goals for care. A comprehensive assessment should include, but is not limited to, the following:

1. Complete history and physical examination:
   a. Medical history (HIV-specific and general history)
   b. Date of HIV infection, recent CD4 count, viral load, and any other recent laboratory test results
   c. History of sexually transmitted diseases (STDs), including herpes and genital and anal warts
   d. Any OIs and their treatment (method and duration)
   e. Surgeries, injuries, hospitalizations, travel history, place of birth, and immunization history
   f. Use of long-term care facility, rehabilitative and support personnel, and home care services
   g. Lifestyle patterns
   h. Current prescriptions, over-the-counter medications, nutritional supplements, and complementary therapies
   i. Prescription adherence
   j. Ongoing clinical needs (e.g., intravenous infusions or tube feeding)
2. Complete psychosocial history
   a. Previous psychiatric condition, treatments, and therapists
   b. Current psychiatric medications
   c. Use of alcohol and recreational drugs
   d. Relationships with family members and significant others
   e. Use of support systems or community resources
   f. Use of psychological testing (if depression, HIV-related cognitive changes, or both are suspected)
3. Assessment of home and community environment
4. Functional status of the client
5. Economic assessment
6. Nutritional assessment
7. Legal issues, including advance directives

CARE PLANNING

The cardinal rule in developing the care plan is that the client and significant others must actively participate in its development. Goals must be mutually agreed on and attainable. The plan of care should include measurable objectives, types of services required, responsible parties (provider, agency, client, family, or other), and a time frame. Ongoing monitoring and evaluation of the plan of care are essential.

ADHERENCE ISSUES ASSOCIATED WITH HAART
Definition

Adherence is a recently identified term that is being used to construct an understanding of the domains and dimensions of behaviors and activities essential in the management of the current multidrug regimens for the treatment of HIV disease. The previously used term was *compliance*. According to Bradley-Springer (1998), the term *compliance* denotes "a paternalistic ethic of a client's requirement to yield to the will of the provider," and that *adherence* "implies consistency and a steady propensity to stick to a prescribed regimen." Chesney (1997) defined *adherence outcomes* as not only taking medications as prescribed, but also remaining in treatment and keeping appointments. Frank and Miramontes (1999) considered the various definitions of *compliance* and *adherence* and attempted to frame adherence within a conceptual context of the partnership between the client and provider and the shared decision-making process that occurs in the relationship. It has become obvious that the conceptual framework of adherence is evolving and will continue to evolve as more providers attempt to facilitate clients' ability to manage these complex regimens.

Background and Historical Perspective

Noncompliance or nonadherence has been a problem for a long time. Sackett and Snow's study (Steels, Jackson, Gutmann, 1990) estimated that 20% to 80% of clients fail to follow treatment recommendations, and DiMatteo et al (1993) stated that 30% to 60% of clients failed to take their medications. A review of the literature on medication treatments for other diseases identified that clients have had difficulty managing regimens that involved fewer medications and simpler regimens. These diseases include hypertension (Caldwell et al, 1983), insulin-dependent diabetes mellitus (Burroughs, Pontious, Santiago, 1993), and asthma (Brooks et al, 1994). Chow et al (1993) found that before the advent of PIs in treatment of HIV disease, clients on antiretroviral drugs omitted over 70% of their medication doses. Before the addition of PIs to the recommended regimens, clients may have been taking two antiretroviral drugs plus prophylactic medications to prevent OIs. Currently the recommendations are that client regimens include at least three drugs (two antiretrovirals that inhibit reverse transcriptase and one PI) (Goldschmidt et al, 1998; Appendix C). Some clients may be taking four or more antiretroviral drugs, two transcriptase inhibitors, and two PIs, in addition to their prophylactic medications to prevent OIs. The complexity of these regimens continues to grow with no end in sight, exacerbating the difficulty for clients to manage their medications.

Scientific Rationale for Maintaining Adherence to Medication Regimens

Data from seminal research in the pathogenesis of HIV show that HIV replicates rapidly and mutates frequently with a rapid turnover of plasma virions (Ho et al, 1995). The frequent mutation potentiates the development of drug-resistant strains of the virus, particularly if clients are not taking their antiretroviral drugs at the optimal doses, at the recommended frequency, and in the prescribed method. Resistance to the current regimen may occur quickly, and cross-resistance to other medications in the same classification may develop (Bartlett, 1998). Recent studies have found that even in clients on HAART, replication-competent virus had been recovered despite prolonged suppression with drugs (Finzi et al, 1997; Wong et al, 1997), which supports the need to continue adherent practices to HAART. The critical threshold of drug taking that is required to maintain effectiveness and prevent treatment failure is not known, so the recommendation at this time is that all antiretroviral medications be taken exactly as prescribed, 100% of the time, without missed doses or drug holidays.

Factors Influencing Adherence

The factors that impact and influence a person's ability to adhere to these complex regimens are multidimensional and can be identified within the context of a person's life (Crespo-Fierro, 1997). Chesney (1997) has identified five domains of influence: client characteristics, characteristics of the regimen, the client-provider relationship, the clinic setting, and the characteristics of HIV disease. Client characteristics include sociodemographics and psychosocial factors.

A client's cultural framework may have a significant impact on his or her ability or desire to take medications. Cultural values about health beliefs and practices, illness beliefs, symptom management, and care-seeking behavior can determine whether or not a client with HIV or AIDS is willing or able to adhere to these regimens (Lipson, Dibble, Minarik, 1996). A client's younger age may affect his or her ability to perceive the importance of maintaining the drug regimen; undeveloped coping skills may not allow a client to deal with the realities of a complex drug regimen associated with a life-threatening illness (Chesney, 1997). Lack of sufficient income or health insurance may also influence adherence. Homelessness or unstable housing can also set up barriers to appropriate storage of medications and impact maintenance of drug regimens.

Substance abuse may interfere with the person's ability to make decisions about care and treatment, yet not all substance users are nonadherent. Assuming lack of commitment to maintaining the medication regimen simply because the client is an active drug user is not supportive and often inaccurate. Depression and stress are also correlates of nonadherence influencing a person's desire to adhere and contribute to the delay to seek care and treatment. Social support or lack of social support is a significant factor in a client's ability and intent to adhere to a medication regimen. Family structure and dynamics and beliefs about sexuality all impact the social structure and support (Chesney, 1997; Chesney, Folkman, 1994; Crespo-Fierro, 1997; Lipson, Dibble, Minarik, 1996).

Knowledge about the regimen, the perceived cost and benefits of the medications, and adherence to the regimen are major factors that are not always explored with the client. To continue to maintain adherence, the client must believe that the benefits of the drugs outweigh the problems associated with taking the drugs. Most of these antiretroviral medications have significant side effects that may interfere with the lifestyle of the client. Aspects of the disease process also influence the client's commitment to a complex drug regimen. Symptoms from taking the drugs, manifestations of OIs, or the status of the client's immune system may interfere with the desire to continue these regimens. Competing activities are also a major barrier. Clients may become busy and forget to take their drugs, or the complexity and duration of the regimen proves to be too much of a burden (Chesney, 1997).

Studies have demonstrated that the client-provider relationship is a major factor in the client's adherence to both medication regimens and staying in treatment (Chesney, 1997). A supportive, empathetic provider with HIV and AIDS expertise and good communication skills increases a client's satisfaction with his or her care and facilitates appropriate medication-taking behavior. Clinic settings that are conducive to confidentiality, flexible scheduling, and childcare and are easily accessed by various modes of transportation also facilitate better adherence to

treatment and care and enhance the client's satisfaction with the provider and the setting. The complexity of the issues that impact the client's medication-adherent behavior requires that providers conduct appropriate and comprehensive assessment of all those influential factors.

Strategies for Home Care Nurses to Facilitate Adherence

The overall goal of initiating adherence interventions by the home care nurse is to facilitate the client's skills and behaviors in fitting these very complex medication regimens into his or her life. Working with the client to identify the potential barriers to success in this activity is essential. Comprehensive assessment in a shared process by the client and the nurse is the first phase of this process. Stressing the need to fit these regimens into the client's life rather than fitting his or her life around the regimen is a primary component of this process. Adherence is a skill to be learned, and similar to any behavioral change, it is a gradual process and influenced by multiple factors as discussed previously. The nurse's support and skill in guiding and facilitating the client's examination of his or her readiness for treatment and supporting the client's decision about treatment are vital to the success of any intervention focusing on adherence. Identifying the necessary resources is part of the assessment process once the client has decided to begin drug therapy. The nurse has the skill and expertise to identify strategies aimed at initiating and maintaining optimal adherence.

Strategies include ensuring that the client has the knowledge and understanding about the prescribed medications, including the scheduling and special conditions of the regimen. Another strategy is teaching the client the importance of adhering to the drug regimen. Assisting the client to identify reminders that will facilitate pill taking and providing tools, such as pillboxes, charts, clocks, and alarms, that will assist tracking these difficult regimens, are part of the nurse's role in providing appropriate intervention. It is important that the client understand the need to develop a routine that fits into his or her life so that medications can be taken on an established schedule and so that advanced plans can be made for potential changes in routine. Holidays, weekends, and trips away from home can be potentially major deterrents to adherence. Some clients may want to keep medication diaries; others may benefit from having family members, partners, or friends provide reminders to follow their schedules. Strategies must be individualized based on the ongoing assessment process of the nurse and the client. Routine follow-up enhances the support needed to maintain the regimen and will also alert the nurse to early signs of treat-ment fatigue, depression, stress, or other factors that may impede adherence.

SUMMARY

Advances in HIV treatment have enhanced the quality of life for people with AIDS. These advances have reduced the number of life-threatening infections suffered by PWAs. This improvement

---

CASE STUDY

Michael is a 35-year-old African-American man referred to a home health care agency by his nurse practitioner. Orders include starting induction therapy for CMV retinitis with ganciclovir 5 mg/kg twice daily for 21 days, followed by maintenance therapy of 5 mg/kg daily. Orders also include placing a peripherally inserted central catheter (PICC line) for IV infusions. Mary, the nurse assigned to Michael, calls to set up an appointment for that day since she knows that CMV retinitis therapy should be started as soon as possible. Michael is only available at 8 o'clock that evening, and luckily Mary is able to meet this requirement , since the agency has evening hours available. Since Mary is certified to insert the PICC line, she gathers the required supplies, orders the medication (which she will pick up on the way) from the pharmacy, and orders the x-ray van for catheter placement check for 9 PM at Michael's address. Finally, Mary gathers the intake paperwork needed to initiate care for Michael and sets out on her afternoon rounds.

Mary reaches Michael's home at 8 PM, and he is there to meet her. To get the infusion going, Mary completes a quick initial assessment, places the PICC line, confirms placement with the x-ray, and starts the first ganciclovir infusion by 9 PM. While the infusion is running, Mary sits down to do the intake interview. She soon learns that Michael is not happy to be doing these infusions and states that he does not think he will take his recently prescribed antiretroviral medications. As a diligent home care nurse, Mary begins a comprehensive history and soon finds out that Michael moved to town only 3 months earlier. He does have a sister in the area; however, she is actively using drugs and is unreliable. Michael relocated for a job that has kept him very busy—too busy, in fact, to develop any friendships. He is not really interested in developing a support network in this city, since he plans to be here only 3 months more before returning to his hometown.

Mary discovers that Michael was diagnosed with HIV only 2 weeks ago. He had suspected he was posi-tive because he had been experiencing significant fatigue over the last year and had unintentionally lost 20 lb. He believes himself to have been positive for at least 10 years. His CD4 count is 9/mm³, and his viral load is over 1 million copies/ml. Michael was prescribed a triple antiretroviral regimen, but he is leery of starting and has not yet done so. He states that his nurse practitioner (NP) talked a long time with him regarding HIV and the importance of treatment, but that it was too much information at one time and he actually remembered little of what he was told. He does have some written information provided by the NP.

Michael's NP sent him for a baseline eye examination, from which the CMV retinitis was diagnosed and the plan for ganciclovir initiated. Michael has private insurance through his job and has not experienced any problems with coverage. He is sexually active with men only and reports only safer sex for the past 5 years. He lives in a small, one-bedroom apartment in a safe part of town. He is willing to learn self-infusion over time but is not willing to interrupt his work schedule for his infusions.

As an astute home care nurse, Mary realizes that for Michael, the process of learning to do his infusions, learning about his disease, and beginning his antiretroviral medications will take some time. Mary knows the importance of making the regimen fit into Michael's schedule to increase his acceptance of treatment and improve adherence. As a result, she plans to return tomorrow before Michael's departure for work at 10 AM to teach him about his infusion and draw the required blood for the biweekly complete blood counts necessary during induction of ganciclovir therapy. As she disconnects the infusion, Mary takes the time to run through PICC line–site care and asks appropriate questions to ensure Michael understands her teaching. Mary completes this visit with a physical examination, which reveals no abnormalities.

The next morning, Michael is happy that Mary has returned and she begins to feel a sense of trust developing in the relationship. Michael states that he had no problems with the PICC line during the night.

Continued

CASE STUDY—cont'd

Mary begins by teaching Michael the proper technique to assess the catheter site and change the dressing. She demonstrates how to set up the 1-hour infusion of the ganciclovir and how to check that the medication is the correct dosage. Michael is able to return a demonstration of the infusion process and assures Mary that he will call the on-call nurse if he experiences any difficulty with his evening infusion dose. Mary draws the required blood and plans to return in 2 days to draw the ongoing blood samples. In addition, Mary will begin her plan of care regarding Michael's other needs.

In this case, the home care nurse correctly assessed that Michael was not yet ready to discuss the possibility of starting the antiretroviral medication. She prioritized the current need of getting the ganciclovir treatment underway and teaching Michael to manage his infusions on his own. Mary's positive reinforcement of his abilities to manage his infusion provided Michael a belief that he could manage all the life changes required by his diagnoses. Mary knows that it is never an "emergency" to begin antiretroviral therapy but that untreated CMV retinitis may rapidly lead to blindness

if not immediately treated. However, she knew she would be visiting twice weekly to begin the longer process of adherence management with Michael and to deal with his social isolation issues and lack of support network.

Over the next 2 weeks, Mary provides Michael with the information he needs to believe that antiretroviral therapy is important for him. She also provides a pillbox and helps Michael set up his medications for 1 week. This pillbox includes the medications he was prescribed for MAC prophylaxis. Mary knows that her biweekly visits will provide the perfect opportunity for ongoing adherence counseling now that Michael is going to undertake antiretroviral therapy. In addition, Mary is successful in engaging Michael to use community resources and join a support group that decreases his social isolation. At first reticent to develop friendships, Michael soon begins to socialize with friends from the group and develop a supportive network. This network assists with Michael's adjustment to his treatment requirements and is instrumental in his decision to stay in the area and work for the company permanently.

---

in health has been evidenced by drastic decreases in the use of home care services by PWAs in the past several years. However, this may be a temporary respite in the onslaught of opportunistic disease. Complex medication regimens are beginning to fail at an alarming rate. Unfortunately, incidence of new opportunistic disease could once again rise and require significant home nursing intervention. In addition, other people with HIV for whom treatments are not successful will usually require home health care some time during the course of their disease. The needs of clients with AIDS requiring home health care services are often complex and multidimensional. It is essential that professional home care nurses are prepared with the required current information and skills to comprehensively assess the needs of HIV home care clients and provide necessary services to meet those needs.

In addition, although these advances have enhanced the quality of life for PWAs, an overriding concern has been the potential for resistance to these drugs to develop as a result of nonadherence in taking the medications. Adherence is really a nursing issue, and the home care nurse is in an ideal position to facilitate successful initia-

tion and maintenance of these complex regimens. Establishing and maintaining supportive relationships, providing ongoing assessment and follow-up, and individualizing strategies to enhance the client's adherence behaviors are skills well integrated into the role of the home care nurse. Perhaps a new role for home health care nursing for people with HIV will be medication-adherence management. Nursing skills and expertise are essential if nurses are to achieve success in facilitating clients' abilities to manage their medication regimens.

REFERENCES

Agency for Health Care Policy and Research (AHCPR): Use of formal home care is concentrated at later stages of HIV infection, *Online Publication of AHCPR* (on-line) 208:8-9, 1997, http://www.ahcpr.gov/.

Bartlett JG: *Medical management of HIV infection*, Baltimore, 1998, Port City Press.

Bradley-Springer L: Adherence: Not a new problem, *AIDS Newslink* 1-5, Winter 1998.

Brooks CM et al: Assessing adherence to asthma medication and inhaler regimens: A psychometric analysis of adult self-report scales, *Medical Care* 32(3):298-307, 1994.

Burroughs TE, Pontious SL, Santiago JV: The relationship among six psychosocial domains, age, health care adherence, and metabolic control in adolescents with IDDM, *The Diabetes Educator* 19(5):396-402, 1993.

Caldwell JR et al: Psychosocial factors influence control of moderate and severe hypertension, *Social Science Medicine* 17(12):773-782, 1983.

Carr A, Cooper DA: Primary HIV infection. In Sande MA, Volberding PA, eds: *The medical management of AIDS,* ed 6, Philadelphia, 1999, WB Saunders.

Casey KM, Cohen F, Hughes A, eds: *ANAC's core curriculum for HIV/AIDS nursing,* Philadelphia, 1996, Nursecom.

Centers for Disease Control and Prevention (CDC): *HIV/AIDS Surveillance Report* 11(1):1999.

Chesney MA: *New antiretroviral therapies: Adherence challenge and strategies,* Paper presented at the meeting of The International Center for HIV/AIDS Research and Clinical Training in Nursing, San Francisco, 1997.

Chesney MA, Folkman S: Psychological impact of HIV disease and implications for intervention, *Psychiatric Clinics of North America* 17(1):163-182, 1994.

Chow R et al: Medication use patterns in HIV-positive patients, *The Canadian Journal of Hospital Pharmacy* 46(4):171-175, 1993.

Crespo-Fierro M: Compliance/adherence and care management in HIV disease, *Journal of the Association of Nurses in AIDS Care* 8(4):43-54, 1997.

daSilva BA, Lowe WL: Metabolic complications associated with antiretroviral therapy of HIV, *Northwestern University Reports on HIV/AIDS* 3(1):1-12, 1999.

Deeks S: Managing ARV resistance-options for salvage therapy. In Sande MA, chair: *The medical management of AIDS: A comprehensive review of HIV management,* Symposium presented at conference, San Francisco, December 1999.

Department of Health and Human Services (DHHS), Kaiser Family Foundation: Panel on clinical practices for the treatment of HIV infection, 2001, (on-line) http://www.hivatis.org. Also available at 1-800-448-0440.

DiMatteo MR et al: Physicians' characteristics influence patients' adherence to medical treatment: Results from the medical outcomes study, *Health Psychology* 12(2):93-102, 1993.

Finzi D et al: Identification of a reservoir for HIV-1 in patients on highly active antiretroviral therapy, *Science* 278:1295-1300, 1997.

Flaskerud JH, Ungvarski PJ: Overview and update of HIV disease. In Ungvarski PJ, Flaskerud JH, eds: *HIV/AIDS: A guide to primary care management,* ed 4, Philadelphia, 1999, WB Saunders.

Folks TM, Hart CE: The life cycle of human immunodeficiency virus type 1. In DeVita VT, Hellman S, Rosenberg SA, eds: *AIDS: Etiology, diagnosis, treatment and prevention,* Philadelphia, 1997, Lippincott-Raven.

Frank L, Miramontes HM: *Health care provider adherence training curriculum,* Washington, DC, 1999, National AIDS Education & Training Center, Health Resources and Services Administration (HRSA), US Department of Health and Human Services.

Goldschmidt RH et al: Individualized strategies in the era of combination antiretroviral therapy, *Journal of the American Board of Family Practice* 11(2):158-164, 1998.

Ho DD et al: Rapid turnover of plasma virions and CD4 lymphocytes in HIV-I infection, *Nature* 373:123-126, 1995.

Kocurek K, Hollander J: Primary and preventive care for the HIV-infected adult. In Sande MA, Volberding PA, eds: *The medical management of AIDS,* ed 6, Philadelphia, 1999, WB Saunders.

Lipson JG, Dibble SL, Minarik PA, eds: *Culture and nursing care: A pocket guide,* San Francisco, 1996, UCSF Nursing Press.

Palella FJ et al: Declining morbidity and mortality among patients with advanced human immunodeficiency virus infection, *The New England Journal of Medicine* (on-line) 338(13):1998, http://content.nejm.org/.

Perlman D: Study shows flaws of new AIDS drugs, *San Francisco Chronicle,* Sept 30, 1997.

Phair JP, Murphy RL: *Contemporary diagnosis and management of HIV/AIDS infections,* Newtown, Penn, 1997, AMM.

Schoofs M: The AIDS epidemic isn't over, *Washington Post,* Dec 15, 1996.

Shilts R: *And the band played on,* New York, 1987, St. Martin's.

Steele DJ, Jackson TC, Gutmann MC: Have you been taking your pills? *The Journal of Family Practice* 30(3):294-299, 1990.

United Nations AIDS (UNAIDS)/World Health Organization (WHO): *AIDS epidemic update: December 2001,* Geneva, Switzerland, 2001, UNAIDS/WHO, (on-line) http://www.unaids.org.

Weiss R: HIV's spread is unchecked, *Washington Post,* Apr 24, 1998.

Wolbach J et al: *A pharmacist's guide to antiretroviral medications,* Denver, 2001, Mountain-Plains AIDS Education and Training Center, University of Colorado Health Sciences Center.

Wong JK et al: Recovery of replication-competent HIV despite prolonged suppression of plasma viremia, *Nature* 278:1291-1295, 1997.

A Current Antiretroviral Medications

For comprehensive information, HIV Telephone Consultation Service Warmline, 1-800-933-3413, Community Provider AIDS Training, Pacific AIDS Education and Training Center, San Francisco General Hospital; web site: http//itsa.ucsf.edu/warmline.

Chemical Name	Generic Name	Brand Name	Recommended Dosages	Common Adverse Reactions	Potential for Interactions
NUCLEOSIDE REVERSE TRANSCRIPTASE INHIBITORS					
AZT	Zidovudine (ZDV)	Retrovir	200 mg three times daily 300 mg twice daily	Anemia, neutropenia, headaches, nausea	Is minimal except for other bone marrow toxic medications
	ZDV + lamivudine	Combivir	150 mg Epivir + 300 mg Retrovir		
ddI	Didanosine	Videx	200 mg twice daily on an empty stomach	Peripheral neuropathy, pancreatitis	Is significant with medicines for which absorption is decreased with buffers
ddC	Zalcitabine	Hivid	0.75 mg three times daily	Peripheral neuropathy, oral ulcers	Is minimal except for other medicines with neuropathic effects
d4T	Stavudine	Zerit	20 to 40 mg twice daily	Peripheral neuropathy	Is minimal
3TC	Lamivudine	Epivir	150 mg twice daily	Headaches, nausea	Is minimal
ABC	Abacavir sulfate	Ziagen	300 mg twice daily	Nausea, vomiting, severe hypersensitivity reaction with fever	Is minimal
NONNUCLEOSIDE REVERSE TRANSCRIPTASE INHIBITORS					
	Nevirapine	Viramune	200 mg twice daily Start 200qd × 2s weeks	Rash	Is both a substrate and inducer of P-450 system
	Delavirdine	Rescriptor	400 mg three times daily	Rash, LFT increases	Inhibits P-450 system
	Efavirenz	Sustiva	600 mg every HS	Rash, central nervous system changes	Induces P-450 system

Generic Name	Brand Name	Recommended Dosages	Common Adverse Reactions	Potential for Interactions
PROTEASE INHIBITORS				
Saquinavir	Invirase Fortovase	600 mg three times daily 1200 mg three times daily (soft gel caps)	Diarrhea, nausea, abdominal pain	Should be taken with high-fat meal, inhibits P-450 system, has poor bioavailability
Ritonavir	Norvir	Start with 300 mg twice daily with increase to 600 mg twice daily over one week	Nausea, vomiting	Causes significant drug interactions as a result of inhibition of P-450 system
Indinavir	Crixivan	800 mg every 8 hours on an empty stomach	Asymptomatic hyperbili-rubinemia, nephrolithiasis	Inhibits P-450 system
Nelfinavir	Viracept	750 mg three times daily with food	Diarrhea, nausea, vomiting	Inhibits P-450 system; decreases ethinyl estradiol by 42%, use alternative contraceptive.
Amprenavir	Agenerase	1200 mg twice daily	Nausea, vomiting, severe rash	Inhibits P-450 system
Lopinavir + Ritonavir	Kaletra*	400 mg lopinavir + 100 mg ritonavir twice daily	Gastrointestinal in-tolerances (nau-sea, vomiting, diarrhea) Hyperglycemia Lipid abnormalities Fat maldistribution	Concomitant use with rifampin should be avoided. Rifabutin dose should be lowered (see above) Decreases ethinyl estradiol by 42%; use alternative contraceptive.

*Special instructions: take with food with moderate fat content; refrigerated capsules are stable until date on label; capsules stored at room temperature are stable for 2 months.

Medications for Common Opportunistic Infections

For comprehensive information on treatment regimens and symptomatology, see Casey, Cohen, and Hughes (1996) and Bartlett (1998).

Common Opportunistic Infections (OIs)	Medications
***Pneumocystis carinii* pneumonia (PCP)** A protozoal infection of the lungs seen in clients with severely suppressed immune systems. In HIV infection, clients are treated both prophylactically and in acute stage.	**Medications Preferred Regimen:** Trimethoprim/sulfamethoxazole (TMP/SMX) (For both acute treatment and prophylaxis) **Alternate Regimen:** Pentamidine or clindamycin (acute treatment) Aerosolized pentamidine Dapsone
***Toxoplasma* encephalitis** A protozoal infection of the brain. In HIV and AIDS, most disease is due to reactivation of dormant tissue cysts. Symptoms may include headaches, fever, altered level of consciousness, and seizures.	**Suppressive Therapy:** Pyrimethamine **Prophylaxis Regimen:** TMP/SMX Dapsone
Cryptosporidiosis A protozoal infection of the gastrointestinal (GI) and biliary tracts. It is commonly transmitted through contaminated food and water.	**Preferred Regimen:** Paromomycin Azithromycin Nutritional supplements Nitrazoxanide **Alternate Regimen:** Octreotide Azithromycin Atovaquone
Candidiasis Yeastlike fungi commonly observed in the majority of HIV and AIDS clients. Infection can be oral, bronchial, tracheal, pulmonary, esophageal, vaginal, and rectal.	**Preferred Regimen:** Fluconazole Clotrimazole Nystatin **Alternate Regimen:** Amphotericin B Itraconazole
Cryptococcosis A yeastlike fungus found naturally worldwide. It can occur in the pulmonary and central nervous systems. Also occurs in bone marrow, kidneys, liver, spleen, lymph nodes, heart, oral cavity, prostate, skin, bones, adrenal glands, and thyroid.	**Preferred Regimen:** Amphotericin B (meningitis) Fluconazole **Alternate Regimen:** Fluconazole Itraconazole **Prophylaxis Regimen:** Fluconazole Itraconazole

Common Opportunistic Infections (OIs)	Medications
***Mycobacterium avium* complex (MAC)** A bacterial infection of two or more organisms. Disseminated MAC commonly occurs in PWAs.	**Preferred Regimen:** Clarithromycin + ethambutol + rifabutin **Alternate Regimen:** Azithromycin + either ethambutol or rifabutin **Prophylaxis Regimen:** Clarithromycin (preferred) Rifabutin (alternate)
***Mycobacterium* tuberculosis (TB)** A bacterial infection of the lungs. It can occur in other organs. Multidrug cases have been identified.	**Preferred Regimen:** Complex regimens of several medications given daily through directly observed therapy (DOT) for 6 months **Alternate Regimen:** Second-line drugs, as well as experimental drugs **Prophylaxis Regimen:** Usually two medications
Cytomegalovirus (CMV) infections A viral infection of the herpes group of viruses. It can be manifested in different organ systems. A common manifestation is retinitis.	**Preferred Regimen:** Foscarnet Ganciclovir Cidofovir **Prophylaxis Regimen:** Oral ganciclovir
Herpes simplex virus (HSV) A viral infection that may be latent and manifests when the human immune system becomes suppressed. It can be mild to severe.	**Preferred Regimen:** Acyclovir Famciclovir Valacyclovir **Prophylaxis Regimen:** Same medications as preferred regimen

APPENDIX
C
Clinical Guidelines

DEPARTMENT OF HEALTH & HUMAN SERVICES

Office of Communications
Bldg. 31, Room 7A-50
(301) 496-5717
Fax (301) 402-0120
Press Line (301) 402-1663

November 13, 1997

To: Editors, Producers and Reporters

From: Patricia Randall
    Director, NIAID Office
    of Communications

Re: Revised HIV Treatment *Guidelines* Available on Web Site

Revised Guidelines for the Use of Antiretroviral Agents in HIV-Infected Adults and Adolescents are now available on the Web site of the HIV/AIDS Treatment Information Service (ATIS) and can be reached at (http://www.hivatis.org).

The Guidelines were developed by the Panel on Clinical Practices for the Treatment of HIV Infection, which was convened jointly by the Department of Health and Human Services (DHHS) and the Henry J. Kaiser Family Foundation. The Panel was charged with developing recommendations for the clinical use of antiretroviral drugs and laboratory monitoring methods in the treatment of HIV-infected individuals. These recom-

mendations were based in part on a companion document, *Report of the NIH Panel to Define Principles of Therapy of HIV Infection.*

HHS released the draft *Guidelines* to the public in June and requested comments. The revised *Guidelines* are based on feedback received during the 30-day comment period and further discussions among Panel members. As research provides new information about the treatment of HIV disease, the *Guidelines* on the ATIS Web site will undergo further revision to include state-of-the-art knowledge. The current revised *Guidelines* are being submitted to the Centers for Disease Control and Prevention (CDC) to be considered for publication in the *Morbidity and Mortality Weekly Report.*

The Panel is co-chaired by Anthony S. Fauci, M.D., director of the National Institute of Allergy and Infectious Diseases, National Institutes of Health, and John G. Bartlett, M.D. Dr. Bartlett is professor of medicine and chief of infectious diseases at Johns Hopkins University School of Medicine. The Panel also includes federal, private sector and academic experts in the clinical treatment and care of HIV-infected people, as well as representatives of AIDS interest groups, health policy groups and payer organizations.

The most current revision of the treatment guidelines (August 8, 2001) can be found at http://www.hivatis.org.

(Courtesy Midwest AIDS Training and Education Center and Renslow Sherer, MD, 1998.)

26 Psychiatric Home Care Nursing

Pamela Kees Parlocha and Linda Chafetz

Psychosocial issues have always occupied a prominent place in home care nursing. Other chapters in this book devote extensive attention to helping individuals and families cope with crises and concerns related to changes in their health status. However, several recent trends have converged to expand the demand for psychiatric home care services or interventions that target problems specific to mental disorders. In psychiatry, as in other areas of health care, cost-containment policies have shortened the duration of inpatient care. As a result, psychiatric clients are discharged from acute care settings at earlier points in their treatment, with the subsequent transfer of some acute care functions to the home setting. The aging of the general population also contributes to the demand for home care, since it increases the numbers of frail or medically ill elderly people with concurrent psychiatric problems. These problems include severe and persistent disorders that typically begin in adulthood, such as schizophrenia. These problems also include psychiatric disorders with late-life onset, such as dementias and confusion states, as well as the depression and anxiety disorders that affect many medically ill elderly people. With increased demand, psychiatric home care services have become highly visible within managed care systems and more accessible to clients and their families.

This chapter will review the evolution of psychiatric home care services as delivered by visiting nurses, public health nurses, and psychiatric clinical nurse specialists. It will provide an overview of the literature on psychiatric home care, consider the ways that it has been conceptualized and evaluated since the early 1970s, and describe the major client groups receiving these services. The chapter will conclude with a discussion of future trends in psychiatric home care nursing and recommendations for nursing research, including defining pertinent variables and measuring their effects on client outcomes.

DEFINITION OF PSYCHIATRIC HOME CARE

The phenomenon of psychiatric home care may be conceptualized from several perspectives; it may be defined as an environment, as the treatment of specific types of clients, as a nursing specialty or treatment process, or as some combination thereof. As a treatment environment, or a place where services are delivered, home care differs substantially from settings such as inpatient units or long-term care facilities. Nursing care delivered in the home is less structured and allows for more individual client control and autonomy. Interventions that promote self-care, rehabilitation, or symptom management may be implemented in the same situations in which new skills will be applied. The home environment can be adapted to accommodate the care of individuals. Coulton, Holland, and Fitch (1984) use the term *person environment congruence* to describe matching of clients' capabilities with the resources and demands of their living environments. They note that psychiatric clients may have difficulty adapting to changing environments, feeling safer and more comfortable with a predictable schedule or routine. They state, "patients may be helped to learn new skills or behaviors that are demanded by their environments. Alternatively, the demands and resources of the home may be the target of change efforts in order to match patients' perceptions of what they need."

Home care can also be defined in terms of the specific types of clients that it serves. Although no large-scale surveys have addressed this issue, it is clear that certain clinical groups predominate in home care populations. In 1985, Soreff listed the following client groups: chronically mentally ill clients living with family, elderly people with psychiatric diagnoses, and agoraphobics. Klebanoff and Casler (1986) developed a slightly different categorization, including clients with a primary psychiatric diagnosis; those with secondary psychiatric problems, such as anxiety and depression among the medically ill; and individuals and families experiencing difficulties coping with a health crisis. Today these categories would still apply, but the most marked expansion of services has occurred among medically ill elderly people, most of whom receive psychiatric interventions within a larger plan of home-based care. Parlocha (1995), in a survey of one northern California home care population, found psychiatric diagnoses generally co-occurred with one or more medical problems.

Finally, psychiatric home care can be considered as a type of advanced-practice nursing. Although home-based mental health services have been provided by staff nurses in home care and public health agencies, they are increasingly recognized as a clinical specialty (Carson, 1994, 1996; Felten, 1997; Mayo, 1997; Poduska, 1997; Quinlan, 1995). In this sense, psychiatric home care draws on knowledge and skills from several areas. It is based in advanced-practice psychiatric nursing and in expertise in assessment and management of problems associated with mental disorders. However it requires additional skills and knowledge from areas of community health nursing and family care. Psychiatric clinical specialists in the home care setting must be able to implement the assessments and interventions that promote a fit between person and environment and to coordinate and manage care from community services. Moreover, they must be able to integrate psychiatric and gerontological care and to communicate effectively with elderly clients. Their role is complex, as a reflection of both the home setting and the special populations requiring home-based psychiatric care.

HISTORICAL PERSPECTIVES

Home care was the predominant mode of psychiatric care from colonial times until the nineteenth century in the United States. If the men-tally ill were confined to institutions, it was generally because of their poverty (e.g., poorhouses and alms houses) or deviance (e.g., jails and prisons). Actual treatment resources were few, with caregiving contained within families, sometimes with private nursing care to deal with acute episodes in the home (Alexander, Selesnick, 1966). With the advent of "moral treatment" and the state mental hospital movement in the nineteenth century, long-term hospitalization became the typical treatment for serious psychiatric illnesses. Psychiatric home care did not reemerge as a treatment modality until the transition from institutional to community-based care that occurred after the second World War.

The deinstitutionalization process in the United States began in the 1950s with the introduction of neuroleptic medications that permitted control of acute psychotic symptoms, such as hallucinations and delusions. This development led to the possibility of treatment and discharge of previously "untreatable" clients. The movement gained its impetus in the 1960s, in the context of federal legislation to promote development of community mental health services. Deinstitutionalization continued at various rates in different geographical regions with varying speed and according to regional policies. By the 1980s, the majority of mentally ill adults resided in communities, with most spending no more than brief periods in hospitals (Chafetz, Goldman, Taube, 1983).

HOME CARE FOR THE SEVERELY AND PERSISTENTLY MENTALLY ILL

State mental hospital populations were heterogeneous, but a large proportion of institutional residents suffered from severe and persistent disorders that implied long-term or intermittent disability. Today, although these same disorders have a more favorable prognosis, the absence of treatment may be expected to result in some level of disability. Some of the most prevalent diagnoses among this population are schizophrenic disorders, bipolar affective disorders, and recurrent major depressions. Smaller numbers of people with less common diagnoses may also experience considerable psychiatric disability, including people whose severe anxiety disorders (e.g., panic with agoraphobia) contribute to homebound status and require home-based services.

During the transition to community-based care, researchers began to study the home environment as an alternative to the long-term psychiatric institution. Visiting nurses and public health nurses provided follow-up to the chronically mentally ill discharged to communities, supporting their adaptation to community living and promoting their compliance with other outpatient care (Heymann, Stanton, 1977; Hildebrandt, Davis, 1975; Keener, 1975). A pioneering study by Pasamanick, Scarpitti, and Dinitz (1967) showed that home nursing visits were as effective as hospital care in managing symptoms of schizophrenia, establishing home treatment as a feasible alternative to inpatient hospitalization. A group of Canadian researchers applied an experimental design similar to Pasamanick, Scarpitti, and Dinitz's to compare home and hospital psychiatric treatment (Fenton et al, 1982) for clients with major affective disorders and schizophrenia. Their findings also confirmed that home care was as effective as hospital care and less costly.

Studies until now tend to support the benefits of psychiatric home care, particularly to clients residing with family. For example, in a recent clinical trial in Toronto, Wasylenki et al (1997) found that acute care in the home compared favorably with hospital care in terms of effectiveness and cost. A large study in the United Kingdom has examined the value of training community nurses to care for families of people with schizophrenia (Brooker et al 1994). In this study, families receiving their services were compared to control cases receiving the usual treatment. Although there is some disagreement about whether the family nursing model actually cuts costs, it has been effective in clinical terms. In terms of individual outcomes, people with schizophrenia showed improved social functioning and decreased levels of symptoms. Benefits to families included decreased minor psychiatric morbidity and increased knowledge of psychotropic drugs.

Many severely mentally ill adults have limited access to family support and reside in nontraditional housing, such as group homes or hotels. Home visits may constitute one component of the multiservice community programs that provide care to these populations. Although programs such as these are not limited to home care and although they do not necessarily involve nursing visits, they are important to mention in any discussion of the severely mentally ill in the community because they demonstrate the value of service delivery in the client's natural environment. This "in vivo" service delivery derives from a substantial body of research on assertive community treatment models that carry services to clients (Burns, Santos, 1995; Olfson, 1990). The success of these assertive programs is attributed in part to the fact that they teach living skills in the settings where they will be applied. Assertive programs also reach out to individuals whose needs exceed the resources of conventional outpatient clinics, such as the homeless mentally ill or residents of single-room housing in urban areas. In these cases, outreach and intensive case management provide some of the support that other clients receive within natural social networks and families (Meeks, Murrell, 1994).

GEROPSYCHIATRIC STUDIES

Other kinds of psychiatric problems are highly prevalent among elderly medically ill clients who predominate in home care populations. Kennedy, Polivka, and Steel (1997) found at least mild to moderate psychiatric symptoms among 74% of their sample of home care clients, including problems such as somatic concerns, anxiety, depressed mood, and feelings of tension, helplessness, and hopelessness. In a review of the psychiatric home care literature from 1986 to 1994, Kozlak and Thobaben (1994) note that a majority of reports concern medically ill elderly people with concomitant psychiatric symptoms. As noted previously, Parlocha (1995) found that psychiatric diagnoses within a home care population were usually associated with the older, multidiagnosis clients requiring coordination of multiple services in the home.

The most salient psychiatric diagnosis within this group may be depression. Dalton and Busch (1995) administered the geriatric depression scale to 40 elderly clients in an urban home care agency. They noted that although 11 (25%) clients in their sample scored in the depressed range on the scale, the visiting nurses identified only 5 of these clients as depressed, and the nurses failed to include any depression-related nursing diagnoses in the clients' charts. Farran et al (1997) collected retrospective data on a home care sample in Chicago. Of 234 elderly clients, 85% were diagnosed with depression, with diagnoses of psychoses, paranoia, anxiety disorders, and dementias distributed among the remaining clients. Chart audits of 20 randomly selected cases indicated considerable medical comorbidity, as well as functional and behavioral problems. The duration of home care was long (55% of clients received services for 8 to 10 months), but outcomes were positive, with 75% of clients discharged from home care because of clinical improvement (versus services terminated because of nursing home or hospital admission or death).

Research conducted in England suggests that elderly clients with depression may benefit significantly from psychiatric home care; Banerjee et al (1996) reported on a study in which 69 depressed clients 65 years of age and older and receiving home care were randomly assigned to a control or a treatment group. The control group received "normal general practitioner care," while the treatment group received a "package of care" developed and implemented by the community psychogeriatric team. The outcome measure was recovery from depression as defined by a score on a standardized rating scale. Among the intervention group, 58% recovered, compared with 25% of the control group. These powerful results indicate that late-life depression is treatable via home care, even for clients who are socially isolated and disabled.

McDougall, Blixen, and Suen (1997) studied the results of a "life review therapy" intervention for older psychiatric home care clients. The treatment goals included freedom from suicidal or homicidal plans, the ability to verbalize feelings of loss of significant others, and the ability to identify prescribed medications and their purposes. The manifest and latent themes of the data were analyzed. After a series of life-review therapy sessions, a significant decrease ($p < 0.0001$) was found in the expression of the disempowerment themes of denial, despair, helplessness, isolation, loneliness, and loss. This kind of therapy, delivered by advanced-practice nurses, is considered to be cost effective for homebound elderly clients with depression.

ROLES OF THE PSYCHIATRIC HOME CARE NURSE

The nursing literature provides a number of accounts that clarify the roles of psychiatric home care nurses. These roles have been heavily influenced by funding regulations, with Medicare regulations having an important impact on current and future practice. Hellwig (1993) specifies the following functions of psychiatric home care nurses: collaboration with psychiatrists and liaison with nonpsychiatric physicians, assessment and intervention for individual clients, client and family education regarding psychopathological processes and medication, provision of support to enhance self-esteem and feelings of control, and monitoring of medication compliance. Hellwig describes care to clients with a broad range of psychiatric diagnoses, usually provided up to 3 times per week for 4 to 8 weeks. Cases of clients on injectable medications are kept open until the clients are no longer homebound or begin to take oral medications.

Blazek (1993) provides another view of the role of the psychiatric home care nurse, including program development. She defines *psychiatric home care* as "the provision of psychiatric services made available in the home on an intermittent basis to individuals who are homebound secondary to their psychological or medical status." She lists the following types of clients as appropriate for psychiatric home care: those who suffer from reactive depression in response to trauma, loss, or diagnosis of a terminal illness; those with bipolar disorder or schizophrenia who are homebound; acquired immunodeficiency syndrome (AIDS) clients who are not yet eligible for hospice; and clients who are referred from crisis clinics or physicians for psychiatric assessment. Blazek recommends that advanced-practice psychiatric nurses (clinical nurse specialists) provide home-based services to these groups.

REIMBURSEMENT ISSUES AND NURSING ROLES

Medicare regulations also emphasize advanced practice. Psychiatric nursing constitutes the sole specialty area in which reimbursement requires special qualifications for the nurse making home visits. Psychiatric home care nurses must have a master's degree in either psychiatric or community mental health nursing, a bachelor's degree and 1 year of related work experience, a diploma or associate's degree and 2 years of related work experience, or American Nurses Association (ANA) certification of community health nursing (Health Care Financing Administration [HCFA], 1989).

Crisis Intervention Theory	Orem's Self-Care Requisites	Behavioral Techniques
Precipitating or stressful event Perception of event Situational support Coping mechanisms	Sufficient intake of air, water, food Elimination Activity and rest Solitude and interaction Prevention of hazards Promotion of normal human functioning	Guided imagery Biofeedback Relaxation Role playing Diary writing Desensitization Assertiveness Psychoeducation Skills training Feedback Homework

Figure 26-1   Components of the psychiatric home care nursing model.

Medicare regulations also strongly influence which groups will receive psychiatric home care services. Although a number of funders, including Medicare, Medicaid, private managed-care organizations (MCOs), and other private sources, pay for psychiatric home visits, a recent survey (National Association for Home Care, 1996) confirms that Medicare remains the most important payor. Medicare reimburses services to *homebound clients,* defined as clients unable to leave home without assistance to obtain care or unable to do so without considerable effort. Conditions such as severe depression, agoraphobia, paranoia, and confusion states can be used as justification for a client's homebound status. Failure to adequately document the homebound status of any client could result in the failure of Medicare to reimburse the providing agency for services.

Carson (1994) points out that psychiatric interventions written in "medical-surgical" language may be preferred by Medicare reviewers who place less value on terminology such as strategies for "expression of feelings," "resistance," and "support." The following skills are considered reimbursable by Medicare and apply to psychiatric home care: assessment and evaluation, teaching, medication management, and management of a care plan. Since teaching is considered a reimbursable skill by Medicare, Carson recommends couching almost everything the psychiatric home visiting nurse does in teaching terms. She states that using teaching as the main nursing intervention will help to span the communication gap between Medicare and psychiatric home nursing. Thus home health care agencies will avoid further Medicare reimbursement denials.

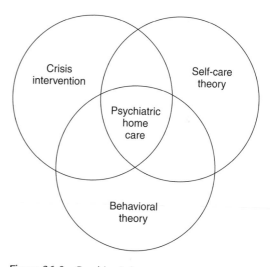

Figure 26-2   Psychiatric home care nursing model.

CONCEPTUAL FRAMEWORK

Duffy, Miller, and Parlocha (1993) have published a conceptual framework to guide practice in psychiatric home care nursing. The framework incorporates concepts from crisis intervention, self-care theory, and behavioral therapies (Figs. 26-1 and 26-2).

According to crisis theory, individuals are confronted by threats that exceed the effectiveness of their usual coping mechanisms (Caplan, 1974). When a person is confronted by a stressful event that is perceived as a threat, a state of imbalance or disequilibrium is precipitated. The presence or absence of certain balancing factors determines whether the state of disequilibrium will continue or resolve. Balancing factors include perception of the stressful event, the presence or absence of

CASE STUDY

The following case study applies the conceptual framework described. Mrs. Stone is a 76-year-old widow who lives alone and has recurrent major depression and congestive heart failure. The mental status assessment on the initial home visit showed Mrs. Stone to be alert and oriented, with no suicidal ideation, but with an affect that ranged between anxious and tearful. She complained of the vegetative signs of depression, such as loss of appetite, weight loss, and difficulty sleeping. She had been noncompliant with her prescribed antidepressant, saying that she kept "forgetting to take it." Her physical assessment showed borderline hypertension, shortness of breath on exertion, and constipation.

Further assessment revealed a psychosocial crisis that influenced Mrs. Stone's condition. She reported losing her husband to cancer 6 months before the initiation of home care services. Her perception of the event was that it was overwhelming and catastrophic, exceeding her usual ability to cope. She became withdrawn and regressed, and consequently gained little benefit from a support system of concerned children and grandchildren who lived in the area.

A self-care assessment indicated functional limitations in the areas of activity and rest, food intake and elimination, and solitude and social interaction. These self-care deficits combined to have a very serious impact on her health and her adjustment to her situation. Intervention included referral to the home care agency dietitian and a plan to incorporate small servings of high-

calorie foods with liquid supplements to replace lost weight. High-fiber foods and increased fluid intake would address the problem of constipation. The nurse introduced a medication planner to help the client to remember when to take her medications.

To address the problems of sleep disturbance and withdrawal, the nurse devised a behavioral contract in concert with the client. The behaviors agreed on included no more than two short naps per day, calls to a friend or relative twice per day, and the assignments of self-care activities, such as bathing and grooming. The nurse offered concrete suggestions for behavioral change and reinforcement for improvement in behaviors. Relaxation techniques were taught as coping mechanisms to decrease anxiety.

After a course of three nurse visits per week for 4 weeks, Mrs. Stone showed considerable improvement. Her affect was less anxious and she became tearful less often, usually when discussing feelings of grief over the loss of her husband. She had gained back 10 pounds, was sleeping better, and was only rarely troubled by constipation. She was able to take medications as prescribed and adhered to the contract to call family and friends, several of whom visited each week. She was still borderline hypertensive, and she was placed on an antihypertensive medication by her physician. When she was able to go out for walks without becoming short of breath, and thus was no longer homebound, the case was closed to further psychiatric home care visiting services.

adequate support systems, and the quality of coping mechanisms. Psychiatric home care nurses identify crises to assess their impact on functional ability. Their goal is to help to restore clients to their precrisis level of functioning as quickly as possible.

The second component of the conceptual framework is Orem's self-care nursing theory (1991). Orem's self-care requisites include maintenance of a sufficient intake of air, water, and food; adequate elimination; maintenance of a balance between activity and rest and solitude and interaction; prevention of hazards; and promotion of normal human functioning. Functional assessment of psychiatric home care clients focuses on the behavioral impacts of psychiatric illness. For example, clients with depression tend to suffer from im-

balances of activity and rest as demonstrated by sleep disorders, vegetative signs, and lack of motivation. Clients with paranoid delusions or fears may be unable to use public transportation to function optimally. Agoraphobic clients' isolation at home interferes with the normal balance between solitude and social interaction. Thus dimensions of Orem's self-care model provide additional parameters for the functional assessment of psychiatric clients in the home environment.

Finally, whereas costly, long-term psychoanalytic approaches are of limited usefulness in the home care setting, behavioral approaches provide helpful assessment parameters and guidance in choice of interventions. Behavioral therapy focuses on behavioral change on the part of the client, the goals of which are chosen and agreed on by both nurse and home care client. Treatment approaches for functional problems are generally oriented toward "here and now" problems and client participation in managing illness. They focus on behavioral changes based on mutually agreed-on goals identified by nurse and client. Behavioral intervention techniques that can be used in home care nursing include, but are not limited to, guided imagery techniques, biofeedback, relaxation training, role playing, diary writing, systematic densensitization techniques, assertiveness training, psychoeducation, social skills training, feedback, and homework assignments. Psychiatric home care populations have multiple and interacting problems with comorbidity more often than not. It follows then that crisis intervention, self-care assessments, and behavioral treatments occur in the context of medical problems and treatment.

A study by Parlocha (1995) clearly illustrates the comorbidity and complexity of treatment planning. In her chart review of 32 psychiatric home care clients from one visiting nurses' association, Parlocha found that more than 80% had at least 1 medical diagnosis in addition to a psychiatric diagnosis, that over 50% had 2 additional medical diagnoses, and that 28% had 3 or more additional medical diagnoses. The mean age of the sample clients was 75 years. These frail elderly clients had lived long enough to develop chronic medical illnesses that extended their needs for home care nursing. This was particularly true of the large subgroup with cardiac problems, who required a longer duration of home care and more visits than others. Elderly psychiatric home care clients, especially those with multiple comorbidities, must receive prompt attention when developing care paths or treatment goals.

FUTURE TRENDS

Carson (1996) summarizes the history of psychiatric home care from the 1960s, a decade when she claims that both psychiatric care and home care were reinvented. Carson first describes how, in the 1960s, multidisciplinary teams of physicians, nurses, and other disciplines "laid the groundwork for the intersection of home care and psychiatric care." By the early 1980s, funding factors dictated that most mental health outreach to the severely mentally ill occurred via psychiatric programs. Psychiatric home care nursing depended primar-

ily on funds from Medicare and targeted clients meeting criteria for homebound status. The largest single subgroup in psychiatric home care became medically ill elderly clients. Their most prominent psychiatric diagnosis was depression.

As health care moves into the new millennium, psychiatric home care is increasingly integrated into emerging models of managed care and case management. This shifts the emphasis of administrators and regulators to new practice issues, such as development of clinical pathways and assessment of outcomes. In April 1996, Medicare removed the requirement for a psychiatrist referral for psychiatric home care, expanding the integration of mental health and physical care. With this integration comes a demand for clinical outcomes of psychiatric home care based on functional status and a developing need for standards that would allow for comparisons of psychiatric home care processes and outcomes across agencies.

Carson (1996) predicts that a combination of national trends will have an impact on the future of psychiatric home care. For example, Congressional actions are moving us toward parity in insurance for mental health insurance coverage. This may effectively prevent refusal of care to severely and persistently mentally ill clients. As the mentally ill become integrated into large health plans, insurers and providers will be strongly motivated to look at cost-effective alternatives for mental health service delivery, including home care. As managed care companies increase their role in providing psychiatric home care, they will want evidence of value and cost effectiveness. A key issue in the future will be identification of functional and clinical outcomes that can be used to gauge efficacy of services.

In a 1997 report, Blazek lists the following as possible outcomes to demonstrate quality client care: client stability, client progress, shorter or less frequent hospital stays, client satisfaction, and cost containment. She considers the development of care paths for psychiatric home care as an essential tool in documenting positive outcomes of care. She lists the following recommendations for care-path development:

- Integrate Joint Commission on Accreditation of Healthcare Organizations (JCAHO) requirements for specific client populations into the path.

- Design care paths so that the problem terminology is the same on all forms used.
- Include a form that allows the nurse to prioritize goals.
- Use an intervention form to track the number of visits needed to reach a specific goal.
- Create an outcome form that includes the dates of goal achievement or reason for variance.

RECOMMENDATIONS FOR FUTURE RESEARCH

In view of current trends in the organization and funding of psychiatric home care services, it is clear that outcomes research will shape the future. To develop a solid research foundation for evidenced-based practice, nurse investigators will need to first accomplish the following:

- Develop clear operationalized definitions of variables and outcomes.
- Test various models of care delivery.
- Study large samples, focusing on differing diagnoses, such as schizophrenia and bipolar disorders.
- Look for links between nursing interventions and client outcomes.
- Design care paths and test them for usefulness.
- Compare the usefulness of care paths based on medical diagnoses with those based on functional status.
- Test existing coding systems of nursing diagnoses, client outcomes, and nursing interventions for their usefulness in documenting the effects of interventions on client outcomes (Parlocha, Henry, 1998).
- Through observations and medical record audits, compare the nursing care actually delivered with the care that is documented.
- Compare the outcomes of clients receiving care from advanced-nurse practitioners versus experienced psychiatric home care nurses versus other home health care nurses.

SUMMARY

Psychiatric home care nursing has undergone a significant evolution from the 1960s to the present. Current trends in health care delivery will not only increase the importance of these services, but also increase the need for outcomes studies that can shape innovative practice. A number of program descriptions are already available in the literature, and the research base in psychiatric home care is expanding. It is hoped that this movement toward evidence-based practice will increase in the future.

REFERENCES

Alexander FG, Selesnick ST: *The history of psychiatry,* New York, 1966, New American Library.

Banerjee S et al: Randomized controlled trial of intervention by psychogeriatric team on depression in frail elderly people at home, *British Medical Journal* 313:1058-1061, 1996.

Blazek LA: Development of a psychiatric home care program and the role of the CNS in the delivery of care, *Clinical Nurse Specialist* 7(4):164-168, 1993.

Blazek LA: Psychiatric home care and care paths: Step by step, *Caring* 16(2):82-84, 1997.

Brooker C et al: The outcome of training community psychiatric nurses to deliver psychosocial intervention, *British Journal of Psychiatry* 165:222-230, 1994.

Burns B, Santos AB: Assertive community treatment: An update on randomized trials, *Psychiatric Services* 46(7):669-675, 1995.

Caplan G: *Principles of preventive psychiatry,* New York, 1974, Basic Books.

Carson VB: Psychiatric home care documentation: Doing psych but talking med-surg language, *Caring* 13(6):32-38, 40-41, 1994.

Carson VB: Psychiatric home care: Reflecting on the past, evaluating the present, envisioning the future, *Caring* 15(12):34-39, 1996.

Chafetz L, Goldman HR, Taube CA: Deinstitutionalization in the United States, *International Journal of Mental Health* 11(4):48-63, 1983.

Coulton DJ, Holland TP, Fitch V: Person-environment congruence and psychiatric patient outcome in community care homes, *Administration in Mental Health* 12(2):71-88, 1984.

Dalton JR, Busch KD: Depression: The missing diagnosis in the elderly, *Home Healthcare Nurse* 13(5):31-35, 1995.

Duffey J, Miller MP, Parlocha P: Psychiatric home care: A framework for assessment and intervention, *Home Healthcare Nurse* 11(2):22-28, 1993.

Farran CJ et al: Psychiatric home care for the elderly, *Home Health Care Services Quarterly* 16(1/2):77-92, 1997.

Felten BS: The geropsychiatric clinical nurse specialist in home care, *Home Healthcare Nurse* 15(9):635-638, 1997.

Fenton FR et al: *Home and hospital psychiatric treatment,* Pittsburgh, 1982, University of Pittsburgh

Press.

Health Care Financing Administration (HCFA): *Medicare home health agency manual,* HCFA Pub No 11, Revision 222, Washington, DC, 1989, US Department of Health and Human Services.

Hellwig K: Psychiatric home care nursing: Managing patients in the community setting, *Journal of Psychosocial Nursing* 31(12):21-24, 1993.

Heymann GM, Stanton LM: A pilot study to evaluate visiting nurses services to chronic psychiatric patients, *Hospital and Community Psychiatry* 28(2):97-101, 1977.

Hildebrandt DE, Davis JM: Home visits: A method of reducing the pre-intake dropout rate, *Journal of Psychiatric Nursing and Mental Health Services* 13(5):43-44, 1975.

Keener ML: The public health nurse in mental health follow-up, *Nursing Research* 24:198-201, 1975.

Kennedy CW, Polivka BJ, Steel JS: Psychiatric symptoms in a community-based medically ill population, *Home Healthcare Nurse* 15(6):431-441, 1997.

Klebanoff NA, Casler CB: The psychosocial clinical nurse specialist: An untapped resource for home care, *Home Healthcare Nurse* 4(6):36-40, 1986.

Kozlak J, Thobaben M: Psychiatric home health nursing of the aged: A selected literature review, *Geriatric Nursing* 15(3):148-150, 1994.

Mayo TL: Mental health services in the home: A balance of sophistication and caring, *Home Healthcare Nurse* 15(4):271-274, 1997.

McDougall GJ, Blixen CE, Suen LJ: The process and outcome of life review psychotherapy with depressed homebound older adults, *Nursing Research* 46(5):277-283, 1997.

Meekes S, Murrell SA: Service providers in the social networks of clients with severe mental illnesses, *Schizophrenia Bulletin* 20(2):339-406, 1994.

National Association for Home Care: *Basic statistics about home care,* Washington, DC, 1996, The Association.

Olfson M: Assertive community treatment: An evaluation of experimental evidence, *Hospital and Community Psychiatry* 41(6):634-641, 1990.

Orem D: *Nursing: Concepts of practice,* ed 4, St Louis, 1991, Mosby.

Parlocha PK: *Defining a critical path for psychiatric home care patients with a diagnosis of major depressive disorder,* unpublished doctoral dissertation, San Francisco, 1995, UCSF School of Nursing.

Parlocha PK, Henry SB: The usefulness of the Georgetown Home Health Care Classification System for coding patient problems and nursing interventions in psychiatric home care, *Computers in Nursing* 16(1):45-52, 1998.

Pasamanick D, Scarpitti FR, Dinitz S: *Schizophrenics in the community,* New York, 1967, Appleton-Century Crofts.

Poduska DD: Development of a psychiatric home care program, *Caring* 16(6):36-39, 1997.

Quinlan J: Psychiatric home care: An introduction, *Home Healthcare Nurse* 13(4):20-24, 1995.

Soreff SM: Indications for home treatment, *Psychiatric Clinics of North America* 8:563-575, 1985.

Wasylenki et al: A home-based program for the treatment of acute psychosis, *Community Mental Health Journal* 33(2):151-162, 1997.

PART V

Professional
Challenges in
Home Health
Care Nursing

27 Home Care: The Ethical Challenges

Mila Ann Aroskar

Ethical challenges confront home care nurses daily in their practice. Use of sophisticated technologies and cost-containment efforts that seem to dominate other goals in health care, such as provision of quality care, create troubling questions about professional obligations and rights of staff nurses and administrators. Ethical concerns and questions arise both in direct client-care situations and in the development of agency and related public policy for tough choices involving ethical and economic values.

This chapter provides examples of ethical problems and concerns in home care agencies, a process for thinking through and responding to ethical issues and problems, institutional strategies for dealing with ethical problems, and future ethical challenges in home care.

Ethical dimensions (i.e., looking at how health care professionals *ought* to conduct their personal and professional relationships with one another) are integral to the delivery of quality home care as they are a part of all client situations. When nurses consider their moral obligations and duties to themselves, clients, colleagues, employing agencies, and the profession, they are considering the ethical dimensions of their practice. These are situations that nurses struggle with when there are no ready-made answers. Laws and policies are nonexistent or inadequate as nurses and home care agencies seek to respond with integrity.

Ethical problems occur in home care populations across the life span, from ventilator-dependent infants to elderly clients who may not have the capacity to make health decisions in their own best interests. Some clients are able to pay, but others have no medical insurance to cover reimbursement for home care over an extended period of time, or available payment systems are inflexible. There may be disagreements about

treatment and concerns about the ability of informal caregivers to provide needed care, similar to the situation of Mrs. P.

Examples of other ethically troublesome situations include contracting with clients for adherence to treatment regimens, "enforcement" of client rights and responsibilities, rights and obligations of nurses to reject a specific client assignment in which they feel endangered, early discharge of hospital clients who are sicker than in the past and require complex nursing care outside of the hospital, protection of client confidentiality, use of chemotherapies in the home, adequate pain management, impact on caregivers of caring for disabled family members in the home, quality assurance and home care standards, and treatment of home care solely as a commodity to be sold like anything else in the marketplace. These ethical problems often confront staff nurses, administrators, and managers directly or indirectly on a daily basis.

Ordinarily health care professionals do not think explicitly of the ethical aspects of these situations. A focus on identification of clinical, legal, political, and economic factors usually dominates problem-solving activities in today's turbulent health care scene. Yet each of these areas has ethical dimensions fundamental to home care nurses and to agencies as both make decisions that have moral aspects and consequences. Technical expertise alone is not sufficient to deal with the ethical aspects of nursing practice when moral principles and values, such as fidelity to clients, respect for persons, nonmaleficence (avoiding harm), beneficence (doing good), and distributive justice are at stake and staff nurses are struggling to decide what they ought to do in client care. Managers and administrators are trying to develop more ethically supportable policies that reflect a home care agency's mission and values.

CASE STUDY

Mrs. P. is a 65-year-old retired secretary and former heavy smoker with cancer of the lung. She had surgery and chemotherapy for the initial course of treatment. She now receives intravenous (IV) chemotherapy (for metastasis) and total parenteral nutrition at home. Her husband is 75 years of age and a former high school teacher. He is able to take care of their small apartment located in a daughter's home and provide some of Mrs. P.'s care with assistance from the daughter who works part time. For 2 weeks, the family has been able to manage Mrs. P.'s care with visits every other day from an agency nurse. When the nurse visited today, he learned that the family is unable to provide adequate care for Mrs. P., who has developed pneumonia, is sometimes confused, and has reddened areas at several pressure points. The daughter thinks that Mrs. P. should return to the hospital, at least temporarily, because she is unavailable to care for her mother during part of the day. Mrs. P. wants someone with her constantly and does not want to return to the hospital. Mr. P. is somewhat forgetful and often leaves his wife alone to pursue his own activities outside of the apartment.

This client and family situation was discussed recently in a conversation between the nursing director and a staff nurse in a nongovernmental home care agency. The staff nurse and the nursing director wonder what their obligations are to the client, the agency, and the community in today's competitive managed-care environment. Both individuals have strong personal and professional values, such as fidelity to clients, that support provision of care to meet client needs. At the same time, they share concerns about who should pay for care when reimbursement is inadequate or not available. Mrs. P.'s daughter has told the staff nurse that she is concerned about her parents' financial situation, that she knows that their insurance reimbursement for home care is about to end, that she is worried about her father's increasing forgetfulness, and that she is seeking full-time employment because of the family's financial circumstances.

Box 27-1 Process for Responding to Ethical Problems

1. Identify the ethical problems and issues in the situation.
2. Gather as complete an information base as possible (e.g., the client's clinical situation and key people involved with the client).
3. Determine all possible options for action.
4. Determine what ethical values and principles of the nurse and the agency are enhanced or negated in the identified options.

5. Decide on recommendations or actions and implement them based on responses to Items 1 through 4.
6. Evaluate the process by which the decisions were made.
7. Incorporate new learning into similar situations that raise difficult ethical problems and questions in home care.

Home care nurses in urban, suburban, and rural areas manage care of terminally ill clients at home. These clients often need 24-hour nursing care. When agency rules and regulations do not include the provision of such care because of lack of reimbursement or unavailability of staff, nurses wonder what they ought to do when family members are unavailable or unable to provide the necessary care and local hospice staff are unavailable or inadequate to meet client needs. Nurses then question who is ultimately responsible for the client's care and who should pay for needed care if the client has inadequate or no insurance coverage. For example, a family agrees to take an elderly stroke victim home from the hospital and then refuses to provide ongoing care for a variety of reasons, or a nurse is concerned that young parents with a ventilator-dependent infant at home are showing signs of neglect in caring for their infant. Nursing care standards, principles and values of client safety, provision of care to all in need, nonabandonment of clients, and stewardship of agency resources are all at stake. There are no ready-made or easy answers to such frustrating situations. A decision-making process that incorporates ethical dimensions is helpful to assist the nurse, client, and agency to make the difficult choices required in such home care situations and considering the ethical "trade-offs." See Box 27-1 for the elements of this decision-making process.

COMPONENTS OF A PROCESS FOR RESPONDING TO ETHICAL PROBLEMS IN HOME CARE

The first component in the ethical problem-solving process is distinguishing the ethical problem in a situation from other legal, clinical, sociocultural, or communication problems. Inadequate communication is often a major issue in dealing with ethical and other client-care problems. The identification of the correct dosage of drugs for a client who is receiving home chemotherapy is primarily a technical question. Obtaining an interpreter for a client who does not speak English is primarily a sociocultural issue. Determining relevant state rules and regulations regarding home care is a legal question. Although laws tell nurses what is permitted or prohibited, or, in some instances, what is required, ethics is the study of how nurses *ought* to conduct themselves. It is determining what is morally right in a situation in which individuals interact and difficult decisions affecting human welfare are required. Ideally, law and ethics are congruent, but this is not always the case. For example, Medicare rules and regulations for home care reimbursement allow a limited number of home visits, but the professional ethic of nursing does not permit a nurse to simply abandon a client.

CHARACTERISTICS OF AN ETHICAL PROBLEM OR SITUATION

Determining whether a situation presents an ethical dilemma has the following four components, as illustrated by Mrs. P.'s situation discussed in the case study:

1. There is a conflict of values, obligations, loyalties, interests, or needs in the client-care situation or in a related agency or policy issue.
2. There are ethical principles at stake, such as respecting people, doing the least harm, providing benefits, keeping promises, telling the truth, or being fair to all involved.
3. The situation requires a reflective thinking process to determine what ought to be done.
4. The values and feelings of all involved, such as staff nurses, clients, families, and administrators, are a part of the context in which the decision is made, and they affect the decision makers and their perspectives.

The identification of ethical characteristics is also useful in the development and evaluation of agency policy that impacts directly or indirectly on the welfare of clients, staff, and the agency. Using such a process should lead to more reasoned policies that incorporate ethical considerations.

Identifying the database necessary for making difficult ethical decisions is another major component in dealing with ethical problems and concerns in home care. An assumption is often made that this is the easy part of dealing with ethical problems in clinical care or policy development. In fact, this component often takes more time than expected as all the involved individuals seek to reach agreement on a common information base. The information base should include such data as the medical "facts"; the client's prognosis; the client's goals and values for treatment and the client's capacity or incapacity to make decisions or to participate in the decision-making process; sociocultural information, such as the education, ethnic, and religious background of clients and families; financial information relevant to client care; and pertinent legal information.

The information base should also include all possible available options for the specific client involved and the intentions of each of these options, such as reducing suffering of a client or easing burdens on family caregivers. The interests of the identified client, Mrs. P. in this instance, should be considered as primary, with the interests of others as secondary. It is not always easy to keep the interests of individual clients and family caregivers separated because they are usually interconnected and interdependent. Nevertheless, the interests of the identified client should always be an explicit priority for caregivers, particularly when individual clients are unable to speak for themselves and need an advocate.

ETHICAL VALUES, PRINCIPLES, AND CONCEPTS

Another important component is determining what ethical values, principles, and concepts are enhanced or negated in the choices identified for action. In any home care situation, the principle of respect for individual autonomy and self-determination must always be considered (Davis et al, 1997). The principle of respect for people, in which individual moral autonomy and self-determination are based, is broader than only individual autonomy. Respect for people also recognizes that individuals are interconnected members of the human community at the same time that individual autonomy is considered. Most of the decisions that individuals make affect the welfare of others to some degree. Nurses are poignantly aware that this is so in the decisions made by them and their clients. Many decisions made by Mr. and Mrs. P. affect their daughter and caregivers and vice versa.

Home care nurses, in maintaining respect for people as unique human beings, must provide special justification if, for example, they are to interfere with the autonomy of clients such as Mr. and Mrs. P. Honoring this principle means that individuals must have their goals and values taken into account in any decision-making that affects them if they are unable to make these decisions themselves or to participate in the process. In home care, this means that individuals must be involved in major decisions whenever they are capable of making or participating in those decisions. Special justification is required to exclude Mrs. P. from decision-making. This special justification requires an assessment that Mrs. P. clearly cannot make decisions in her own best interests or that her decisions will clearly have dangerous or harmful consequences for her, and possibly for others. A surrogate decision-maker may then be appointed to make decisions.

Home care nurses are in a unique position to ensure that client values and goals are taken into account in decision-making because they often come to know a client intimately, sometimes more intimately than family members or loved ones. Nurses who care for hospice clients in home settings are clearly in such a position. Commitment to respect for people and their autonomy by home care nurses means that the goals and values of individual clients must be taken into account in any decisions that are made with, or in some instances, for a client. This principle is fundamental to relationships between all health care professionals and other caregivers, such as family members. Individual interactions and agency policies can be examined from the perspective of this principle as to whether or not respect for people is enhanced or negated by a

particular decision, action, or policy. Home care nurses may find their own personal and professional values, such as avoiding or preventing harm, conflicting with those of respect for clients.

In an effort to enhance respect for individuals, nurses and other caregivers frequently invoke the idea of rights of individuals in and to health care. *The Standards of Community Health Nursing Practice* (American Nurses Association [ANA], 1986) incorporates a discussion of the ethical responsibilities of nurses from the perspective that nurses working "in the community may encounter situations in which human rights and freedoms are in jeopardy." In this document, health care is assumed to be a right of clients from which responsibilities flow for community health nurses (and home care agencies). Many home care nurses identify themselves as community health nurses; thus they have community health nursing responsibilities. These responsibilities include "responsibility to advocate for individuals and families, to identify and rectify gaps in health care services, and to influence health and social policies that are inconsistent with this basic right" (ANA, 1986).

Fundamental human rights, such as a person's right to make decisions about his or her own body, are based on respect for people and are shared equally by all people (Bandman, 1978). They are rights that transcend, override, or cancel other rights, such as "special rights" or privileges of health professionals to practice their profession. Fundamental human rights are independent of legal or institutional norms. If nurses accept that a basic right to nursing and health care is a fundamental right, then the abridgement of such a right by an individual, agency, or society will strike morally sensitive nurses as unjust.

Home care nurses may find themselves in situations in which what they consider to be a basic right to nursing and health care is in jeopardy. For example, an individual such as Mrs. P. may no longer be able to pay for nursing services that are still required from a health and safety perspective. If they are unable to provide care themselves or be assured that care is available from another source, such a situation creates a great deal of tension and frustration for nurses who feel that they are powerless and caught in the middle. This same frustration and tension will probably not be experienced by a nurse who makes judgments based primarily on "the rules" rather than judgments based primarily on ethical principles and values.

The *National Association for Home Care Code of Ethics* incorporates a section on client rights and responsibilities but is not explicit about responsibilities. All home care nurses should be knowledgeable about this document because it indicates what home care agencies consider to be their ethical responsibilities to clients and should be discussed with clients and their families.

Client rights include full information about rights and responsibilities (Box 27-2). Client rights include a right to appropriate and professional care, information about agency policy and charges for services, choice of care providers, informed decision-making about procedures or treatments, reasonable continuity of care, the right to refuse treatment within the limits of the law and information about the consequences of such a decision, timely response to a request for service, service from an agency that has the capabilities to meet the client's specific needs, timely information about anticipated termination of service, a right to voice grievances without fear of reprisal, and referral when the client is denied service by an agency solely on his or her ability to pay.

The National Association for Home Care continues to use a code of ethics adopted in 1982, which includes client rights and responsibilities with a focus on rights (2000).

Box 27-2 Examples of Home Care Client Rights and Responsibilities

RIGHTS

Appropriate and professional care
Information on agency policy and charges for
   services
Informed decision-making about procedures and
   treatments
Reasonable continuity of care

RESPONSIBILITIES OF CLIENT AND FAMILY

Client and family participation in the plan of care
Provision of a safe environment to the highest
   degree possible
Accountability if the plan of care is not followed

Client responsibilities are identified in documents such as the Minnesota Assembly of Home and/or Community Health Nursing Agencies' *Code of Ethics* (1984). They include participating in the plan of care by the client and family, assisting in provision of a safe environment to the highest degree possible, providing accurate and complete information about the client's health, taking responsibility if the plan of care is not followed, and informing the nurse or agency when instructions are not understood or cannot be followed by the client or family. Clients' bills of rights in health care generally incorporate client responsibilities.

Respect for clients and their rights and responsibilities includes respect for all the individuals involved in a client-care situation. Involved individuals will usually be clients, families, significant others, and caregivers who are affected directly or indirectly in the provision of care to a specific client. Respecting people as individuals and as members of families, groups, and communities means that nurses and other health professionals must justify, for example, why clients do not participate in major decisions concerning their care, if this occurs. Decisions made for home care clients in a paternalistic mode would not be acceptable without such justification. Decision-making may become more burdensome in terms of the time and effort required. At the same time, it can be argued that decisions made in this way are more ethically adequate, take into consideration client rights in health care systems, and are congruent with standards of the American Nurses Association, which supports joint planning of care with clients and families.

Ethical principles and values that should be considered in addition to respect for the moral autonomy of individuals include avoiding harm, alleviating suffering, providing benefits, and being fair to individuals. Consideration of these principles and values will not automatically provide home care nurses or agencies with an ethically appropriate decision or action but will generally rule out certain decisions and actions, such as ignoring clients' goals and values when they have been identified.

Nonmaleficence, or avoiding and preventing harm, is always an obligation that home care nurses should attempt to enhance in any client-care situation. In the discussion of Mrs. P., the available options should be considered in light of how they enhance or negate the avoidance of harm and the alleviation of suffering for Mrs. P. Consideration of this principle and home care client rights rule out the abandonment of Mrs. P. This could not be justified ethically, although it might be justified solely on the basis of economic values of agency survival. This would be a situation in which ethical and economic values are in fundamental conflict, difficult choices are required, and the options for choice seem equally unattractive.

The principle of beneficence, or doing good, requires the provision of benefits and a balancing of harms and benefits (Beauchamp, Childress, 1994). Although the provision of benefits is considered by some to be a moral requirement, others argue that it is a virtue of practicing charity and should not be viewed as a moral obligation. Discussion of the harms, costs, and benefits of the different options in Mrs. P.'s situation should take place to consider how identified options will enhance or negate Mrs. P.'s welfare, the primary consideration.

Benefits are considered to have a positive value on stakeholders, whereas costs or harms are usually considered to have a negative effect (Beauchamp, Childress, 1994). Costs are usually thought of in financial terms but should also be considered from the perspective of physical, psychological, spiritual, and emotional pain as well. Since it is often difficult, if not impossible, to quantify all the costs and actual or potential harms in a client situation, they may be referred to as risks that are considered to be potential harms. Explicit consideration of risks and benefits of the available options for Mrs. P.'s care is part of the thoughtful and careful action required by the principle of nonmaleficence.

Home care nurses and administrators should recognize that consideration of costs, risks, and benefits in a client-care situation or in the development of agency policy takes place against a background of varying degrees of uncertainty and profound changes in the financing and delivery of health care services, including home care. Some would even argue that cost containment, rather than quality or access, is now the major goal in health care. However, nurses and administrators should be able to recognize that actions such as abandonment of a client by an agency without appropriate planning for needed care will result in identifiable harm to the client in many instances. For example, in Mrs. P.'s situation, it may become clear with consideration of the risks and benefits of the available options that hospitalization is an ethically justifiable decision, at least temporarily.

Considering principles of autonomy, nonmaleficence, and beneficence in decision-making usually will point to certain decisions and actions as more ethically justifiable or as unjustifiable in an individual client-care situation. Consideration of these principles related primarily to individual welfare will not automatically resolve questions as to what moral obligations an agency has to continue care of a client when insurance benefits have ceased. Such questions fall under the principle of distributive justice, which is concerned with how costs and benefits are fairly distributed among individuals, groups, communities, and so forth. Nurses deal with issues of distributive justice in individual client-care situations when they decide how to allocate their time for client visits. This might seem to be solely a professional judgment, but it also incorporates implicit considerations of distributive justice, such as need. Although our society does not have a consensus on the ethical criteria for distributing cost or risks and benefits, equity and fairness are still considered to be important social ideals. At the same time, nursing and health care needs are not the same for everyone. How then can treating people differently be justified ethically?

Without an overall consensus on the basis for distributive justice in a pluralistic society, it is difficult to agree on how the costs and benefits of nursing and health care ought to be distributed. There are several ways that treating people differently might be justified. Health care professionals most often argue that the benefits of health care should be distributed on the basis of medical need. Certainly, individuals who are acutely or chronically ill should receive the care they need to restore them to the greatest degree of health possible. When return to health is no longer the goal, appropriate care and comfort to reduce physical, emotional, and spiritual suffering become the goals.

One problem with a needs approach to justice is that needs are determined differently by different individuals, even health professionals. Some individuals may argue that they should have every available option in health care, regardless of their ability to pay. Some would consider this to be extreme and argue that a minimal level of care is what should be available to everyone, regardless of ability to pay. Access to emergency care might be one example of a minimal level of care. Others argue that an individual is entitled to whatever he or she can pay for through insurance or other payment mechanisms. Some visions of distributive justice include combinations of criteria such as need, vulnerability, and age, which is a very controversial criterion.

The President's Commission for the Study of Ethical Problems in Medicine and Biomedical and Behavioral Research (1983) based its recommendations for access to health care (including home care and mental health care services) on consideration of society's ethical obligations, rather than rights. The Commission concluded that society has an ethical obligation to ensure equitable access to health care for all, which is balanced by individual obligation; that all citizens should be able to secure this adequate level of health care without excessive burdens; that costs ought to be shared fairly; and that efforts to contain health care costs should not focus on limiting equitable access to health care for the least well-served individuals and groups, such as those dependent on public programs. The federal government, according to the Commission, has the ultimate responsibility to ensure that society's obligation is met. To date, this obligation is far from being met, even with health care reform efforts by federal and state governments. Although each individual is not automatically ensured access to every available option in health care, an individual should never be denied necessary care solely because of inability to pay.

Determining an adequate level of health care is relative to an individual's health condition but would not automatically mean that society has an obligation to provide whatever care individuals think they need or that might be of marginal benefit. The societal obligation is to ensure adequate health care for everyone, delivered with respect.

Explicit consideration of these principles in decision-making will assist home care nurses and administrators in efforts to make more ethically adequate decisions. Difficult choices will still be required, and everyone may not agree with the choices (e.g., when respect for client autonomy and concerns for client safety conflict). Choices should reflect an ethical rationale that the decision-makers are aware of and can articulate to others, such as clients, families, agency staff, administrators, payors, and even legislators, in a clear and consistent way.

ETHICAL THEORIES: THEIR PLACE IN "REAL-LIFE" SITUATIONS

A purpose of ethical theories is to explain and justify concepts of what is good and right. Philosophers have argued about what is good and right for centuries. Ethical theories per se are not particularly helpful in resolving ethical dilemmas in client care or policy situations because they are too abstract for such purposes. This might be said of theories in general. Theories do lead in particular directions and provide specific frameworks for analysis of problems, but their purpose is not to provide concrete solutions. It is useful for home care nurses to be aware that ethical theories exist and are represented in a general or implicit way in the arguments, disagreements, and proposed resolutions to ethical problems and questions. Consideration of ethical principles and theories in decision-making may rule out actions that might be taken when decision-makers focus primarily on economic consequences.

In the bioethics literature, there has been a major emphasis on two families of ethical theory. One is deontology and the other is utilitarianism. Deontology emphasizes duties and obligations and argues that decision-makers should be able to universalize their actions and should never treat people solely as means to ends, such as viewing potential clients only as means to financial solvency of an agency. This theory also emphasizes that certain actions or rules and principles are considered to be inherently right or wrong without regard to consequences, such as respect for autonomy.

A second set of theories, including utilitarianism, focuses on consequences of rules or actions and is more community oriented. Consequence-based utilitarians argue that the greatest utility or good will be obtained by making decisions that seek to enhance the greatest amount of happiness or the least amount of unhappiness for the greatest number of people. Administrators often use this theory implicitly in their decision-making. A limitation of using this theory is that an individual client who lacks payment for home care may not get needed care, since more people will benefit from agency survival in the long run. Generally, in health care situations, decision-makers use a combination of the two theories described or these two sets of theories in combination with others, such as feminist ethical theory, which focuses on responsibilities to specific people and relationships to determine the right decisions and actions. For example, the nurse working with Mr. and Mrs. P. would encourage Mr. P. to consider both his obligations to Mrs. P. and their daughter and the probable consequences of his decisions before taking action. The nurse would also consider the consequences of different options for future relationships within the P. family and discuss the options with all of the family members.

In summary, after consideration of these ethical values, principles, and concepts and careful assessment and discussion with Mrs. P., her family, and her physician, the nurse determines that Mrs. P.'s medical condition and home circumstances require hospitalization for treatment of her pneumonia. Not everyone will agree with this decision, but an ethically supportable rationale exists for such action.

INSTITUTIONAL MECHANISMS FOR RESPONDING TO ETHICAL PROBLEMS

A reasoned decision-making process is necessary for dealing with ethical problems related to client care and agency policy in any setting. A process such as the one discussed in this chapter can be used by home care nurses to respond to ethical problems in individual client-care situations and by agency administrators to develop, review, and evaluate agency policy. There are several institutional mechanisms for dealing with ethical problems, such as ethics rounds, nursing ethics committees, and agency ethics committees.

Ethics rounds provide a forum similar to client-care conferences. The major focus is on the ethical problems in the situation rather than on the client's medical problems and prognosis, which are included here as a critical part of the information base. Participants would include all of those involved in the care of the client and the client and family, if they are able and wish to participate to ensure adequate consideration of the client's goals and values. Discussion would focus on the ethical principles and values at stake, duties and obligations of the client (if appropriate), family, home care nurses, and the agency and ways that relevant ethical principles and values, such as respect for people, avoidance of harm, and protection of family relationships, would be enhanced or harmed by the identified options. In addition, there would probably be some discussion of the issue of paternalism and the person who should make major decisions if Mr. and Mrs. P. are unable to do so by identified criteria.

One criterion might be that both Mr. and Mrs. P. are unable to make major decisions that are clearly in their best interests. For example, Mrs. P. might insist that she wants only her husband to care for her, but her condition rapidly deteriorates when her husband is the only one providing her direct care. Such a situation might justify a position known as *weak paternalism,* which allows intervention based on a client's defects or limitations, such as an inability to consider alternative choices or choices that clearly put others in jeopardy or do not reflect his or her own previously stated goals and values related to health and nursing care—a substantially nonautonomous decision. *Strong paternalism* would allow interventions based on probability of harm even though the client's choices are considered to be informed, voluntary, and autonomous (Beauchamp, Childress, 1994). The home care nurse might assess that Mrs. P. is able to make informed and voluntary choices but arrange for other types of care based on the avoidance of further harm and deterioration of Mrs. P.'s physical condition.

Ideally, ethical dimensions would be considered as an integral part of a comprehensive client-care conference for all clients as one example of preventive ethics. Such discussion has a goal of modifying or preventing "ethical crises" for clients, families, and caregivers. Conferences could probably not be done in every instance because of time pressures and other practical constraints, but they have the potential for improving care of home care clients through anticipation of possible ethical problems. Examples might include terminally ill clients who have expressly stated that they wish to die at home although family members may want them in the hospital or a hospice when they are imminently dying. Such an approach could also be used in developing or modifying agency policy for recurring ethical problems, such as withdrawal of specific medical interventions (e.g., artificial nutrition and hydration) and termination of client care for considerations of reimbursement or safety of staff members who have 24-hour responsibility for client care in unsafe areas.

A second possible institutional mechanism is a nursing ethics committee, which might be more appropriate in a large home care agency with a variety of services. Purposes of such a committee include educating nurses about the ethical dimensions of their practice, delineating types of ethical problems that confront home care nurses, and formulating a decision-making process for dealing with these problems. Such a committee could also be used for orientation of new agency nurses and for retrospective and prospective review of an agency's caseload to determine how best to resolve the ethical problems that have been and are currently in the agency caseload. A major goal would be to ensure that decisions and actions by nurses and agency policy are taking into explicit account the conflicting ethical principles and values in any given situation and that the goals and values of clients, to the degree that they can be determined, are always considered in planning nursing care. Small agencies might wish to join with other agencies to pool their resources for ethics-education purposes. This possibility would be applicable to a third mechanism for dealing with ethical problems in home care.

A third institutional mechanism is an agency or system-wide ethics committee that would be representative of the agency staff and community served. Such a committee has as its major purposes ensuring more reasoned decision-making in client care, education, and policy development that takes the ethical aspects of practice into explicit account. Ensuring that the best interests of clients are served is the major reason for such a committee to exist. This is not always easy to do in the present era when cost containment is an overriding concern and agencies are struggling to survive under greater legal and economic constraints. Such a mechanism does provide a place where ethical tensions can be discussed from a variety of perspectives in a sympathetic forum. Such a committee might develop policies or guidelines for consideration in situations similar to that of Mr. and Mrs. P. An agency ethics committee could also serve as a forum for a prospective consultation on client-care situations that present ethical problems to individual nurses and to the agency. Discussion that takes the ethical aspects of practice into explicit account will not provide ready-made answers, but it does begin to rule out certain actions and point to more ethically justifiable decisions and actions. These decisions and actions should be congruent with an agency's mission and goals. Another function is to discuss and reflect on home care codes of ethics and their meaning in the context of individual nursing practice and agency culture. Another option is to make available an individual with expertise in clinical and organizational ethics, an ethics consultant, who can serve as a resource in dealing with ethical problems in a home care agency or group of agencies.

Nurses in home care agencies can provide the leadership necessary to ensure that mechanisms for discussion and resolution of ethical problems exist, as they have done in many acute-care settings. Nurses do not have to remain totally frustrated or isolated in dealing with the ethical problems that confront them. At the same time, nurses must recognize that dealing with ethical problems in home care agencies requires sensitivity to the political, cultural, legal, and economic realities within which nursing and health care are delivered. These realities will always be in conflict with the ethical and moral dimensions of care delivered by individual nurses and by agencies, who may themselves hold differing personal or professional values in a given situation. Forums for sensitive discussion of such tensions and conflicts are an achievable reality. Through such discussions, nurses and other participants have a better understanding of what is at stake from an ethical or value perspective that is critical to the moral integrity of individuals and agencies.

FUTURE CHALLENGES

Dealing with ethical problems in home health care in turbulent environments in which a cost-containment mentality prevails is a major challenge for nurses who are committed to client advocacy and justice in the delivery of needed home health care. The integrity of individual nurses, the nursing profession, client health and safety, and quality of care are at stake as efforts are made to learn to deal with the ethical questions and problems in home care settings created by cost containment and new technologies. A new ethic is needed in nursing and health care that is adequate to the situations confronting society, organizations, caregivers, families, and clients. The development of an adequate ethic for nursing and health care delivery in the present and future must be part of the agenda for the nursing profession and for public policy decision-makers—an ethic that considers individual, organizational, and social aspects. The integrity of health care systems and of home care as a system component is at stake.

REFERENCES

American Nurses Association (ANA): *Council of community health nurses: Standards of community health nursing practice,* Kansas City, 1986, The Association.

Bandman B: The human rights of patients, nurses, and other health professionals. In Bandman EL, Bandman B, eds: *Bioethics and human rights,* Boston, 1978, Little, Brown.

Beauchamp TL, Childress JF: *Principles of biomedical ethics,* ed 4, New York, 1994, Oxford University Press.

Davis AJ et al: *Ethical dilemmas and nursing practice,* ed 4, Norwalk, Conn, 1997, Appleton-Century-Crofts.

Minnesota Assembly of Home and/or Community Health Nursing Agencies: *Code of ethics,* Roseville, Minn, 1984, Minnesota League for Nursing.

National Association for Home Care: *National Association for Home Care code of ethics, Caring* 19(8):26-27, 2000.

President's Commission for the Study of Ethical Problems in Medicine and Biomedical and Behavioral Research: *Securing access to health care: The ethical implications of differences in the availability of health services,* vol 1, Washington, DC, 1983, US Government Printing Office.

28 Stress and Burnout in the Home Health Care Professional

Ann G. Widmer

Stress, stated simply, is the way an individual interprets and responds to an event. What is perceived to be stressful to one person may be challenging and exciting to another. Not all stress is bad. Weddings, job promotions, and vacations can all produce stress, but most identify these as harmless stress events. However, the stress of caregiving in an imperfect system can be fatiguing. Such emotional fatigue can result in burnout.

Burnout is the progressive process of fatigue and depletion of resources; energy is reduced, and the possibility of investing in others is diminished. Nurses who experience burnout most often use the adjectives *stagnant, ineffective, bitter, visionless, tired,* and *resigned* to describe their state. Burnout is a syndrome of emotional exhaustion and cynicism that occurs among individuals who do "people work" when the worker's emotional resources are depleted (Toscano, 1998). Perhaps the opposite of burnout is vitality. The word *vitality,* as used in this context, means a sense of aliveness, optimism, and well-being. According to Hover-Kramer, Mabbett, and Shames (1996), "vitality engenders a feeling of positive energy, whereas burnout is the depletion of energy." The individual with vitality will find meaning in a task and will be motivated and enriched through caregiving. In contrast, "an individual without vitality will experience a similar situation as impossible, demoralizing, and depleting." McConnell (1981, 2000) reminds us that burnout is not the result of an occasional "bad day"; it is the product of constant emotional stress over time, combinations of stressors, and the individual's ability to cope. It may be a state of fatigue and frustration brought about by devotion to a cause, task, or relationship that fails to produce the expected reward. Those most likely to experience burnout share certain personality characteristics: unassertiveness, submissiveness, anxiousness, and fearfulness (Toscano, 1998). Maslach (1982) describes these same people as being, in addition, intolerant and lacking in confidence. They exhibit little ambition or sense of personal accomplishment.

Stress is produced in response to a crisis. Energy levels rise rapidly and remain elevated to provide the mental and physical strength necessary to work the problem through. As the situation is resolved, the stress is reduced, and the body returns to normal. Such resolution is usually achieved in 1 of 3 ways: (1) goal-directed action is taken, (2) insight or learning is gained, or (3) closure is achieved conceptually (in other words, "It is over"). Staying at the resistance stage can produce exhaustion, whereas resolution allows rest (Bandler et al, 2000).

Chronic stress, rather than acute crisis, appears to bring about the highest degrees of burnout (Toscano, 1998). Caregivers are under constant pressure, yet may rarely see the problems with which they deal resolved. According to Bramhall and Ezell (1981a), people working in stressful situations "may not be able to rest, physically or emotionally, after the stress of the day—or even the previous hour. They do not return to the stage of resolution and, as a result, find themselves operating with less and less energy." The end stage of this loss of energy is burnout. As a note, nurses are not alone in experiencing burnout. During the first quarter of 1998, Aon Consulting interviewed a broad set of workers nationally and found that 53% of employees were feeling some degree of burnout, up dramatically from 39% in 1995, when they did a similar survey (Coutu, 1998).

CAUSES OF STRESS

The first step in preventing burnout is recognizing the stressors that are draining on emotional reserves. Causes of stress can be either system-generated or self-generated.

System-Generated Causes

System-generated causes of stress that originate in the work or professional setting include working conditions, supervisory and administrative styles, communication structures, relationships with colleagues, appropriateness of position, politics, and pay scale and advancement opportunities.

Changes in the home care industry during the last decade have been rapid and intense. There have been increases in client activity levels, skill expectations, and care requirements (Potter et al, 1998). These changes have had a major impact on the delivery of services and working conditions. As efforts to reduce inpatient lengths of stay grow, the "quicker-but-sicker" client discharge will continue to spur the growth of home health care (Murray, 1998). Home health care nurses also have felt the effects of the interim payment system (IPS), the advent of the Outcomes Assessment and Information Set (OASIS), and the pressure of scrutiny from payor sources and regulatory agencies (Haydel, 1998). The prospective payment system (PPS) requires nurses to work proactively and develop solid strategic plans.

More generally, the environment in which a health care professional works can be either barren or nurturing. Although workplace stresses often flow from social, economic, or political conditions beyond agency control, some improvements usually can be made (Bramhall, Ezell, 1981b). Heading the list of stress factors in the work situation are shortages of supplies, personnel, or both, which make it impossible to provide the quality of care with which the health care provider can be satisfied. Staffing conflicts, particularly those caused by widespread agency changes, including the addition of new components, such as computer systems or community partners, can create role instability (Potter et al, 1998). Moreover, an office that has high noise levels, inadequate telephone connections, or poor clerical support can escalate otherwise tolerable tension.

Supervisory and administrative styles Supervisors can also be potential sources of stress (Hemingway, Smith, 1999). A director or supervisor whom the staff perceives as clinically in-competent, weak in leadership, too demanding, or unappreciative is a stressor. One management style that creates widespread stress pits one employee against another in a competitive environment as a way of stimulating productivity. Leaders who are confused about goals or unrealistic about expectations or who pass down their own mistakes or errors in judgment also create employee dissonance, and eventually, stress. Still, secure professionals can function capably and even transcend such stress by setting, accomplishing, and documenting personal goals.

Communication structures Burnout occurs most often when a person senses a lack of control over the care he or she is providing. Such lack of control occurs when superiors dictate all decisions and plans cannot be changed even in positive ways. It also occurs when a person does not know how or if he or she is being evaluated. It is frustrating to be part of a system in which feedback is given to staff only when something goes wrong (Bramhall, Ezell, 1981b). The results of a study by Landsbergis (1988) provide evidence that burnout is significantly higher in jobs that combine high workload demands with low decision latitude. At a more tangible level, stress occurs in the management of information and messages. Delays in obtaining information from physicians and getting messages from the office and at the client's home and breakdowns in computer and telephone lines can be incredibly frustrating.

Relationships among colleagues Sometimes relationships among colleagues can be even more stressful than client needs. A lack of rapport with peers robs a person of the support group to whom he or she could otherwise turn for advice, praise, or comfort. Constant competition with co-workers for promotions, raises, and recognition also creates tension. Competition keeps staff members from sharing problems or revealing any doubts, which could be interpreted as weakness or incompetence and used against them. According to Maslach (1982), the lack of trust that exists in such settings can put invisible walls between potential allies. Failure to recognize and value expertise in colleagues is both a cause of and a symptom of burnout. An environment of derogatory comments regarding the perceived flaws, omissions, and failures of other nurses erodes self-esteem and decreases job satisfaction (Thomas, Droppleman, 1997).

Appropriateness of position   Jobs comprise many tasks, some of which may not be matched to an individual's training and experience. If a person is asked, for instance, to fulfill a role that requires more or less decision-making skill than he or she has acquired, pressure builds. Competencies and skills should be commensurate with work tasks because skills that are either underused or overestimated can cause stress at all levels. Nurses new to home health care, even if they have considerable nursing experience elsewhere, may be unfamiliar with community resources, care management, reimbursement, or the paperwork. Careful orientation and mentoring of new employees can decrease the stress of the unfamiliar (Murray, 1998).

Politics   Power struggles for positions and leadership roles are almost as frequent in nursing and its organizations as in other "miniempires," and nurses need practical approaches to handling such pressure. Leadership courses need to address the role of politics within nursing. Understanding lines of authority and job boundaries keeps politics in check, and an open management style among supervisors usually limits the effectiveness of negative political manipulations.

Pay-scale advancement and social rewards   Low pay for work that is comparable in responsibility and effort to higher-paying work can seem degrading. Even more discouraging is the perception that there are few or no opportunities for advancement. Well-designed and fairly-administered career ladders can provide necessary incentives. Nurses also tolerate stress better if they receive supportive social rewards (Visintini et al, 1996) and if their value is acknowledged periodically.

Self-Generated Causes

Age, sex, marital status, and educational levels
Stress can also be self-generated. Causes may be associated with a person's perceptions of and responses to tensions in his or her work or personal life (Tarolli-Jager, 1994).

The demographic characteristics of those who burn out can be discussed in general, even though there are specific exceptions. Both men and women seem to burn out in equal numbers, although they may respond to stress in different ways (Bennett, Michie, Kippax, 1991). Single people and those without children experience more burnout. Even though there are additional burdens in having a family, the support and self-esteem it adds counteract much of the emotional exhaustion at work. Younger, less-experienced workers are more susceptible to stress, and sadly, some even leave the profession as a result (Bennett, Michie, Kippax, 1991).

It is hard to separate the variables of education and job because education and the work available to people are so highly interrelated. People with higher levels of education do seem to have higher expectations, are more idealistic, and assume they will accomplish a great deal in life. Thus, while they also have greater opportunities to achieve fulfillment through more varied and responsible contributions, they risk falling short of their high goals. It has been suggested that, in fact, a nurse who identifies with and values the goals of the nursing profession may react more strongly and with greater stress when distracted from its ideals (Reilly, 1994).

Self-concept and coping strategies   Perhaps one of the variables most closely associated with high levels of stress is self-concept. A poor self-concept and lack of self-esteem cause a person to have little faith in overcoming difficulties, be less assertive in frustrating situations, and focus selectively on failures rather than successes (Maslach, 1982).

Stresses in an individual's personal life do affect productivity and satisfaction in the work setting. Marital problems, loneliness, parenting difficulties, financial strains, or even a lack of centeredness in an individual's personal life can seriously compound job-related frustrations (Patrick, 1979).

The loss of a significant partner through death, separation, or divorce can unravel the most carefully knitted professional role. When such a loss occurs, there is likely to be a loss of one or more functions that contribute to an individual's person identity (e.g., mother, wife, or lover). The loss must be compensated for in some way that restores that person's sense of well-being and identity. Such devastating separation from self can make functioning well in the work setting virtually impossible; this leads to the additional anxiety of not performing well and the erroneous guilt of "becoming a failure" in yet another area.

Personal motivations for becoming a health care professional   Although the motives of most caregivers are admirable, altruistic, and selfless, there are other reasons that people choose such careers. Some want to boost their self-esteem through doing what they consider to be "good deeds." This is not necessarily a bad motive; feeling good about one's work is essential, but expecting the client to provide such personal gratification leads to disappointment. Also, emotional empathy has been found to correlate positively with both emotional exhaustion and personal accomplishment. Stress is mediated by this sense of personal accomplishment (Williams, 1989). Others have found that compassion, rather than leading to burnout, actually helps prevent it (Lamendola, 1996).

The nurse believes that competent caring matters and that being sensitive to client needs is what nursing is all about. He or she hopes to help people to heal and to be cured. The relationship of hope to three of the components of burnout—depersonalization, emotional exhaustion, and personal accomplishment—has been assessed by Sherwin et al (1992). Higher levels of hope were significantly associated with lower emotional exhaustion and depersonalization and greater accomplishment. This commitment to good care clashes with the reality of a health care system that demands financial cost effectiveness or an unrealistic standard of productivity. The perfectionist who cannot compromise (in productive ways) and remain flexible will encounter extreme stress in the face of the constantly shifting health care–system regulations and demands (McConnell, 1981).

Professional goals and personal needs   Nurses continually face highly stressful client-care and decision-making situations. They expend personal emotional resources, sometimes for weeks and months, as they maintain high levels of emotional involvement with clients and families. Stress also occurs when nurses feel inequitably treated in their relationships with clients who either do not, or cannot, have positive emotional responses (VanYperen, 1996). They may feel inadequate when they want to "distance" themselves emotionally so that they can continue to function. This is not an abnormal reaction because there are basic psychological needs (Maslow, 1954) that include the following:

- The need to be respected
- The need for approval and recognition
- The need for independence and autonomy
- The need for control
- The need for affection and love

The degree to which these are important and the extent to which they are satisfied are related to burnout. The individual who seeks all of these in the work setting because there are few sources in his or her personal life may be headed for disillusionment. Also, if needs such as those for recognition, achievement, and control are excessive, the person may be in a no-win situation. He or she will become exhausted pursuing such ultimates.

Grief and work-related loss   The aged or dying client can force a person to deal with fears about dying or aging or to bring back unresolved grief over lost loved ones. Individuals who work in health-related fields often have a need to "make things better," giving to the elderly a sense of decreased vulnerability. It is impossible, however, for professionals to work in health care for very long without realizing their own vulnerability to illness, tragedy, and death. Acknowledging and responding to this awareness are nearly always stressful.

One of the most difficult problems in working with the dying is the constant need to establish and then relinquish relationships with people. No matter how committed a nurse is to the value of comforting care, the intensity of dying clients' daily circumstances is highly stressful for the nurse to witness. The situation often requires a nurse to meet the broad-spectrum needs of an entire family and to explore his or her own unresolved personal pain of loss.

General health   It is not always understood that the circle of fatigue, lack of exercise, and poor nutrition can be a cause of burnout as well as a symptom (Schneider, 1998). Habitually ignoring the need for rest will weaken the immune system and may lead to lost work time and low energy levels. Such fatigue will make difficult situations seem overwhelming (Bramhall, Ezell, 1981a). The immoderate use of alcohol, tranquilizers, or smoking to unwind and relax can seriously impair the caregiver's ability to handle work assignments, ultimately creating more tension. Conversely, the integration of Western techniques with alternative therapies is becoming the model for the twenty-first century. Nutritious diet, meditation, and exercise converge in stress management (Jordan, 1998).

STRESS AS IT RELATES TO HOME CARE

Each specialty in nursing, such as pediatrics, hospice, or emergency department, has its own brand of stress, and home health care is no exception. Home health care is a general practice that encompasses concepts from mental-health nursing, parent-child nursing, and gerontological, medical-surgical, and community health nursing. Spending cutbacks have threatened the system as it strives to cope with an increasingly elderly and disease-prone population (Nichols, 2001). Home health care nurses are often challenged to care for clients from various clinical practices. Because clients may be assigned based on geographical boundaries, the coverage area may include clients with problems as diverse as congestive heart failure, insulin-dependent diabetes mellitus, and schizophrenia or cystic fibrosis (Murray, 1998). Although such variety certainly prevents boredom, having to devote personal time to find resources for clients who never have the same needs can be frustrating (Murray, 1998).

Working in the Client's Home

It takes real improvisational skills to find and use equipment and resources available in the client's home. It may also be difficult to work in a less than hygienic environment. Clients cannot always afford to order appropriate equipment. The control that comes with working in a professional facility may not be shared by the home health professional, who is viewed as a guest in the client's home. Being on the client's "turf" may create difficulties in compliance. For example, a client who conscientiously followed a diet, took medications, or completed exercises in the hospital may become less compliant when he or she is home.

Additional responsibilities include coordinating with the social worker what is and is not covered by Medicare, Medicaid, and private insurance and finding community groups that lend equipment or furnish supplies to people in financial need (Sherry, 1985). In "On the road with a home health nurse" (Senapatiratne, Venture, 1996) a typical working day is described. From the loading of five bags of medical supplies through a day of medicating, counseling, educating, treating, and doing paperwork, a picture emerges of multiple responsibilities. The day ends with reams of paperwork and calls to a physician, social worker, and adult protective services.

Placing Responsibility for Follow-Through in the Hands of Nonprofessionals

Family members who are concerned, supportive, and receptive to being trained can provide the most conscientious and loving care imaginable. Sometimes, however, the members of a support system are irresponsible, uninterested, or even actively resentful of their new roles as care partners. The counseling and affirmation it takes to keep such care providers stable and compliant are draining. Demonstrations may need to be repeated and care plans closely monitored. There may be a feeling of uneasiness with the extent to which care providers are actually doing what they report they are doing, and deciding whether and how to intervene is difficult.

Time, Distance, and Travel Schedules

Sometimes getting to the client is half the work. Time at each home, the distance between visits, and the traffic must all be considered if a reasonable schedule is to be maintained. In addition, as the day unfolds, new needs arise, or there may be changes in the planned daily schedule. Not having everything necessary for client care on arrival or having a car that is not in good running order can cause overwhelming frustration.

Status of Home Care Position

Although nursing as a profession has always been held in high esteem for its contributions to humanity, home care nurses have been viewed by some as providing less-sophisticated or less-specialized care than the nurse in the acute care setting. This is rapidly changing as heavier levels of care are being maintained in the home setting, but the home care nurse's felt need to justify this creative, sophisticated branch of nursing is often damaging to his or her self-esteem. Add to this the erroneous view that nursing in general, and home care specifically, is a nurturing "woman's work" role, and esteem is, for some, eroded even further. Thomas (1997) found that this societal lack of regard for nursing practice contributes to workplace anger and frustration.

Compensation and Quality Care

A primary interest of agencies must be their own financial stability. In times of growth, the interests of agencies and clients frequently coincide, since both the agency's and client's main concern is with more and better services. However, in a period of reduced reimbursement or limited funding, the agency's attention will shift from growth to maintenance. Such attempts to stabilize, or even cut back, may diverge from the best interests of both client and staff. Salaries may not keep up with inflation, programs may become short-staffed, and client services may be reduced. Productivity standards are receiving increased emphasis. All of this leads to stress for the nurse trying to maintain a high quality of care.

Continuous On-Call Status

Some home care nurses prefer to give clients their home phone numbers for use in emergencies. Unlike the facility nurse who knows his or her role is filled when he or she is not there, some home care nurses live in a 24-hour-a-day, 7 day-a-week, on-call situation with frail or very dependent clients. Such permanent, constant responsibility is cumulatively stressful. In the majority of home care agencies, the policy is to not give beeper numbers to clients so that a nurse can be called after hours. On-call nurses should fill this role for several very good reasons. When a nurse gives a beeper or home number, it may reflect a problem with co-dependence; this nurse may not want other nurses to visit the client. It also creates a liability issue for the home health agency if, when that nurse can't be reached, the client has not learned the correct way to contact the agency or does not feel comfortable using other nurses.

Degree of Isolation

Home care nurses may feel that there is a greater degree of isolation from outside ideas in the less academic or research-oriented home setting. Some home care nurses have little interaction with colleagues and pursue their day's work without substantial interface with other nursing professionals. Worthwhile and stimulating professional or educational opportunities can and need to be incorporated into home care agencies, or the brightest and most involved nurses will soon be bored and dissatisfied. If there are few opportunities for educational advancement, professional satisfaction levels will fall.

Client Dependency

Clients have the potential to become far more dependent in the home-care setting than in the multistaffed institutional setting. The visiting nurse becomes the primary link and conduit to most, if not all, facets of health care for the client, the most accessible "ear," and the focus of problem resolution. Nurses experience less stress when they are able to be engaged and caring without becoming overwhelmed by another's needs (Carmack, 1997).

Truth-Telling Issues

The home care nurse is often the focus of the client's requests for information. The client's legal and ethical rights to information may conflict with the nurse's directions for disclosure. It is sometimes difficult to coordinate the communication that should be taking place among physician, client, family, and counselor. Because the nurse is in and out of the home regularly, the client relies on him or her for the truth. Although it can seem quite rewarding and flattering to be so needed, it can also drain a nurse's emotional resources. A co-dependency or confidant relationship may develop, which would defeat any of the supportive team or group interactions that might be in place.

Difficult Clients

Difficult and violent clients take on a whole new dimension in the home setting. There is seldom an observer of client hostility or accusations, so there may be no backup for the home care nurse's position or decision. Issues of noncompliance, active or passive aggression, or fear and depression, which might be difficult to handle in the home setting, should be discussed by the health care team (Jones, 1986). The client may need to be transferred to a facility before proper care can be administered. Situations may be discovered in which a client is being neglected or abused or having medications stolen and sold that are out of the realm of nursing management. Yet it may be the home care nurse who first confronts and directs attention to these problems. A crisis must sometimes be handled quickly and decisively without the benefit of a team conference. As protection, nurses need to be aware of the policy an agency has in place to address this. If policies do not exist in the agency, a request for the development of a standard procedure should be made. Ordinarily, potential dangers would have been assessed, and the nurse would not be in the position of handling them, but sometimes knowing that such possibilities exist creates tension.

The client who will not allow himself or herself to be helped or who either actively or passively rejects help to the point that it becomes life-threatening can be discouraging. All the nurse's skills and energies will go into reversing such a situation.

When clients refuse to self-manage or work with the health care team, there can be a variety of consequences. A client's condition can worsen if he or she underuses his or her medications. A physician, not realizing that a client has not been taking his or her medication, may prescribe a larger dose. Clients with chronic diseases are likely to become less willing partners in care as they grow discouraged with extended therapy programs that do not produce a cure. Clients may conceal an alcohol problem or self-medicate. Combinations of confusion and fear may keep clients from following orders. It takes additional effort to monitor and encourage positive behaviors (Hitchcock, Schubert, Thomas, 1999).

Family Interactions

The home care nurse provides care in an arena of family interaction. The family may be the client's best support system, and the nurse's role becomes one of teacher and facilitator. In other cases, the family is absent or all efforts at engaging those present seem to fail. Few families are without some disagreement about the client's needs and may constantly hint or complain that the nursing care is inadequate. They may change care plans or refuse to comply with instructions between visits. They may quite honestly be grieving over or be frightened by the client's status. They may try to move the client to a facility to decrease their own responsibility. Their constant dissonance can be upsetting to the client, slowing the healing process.

Years of family problems cannot be resolved in a few weeks. Counseling is often the best ad-junct to care if family members will consent. It is sometimes next to impossible to remove the source of family stress, no matter how disabling the home health care team perceives it to be for the client. Some evidence suggests that home care nurses experience severe stress because they have heavy decision-making and leadership responsibilities (Patrick, 1979). As clients are discharged earlier with more complex care needs, this stress will increase.

Safety

The nurse is somewhat less safe in the home care setting. Automobile time, exposure to neighborhood dangers, and lack of proper equipment increase the chances for accidents. Hemingway and Smith (1999) report that nurses who experience role ambiguity were more likely to have a reportable accident at work. Associated with these accidents were also the variables of deficient training and working in unfamiliar settings. Every occupation has its hazards, but these dangers can increase the home care nurse's daily stress levels.

Paperwork

Reimbursement and legal requirements continue to increase the amount of nonclient contact hours with which home care nurses must contend. It is not unusual to find some nurses who feel that they spend more hours filling out forms and reports than they spend providing care. Not being prepared for this reality can cause frustration.

Long-Term Care

Many home care clients have long-term care needs. Professionals can become frustrated when their expectations for these clients are not met—and often they are not. For a sizable percentage of long-term clients, an important role of the nurse may be to provide support in the form of a personal relationship. Clients may feel less need for productively pursuing therapy or staying on medications or a proper diet. It is stressful to sort out just what a nurse does that is truly helpful in such cases (Lammert, 1981).

Some clients, particularly the elderly, will never get well, and many die while being cared for, and this can cause feelings of inadequacy

STRESS AND THE HOME HEALTH CARE NURSE

The following case addresses not the clinical management of clients, but the expectations, management, and organization related to stress in providing home care.

The day begins for Liz at 7:30 AM. The car needs to be loaded with four bags of medical supplies, including liquid nutritional supplements, charts, a nursing bag, and a venipuncture bag. There are seven clients to visit; two of them are beginning home care today.

The first client, a frail 87-year-old woman, is doing well. It is obvious she enjoys Liz's visits, and the dressing change she requires is completed quickly. Her only problem is a recurring nightmare that she would like to talk about. Liz listens for as long as she can, tries to reassure her, and makes a note to call the social worker. She realizes that she seems hurried and regrets the impression of her haste to leave.

The second and third clients, both new to home care, require extra time. Liz has been given incorrect information by the office staff, of whom Liz has been openly critical. The next new client, just home from the hospital, is up and doing well. He seems surprised by Liz's visit and perplexed by her procedures. By 10 AM, Liz is running 30 minutes behind, and the traffic is not cooperating. Hungry, she eats half of her lunch sandwich and drinks her thermos of coffee on the way to drop off blood work at the hospital.

The husband of the fourth client meets Liz in the entry hall and explains that his wife has soiled herself and will not dress or let him help her. He has not spoken to his wife since the night before when she angrily flushed her medication down the toilet. He wants Liz to confirm his opinion that his sons should help him put his wife in a nursing home.

The fifth client has had a coronary bypass graft, and his wife is also ill with a bad cold. Both speak only a little English, and Liz determines that he is experiencing some respiratory distress and is frightened. A call is made to his physician, who is in surgery, and

a message is left for a daughter who has previously indicated an interest. It is 3:00 in the afternoon, and Liz is now almost an hour behind schedule. A call to the office while driving to the home of client six results in being put on hold until Liz is in the next driveway. She leaves a message that she is running late. Angry, she enters the home of an 80-year-old woman who listens to her complaints and makes her a cup of tea to go with the other half of her sandwich, the first thing she has had to eat since 10:30. Liz receives a page that her seventh client has had her appointment moved to the next morning. "She will not be happy about that," Liz thinks. "I will call her when I get home."

It is 5:15 PM. There is still a report to be given to the supervisor, paperwork, and calls to be made to the pharmacist and social worker. Dinner will be a little late for the family, who will have probably already scattered to various activities. Liz thinks, "Why do they put up with me?"

CASE DISCUSSION

Liz is clearly approaching burnout. She exhibits many of the classic signs, as follows:

- *She is angry and frustrated, yet at times feels sad and guilty.*
- *She is cynical and critical of the work she and others are doing.*
- *She evaluates herself negatively.*
- *She is emotionally depleted.*
- *She has developed unhealthy patterns of eating and an unsatisfactory home life.*

A number of the stressful factors associated with burnout presented earlier in the chapter are evident in this case. Both unrealistic client load and time-management issues seem likely. There is perhaps an unwillingness to or lack of knowledge about how to share responsibility for clients. Work and home have merged into an unhealthy work continuum. The first step in reversing this process is for Liz to recognize these symptoms of stress.

(Ufema, 1999). The client who makes little or no progress despite high-quality nursing and the client who returns to the hospital or to a long-term care facility can, if the nurse is not equipped to deal with the realities of the life continuum, lead to a sense of failure and despair (Lamb, 1979).

RECOGNITION OF SYMPTOMS OF STRESS AND BURNOUT

If burnout is to be prevented, its symptoms must be recognized. Stress to the point of burnout is an emotional, mental, and physical condition that is manifested in an array of symptoms. Burnout should be distinguished from general depression. Although burnout may look somewhat like depression, its symptoms are very different and can be defined more specifically (Bramhall, Ezell, 1981). It has basic, consistently identifiable elements, such as emotional exhaustion, shift toward negative attitudes, and a sense of personal devaluation that occur over time (Patrick, 1979).

Physical Symptoms

Many of the first symptoms of burnout are physical—increasing levels of fatigue, easy tiring, sleep disturbances, low levels of energy, and changes in appetite and weight. There may be lowered resistance to infection, and a variety of physiological dysfunctions, such as gastrointestinal disturbances, headaches, and neckaches. In many cases, the major physical consequence of stress is a tiredness even before work begins and a sense of physical depletion.

Emotional Symptoms

Emotional exhaustion also occurs, and the care provider experiences a sense of being drained by interpersonal contact, first with clients and then with families. Such emotional exhaustion can contribute to negative thinking and generally uncharacteristic emotions, such as inappropriate anger, fault finding, depression, or withdrawal. Key aspects of the burnout syndrome are increased feelings of cynicism and the development of negative self-concept. Burnout has also been equated with loss of idealism and loss of spirit. Experiencing these occasionally is normal, but their increasing frequency may indicate increasing stress.

Psychological Symptoms

One of the chief symptoms of burnout is a declining ability to make decisions. As the health care professional who is experiencing burnout tries to maintain order and control over surroundings, tolerance for ambiguity decreases. There may be a sense of alienation. According to Patrick (1979), "decision making within multiple-option situations becomes more difficult." Thus the person may categorize options and see things as black and white or right and wrong. He or she loses the flexibility necessary to consider alternatives and stay open to creative resolutions.

When things do not go as desired, a shift in attitude may take place regarding both colleagues and clients. "Colleagues may be viewed as adversaries" and clients as "difficult" or "complainers" to maintain the negative viewpoint (Patrick, 1979).

Social Symptoms

Symptoms of job-associated stress also affect a person's personal and social life. Unhappiness, negative opinions, or withdrawal may alienate friends and family when an individual needs them most. At the same time, he or she may be attracted socially to people who are also experiencing severe stress and share the negative attitudes, dissatisfactions, and common problems. Rather than being supportive, the social life may actually contribute to the debilitation.

Stress that cannot be resolved while on the job is often resurrected at home. Sometimes the health care professional is unaware of the job-related causes and wrongly attributes the dissonance to something in the family relationship. Furthermore, according to Maslach and Leiter (1997), burnout correlates with other damaging indices of human stress, such as alcoholism, mental illness, marital conflict, and suicide.

Although there is no definite point at which people burn out from stress, patterns can be spotted that might indicate the beginnings of burnout. One scale that considers not only the symptoms of stress but also the duration, frequency, and intensity is shown in Fig. 28-1. Having a close working partner fill this form out can also reveal discrepancies in areas a stressed person has preferred to overlook. The more overstressed an individual is, the more difficult it is to recognize a problem (McConnell, 1981).

SYMPTOMS PHYSICAL	Duration				Frequency			
	1 Mo.	6 Mo.	1 Yr.	Sev. Yrs.	Mnthly	Wkly	Daily	Con-stantly
Fatigue/lethargy								
Depression								
Insomnia/sleepiness								
Headaches/neckaches								
Gastrointestinal problems								
Lingering minor illness								
Weight loss or gain								
Shortness of breath								
Tightness in throat								
Crying easily								
Dependence on alcohol								
Dependence on drugs								
INTERPERSONAL & BEHAVIORAL								
Bored								
Anxious								
Discouraged								
Resentful/bitter								
Irritable								
Fault-finding								
Quick to anger								
Resistant to change								
Work harder/enjoy less								
Pass up breaks								
Live for breaks								
Careless								
Defensive								
Resigned								

Fig. 28-1   Burnout symptoms.

DECREASING STRESS

As is exhibited by the case study, stress can be an "inside job." The way a person responds and the extent to which stressors impact a person depend on his or her environment and development history, because each person has unique adaptive habits that have been selected and reinforced by life experiences (McConnell, 1981). People have two kinds of adaptive systems to deal with emotional stress: noncognitive and cognitive. Noncognitive strategies, some healthy, some not, include efforts to get relief without resolving or clarifying the problem. Examples include jogging, letting off steam to a coworker, or eating a banana split. Studies of the relationship between exercise activity and stress often reveal that individuals with higher exercise levels reported higher feelings of personal accomplishment that correlated negatively with emotional exhaustion. In other words, more exercise equals less burnout. Electronic sources of stress relief also exist; in MacUser, nine stress-relieving software programs are reviewed from CD calisthenics to meditations in Kyoto Gardens (Breen, 1997).

Stress-reduction educational materials frequently suggest finding ways to meditate: breathing deeply with the eyes closed and visualizing a peaceful favorite scene. Almost all advise searching for humor, since almost any situation contains comic elements (Thomas, 1997). In the article "Being centered, setting limits and having fun," Scott (1997) suggests that when faced with multiple responsibilities and fierce ambitions, many individuals fail "to keep life in its proper perspective by having fun." Being able to laugh at stressors is important also. One nursing periodical (You're obsessed with home health care if . . . , 2000) has published a humorous "How to know if you're obsessed with home health care" list. It pokes good-natured fun at nurses who automatically do a home-safety assessment while having dinner at a friend's house, feel guilty about staying anywhere longer than 25 minutes, or are only comfortable eating if they are in a car. Taking time to relax with recreational activities also balances out demanding work schedules.

The second type, cognitive strategies, includes conscious adaptive and problem-solving techniques, such as brain-storming alternative solutions, seeking specialized help, planning new courses of action, analyzing responses and feelings, and establishing support systems. It has been demonstrated that support groups can help nurses feel less isolated and allow them to share feelings regarding death, anger, helplessness, and loss. Just developing rapport with colleagues can relieve a tense environment (Willard, 1999). Support groups that focus on awareness and shared experiences and that help participants identify the emotional consequences of their work are most helpful (Grossman, Silverstein, 1993).

One unexpected finding in a study of stress and burnout in oncology was that the greater a

person's perception of himself or herself as religious, the lower the level of burnout (Kash, 2000).

There are many ways to use adaptive habits more effectively or learn new, more successful ones. Techniques that promote physical and psychological well-being can do much to offset the negative costs of burnout. Because burnout is treatable, human professional potential need not be wasted (Andrica, 1996). A "tend or befriend" response rather than the traditional "fight or flight" response may promote safety and reduce distress (Taylor et al, 2000).

Maslach, in her historical book, *Burnout: The Cost of Caring* (1982), outlines techniques that are still used for handling stress independently and through social and organizational approaches.

There are a number of things the individual can do to develop techniques to cope with stress. Some involve simply becoming aware of problem areas and truly understanding their sources (Siska, 1997). Evidence supports the assumption that appropriate training also decreases the level of response to stressors (Demmer, 2000). Such understanding can often eliminate the frustrations of tasks or interactions that previously seemed threatening, useless, or burdensome. Other techniques for coping are extremely difficult to cultivate, since they may represent considerable learning or attitude changes.

The first category focuses on changing things about the work setting itself and includes the following:

- Setting realistic goals and evaluation methods
- Creating work variety and respite
- Performing more efficiently
- Reviewing lines of control, responsibility, and communication

Although an ideal such as improving the quality of health care for all is advisable, it is virtually impossible for an individual to achieve. Ideals should act as guiding principles or beliefs that encourage, stimulate action, and provide hope. Objectives, on the other hand, are specific, concrete, and measurable. For example, it is idealistic to believe that the grief an elderly person is experiencing in losing his or her health, spouse, and independence can be removed. The powerlessness to take away such grief will overwhelm the care provider. However, objectives for providing support, comfort, activity, and independent function can be implemented, and satisfaction can be experienced by both client and provider. According to Carmack (1997), people who balance engagement with detachment learn how to set limits and boundaries. A sense of personal control is fundamental to this balance.

This ability to "let go" is essential when a nurse has done all that can be done (Arnold, 1990). Not everything can be done alone, and everything cannot be changed immediately, yet many people feel extremely guilty when they say "no" to unrealistic requests or demands others make of them.

Devising new ways of doing things can occur even in relatively rigid and routine jobs. It may be possible to reschedule the order of tasks for efficiency, repace particularly distressing tasks, or group boring chores to cut down on the time spent doing them. It can be useful to reevaluate the reasons things have always been done a certain way (Maslach, 1982). It is important to take real, not partial, breaks from the pressures of the job. Returning telephone messages on break or calling the office to direct the writing of a grant or budget every day of vacation is not respite.

Sometimes a thorough reassessment of the job description or the ways communication does or does not work in favor of productivity and cooperation can help. If it is difficult for supervisors and staff to get time together because they are in and out of the agency at opposite times, just rescheduling a morning or two a week so that schedules intersect might ease the pressure.

The second category of things that can be done individually includes changes in general attitudes and behaviors, such as the following:

- Developing problem-solving skills
- Improving interpersonal and communication skills
- Taking care of physical health through rest, exercise, and sensible nutrition
- Assessing ambitions and ideals and developing a realistic career plan
- Understanding personal needs
- Discovering and using relaxation and decompression techniques
- Cultivating a social life apart from work
- Working on constructive assertive techniques, self-esteem, and confidence

These include some of the most important of life's tasks. Most people continue to work on

them throughout their careers, but improvement in these areas can be a positive step in both personal growth and stress reduction. Those who are sensitive to their personal reactions and are willing to attempt to understand the underlying reasons for them frequently find they are far more able to cope with stress (Maslach, 1982). Relaxation techniques help almost as soon as they are begun. They include muscle relaxation, mental relaxation, and mental imagery. Books, video and audio cassettes, and classes exist to guide those who want to learn more about them and practice their benefits (Maslach, 1982).

Those who have good problem-solving skills and confidence can frequently restructure a situation into a more positive experience. Assertiveness training is recommended as a valuable tool in decreasing emotional exhaustion by increasing perceived personal control over decision-making in the workplace (Ellis, Miller, 1993). According to Thomas (1997), the ABCs of effective action are assertiveness, bargaining, and coalition-forming. Specific actions include translating anger into an assertive request (clearly stated as "I need—"), bargaining to obtain better conditions, and forming a coalition with other nurses to tackle a common problem. Making good things happen begins with a nurse understanding his or her own needs (Hamilton, 1986). In addition, it is essential to maintain a balanced social life and to associate with committed, concerned colleagues.

One important step is recognizing the need for additional support or counseling (Buechler, 1985). Too many people in the caring professions feel that because they have been trained to care for the problems of others in an effective way, they can handle their own problems without help. An objective friend or professional can provide help in the forms of comfort, insight, comparison, rewards, humor, modeling, and escape. A supportive workplace can protect against burnout, particularly during times of change and uncertainty in the work environment (Garrett, 2001).

Administrative Changes

Administrative changes in the way an agency, program, or organization functions can also reduce stress. These changes may include the following:

- Redividing work tasks
- Making changes in work environment

- Balancing working, on-call, and off hours
- Providing continuing education
- Fostering peer support
- Providing positive evaluation and feedback
- Pacing work concentration and deadlines
- Balancing responsibility and compensation
- Rewarding achievement
- Handling dissonance professionally
- Providing channels for complaint and remedy

Administrators who practice good management skills will decrease stress in the agency for which they are responsible. Understanding and facilitating such management styles as a staff member will improve job satisfaction for all those involved. Staff meetings that focus on perhaps one or two of the tasks just mentioned are far more productive in the long run than weekly gripe sessions, although there should be also a time for regular airing of difficulties. Before change is made, it should be carefully analyzed; simply changing things does not always improve anything. Moving in conscientiously planned directions, however, often provides far-reaching improvement in stress levels. The changes may be as simple as providing reasonably quiet, private space for deskwork; organizing the storage of supplies; or improving lighting and ventilation. It may be necessary to reduce or rearrange on-call hours. Management's recognition of personal and family life ranked first, above salary, in importance for employee satisfaction (Coutu, 1998). It is important for staff first to define the source or sources of stress as specifically and professionally as possible if requests or plans for reduction are going to be accepted. Benefits such as a lowering of absentee rates, a decrease in health insurance claims, and greater productivity can be cited as incentives to administration to hasten the improvements.

SUMMARY

The costs of burnout can be high; both the caregiver and the client are negatively affected by it, and the home health care agency with which they are associated becomes less effective. Personal incidents, turnover, nurse injuries, and client incidents all may increase. Families and programs can be the victim of the helper's negative, isolated, and depersonalized view of the world. Helping and caring for other people is highly de-

manding work. Meeting these demands without falling victim to burnout can best be done by people who are strong in both body and spirit and who make sure they stay that way. It is well worth both the personal and professional effort it may take to reduce stress in the job setting.

REFERENCES

Andrica DC: Burnout: Is it happening to you? And what to do? *Nursing Economics* 14(5):313-314, 1996.

Arnold LJ: Codependency. Part III: Strategies for healing, *AORN Journal* 52(1):85-89, 1990.

Bandler R et al: Active vs. passive emotional coping, *Brain Research Bulletin* 53(1):95-104, 2000.

Bennett L, Michie P, Kippax S: Quantitative analysis of burnout and its associated factors in AIDS nursing, *AIDS Care* 3:181-192, 1991.

Bramhall M, Ezell S: How burned out are you? I. *Public Welfare* Winter:23-27, 1981a.

Bramhall M, Ezell S: Working your way out of burnout. II. *Public Welfare* Spring:32-39, 1981b.

Breen C: The laid-back mac, *MacUser* 13(4):155-175, 1997.

Buechler DK: Help for the burned-out nurse? *Nursing Outlook* 32(4):181-182, 1985.

Carmack B: Balancing engagement and detachment in caregiving, *Image: Journal of Nursing Scholarship* 29(2):139-143, 1997.

Coutu D: Human resources: The wages of stress, *Harvard Business Review* 76(6):21-24, 1998.

Demmer C: Relationship between death-related experiences, death anxiety among AIDS nursing staff, *Journal for Nursing Staff Development* 16(3):118, 2000.

Ellis BH, Miller KI: The role of assertiveness, personal control, and participation in the prediction of nurse burnout, *Journal of Applied Communication Research* 21(4):327-342, 1993.

Garrett DK, McDaniel AM: A new look at nurse burnout, *Journal of Nursing Administration* 31(2):91, 2001.

Grossman AH, Silverstein C: Facilitating support groups for professionals working with people with AIDS, *Social Work* 38(2):144-151, 1993.

Hamilton JM: You're not an angel, you're a nurse, *Nursing* 16(5):113-115, 1986.

Haydel J: Help for home health strategies, *Nursing Management* 29(12):30-32, 1998.

Hemingway M, Smith CS: Organizational climate and occupational stressors as predictors of withdrawal behaviors and injuries in nurses, *Journal of Occupational and Organizational Psychology* 72:285-299, 1999.

Hitchcock JE, Schubert PE, Thomas SA: *Community health nursing,* Albany, 1999, Delmar.

Hover-Kramer D, Mabbett P, Shames KH: Vitality for caregivers, *Holistic Nursing Practice* 10(2):38-49, 1996.

Jones MK: For the patient who makes caring difficult, *Nursing* 16(5):45-46, 1986.

Jordan P: A prescription for good health, *American Fitness* 16(5):5-6, 1998.

Kash KM et al: Stress and burnout in oncology, *Oncology* 14(11):1621-1633, 2000.

Lamb HR: Staff burnout in work with long-term patients, *Hospital Community Psychiatry* 30(6): 396-398, 1979.

Lamendola F: Keeping your compassion alive, *American Journal of Nursing* 96(11):16, 1996.

Lammert M: A group experience to combat burnout and learn group process skills, *Journal of Nursing Education* 20(6):41-46, 1981.

Landsbergis PA: Occupational stress among health care workers, *Journal of Organizational Behavior* 9(3):217-239, 1988.

Maslach C: *Burnout—The cost of caring,* Englewood Cliffs, NJ, 1982, Prentice-Hall.

Maslach C, Leiter MP: *The truth about burnout: How organizations cause personal stress and what to do about it,* New York, 1997, Josey-Bass.

Maslow A: *Motivation and productivity,* New York, 1954, Harper & Row.

McConnell EA: How close are you to burnout? *RN* 11(5):29-31, 1981.

McConnell EA: Myths and facts about stress, *Nursing* 30(8):82, 2000.

Murray T: From outside the wall, *Journal of Continuing Education in Nursing* 29(2):55-59, 1998.

Nichols M: At the breaking point, *Maclean's* Jan 8, 2001.

Patrick P: Burnout: Job hazard for health workers, *Hospitals* 53(27):90-92, 1979.

Potter et al: Change. . . . ouch! *Nursing Management* 29(11):27-29, 1998.

Reilly NP: Exploring a paradox: Commitment as a moderator of the stressor-burnout relationship, *Journal of Applied Psychology* 24(5):397-414, 1994.

Schneider P: Staying healthy on a healthy schedule, *Nursing* 28(12):62-63, 1998.

Scott M: Being centered, setting limits and having fun, *Association Management* 49(3):55-57, 1997.

Senapatiratne L, Venture MJ: On the road with a home health nurse, *RN* 59(4):54-58, 1996.

Sherry D: The incredible, flexible nurse, *Nursing* 15(12):72, 1985.

Sherwin ED et al: Negotiating the reality of caregiving: Hope, burnout and nursing, *Journal of Social and Clinical Psychology* 11(2):129-139, 1992.

Siska N: Heart failure in a health care organization, *Nursing Management* 28(4):54-55, 1997.

Tarolli-Jager K: Personal hardiness: Your buffer against burnout, *American Journal of Nursing* 94(2):71-72, 1994.

Taylor SE et al: Biobehavioral responses to stress in females, *Psychology Review* 107(3):411-429, 2000.

Thomas SP, Droppleman P: Channeling nurses' anger into positive interventions, *Nursing Forum* 32(2):13-21, 1997.

Toscano P, Ponterdolph M: The personality of buffer burnout, *Nursing Management* 29(8):32-33, 1998.

Ufema J: Never forgive—Or never forget? *Nursing* 29(9):24-25, 1999.

VanYperen NW: Communal orientation and the burnout syndrome among nurses, *Journal of Applied Social Psychology* 26(4):338, 1996.

Visintini R et al: Psychological stress in nurses' relationships with HIV-infected patients, *AIDS Care* 8(12):183-194, 1996.

Willard J: Round the clock, *Nursing* 29(9):68, 1999.

Williams CA: Empathy and burnout in male and female helping professionals, *Research in Nursing and Health* 12(3):169-178, 1989.

You're obsessed with home health care if . . . , *Nursing* 30(1):84, 2000.

29 Advanced-Practice Nursing in Home Care

Karen L. Schumacher and Carmen J. Portillo

The emergence of advanced-practice home care nursing was one of the most significant developments in home care in the 1990s. The increasing complexity of acute- and chronic-illness care at home makes access to advance-practice nurses (APNs) imperative. Thus graduate education in home care is increasingly available and descriptions of the role of advanced-practice home care nurses are increasingly found in the literature.* In spite of these developments, however, the full potential of advanced-practice home care nursing has yet to be realized. Historically, constrained by reimbursement, organizational, and regulatory barriers, advanced-practice home care is too often invisible and underused (Scannell, 1995), and consumer access to the expertise of APNs currently is limited. The challenge for the future will be to build on the foundational work of recent years and make advanced-practice home care nursing more readily available to consumers who need it. Clearly articulating the nature of advanced-practice home care nursing will be central to this endeavor.

In this chapter is a brief historical overview of the development of two advanced-practice roles with great potential for home care: the clinical nurse specialist (CNS) role and the nurse practitioner (NP) role. Then the current status of advanced-practice home care nursing is described, and barriers to realizing the full potential of the role are analyzed. Finally, a model of advanced-practice home care nursing is proposed, and an agenda for further implementation of this level of nursing practice in home care is presented.

---

*Beuscher, 1991; Cyr, 1990; Hackbarth, Androwich, 1989; Miller, 1995; Milone-Nuzzo, 2000; Mitty, Mezey, 1998; Neal, 1995; Pierson, Minarik, 1999; Portillo, Schumacher, 1998; Scudder, 1996.

ADVANCED-PRACTICE NURSING

What is *advanced-practice nursing?* The answer to this question has been a matter of considerable debate over the past decade. Some use the term to describe the merger or fusion of the CNS and NP roles (Mezey, McGivern, 1993; Snyder, Mirr, 1995), whereas others use it broadly to describe a level of practice that can be operationalized through a variety of nursing roles, including CNS, NP, nurse anesthetist, and certified nurse midwife (Hamric, Spross, Hanson, 2000). The latter usage assumes that these roles have unique functions, as well as a common core of knowledge and practice. This chapter uses Hamric's definition: "Advanced-practice nursing is the application of an expanded range of practical, theoretical, and research-based therapeutics to phenomena experienced by patients within a specialized clinical area of the larger discipline of nursing" (Hamric, 2000). The primary defining criteria for advanced-practice nursing are (1) an earned graduate degree with a concentration in an advanced-nursing practice category, (2) professional certification of practice at an advanced level within a specialty, and (3) a practice focused on clients and their families (Hamric, 2000).

To understand advanced-practice nursing, it is helpful to distinguish between the terms *specialization, role expansion,* and *advanced practice* (Hamric, 2000), because these terms are often used incorrectly. They are not interchangeable terms. *Specialization* is concentration or delimitation of focus to part of the whole field of nursing. A nurse can specialize without graduate education. Specialization can occur through experience or through continuing education and certification in a delimited area of nursing, such as enterostomal therapy or intravenous therapy. Expansion is the acquisition of new practice knowledge and skills, including the knowledge and skills that legitimize role autonomy within areas of practice that overlap traditional boundaries of medical practice. Role expansion also can occur without graduate education. For example, many NP programs originally were certificate rather than degree programs. However, nurses completing certificate programs could properly be described as functioning in an expanded role. Advancement involves both specialization and expansion and is characterized by the integration of a broad range of theoretical, research-based, and practical knowledge that occurs as a part of graduate education (American Nurses Association [ANA] Social Policy Statement, 1995; Hamric, 2000).

All APN roles are characterized by skills that constitute the core competencies of advanced practice. First and foremost is the central competency of direct clinical practice. Skill in direct clinical practice is central to and informs all other APN core competencies, as follows (Hamric, 2000):

1. Expert guidance and coaching of clients, families, and other care providers
2. Consultation
3. Research skills, including utilization, evaluation, and conduct
4. Clinical and professional leadership, which includes competence as a change agent
5. Collaboration
6. Ethical decision-making skills

These core competencies form the common foundation upon which role-specific skills are built. Role-specific knowledge, such as knowledge about primary care for NPs and knowledge about disease-specific pathophysiology for CNSs, builds on this foundation.

Although all APNs share the primary defining criteria and core competencies, advanced-practice nursing is operationalized through a variety of roles, including CNS, NP, a blended CNS/NP acute-care NP, case manager, nurse midwife, and nurse anesthetist (Hamric, Spross, Hanson, 2000). The particular role through which advanced-practice nursing is operationalized depends on the needs of the client population and the organizational structure in which the APN is working. New roles or new combinations of these roles may arise according to the needs of society and the health care system.

The advanced-practice roles implemented to date in home care are the CNS and NP. Case management, although now often identified as an advanced-practice role (Mahn, Zazworsky, 2000; Schroer, 1991; Wells, Erickson, Spinella, 1996), has derived its conceptualization in home care from community-health nursing and typically refers to the level of care delivered by Bachelor of Science in Nursing (BSN)–prepared nurses. Case managers in home care conduct comprehensive assessments, coordinate multidisciplinary care, and work collaboratively with community resources. Although an advanced-practice component of case management in home care may be identified in the future, distinguishing between BSN and advanced-practice case management is beyond the scope of this chapter. Thus discussion is limited to the CNS and NP roles.

To place roles in advanced-practice home care nursing into a historical context, the origins and evolution of the CNS and NP roles will be described briefly. Understanding the historical evolution of these roles makes possible a more informed appreciation of their potential contributions in home care. A historical perspective also allows the anticipation of potential barriers to role implementation that may arise in home care as they have in other settings. Anticipatory awareness of such barriers is needed to deal with them proactively.

CNS Role

The CNS role was originally conceptualized in the 1940s and was put into practice in the 1950s and 1960s (Peplau, 1965; Reiter, 1966; Smoyak, 1976). Although the earliest writing about clinical specialization did not specify the master's degree as the required educational credential (Reiter, 1966; Smoyak, 1976), the CNS role soon became associated with graduate education at the master's level (Harper, 1996; Peplau, 1965). The CNS role originated in the context of a health care system undergoing profound change after World War II (Montemuro, 1987). During this era, tremendous expansion of hospital facilities, accompanied by increasing specialization in medical care, occurred in the United States. Nursing care within hospitals became fragmented, with care delivery organized around nursing functions, such as medication administration, rather than around total client care. Nurses who chose to advance professionally through graduate education specialized in administration, teaching, or supervision, since clinical specialization at the graduate level was not available at the time (Smoyak, 1976). The combination of fragmented care at the bedside and movement away from clinical practice by master's-prepared nurses created concerns among nursing leaders about the quality of nursing care provided in hospitals (Reiter, 1966). Early calls for expert nurses to stay involved with direct care, found in Reiter's description of the nurse clinician, evolved into graduate programs to prepare clinical specialists. The first such program prepared psychiatric CNSs and was begun at Rutgers University in 1954 under the direction of Dr. Hildegard Peplau. Programs in other specialties, such as medical, surgical, and pediatric nursing, soon followed. In the 1970s and 1980s, further subspecialization occurred with the emergence of master's programs in cardiovascular, oncology, and acute-care nursing.

The original purpose of the CNS role was to improve the quality of nursing care through role-modeling, consulting with other staff members, applying research findings to practice, and functioning as a change agent (Bullough, 1992; Georgopoulos, Christman, 1970). As the role became clarified and formalized, the CNS subroles of direct care, consultation, teaching, and research were increasingly well-defined and integrated with APN core competencies (Boyd et al, 1991; Boyle, 1996; Sparacino, 2000; Sparacino, Cooper, 1990). The goal of CNS practice is to improve client care through the judicious application of each subrole. For example, the CNS may provide direct care for particularly complex individual clients. In addition, he or she promotes high-quality care indirectly for client aggregates by consulting with other nurses and with other members of the health team, conducting educational programs, and engaging in research. Through consultation, education, and research, the CNS intervenes at the system level with a focus on aggregates or client populations, rather than on individuals. Which of the four role components receives priority in any given situation is a matter of judgment based on assessment of both clinical and organizational needs. The integration of multiple subroles with an emphasis on systems-level intervention and

mentoring of staff nurses distinguishes the CNS role from other advanced-practice roles (Boyle, 1996; Page, Arena, 1994).

Over the years, CNSs have encountered a number of difficulties with the role that have threatened its viability (Hamric, 1992). One of the most serious difficulties has been the perceived ambiguity of a role with diverse components (Harrel, McCulloch, 1986; Rasch, Frauman, 1996). CNSs have often faced the question, "Just what exactly is it that you do?" The flexibility inherent in the enactment of multiple subroles and the option of intervening at either the system level or the individual level are both strengths and weaknesses of the CNS role. The focus on system-level intervention is a strength in that improvements in care can be institutionalized through consultation, education, and research more broadly than is possible with intervention solely at the individual client level. The CNS's knowledge thus can have a ripple effect throughout an institution through staff development, policy formulation, and formalization of practice innovations into standard procedures. On the other hand, the option of creatively enacting multiple subroles has made it difficult to demonstrate the core contributions of the CNS and has resulted in considerable ambiguity about the role.

Another challenge faced by CNSs has to do with the type of authority vested in CNS practice (Harrell, McCulloch, 1986). This issue is tied to the question of whether a CNS should occupy a line (managerial) position or a staff position. The pros and cons of each have been debated at length and a detailed analysis is beyond the scope of this chapter.* Nevertheless, the issue of authority is important because it influences the effectiveness of the role.

In spite of these difficulties, the CNS role remains needed in health care as a means of introducing innovations into practice, implementing an aggregate or population focus, and creating systems of care for enhancing quality. These important functions of the CNS require cutting-edge clinical practice expertise, as well as change-agent and organizational skills. Such a broad

---

*Beeber, 1980; Blount et al, 1981; Sample, 1983; Scicchitani, 1980; Stevens, 1976; Wallace, Corey, 1983; Williams, Cancian, 1985.

array of skills allows the CNS to contribute to quality of care in a broader way than would be possible through either direct practice alone or management alone.

NP Role

The NP role originated in Colorado in the 1960s in the context of an acute shortage of primary care physicians (Bullough, 1992). The first NP program, developed by Loretta Ford and Henry Silver at the University of Colorado, was based on the premise that public health nurses could significantly improve access to primary care by incorporating into their practices expanded knowledge and skills previously within the domain of medical practice. The curriculum of the first program included history-taking and physical assessment, management of well-child care, and treatment of minor acute illnesses (Ford, 1979, 1997; Ford, Silver, 1967).

Significant resistance to the NP role occurred in nursing education in which NPs were often viewed as physician extenders, functioning within a medical model (Elder, Bullough, 1990; Rogers, 1972). As a result, nursing education was slow to embrace NP education, and for years NPs were trained in certificate programs, rather than in master's-degree programs. Gradually, clarification of the nursing component of the NP role took place. An increasing emphasis on health promotion and illness prevention, psychosocial well-being, and health education quieted concerns about whether nurses were being inappropriately used for medical functions. Growing awareness of the need to standardize the educational preparation of NPs and to incorporate nursing theory and research into NP curricula led to the conclusion that NP education should take place at the master's level parallel to CNS education. Today, most NPs are prepared in graduate programs.

The central function of the classic NP role is to provide primary care to individuals. Primary care is conceptualized as the consumer's first point of contact with the health care system and is characterized by continuity, comprehensiveness, and accountability. Referrals to specialists are made as needed. However, as a primary care provider, the NP has an ongoing relationship with clients and a holistic perspective that integrates health promotion and illness prevention,

psychosocial and developmental care, treatment of acute illnesses, and management of chronic conditions.

Over the years, NPs have confronted a number of serious issues that have limited their ability to practice at their full potential (Safriet, 1992). Included are constraints on the NP scope of practice as defined by state boards of nursing, issues related to prescriptive authority, and reimbursement barriers (Pearson, 1996; Safriet, 1996). With the exception of Medicare and a few other federal sources of reimbursement, these issues are governed by individual states, so their solutions occur on a state-by-state basis (Pearson, 1996; Safriet, 1992). Nevertheless, three decades of collective effort to redress these issues has led to great sophistication among NPs about political and regulatory processes. In all three areas—scope of practice, prescriptive authority, and reimbursement—progress is evident in most states, and in some states NPs function with a great deal of autonomy (Pearson, 2001). However, even with significant progress, new threats to NP practice, such as exclusion from provider panels in managed care organizations (Pearson, 1998), require ongoing political vigilance and activism.

Although the nature of constraints on practice has differed for CNSs and NPs, both groups have faced serious challenges over the years. CNSs and NPs in home care can be expected to face similar issues, and the wise advanced-practice home care nurse will learn from both the mistakes and the accomplishments of predecessors in other settings. The reader is encouraged to consult the sizable collection of literature on the NP and CNS roles to generate strategies for successful role implementation in home care.

Evolution of the CNS and NP Roles into Advanced Practice

A recent development in nursing is the movement toward blending the CNS and NP roles into a unified advanced-practice role (Mezey, McGivern, 1993; Snyder, Mirr, 1995). Early CNS and NP practices differed in many respects, including setting (outpatient for the NP and acute care for the CNS), focus (delivery of primary care for the NP and improvement of quality of care for the CNS), scope of practice (generalist for the NP and specialized for the CNS), and role components (direct care for the NP and direct care, education, consultation, and research for the CNS) (Kitzman, 1983). Early CNSs and NPs also differed in their educational preparation. CNS education traditionally has been at the master's-degree level, whereas early NPs were prepared in certificate or continuing education programs (Elder, Bullough, 1990; Harper, 1996; Kitzman, 1983).

However, beginning in the early 1980s, nursing leaders began pointing out commonalties in practice. In one of the earliest publications on the subject, Kitzman (1983) described similarities in professional attributes, including the shared need for systematic assessment skills, high-level clinical judgment, and interdisciplinary collaboration. She argued that the contributions of the CNS and NP must be combined and that specialization in nursing should not occur by title (e.g., practitioner or specialist), but rather by client need. Building on this premise, Hamric and Spross (1983) proposed a population-based model of practice that combined the assessment skills of the NP with the complex clinical decision-making skills of the CNS.

Subsequent developments in nursing education and health care delivery provided further impetus for merging the CNS and NP roles. For example, studies of master's degree curricula and graduates' practice roles documented commonalties in NP and CNS education and practice (Elder, Bullough, 1990; Forbes et al, 1990). Also, changes in health care delivery began to blur traditional distinctions between settings for NP and CNS practice. The traditional assumption that CNS practice focuses on acutely ill clients in hospitals, whereas NP practice occurs with well individuals in ambulatory care settings began to break down as CNSs and NPs began to cross traditional boundaries (Rasch, Frauman, 1996; Sawyers, 1993). Hastening the breakdown of traditional assumptions about practice settings was the advent of the acute- or tertiary-care NP. Acute-care NPs integrate the acute-care specialty knowledge traditionally associated with CNSs with the assessment and illness-management skills traditionally associated with NPs (Keane, Richmond, 1993; Keane, Richmond, Kaiser, 1994). Acute care NPs provide an expanded range of services across multiple levels of care, coordinating and managing the acute care phase of an illness, facilitating discharge planning, and following the client after discharge. Cutbacks in medical residency programs provided impetus for the development of the acute-care NP role (Knaus et al, 1997). Another change in health care delivery that blurred traditional assumptions about settings for practice was the increasing use of technology in home and other ambulatory settings. The need for nurses with expertise in managing high-tech care further expanded CNS practice to settings other than acute care (Noble, 1988; Rasch, Frauman, 1996).

As role boundaries blurred, the proliferation of roles for master's-prepared nurses became increasingly confusing for the public, including consumers, legislators, and policy-makers (Safriet, 1992). Clearly needed was a unifying term to encompass practice by all master's-prepared nurse clinicians. The term *advanced-practice nursing* is now commonly used to refer to such practice. Support for merging the CNS and NP roles culminated in the merger of the ANA Councils of Clinical Nurse Specialists and Primary Health Care Nurse Practitioners in 1991 (Hawkins, Rafson, 1991).

However, in spite of the benefits of merging the CNS and NP roles, some drawbacks exist. Although many similarities exist between CNS and NP education and practice, significant quantitative and qualitative differences also exist (Elder, Bullough, 1990; Fenton, Brykczynski, 1993; Lindeke, Canedy, Kay, 1997). For example, NPs spend significantly more time in direct care, whereas CNSs spend a considerable amount of time in indirect care, contributing to organizational change and staff development (Williams, Valdivieso, 1994). One of the risks in blending the CNS and NP roles is that the CNS role may be eclipsed (Rasch, Frauman, 1996). If the CNS role is eclipsed, direct care, especially medical tasks associated with direct care, may ultimately overshadow the role-modeling, mentoring, consulting, and organizational work that has been the hallmark of CNS practice (Fenton, 1992; Page, Arena, 1994). In addition, the NP focus on individual clients may supersede a focus on improving the quality of care for aggregates. Furthermore, educating master's students for the merged CNS and NP roles means either that the curricula of graduate programs become significantly more demanding or that depth of content is sacrificed for breadth (Rasch, Frauman, 1996). Finally, although following clients across multiple settings and levels of care is conceptually appealing, the reality of this mode of practice means that time at each setting will be limited. Thus the close working relationships needed with staff and management to influence quality of care and to create systems for care delivery will be less fully developed than is possible in a setting-based practice.

As APN roles have evolved, increasing consensus has emerged about the value of both blended and separate CNS and NP roles (Hamric, Spross, Hanson, 2000). The debates of the 1990s about the merits and limitations of each role have shifted to a focus on the need to clearly articulate the contributions that APNs can make in an increasingly complex health care system. It is imperative that diverse health care constituencies, including consumers, policy-makers, legislators, and health care providers, understand the nature of APN practice and the need to enhance client access to the skills and expertise of APNs. As the health care system undergoes rapid changes, it is important for nursing not to be distracted from the larger advanced-practice agenda by internal debates about one role versus another.

The history of the evolution of the CNS and NP roles has implications for home care. Clearly, both roles have been and continue to be in flux, changing in response to the needs of consumers and evolution of the health care system (Williams, Valdivieso, 1994). Thus, to look for the one best advanced-practice nursing role to apply in home care is to search in vain. Home care is an area of nursing in which advanced-practice roles are just beginning to come into their own. As advanced practice evolves in home care, the experiences of APNs in other settings provide a solid foundation and starting point for understanding the role. Although home care will create variations of the classic advanced-practice roles to meet the needs of this particular setting, advanced-practice home care nursing will be shaped by the primary defining criteria and core competencies characteristic of all APN roles.

ADVANCED-PRACTICE NURSING IN HOME CARE: EMERGING ROLES

The discussion now turns to advanced-practice roles in home care, examining their evolution to date and identifying opportunities for development in the future. Although the need for gradu-

ate education in home care has long been recognized (Beuscher, 1991; Hackbarth, Androwich, 1989), numerous barriers have inhibited the implementation of advanced-practice clinical roles (Scannell, 1995). However, recent changes in home care not only make the need for advanced-practice nursing more compelling, but also provide an opportunity to approach practice in new ways (Mitty, Mezey, 1998). In addressing the need for a multiskilled workforce in home care, Dower et al (1995) observe that as the demands for quality care and the level of client acuity increase, providing an appropriate skill mix from the paraprofessional to the APN is imperative. Their report recommends support for graduate education in nursing to prepare both CNSs and NPs to work in the home health care environment.

Opportunities for graduate education in home care have grown steadily since the first program opened in 1983 at the University of Michigan. In 1989, there were 19 schools of nursing with graduate options in home care, the majority of which were located in departments of community health nursing (Hackbarth, Androwich, 1989). In 1995, the National Association for Home Care (NAHC) listed 106 schools of nursing that offer home care–specialty programs, home health courses, home health content in another specialty, or optional clinical practice in home care (Milone-Nuzzo, 1997; Wills, Delahoussaye, 1998). Although the earliest master's programs in home care focused on management, the need for advanced clinical preparation was recognized also and led to the first home care program for CNS preparation at Azusa Pacific University in 1989 (de la Cruz, Jacobs, McCown, 1992).

Expanded Specialty Practice

In spite of increasing numbers of master's degree programs specifically for home care, the predominant approach to advanced practice in home care has been that of the specialist in another field expanding his or her practice to include the care of clients at home. For example, rehabilitation CNSs are increasingly practicing in home care (Buchanan, 1992; Neal, 1995). Their focus on improving functional status and self-care abilities provides a natural conceptual fit with client needs in home care. Agencies also are increasingly employing CNSs with expertise corresponding to the major diagnostic categories found in home care, such as cardiovascular disease, diabetes, and cancer (Carney, 1997; Dailey, O'Brien, 2000; Milone-Nuzzo, 1996; Thompson, 1996). Other nursing specialties increasingly found in home care include mental health (Felten, 1997; Iglesias, 1998; Mohit, 2000), enterostomal therapy (Robinson, 1996), continence care (Beheshti, Fonteyn, 1998), and critical care (Noble, 1988). These CNSs bring expertise in specific diseases and conditions to home care, thus enhancing the quality of care provided in the home. However, their formal education in home care is variable (Neal, 1996), and they may lack the specific knowledge base needed to practice in the home environment (Nemcek, Egan, 1997).

Home Care NPs

NPs represent another advanced-practice role that is increasingly used in home care. Home care NPs provide primary care and chronic-illness management to clients who are homebound as a result of advanced illness or disability and cannot readily access care in providers' offices (Fried, Wachtel, Tinetti, 1998; Mezey, McGivern, 1993; Mitty, Mezey, 1998). Although home care NPs are not yet widely used (Solheim, Snyder, Mirr, 1995), the Veterans Administration (VA) hospital-based primary care program was one of the first programs in which home care NPs played a key role. The VA program provides in-home primary care to chronically ill veterans who cannot attend outpatient clinics on a regular basis because of functional limitations. Care is delivered by a multidisciplinary team whose members include NPs, registered nurses (RNs), licensed practical nurses (LPNs), nursing assistants, social workers, dietitians, rehabilitation specialists, pharmacists, and physicians. Program goals are to provide primary care that is accessible, comprehensive, coordinated, continuous, accountable, and acceptable to homebound or bedridden veterans and their families. The client and family constitute the unit of care, and education for self-care and caregiving constitute a major focus of the program (Cummings et al, 1990; Hughes et al, 1990; Kubal et al, 1997; Weaver et al, 1995).

Another program that has pioneered the use of NPs in home care is the Community Medical Alliance (CMA) in Boston. In this program, NPs provide in-home care to people with severe physical disabilities and late-stage acquired immunodeficiency syndrome (AIDS) within a prepaid managed-care framework. The CMA program maximizes access to care for participants and provides early intervention and coordination of services (Master et al, 1996). NPs play a pivotal role on the CMA team. By integrating in-home clinical care with case management, they have been able to successfully shift care from a hospital-dependent, specialty focus to a home-based, primary care focus, resulting in cost savings.

A recently inaugurated program is VNA HouseCalls, at the Visiting Nurse Association of Greater Philadelphia (Rinke, Holt, 2000). VNA HouseCalls provides client-driven, comprehensive, collaborative care to homebound Medicare recipients, many of whom have not visited a primary care provider for years. The VNA House-Calls team consists of APNs (in primary care and psychiatric/mental health nursing) and a primary care physician employed by the VNA. As the first modern primary care program in the United States to be housed solely within a home health agency, it is a "back to the future" initiative that recalls the historical provision of primary care services by visiting nurses and physicians in the early days of home care. A significant innovation of the program is reimbursement through Medicare Part B. Changes in APN reimbursement that occurred as a result of the 1997 Balanced Budget Act and changes in the Medicare Part B physician fee schedule (1998) greatly expanded the economic feasibility of the program.

Home Care CNSs

The home care CNS is a third advanced-practice role in home care. The home care CNS has an advanced specialty knowledge base in home care itself. The development of the home care CNS role assumes that home care is a unique specialty with a unique knowledge base, even though the wide range of ages and conditions encountered in practice gives home care a generalist quality. Thus the home care CNS specializes in home care itself, rather than in a specific client population. The role of the CNS in home care is relatively new. However, the needs for critical thinking, role-modeling for clinical practice, and synthesis of information to adapt care to the home setting are characteristics of CNS practice that are needed urgently in home care today (Beuscher, 1991).

According to Scannell (1995), the functions of a home care CNS are (1) directing care by providing, guiding, and evaluating home health nursing practice; (2) coordinating professional home health care by collaborating with interdisciplinary team members; (3) influencing change by swaying attitudes, modifying behavior, and introducing new approaches to nursing practice; (4) teaching new or important concepts and skills; (5) researching clinical nursing problems; and (6) engaging in scholarly work. The home care CNS is most likely to be agency based, although he or she consults with colleagues in other settings. The goal of the home care CNS is to improve client care through direct care, education, consultation, and research, and in some instances, clinical team management.

Of all the advanced-practice nursing roles in home care described in the literature, the role of the home care CNS is the most ambiguous and underdeveloped. Role development has been severely constrained by reimbursement policies and agency organizational structures. Scannell (1995) describes the home care CNS role as a camouflaged practice in which the services delivered by master's-prepared specialists are not formally differentiated from the services of other home care nurses. Master's-prepared home care nurses tend to be unable to function to their full potential and do not, as a group, tend to receive credit for the level of expertise they provide.

In response to the increasing need for high levels of nursing expertise in home care, many agencies have incorporated elements of advanced practice into middle-management positions with various titles, including clinical team leader, client-care coordinator, and manager of skilled services (Buchanan, 1992). These are the positions in home care today that most closely approximate that of the CNS. However, such positions have not been formalized as advanced practice. Rather, they are filled by home care nurses who have distinguished themselves through experience, expertise, natural leadership abilities, continuing education, and perhaps certification as a generalist in home care. Formalizing educational requirements for clinical leadership would provide a standard for the knowledge and skill needed at this level of practice and provide greater uniformity of role expectations across agencies.

BARRIERS TO IMPLEMENTATION OF ADVANCED-PRACTICE ROLES IN HOME CARE

Although various advanced-practice roles in home care are emerging, the actualization of their full potential remains constrained. A host of barriers to full implementation of the advanced-practice role in home care exists and needs to be addressed to improve consumer access to the full range of nursing expertise.

Reimbursement policies constitute one of the most entrenched barriers to advanced practice in home care. Medicare and Medicaid, the traditional sources of revenue for home health agencies, do not recognize APNs in home care. Rather, their reimbursement policies assume an undifferentiated model of practice in which "a nurse is a nurse is a nurse." This assumption is much decried in home care, but it has nevertheless shaped employment and practice patterns. In the fee-per-visit reimbursement model, APNs do not generate any more revenue per visit than other RNs. Thus agencies have been unable to offer a higher level of compensation to master's-prepared nurses, regardless of their advanced knowledge and skill (Milone-Nuzzo, 2000). As a result, agencies have tended to employ nurses with basic educational levels for home visiting and reserve nurses with graduate education for managerial positions. However, as prospective payment capitated reimbursement becomes the norm, the focus on per-visit revenues will become obsolete, and the linkages between knowledge, quality, outcomes, and cost in clinical practice will become paramount.

Home care NPs also have had difficulties with reimbursement. In fact, Scudder (1996) described reimbursement as the Achilles heel of home care NP practice because of the difficulties in billing directly for home care services. Until recently, direct billing by NPs was possible only in limited geographic areas (Keepnews, 1998). Some NPs provided services to home health care agencies on a contractual basis and were reimbursed as consultants. Others were employed in group practices in which they received a salary. Others billed clients directly, or in some instances, could bill Medicaid (Scudder, 1996). Although some home care NPs were able to obtain reimbursement on a limited basis, until recently, the overall effect of reimbursement policies was to restrict access to primary care services among home-bound, chronically ill people. As noted above, the 1997 Balanced Budget Act expanded reimbursement for APNs (Rinke, Holt, 2000) and is likely in the near future to result in widespread improved access to home care NPs among home-bound individuals.

Another barrier to the use of APNs in home care is the typical organizational structure found in home health agencies. Cyr (1990) describes it as a flat organizational structure, consisting simply of geographically assigned client-care staff and one or two levels of management. This undifferentiated organizational structure offers essentially two options for nurses with master's degrees: they can function as staff nurses, carry a geographically determined case load, and serve as invisible APNs, or they can work in managerial positions. Geographical assignment dilutes the benefit of the knowledge and skills APNs bring to home care in that a geographically determined case load contains both complex and routine clients. Because the clinical effectiveness and cost effectiveness of APNs will be most evident in complex cases, making routine visits reduces the impact of advanced practice.

Another barrier to implementation of the home care CNS role is conceptual. Because of the range of ages and clinical conditions seen in home care, it is typically viewed as a generalist practice. As Scannell (1995) notes, to view home care as a specialty when it is a generalist practice seems a contradiction in terms. Articulation of the knowledge base that makes home care a specialty has been slow to develop. Too often when asked what makes home care unique, nurses answer, "the paperwork!" Thus what is believed to make home care unique is practice management, rather than a specialty knowledge base about client needs and nursing interventions.

The ANA scope and standards for home care (1999) and the American Nurses Credentialling Center certification examination for clinical specialists in home care begin to articulate both the role functions and the scope of knowledge of advanced-practice nursing in home care, but there is much work yet to be done. Without this conceptual work, it will remain difficult to articulate the differences in practice between BSN-prepared case managers and the direct client-care activities of the master's-prepared APN. Lack of differentiation of the knowledge base will lead to the assumption that the basic or generalist level of care is sufficient in home care.

The cumulative result of these barriers is limited consumer access to the expertise of advanced-practice home care nurses. However, a confluence of broadly based societal factors has created a rare opportunity to expand advanced-practice nursing in home care and thus to improve consumer access to this level of nursing practice. For example, the increasing numbers of acutely ill people being cared for at home, and technological advances in home care require a level of clinical expertise unparalleled in home care history. As a result, a rapidly growing need for APNs with expertise in adapting complex therapeutic regimens to the home environment has developed. The aging of the population and the clear preference of older adults to remain at home whenever possible are other factors driving the need for advanced-practice home care nursing. As the population ages, more and more families will be providing long-term care at home and will need access to primary care services for their functionally impaired members. Nurses skilled in providing primary care in the home environment will be needed.

Furthermore, the rapidly increasing ethnic diversity of many U.S. communities has created the need for home care nurses with exceptional cultural competence. Home care often means leaving a familiar cultural milieu and going into quite different communities and homes. Thus cultural competence in home care has an additional dimension not found in settings in which the client comes to the nurse's "turf." Home care nurses work on the client's "turf," and to be effective must be able to work with both sensitivity and personal comfort within a wide variety of unfamiliar cultural environments. This requirement of home care presents an enormous challenge to novice home care nurses, and the role modeling of advanced-practice home care nurses can be invaluable in assisting them to tailor care for clients from multiple cultures.

Widely publicized concerns about the quality of home care, warranted or not, provide yet another opportunity to move forward with the implementation of advanced-practice nursing in home care. The original CNS programs were conceived in the context of concern about quality of care in a rapidly changing health care system. Today there is a comparable need for nursing to take a proactive stance with regard to quality in home care. Assurance of impeccable quality is both an ethical and a regulatory mandate in home care. The historical link between advanced-practice nursing and quality of care needs to be brought to home care.

Finally, the shift to prospective payment, integrated systems of health care delivery, and capitated reimbursement provides yet another opportunity to move forward with advanced-practice home care nursing. The greater flexibility inherent in prospective payment and capitated systems potentially frees home care from the restrictive regulations that have impeded the growth of differentiated practice in the past. The demand for clinical effectiveness and cost effectiveness makes the critical thinking skills of APNs highly marketable. Similarly, the requirements for outcomes assessment and evidence-based practice make research and data-management skills essential. In short, numerous sociocultural, demographic, and epidemiological trends and changes in health care delivery have coalesced to provide an unprecedented opportunity to move into a new era in home care. This new era will have a critical need for advanced-practice home care nurses.

MODEL OF ADVANCED-PRACTICE HOME CARE NURSING

The emerging roles for advanced-practice home care nurses described in the literature coupled with new opportunities in a rapidly changing environment suggest a tripartite model of advanced-practice home care nursing (Fig. 29-1). This model encompasses three specific roles: the home care CNS, the home care NP, and the CNS specialized in particular clinical conditions. These advanced-practice roles share a common core of knowledge, skills, and values but also address unique needs in home care and fill particular niches in the current organizational structures found in home care. In proposing this model, it is assumed that home care is a specialty in and of itself and needs APNs prepared specifically in home care. It is believed that specialists prepared in other areas of nursing who expand their practices into the home setting make valuable contributions to home care (Milone-Nuzzo, 1996), but

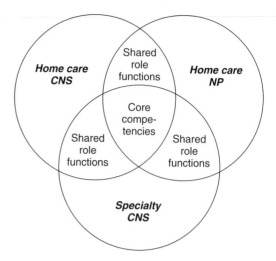

Fig. 29-1   A model of advanced-practice nursing in home care.

they alone cannot meet today's urgent need for advanced-practice home care nursing. The complexities of providing care in the home environment warrant a specialty knowledge base in home care itself. In this model, home care is conceptualized as a subspecialty of community health nursing. It is a synthesis of the community and family orientation of community health with the assessment and illness-management skills traditionally associated with inpatient and ambulatory care settings.

Home Care CNS

The defining characteristic of the home care CNS in our model is in-depth knowledge of health and illness care in the natural environment. The natural environment includes the physical, emotional, and family environment of the home; the wider sociocultural and economic context; and the neighborhood and community in which the home is situated. Clients' environments may well be nontraditional homes, such as foster homes, group board-and-care facilities, and halfway houses.

Included in the home care specialty knowledge base is a solid background in health behavior, including self-care and caregiving, the ability to adapt complex medical regimens to an infinite array of home environments, the ability to work effectively within diverse cultures, and the background needed for sound clinical judgment in highly complex situations. This knowledge base is coupled with the advanced assessment and care-planning skills required for the relatively independent and isolated practice of home care. In addition, home care CNSs need advanced skills in family assessment, an understanding of family dynamics and ways that they influence health and illness care, and familiarity with family-level interventions to intervene effectively in complex family situations. Although Medicare, Medicaid, and other third-party insurers have shifted home care away from the family focus characteristic of community health nursing (Mason et al, 1992), family situations are often what make health and illness care at home complex, and a family-nursing focus must be reclaimed.

Clinical-systems management is another area of knowledge and skill for the home care CNS. The time-honored systems focus of CNSs is greatly needed in home care. An ability to assess aggregate-level outcomes and to design outcome-improvement programs is part of the clinical-systems expertise needed (Wojner, Kite-Powell, 1997). Also, the ability to translate policy and regulatory mandates into practice requires both clinical expertise and up-to-the-minute knowledge of policy changes. Similarly, the ability to assist staff nurses in crafting individualized care plans within a pluralistic reimbursement environment requires detailed knowledge of many reimbursement mechanisms, expertise in staff development and mentoring, and advanced skills with clinical problem-solving.

Finally, home care CNSs need the political savvy to proactively influence policy. The home care CNS must understand how sociopolitical factors influence policy development, which in turn influences clinical practice. The home care CNS must have an appreciation of the macrolevel of health care delivery and must be an active participant in health policy debates (Milstead, 1997). Developing reciprocal linkages between clinical practice and the policy-making arena is part of the CNS role. As translator between the world of clinical practice and the world of policy-making and reimbursement, the home care CNS must have high levels of knowledge about each.

The knowledge base of the home care CNS is implemented in practice through the subroles of direct care, education, consultation, research, and management. Each subrole is approached from the perspective of clinical practice. Through direct care, the advanced health-assessment skills of the home care CNS, in concert with advanced nursing interventions, ensure effective care for complex clients. The home care CNS also introduces innovations into practice, honing them through his or her own practice and gradually integrating them into basic staff-nurse practice. In addition, the home care CNS emphasizes quality improvement through the creation of systems for care involving all levels of nursing and all clients. Other key aspects of the home care CNS role are assessing the needs of and planning programs for specific aggregates or client populations. Role modeling and mentoring nurses are other critical components of the home care CNS role. Finally, the home care CNS has the educational background to be accountable for most aspects of care planning. Although physician gate-keeping in home care is currently the norm (Scannell, 1995), home care was historically an autonomous nursing service, and today home care CNSs are eminently well qualified to function with greater autonomy. For example, a CNS can and should determine the frequency and duration of home visits and much of the visit content, collaborating with physicians on disease management as indicated. Policy and regulatory changes are needed to fully implement this aspect of the home care CNS role.

In the immediate future, the home care CNS role can most efficiently be implemented as an agency-based practice in clinical leadership positions with some degree of middle-management responsibility, such as clinical team leader, client-care coordinator, or clinical manager (Cyr, 1990). This approach would build on familiar organizational structures. An important factor in developing the home care CNS role will be to ensure that the CNS does not become overwhelmed with administrative duties and confined to office work. Clinical leadership positions must be structured so that the CNS can spend some time in the field, managing his or her own caseload of complex clients and consulting and covisiting with other nurses.

Home Care NP

The essential characteristics of the home care NP role is the provision of primary care and chronic-illness management in the home to clients with advanced illness and severe functional impairments. Lacking access to primary care because of inability to easily leave home, such people tend to seek health care only when a problem has become acute or has become an emergency. In-home primary care with a focus on prevention and early detection of acute illness reduces the need for costly inpatient treatment and long recovery periods.

Home care NPs share much of the theoretical and clinical knowledge base described for home care CNSs, but the implementation of the two roles differs in several respects. First, the home care NP can be expected to have ongoing responsibility for clients as primary care providers, whereas the home care CNS is more likely to have short-term involvement with clients while they are receiving services from a home health agency.

Second, at present, home care NPs are less likely than CNSs to be agency based and more likely to work in offices or clinics, in home-based primary-care programs, or in group practices with physicians as described by Kavesh (1993). However, as traditional Medicare agencies expand and diversify their services, the employment of NPs by home health agencies will increase (Mitty, Mezey, 1998; Pierson, Minarik, 1999; Rinke, Holt, 2000).

Third, in a number of states, NPs have prescriptive authority or furnishing privileges, whereas CNSs do not at present (Pearson, 1999). In these states, the NP role currently may include more independence with the pharmacological management of illness. Finally, home care NPs tend to have less responsibility for staff development, quality of care for aggregates, and creation of systems for care delivery than the CNS.

Over time, with changes in the organization and regulation of health care, we expect increasing overlap between the roles of the home care CNS and the NP, with the emergence of a blended role in the future. Descriptions of blended advanced-practice home care nursing roles implemented in home health agencies are beginning to appear in the literature (Pierson, Minarik, 1999). Encompassed in the blended home care APN role are direct primary care and illness-management services, consultation with staff on complex clients, staff development, teaching, and research. Opportunities for expansion of CNS and NP roles and further development of the blended role should be sought. Collaborative relationships between schools of nursing and home health agencies will be a key strategy for seizing such opportunities (Buhler-Wilkerson et al, 1998; Mitty, Mezey, 1998; Pierson, Minarik, 1999).

Expanded Specialty Practice

CNSs specializing in particular clinical populations also make significant contributions to home care. The specialty CNS is the advanced-practice role most widely implemented in home care to date. Specialty CNSs have in-depth knowledge about particular clinical conditions, such as cancer, cardiovascular disease, or psychiatric disorders. Although their education may not have prepared them specifically for work in home care, CNSs today move easily between settings, seeing clients in outpatient settings and at home, as well as in hospitals. Their in-depth knowledge about specific conditions, associated medical therapies, and nursing interventions makes them ideal candidates for collaboration with home care nurses. However, unless an agency is particularly large or has developed specialty programs for target populations, it may not be able to employ multiple-specialty CNSs full time. Thus many agencies may need to collaborate with hospitals or contract independently with CNSs to obtain their services (Cyr, 1990; Milone-Nuzzo, 1996).

The tripartite model is consistent with the conceptualization of advanced-practice nursing in which a variety of roles have both shared and unique areas of knowledge. Furthermore, the model portrays the reality that no one APN can know and do everything for a given population of clients. Needed are collaborative efforts among APNs in which each draws on particular areas of expertise of the others. For example, a home care CNS might collaborate with an oncology CNS with respect to a client and family struggling with cancer at home. In another instance, an agency-based home care CNS might collaborate with a home care NP in private practice who provides ongoing primary care to homebound clients. The home care NP's client may receive intermittent "skilled care" services from a home health agency during an illness exacerbation, providing an opportunity for collaboration with the agency-based CNS. The possibilities for collaborative practice will vary depending on client needs, organizational structures, and the availability of APNs.

The model emphasizes the unique knowledge base required in home care. Although the model acknowledges the important contribution of other specialists working in home care, it highlights the pressing need for specialization and advanced practice in home care per se. Some clients will be so medically complex that they require the services of CNSs in specialties such as oncology, cardiovascular nursing, and acute care nursing. Other clients are less medically complex, but other aspects of their health status or home environment make their care challenging. These clients are ideal candidates for the services of the home care CNS or the home care NP.

IMPLEMENTING ADVANCED-PRACTICE ROLES IN HOME CARE

What is needed to move ahead with implementation of advanced-practice roles in home care? Action is needed on a variety of fronts by clinicians, administrators, policy-makers, researchers, and theorists. Clinicians will need to pioneer new roles in home care by demonstrating the clinical effectiveness and cost effectiveness of advanced-practice nursing. They will need to be visionary, willing to take risks, and able to recognize and seize opportunities. They will need to take off the historical "camouflage" in which advanced-practice home care nursing has been hidden and assert the substantial contribution to client care APNs can provide. They will need to publish descriptions of their practices and increase public awareness of their services. They will need to become key players in policy-making.

Home care administrators will need to create organizational structures that include advanced-practice nursing. Such organizational structures must accommodate differentiated levels of expertise and include creative ways to integrate the system-level interventions of advanced-practice nursing with direct client care. The nature of home care will make this challenging, but it must be done. Lack of role-modeling and insufficient access to consultation about difficult clinical issues lead to high staff turnover and increased agency costs. Finally, administrators must publish models of care delivery and evaluate their outcomes and cost effectiveness.

Nurse policy-makers will need to devise legislation and regulations that allow APNs to function with more authority, accountability, and autonomy in home care. Historically a nurse-driven area of practice, home care has been ceded progressively to medical and corporate interests. Nursing needs to take back a significant proportion of home care to meet client needs to the fullest extent possible. Consumer access to advanced-practice home care nursing is extremely limited, and this will change only through concerted political action and sophisticated policy initiatives by nurses.

Researchers will need to demonstrate the efficacy of nursing interventions in home care and evaluate outcomes of various care processes. Only through such work can evidence be amassed to support the claim that advanced-practice home care nursing contributes substantially to clinical effectiveness and cost effectiveness. Also, research-generated evidence is needed to move claims about the efficacy of nursing interventions from anecdote to science.

Theorists will need to expand the conceptual and theoretical basis for home care nursing. Advanced-practice nurses need more than a set of skills for practice. They need sound theoretical models to guide health and illness care in the natural environment. Such theories need to be behaviorally focused, address the family and other social units, and include the cultural aspects of the client's natural environment. Theories also need to take into account the lived experience of managing health and illness care at home. Developing and organizing the theoretical basis for home care will further the conceptualization of advanced practice in home care and provide structure for educational programs.

With such concerted effort, advanced-practice home care nursing has a bright future. Recent ground-breaking work by APNs in home care, changes in the health care delivery system, and an emerging vision of the future put advanced-practice home care nurses in a position to enter an era in which their full potential can finally be fully realized.

REFERENCES

American Nurses Association: *Nursing's social policy statement,* Washington, DC, 1995, The Association.

American Nurses Association: *Scope and standards of home health nursing practice,* Washington, DC, 1999, The Association.

Beeber LS: Should the clinical nurse specialist be free of administrative responsibility? Point, *Perspectives in Psychiatric Care* 13:250, 264-266, 1980.

Beheshti P, Fonteyn M: Role of the advanced practice nurse in continence care in the home, *AACN Clinical Issues* 9:389-395, 1998.

Beuscher TL: The clinical nurse specialist: A valuable resource in home care, *Caring* 10(4):22-25, 1991.

Blount M et al: Extending the influence of the clinical nurse specialist, *Nursing Administration Quarterly* 6(1):53-63, 1981.

Boyd NJ et al: The merit and significance of clinical nurse specialists, *Journal of Nursing Administration* 21(9):35-43, 1991.

Boyle DM: The clinical nurse specialist. In Hamric AB, Spross JA, Hanson CM, eds: *Advanced nursing practice: An integrative approach,* Philadelphia, 1996, WB Saunders.

Buchanan LC: A rehabilitation clinical nurse specialist: Evaluation of the role in a home health care setting, *Holistic Nursing Practice* 6(2):42-50, 1992.

Buhler-Wilkerson K et al: An alliance for academic home care: Integrating research, education, and practice, *Nursing Outlook* 46:77-80, 1998.

Bullough B: Alternative models for specialty nursing practice, *Nursing and Health Care* 13:254-259, 1992.

Carney K: Clinical nurse specialists: A market advantage, *Caring* 16(6):16, 1997.

Cummings JE et al: Cost-effectiveness of Veterans Administration hospital-based home care: A randomized clinical trial, *Archives of Internal Medicine* 150:1274-1280, 1990.

Cyr LB: The clinical nurse specialist in a home healthcare setting, *Home Healthcare Nurse* 8(1):34-39, 1990.

Dailey M, O'Brien K: Clinical nurse specialists: Key to improving outcomes in home care, *Home Health Care Management and Practice* 12(3):332-342, 2000.

de la Cruz FA, Jacobs AM, McCown D: Home health care nursing: A clinical specialty in need of graduate education, *Home Healthcare Nurse* 10(2):44-51, 1992.

Dower CM et al: *A multi-skilled workforce in geriatric home health care: Issues, models and recommendations,* San Francisco, 1995, Center for the Health Professions, University of California, San Francisco.

Elder RG, Bullough B: Nurse practitioners and clinical nurse specialists: Are the roles merging? *Clinical Nurse Specialist* 4:78-84, 1990.

Felten BS: The geropsychiatric clinical nurse specialist in home care, *Home Healthcare Nurse* 15:635-638, 1997.

Fenton MV: Education for the advanced practice of clinical nurse specialists, *Oncology Nursing Forum* 19(suppl 1):16-20, 1992.

Fenton MV, Brykczynski KA: Qualitative distinctions and similarities in the practice of clinical nurse specialists and nurse practitioners, *Journal of Professional Nursing* 9:313-326, 1993.

Forbes KE et al: Clinical nurse specialist and nurse practitioner core curricula survey results, *Nurse Practitioner* 15:43-48, 1990.

Ford LC: A nurse for all settings: The nurse practitioner, *Nursing Outlook* 27:516-521, 1979.

Ford LC: A deviant comes of age, *Heart & Lung* 26:87-91, 1997.

Ford LC, Silver HK: The expanded role of the nurse in child care, *Nursing Outlook* 15(9):43-45, 1967.

Fried TR, Wachtel TJ, Tinetti ME: When the patient cannot come to the doctor: A medical housecalls program, *Journal of the American Geriatrics Society* 46:226-231, 1998.

Georgopoulos BS, Christman L: The clinical nurse specialist: A role model, *American Journal of Nursing* 70:1030-1039, 1970.

Hackbarth DP, Androwich IM: Graduate nursing education for leadership in home care, *Caring* 8(2):6-11, 1989.

Hamric AB: Creating our future: Challenges and opportunities for the clinical nurse specialist, *Oncology Nursing Forum* 19(suppl 1):11-15, 1992.

Hamric AB: A definition of advanced nursing practice. In Hamric AB, Spross JA, Hanson CM, eds: *Advanced nursing practice: An integrative approach,* ed 2, Philadelphia, 2000, WB Saunders.

Hamric AB, Spross J: A model for future clinical specialist practice. In Hamric AB, Spross J, eds: *The clinical nurse specialist in theory and practice,* New York, 1983, Grune & Stratton.

Hamric AB, Spross JA, Hanson CM, eds: *Advanced nursing practice: An integrative approach,* ed 2, Philadelphia, 2000, WB Saunders.

Harper D: Education for advanced nursing practice. In Hamric AB, Spross JA, Hanson CM, eds: *Advanced nursing practice: An integrative approach,* Philadelphia, 1996, WB Saunders.

Harrell JS, McCulloch SD: The role of the clinical nurse specialist: Problems and solutions, *Journal of Nursing Administration* 16(10):44-48, 1986.

Hawkins JE, Rafson J: ANA council merger creates council of nurses in advanced practice, *Clinical Nurse Specialist* 5:131-132, 1991.

Hughes SL et al: A randomized trial of Veterans Administration home care for severely disabled veterans, *Medical Care* 28:135-145, 1990.

Iglesias GH: Role evolution of the mental health clinical nurse specialist in home care, *Clinical Nurse Specialist* 12:38-44, 1998.

Kavesh W: Physician and nurse practitioner relationships. In Mezey MD, McGivern DO, eds: *Nurses, nurse practitioners: Evolution to advanced practice,* New York, 1993, Springer.

Keane A, Richmond T: Tertiary nurse practitioners, *Image: Journal of Nursing Scholarship* 25:281-284, 1993.

Keane A, Richmond T: Kaiser L: Critical care nurse practitioners: Evolution of the advanced practice nursing role, *American Journal of Critical Care* 3:232-237, 1994.

Keepnews D: New opportunities and challenges for APRNs, *American Journal of Nursing* 98:62-64, 1998.

Kitzman HJ: The CNS and the nurse practitioner. In Hamric AB, Spross J, eds: *The clinical nurse specialist in theory and practice,* New York, 1983, Grune & Stratton.

Knaus VL et al: The use of nurse practitioners in the acute care setting, *Journal of Nursing Administration* 27(2):20-27, 1997.

Kubal JD et al: VA's home-based primary care program, *Federal Practitioner,* 1997.

Lindeke L, Canedy BH, Kay MM: A comparison of practice domains of clinical nurse specialists and nurse practitioners, *Journal of Professional Nursing* 13:281-287, 1997.

Mahn VA, Zazworsky DJ: The advanced practice nurse case manager. In Hamric AB, Spross JA, Hanson CM, eds: *Advanced nursing practice: An integrative approach,* ed 2, Philadelphia, 2000, WB Saunders.

Mason DJ et al: Promoting the community health clinical nurse specialist, *Clinical Nurse Specialist* 6:6-13, 1992.

Master R et al: The Community Alliance: An integrated system of care in Greater Boston for people with severe disability and AIDS, *Managed Care Quarterly* 4(2):26-37, 1996.

Mezey MD, McGivern DO: *Nurses, nurse practitioners: Evolution to advanced practice,* New York, 1993, Springer.

Miller SE: The role of the clinical nurse specialist in home health care, *Journal of Home Health Care Practice* 7(2):62-72, 1995.

Milone-Nuzzo P: A creative way to use clinical nurse specialists in home care, *Home Healthcare Nurse* 14:224, 1996.

Milone-Nuzzo P: Home care and nursing education—Past, present, and future implications, *Home Healthcare Nurse* 15:879-880, 1997.

Milone-Nuzzo P: Advanced practice nurses in home care are essential, *Home Healthcare Nurse* 18:22-23, 2000.

Milstead JA: A social mandate: APN leadership for the whole policy process, *Advanced Practice Nursing Quarterly* 3(3):1-8, 1997.

Mitty E, Mezey M: Integrating advanced practice nurses in home care, *Nursing and Health Care Perspectives* 19:264-270, 1998.

Mohit D: Psychiatric home care and family therapy: A window of opportunity for the psychiatric clinical nurse specialist, *Archives of Psychiatric Nursing* 16:127-133, 2000.

Montemuro MA: The evolution of the clinical nurse specialist: Response to the challenge of professional nursing practice, *Clinical Nurse Specialist* 1:106-110, 1987.

Neal LJ: The rehabilitation CNS in the home health care setting, *Clinical Nurse Specialist* 9:293-298, 1995.

Neal LJ: The clinical nurse specialist: Practice in the home health setting, *Home Health Care Management and Practice* 8(3):64-68, 1996.

Nemcek MA, Egan PB: Specialty nursing improves home care, *Caring* 16(6):12-14, 18, 1997.

Noble MA: The critical care clinical nurse specialist: Need for hospital and community, *Clinical Nurse Specialist* 2:30-33, 1988.

Page NE, Arena DM: Rethinking the merger of the clinical nurse specialist and the nurse practitioner roles, *Image: Journal of Nursing Scholarship* 26:315-318, 1994.

Pearson LJ: Annual update of how each state stands on legislative issues affecting advanced nursing practice, *The Nurse Practitioner* 21:10-16, 21-69, 1996.

Pearson LJ: Annual update of how each state stands on legislative issues affecting advanced nursing practice, *The Nurse Practitioner* 23:14-19, 1998.

Pearson LJ: Annual update of how each state stands on legislative issues affecting advanced nursing practice, *The Nurse Practitioner* 24:16-83, 1999.

Pearson LJ: Annual legislative update, *The Nurse Practitioner* 26:7, 11-16, 2001.

Peplau H: Specialization in professional nursing, *Nursing Science* 3:268-287, 1965.

Pierson CL, Minarik P: APNs in home care, *American Journal of Nursing* 99(10):22-23, 1999.

Portillo CJ, Schumacher KL: Graduate program: Advanced practice nurses in the home, *AACN Clinical Issues* 9:355-361, 1998.

Rasch RFR, Frauman AC: Advanced practice in nursing: Conceptual issues, *Journal of Professional Nursing* 12:141-146, 1996.

Reiter F: The nurse clinician, *American Journal of Nursing* 66:274-280, 1966.

Rinke LT, Holt SW: Primary care in the home: The time is now! *Home Health Care Management and Practice* 12(3):1-9, 2000.

Robinson SM: Advancing home care nursing practice with an ET clinical nurse specialist, *Home Healthcare Nurse* 14:269-274, 1996.

Rogers ME: Nursing: To be or not to be, *Nursing Outlook* 20:42-46, 1972.

Safriet BJ: Health care dollars and regulatory sense: The role of advanced practice nursing, *Yale Journal on Regulation* 9:417-488, 1992.

Sample SA: Justifying and structuring the CNS role in the nursing department. In Hamric AB, Spross J, eds: *The clinical nurse specialist in theory and practice,* New York, 1983, Grune & Stratton.

Sawyers JE: Defining your role in ambulatory care: Clinical nurse specialist or nurse practitioner? *Clinical Nurse Specialist* 7:4-7, 1993.

Scannell A: The camouflaged home health clinical nurse specialist, *Home Healthcare Nurse* 13:62-65, 1995.

Schroer K: Case management: Clinical nurse specialist and nurse practitioner, converging roles, *Clinical Nurse Specialist* 5:189-194, 1991.

Scicchitani BM: Should the clinical nurse specialist be free of administrative responsibility? Counterpoint, *Perspectives in Psychiatric Care* 13:251, 267-269, 1980.

Scudder LE: NPs in home health care, *Nurse Practitioner World News* 1:1, 9, 11, 1996.

Smoyak SA: Specialization in nursing: From then to now, *Nursing Outlook* 24:676-681, 1976.

Snyder M, Mirr MP, eds: *Advanced practice nursing: A guide to professional development,* New York, 1995, Springer.

Solheim K, Mirr M, Snyder M: Settings for care. In Snyder M, Mirr MP, eds: *Advanced practice nursing: A guide to professional development,* New York, 1995, Springer.

Sparacino PSA: The clinical nurse specialist. In Hamric AB, Spross JA, Hanson CM, eds: *Advanced nursing practice: An integrative approach,* ed 2, Philadelphia, 2000, WB Saunders.

Sparacino PSA, Cooper DM: The role components. In Sparacino PSA, Cooper DM, Minarik PA, eds: *The clinical nurse specialist: Implementation and impact,* Norwalk, Conn, 1990, Appleton & Lange.

Stevens BJ: Accountability of the clinical specialist: The administrator's viewpoint, *Journal of Nursing Administration* 6(2):30-32, 1976.

Thompson MW: Clinical nurse specialist: Making the shift from critical care to home care, *Dimensions of Critical Care Nursing* 15:40-47, 1996.

Wallace MA, Corey LJ: The clinical specialist as manager: Myth versus realities, *Journal of Nursing Administration* 13(6):13-15, 1983.

Weaver FM et al: A profile of Department of Veterans Affairs hospital based home care programs, *Home Health Care Services Quarterly* 15(4):83-96, 1995.

Wells N, Erickson S, Spinella J: Role transition: From clinical nurse specialist to clinical nurse specialist/case manager, *Journal of Nursing Administration* 26:23-28, 1996.

Williams CA, Valdivieso GC: Advanced practice models: A comparison of clinical nurse specialist and nurse practitioner activities, *Clinical Nurse Specialist* 8:311-318, 1994.

Williams LB, Cancian DW: A clinical nurse specialist in a line management position, *Journal of Nursing Administration* 15(1):20-26, 1985.

Wills EM, Delahoussaye CP: Home health graduate nursing programs in the United States, *Home Healthcare Nurse* 16:85-93, 1998.

Wojner AW, Kite-Powell D: Outcomes manager: A role for the advanced practice nurse, *Critical Care Nursing Quarterly* 19(4):16-24, 1997.

30 Research in Home Care

Violet H. Barkauskas

IMPORTANCE OF RESEARCH TO HOME CARE

Over the past several decades, research in home care has been accelerated by various changes in the field. In the early to mid-1980s, the emphases on hospital cost savings through early hospital discharges and transfer of care to homes stimulated considerable growth in the field. Substantial increases were seen in numbers of home care agencies, types of services provided, and mechanisms of reimbursement for services. Home care was proposed as a cost-effective alternative to institutional care for both acute and long-term care needs. Concurrently, the aging of the population in the United States and in many other countries substantially increased the need and demand for home care services by the elderly. Key research questions focused on descriptions of clients served by home care, costs of care, resource utilization, and differentiating clients most appropriately served by various long-term care alternatives.

As home care became a more prominent service and represented increasing expenditures of resources, it too became the focus of cost-effectiveness scrutiny and cost-containment regulation. In addition, questions were raised about the quality of care being provided by home care providers. Quality questions were relevant for two major reasons. First, a number of services and treatments, previously provided only in more controlled hospital settings and by professional care providers, were being transferred to homes and to other professional and nonprofessional people. The quality and safety limits of such technology transfers were unknown. Second, home care is a largely invisible service. Care provided in homes is not generally observed by people other than clients, family members, and providers. Thus questions about needs for home care, descriptions of services provided, and benefits and outcomes of services became important research and policy foci. While these questions continue to be explored, scrutiny of and financing for the field continues to be based on incomplete information. Consequently, during the second half of the 1990s, a number of home care agencies closed or were incorporated into large, comprehensive health care systems in response to cost-containment reimbursement policies.

Thus research in the home care field is critical in documenting the particular needs of specific client populations for services, the assets of home care in contrast to alternative forms of care provision, the services themselves, and the outcomes of home care (Balding, 1997; Benefield, 1997). Research findings hold promise for contributing to policies that would ensure rational distribution of services among people needing them and at a fair cost to third-party payors, as well as to providers. Therefore home care agency participation in research is key for documenting the needs for services, the costs of services, service improvements, and access to services for clients and developing the field in numerous other dimensions.

Home care agencies can directly benefit from research participation in several ways. First, discussions about research projects and findings within an agency can stimulate critical thinking about the provision of home care services and encourage exploration of the best evidence-based practices. Second, staff participation in research contributes to staff development and general enrichment. Likewise, contacts with investigators facilitate participation in a larger network of scientists and others interested in home care and often leads to involvement in other creative projects.

Despite the benefits of research participation, the question of who pays for research is important to home care agencies, whose financial reserves may be low. If the research is being led by an outside institution and requires a substantial investment of agency resources (e.g., staff time), the agency should expect to be reimbursed for that participation by the collaborating institution. Agencies initiating projects on their own should carefully itemize the projected full costs of such projects to determine their potential cost benefit before making commitments for implementation.

The interest in home care research has grown as the questions in the field have emerged. Several large home care agencies have reported models for intraagency research-program development.* However, financial constraints and lack of staff prepared in research present obstacles to independent research-project initiation by most home care agencies.

Much of the research in the home care field has been conducted by university faculty. Collaborative research between home care agencies and universities has been common in the field. In a study of home care administrators and staff conducted by the Affiliates of the Visiting Nursing Associations of America, Hekelman et al (1992) documented strong interest of agency personnel in supporting, participating in, and conducting home care research. The authors pointed out that the personnel within home care agencies are well positioned as collaborators in research projects because they have a wealth of experience and knowledge as the bases for identifying key questions and designing innovative interventions. Findings from this study suggest that collaboration between academicians and clinicians can be very effective in addressing both scientific research questions and practical clinical issues. However, although such collaborations make strong objective sense, experience has demonstrated that they require substantial, bilateral negotiation, commitment, communication, and resource sharing over extended periods (McWilliam, Desai, Greig, 1997). Examples of such successful agency-university collaborative projects are demonstrated in studies reported by Feinglass, Slavensky, and Tang (1996) for clients with intermittent claudication; Kelly et al (1996) for

services to children with cancer; and Salesberry, Nickel, and O'Connell (1991) for AIDS care.

Although only some home care agencies are large enough to support a research division, all are consumers of, and are significantly affected directly by, the research conducted by others. In addition, home care agencies are often asked to participate in research projects and use components of the research process as they address clinical questions and develop proposals for funding. Although a comprehensive discussion of the research process is not possible within the context of this chapter, the key issues related to the conduct and use of the research process will be presented as a reference for home care staff who will be participating in research projects, using components of the research process to develop grant proposals, and applying published research findings to practice. The final section of this chapter includes a presentation of the current status of knowledge generated from research in home care and a discussion of priority issues for future research.

PARTICIPATION IN RESEARCH

Home care agencies are frequently asked to participate in research. Therefore home care agency staff need to understand the research process well enough to evaluate the quality of a research proposal submitted to the agency, understand what data would be collected and what data-collection–related resources may be expected of the agency, identify any potential risks to staff or clients, and assess the relative costs and benefits of participation.

Research approaches are of two general types: quantitative and qualitative. Quantitative research is based on deductive thinking and is characterized by large subject groups and heavy reliance on numerical measurement of variables and statistical analysis. Quantitative research can be descriptive, experimental, or quasiexperimental. Qualitative research is based on inductive thinking and is characterized by in-depth exploration of concepts and their relationships. Qualitative research is descriptive. Data are generally collected through extensive interviewing or observational techniques, and data analyses often use nonnumerical techniques for the classification of observations, concepts, and relationships. Sometimes large research projects will include both general types of approaches, with initial phases focused on qualitative approaches

---

*Bowen, LeDuc, 1994; Dellasega, King, 1996; Harris, 1990; Pessin et al, 1993; Raphael, Angelicola, 1993; Stricklin, Hekelman, 1991.

for understanding the phenomena of interest and later phases involving quantitative approaches focused on measuring the phenomena as independent or dependent variables. Qualitative studies are useful for understanding phenomena, (e.g., the process of adapting to a chronic condition), whereas quantitative studies enable hypothesis testing and evaluation (e.g., comparing interventions designed to assist in clients' adaptation to a chronic condition).

When formally requested to participate in a research project, the agency should expect a written proposal from the investigator with the components listed in Table 30-1. Each component is defined in Table 30-1, and questions agency staff can use in evaluating the merits of the proposal

Table 30-1 Components of a Research Proposal and Questions to Evaluate Merit and Participation

Proposal Components	Evaluation Questions
STATEMENT OF THE PROBLEM The central issue or question is addressed by the research.	• Is the statement of the problem clear? • Is the problem significant to the agency or to the field of home care? • Can key questions about this concern be answered by the proposed research?
REVIEW OF THE LITERATURE What is known about the problem from the published literature is discussed.	• Has the investigator presented a comprehensive, up-to-date discussion of the relevant literature? • Does the proposed research logically build on the knowledge base in the field?
THEORETICAL FRAMEWORK The investigator's abstract view of the phenomena to be studied and the relationships among the various concepts important to the phenomena are presented. Sometimes the theoretical framework is a well-known theory proposed by others and applied by the investigator to the particular problem. The theoretical framework can also be the investigator's unique presentation of his or her view of the components and dynamics of the phenomena under investigation.	• Is the presentation of the theoretical framework logical to the problem and to the agency's empirical experiences with it?
IDENTIFICATION OF VARIABLES Variables are characteristics or attributes of people or things that change and that are observed or measured. In quantitative studies, there are two main types of variables: *Independent variables* are those that vary by themselves or are manipulated by the investigator. *Dependent variables* are those that change as some aspect of the independent variables also changes.	In qualitative studies, the exploration may focus on the identification of variables important to a given situation. Thus the investigator may not specify the specific variables of interest, but rather the methods of their identification. The following questions are relevant for quantitative studies: • Is the investigator measuring the variables staff and administrators think are important to the questions? • Are the variables defined both theoretically and operationally? • Are the selected variables congruent to the theoretical framework?

Continued

Table 30-1	Components of a Research Proposal and Questions to Evaluate Merit and Participation—cont'd	
Proposal Components	**Evaluation Questions**
FORMULATION OF HYPOTHESES OR SPECIFIC QUESTIONS TO BE ADDRESSED	
The statements of the proposed relationships among key variables or the specific questions about the relationships between or among the concepts are presented.	• Are the hypotheses and questions logical to the discussions in the proposal up to this point? • Are the hypotheses or questions important to the field?
RESEARCH DESIGN AND METHODS	
The overall plan for the selection of subjects, any interventions subjects may receive, the tools for data collection, and the mechanisms by which data will be collected are presented.	• Is the research design clearly specified? • Is the design logical to the questions or hypotheses? • Is the description of this research proposal design consistent with its specification? • Have the researchers controlled for circumstances or other variables that might positively or negatively affect findings or the generalizability of their findings (i.e., the threats to internal and external validity)? • Can sufficient numbers of subjects be recruited to participate in the study? • What will be expected from the agency in terms of access, support, or direct involvement in the data collection? • Are the proposed data-collection tools and instruments valid, reliable, and reasonable to the questions addressed? • How will the data collection impact clients and staff? • Is there any way the clients or staff can be harmed by the study methods? • Is participation fully voluntary and informed? • Are the limitations in the study known and clearly stated?
DATA ANALYSIS	
The plan for the management, coding and reporting of data is presented.	• Do the researchers have a preliminary plan for the analysis of data? • Will the data-analysis plan address the questions proposed for the study?
DISSEMINATION OF FINDINGS	
The plan for sharing the findings with the participants and with the professional world is presented.	• Is the plan for sharing study findings with the agency and the participating clients and staff clear? • What rights does the agency have to the data? • Will the agency be identified in publications? • Will the agency have a right to review manuscripts before they are submitted for publication?

and the feasibility of participation in it are listed. Most of the components and evaluation questions, except as indicated, are relevant to both qualitative and quantitative studies. Investigators seeking research collaboration with an agency should be fully expected to supply complete information about all of the proposal components listed. If a proposal is incomplete, agency staff should request clarification and additional information before agreeing to participation that is not fully understood and around which there may be future misunderstandings.

Some agencies receive numerous requests for research participation—perhaps more requests than the agency can reasonably manage. Other agencies have sufficient resources to participate in only one project at a time. The following general criteria for prioritization are offered for agencies needing to prioritize participation in collaborative research projects:

- The problems addressed by the research are important and common within the agency and within the field.
- The problems are empirically observable and testable.
- The results are likely to have a direct impact on practices or policies in the agency or the field.

Once the understanding of the research process is mastered, this learning can be applied to various other activities within the agency, specifically the development of grant proposals for new program initiatives and program evaluation. The main components of a research proposal are listed in Table 30-1, along with important questions for developing and evaluating a proposal.

When the agency is developing its own proposal, agency staff should do some preliminary work in matching a desired project to an interested funding source. Roland and Rowland (1997) identified important activities for preparing a successful grant proposal. These are summarized in Box 30-1.

An additional resource for agencies participating in research or related activities is a publication entitled *Home Care: A Research Guide,*

Box 30-1 Tips for the Development of a Research or Program-Evaluation Proposal

1. Identify a funding source that is logical for your project and be prepared to tailor your project to fit the requirements of the funding source.
2. Obtain application materials from the funding source and thoroughly study them before making key decisions about the project. The application should be the guide for designing and presenting the project.
3. Identify the funding agency's essential content for the proposal and note areas in which you need clarification. If the application instructions are not clear, contact the agency with your questions.
4. Follow the application instructions exactly. Do not omit requested information and do not include extraneous, nonrequested information.
5. Be sure the project goals, objectives, implementation strategies, and evaluation are clear.
6. Carefully review a draft of the full application to assess completeness, flow, clarity, specificity, and strength of presentation. Ask peers to review the proposal and to provide honest critiques of it. It is better to know the problems and fix them before submission than to learn about them from the grant reviewers after the proposal has been rejected. Give yourself enough time to do this critique and appreciate that even the most experienced of grant writers

prepare many revisions of a proposal before submission.
7. If possible and permitted, submit a draft of the proposal to presubmission review (i.e., review by the staff of the funding agency with feedback from them regarding how the proposal could be improved).
8. Avoid the following common mistakes:
   - Submitting the proposal after the deadline
   - Omitting literature citations that are needed to support the needs assessment or to document the rationale for an intervention
   - Committing errors in the application forms
   - Omitting required signatures
   - Committing mathematical errors in the budgets
   - Writing inconsistent budget figures or other numbers throughout the proposal
   - Including goals, objectives, or strategies that do not address the stated need or are inconsistent among themselves
   - Using evaluation criteria that are not measurable or do not address desired project outcomes
9. For your and the grant reviewers' convenience, include a table of contents and number the pages.
10. Submit the proposal within the deadline and in a way that will provide you with dated evidence of its receipt.

Modified from Rowland HS, Rowland BL: *Nursing administration handbook,* ed 4, Gaithersburg, Md, 1997, Aspen.

published by the Michigan Foundation for Home Care (Balding et al, 1994). This publication elaborates on the notions presented in this section of the chapter and is recommended as an excellent reference for all home care agencies.

Human-Subjects Projection

Home care clients are especially vulnerable research subjects. Many are in physiologically, emotionally, and sociologically complex and unprotected situations and often are exhausted. All research involving human subjects requires review for the ethical involvement of human subjects by an Institutional Review Board (IRB). University investigators should have completed the IRB review and received approval before submission of a formal proposal to a potential participating agency. This initial safeguard is important, but agency staff need to understand that the review was not conducted with awareness of the specific, proposed context of the research and the idiosyncratic risk that a particular subject group may be experiencing at a given time. Therefore it is recommended that home care agencies establish some type of internal research review board to evaluate the merits of submitted proposals and the risks of participation. Increasingly funding agencies are requiring human subjects reviews by both the academic institutions and the participating clinical agencies. This internal board would address the following general questions and others that may be important to a given agency:

- Is this project important enough for our staff to expend resources for participation?
- Will participation in the study impose significant hardship on or cost to the agency?
- Will the proposed study expose subjects, including clients, staff, and others, to unreasonable risks?

Unreasonable risk to a given client or staff population may relate to unique circumstances in a given agency at a particular time. For example a particular target client group may be atypical and more seriously ill than was earlier anticipated, and the addition of new people and data collection to the home may be unusually stressful. Sometimes changes within an agency can create hardships for staff members who may not be able to participate in research and simultaneously maintain quality care.

Establishment of an agency-based research review board will not only protect the human subjects connected with the agency and facilitate the most efficient use of resources available for research collaboration, but will also keep the idea of research-based practice active in the agency. Staff participating in the reviews will learn much from the proposals submitted for review and from related discussions. Ideas for agency-initiated projects are likely to emerge from discussions of literature reviews and the strengths and weaknesses of proposals.

Research- and Evidence-Based Practice—Applying Research Findings

The ultimate objective of all health care research is the discovery of knowledge that will be used in understanding and improving health. Research applicable to home care is extensive, especially when one considers the multitude of clinical issues related to home care practice. Also, research in areas relating to home care is found in the literature of many disciplines, including nursing, medicine, the therapies, social work, public health, gerontology, sociology, psychology, and administration. Thus user-friendly dissemination of study results is an important responsibility of the scientific community. Today, this responsibility is being operationalized through formal national and international efforts to summarize, analyze, synthesize, and disseminate research results across studies in an effort to publish evidence-based guidelines for practice and the education of health-professional students. These evidence-based guidelines are developed through the synthesis of existing research in combination with the consensus of experts in the relevant fields.

Although the need to keep up with emerging knowledge relevant to home care may appear daunting, assistance is available from various sources. A number of governmental groups, notably the Agency for Healthcare Research and Quality (formerly known as the Agency for Health Care and Policy Research [AHCPR]), has assembled a number of panels focused on establishment of research-based guidelines for clinical practice (AHCPR, 1999). The web address for this agency is http://www.ahrq.gov. Academic groups, such as the Cochrane Collaboration (Jadad, Haynes, 1998), prepare and disseminate up-to-date reviews of research about clinical issues. An example of how AHCPR's pressure ulcer guidelines were actually used to develop a comprehensive skin-care prevention and treatment program across care settings (from acute to home care) for a specific community was published by Suntken et al (1996). Madigan (1998) described how a home care agency applied AHCPR guidelines to its care practices, measured the effectiveness of practice changes, and demonstrated positive outcomes.

These types of research- and evidence-based guidelines will be very useful to home care agencies. However, given the diversity of home care clients and services, published guidelines will never address the full scope of the clinical issues associated with home care. Thus agencies will need to structure mechanisms for identifying research and other evidence relevant to their services and consider the application to their practices.

Various methods have been used in home care agencies to identify current research potentially applicable to practice, to explore the use of research findings in service provision, and to integrate new research into nursing protocols and practices. Successful approaches have included research surveillance systems to identify new information of interest to the staff in an agency, systematic approaches to analyzing promising studies to determine if the findings are generalizable to the agency, and methods for disseminating the findings to staff and integrating them into agencies' procedures and policies.

All of the questions for evaluating a research proposal presented in Table 30-1 are applicable to analyzing research findings for application to practice. However, in the case of a published report, additional attention needs to be paid to the discussions about data analysis and results and their interpretation. Although much of the research on home care is published in peer-reviewed journals or shared through other peer-reviewed mechanisms, some less-than-quality studies and erroneous or misleading results have been published. Therefore the reader must approach all research reports with healthy skepticism. In addition, two rigorous quality studies addressing the same questions may demonstrate apparently contradictory results. Thus agency staff will need to identify and review a full body of literature about a given clinical question to determine the consistent findings applicable to clinical practice.

The data-analysis section of a research report should present results clearly and concisely, including both positive and negative results relevant to the research questions or hypotheses. Information about subjects should be presented in a manner that would provide the reader sufficient information to determine the similarity between the studied sample to the reader's group of interest. The results should be linked to the research questions and hypotheses addressed by the study. Appropriate statistics should have been used for the analysis, and where appropriate, degrees for freedom, actual statistical results, and levels of significance should be presented.

Each research report should have a concluding section in which the results are interpreted and discussed, the limitations of the study presented, and the significance and applicability of the findings critiqued. The practitioner should read this section carefully, considering the following questions:

- Are all the conclusions supported by data?
- Does the researcher discuss both the statistical and the practical relevance of the results?
- Are the results linked back to the questions or hypotheses, the literature review, and the theoretical framework in a coherent way?
- Are the interpretations reasonable and unbiased?
- Are the results useful to the agency?
- In the case of a descriptive study, how can findings be used to better understand the clients, their needs, and their responses to their conditions and home care services? What implications exist for modification of services based on this new information?
- In the case of an experimental study, how can the intervention be considered in the context of current services? Should new services be offered? Has evidence been presented that the agency's current services may not be effective?

The bibliographic search programs used by health science libraries can facilitate self-directed reviews of clinical issues and can link to article abstracts or full-text articles. The good news is that research findings are increasingly accessible and often in review form; however, the availability of increasing amounts of information places more responsibility on agency staff to know, consider, and apply new knowledge.

Once a practice guideline is explored, reviewed, and judged to be solidly evidence based, staff need to consider the incorporation of the practice. Criteria, such as relative advantage; compatibility with resources, values, and priorities; and complexity need to be applied to an evaluation of the potential adoption of the guideline (Madigan, 1998). All changes require planning and communication and often require training. Thus home care agency involvement in the active application and dissemination of research results is likely to increase in the future.

Outcome and Assessment Information Set—A Major Resource for Home Care Data

Outcome and Assessment Information Set (OASIS) is a relatively recent data-reporting requirement of the Centers for Medicare and Medicaid Services (formerly known as the Health Care Financing Administration [HCFA]) for measuring client outcomes in home care (HCFA, 1999). Outcomes are defined as changes in health status between two or more time points. Although this tool was developed to assist home care agencies with quality-improvement activities, its content and administration structure provide standardized clinical data that could be effectively used in agency-based and larger research and evaluation projects. The B1 version of the tool, issued June 1998, contains 79 demographic, clinically focused items measuring variables important to the care of adults. The following variables are measured: medical diagnoses and their severity, concurrent health conditions, home care therapies, prognoses, risk factors, living arrangements, supportive assistance, sensory status, integumentary status, respiratory status, elimination status, neuroemotional status, activities of daily living and instrumental activities of daily living, medications, equipment management, emergency care, and discharge disposition. The website for the OASIS project is probably the best source for up-to-date information on the OASIS tool and its development and application. The site address is http://www.hcfa.gov/medicaid/oasis/newaddre.htm.

The full operationalization of this quality-improvement mechanism across the United States will provide a significant, dynamic database of home care clients and changes in health status from admission to discharge. The tool does not measure home care services or interventions; however, such data would be available in records and in other databases. Several recent publications have discussed the application of the OASIS database to various evaluation home care investigations (Adams et al, 1998; Clark, 1998; Sperling, 1998).

REVIEW OF CURRENT STATE OF HOME CARE RESEARCH

Because the field of home care represents diverse services addressing a range of needs and therapies provided to people across the lifespan and their families, this chapter is insufficient to fully review all of the published research about and applicable to home care. Therefore this section of the chapter focuses on recent reviews of home care research and selected other publications that represent important trends or issues in home care.

As a service, home care was developed over 100 years ago in response to human needs, and its development has been guided, not only by data, but also by a number of strongly held values. Data are important as the scientific bases for practice and the base from which new knowledge will be built. Values guide the selection of research priorities and decisions in the absence of data or in conjunction with data. In a recent discussion, Val Halamandaris, President of the National Association for Home Care, outlined 20 reasons for home care (Navarra, Ferrer, 1997). The following statements about home care are reasons that exemplify the intermingling and interrelationship of the information base and the values that guide current home care practice and implicitly provide a framework for a home care–research agenda.

1. It is delivered at home.
2. It represents the best tradition in American health care.
3. It keeps families together.
4. It serves to keep the elderly independent.
5. It prevents or postpones institutionalization.
6. It promotes healing.
7. It is safer than care in other settings.
8. It allows a maximal amount of freedom for the client.
9. It is personalized care.
10. It, by definition, involves the client and the family in the care that is delivered.

11. It reduces stress for the client.
12. It is the most effective form of health care.
13. It is the most efficient form of health care.
14. It is performed by special people.
15. It is the only way to reach some clients.
16. There is little fraud and abuse associated with home care.
17. It improves the client's quality of life.
18. It is less expensive than other forms of care.
19. It extends life.
20. It is the preferred form of care, even for clients who are terminally ill.

This list includes facts, beliefs, hypotheses, hopes, and values and can serve as a rich source of assumptions that could form the basis of a home care–research agenda.

Because of the breadth of home care services and related practice and administrative issues, several research reviews have been published since 1990. Key conclusions from these reviews will be discussed throughout this chapter. The reader is referred to the original articles and reference lists for additional information and the evidence supporting the conclusions.

In an early, comprehensive review of the research in home care published until 1990, Barkauskas (1990) concluded the following:

1. The foci of home care research reflect the multiple and diverse client groups served by professional nurses.
2. Care provided in the home has a unique treatment effect over care provided in other settings.
3. The need for home care services and their effectiveness across diverse populations is well documented.
4. The elderly ill are and will be a major client group within home care.
5. The following factors influence the initial use of home care services and the amount of services received: geographical residence, functional status, sex, economic situation, recent medical history, living arrangements, treatment needs, referral source, source of care, and type of payment.
6. Home care for health-promotion and risk-reduction services has demonstrated effectiveness when targeted, high-intensity services are provided to high-risk clients and families.
7. The home can be a safe environment for the provision of numerous treatments and care

regimens by health care providers, by informal care givers, and by the clients themselves.
8. The home is the preferred source of care by the majority of people needing care.
9. Clients and families often have unmet needs for information, guidance, and assistance with coping strategies during their transition from acute care to home care.
10. Findings across studies of the cost effectiveness of home care, as an alternative method of care for chronically-ill people, are inconsistent when cost is the dependent variable.

This review documented the high interest in home care research across a number of constituencies, including university faculty, governmental agencies, home care agencies, and consumers.

Ciliska et al (1996) conducted a general review of the evidence for the effectiveness of public health–nursing interventions provided through home visits. No negative results of home-visiting interventions were identified, and positive outcomes included improvement in children's health status, improvement in maternal health and health behaviors, health care–expenditure cost savings, and improvements in the functional status of elderly people.

In general, the conclusions of general reviews of home care research are positive and provide useful data for practice, as well as raise questions for future studies. The following sections of this chapter will present summaries of home care–related research according to specific topics.

High-Tech Home Care

As more and more high-tech therapies have been integrated into the home, important questions about the abilities of clients and their families, as well as home care agency staff, to adequately manage complex therapies in homes motivated this area of research. The findings of most studies have reported optimism about the safety of home-based use of medical technology and the satisfaction of clients and families with the option to provide care at home (Smith, 1995, 1996). Most negative findings have emanated from care-giver issues when high-tech interventions needed to be maintained over long periods. Most studies demonstrated cost savings over hospital care, but many of the costs were shifted to families (Chiu, Shyu, Chen, 1997). Caregivers reported limited social lives, loss of privacy, disruption of sleep, difficult schedules, demanding physical care, and curtailed activities. However, findings of studies regarding caregiver and client education indicated that educational and related supportive interventions served to relieve anxiety and increase confidence in managing home care. Several specific studies are highlighted in this section.

Smith (1995, 1996) conducted two recent reviews on research related to the application of technology to home care and the quality of life and caregiving in technological home care. She reviewed the literature on home mechanical ventilation, apnea monitoring, oxygen therapy, assistive-device technologies, nutrition support, hemodialysis, peritoneal dialysis, infusion therapies, and automatic external defibrillation. Smith (1995, 1996) observed that, across studies, the prevalence of technology home care is increasing and that, overall, the clinical outcomes have been positive. She cautions, however, about the paucity of published data on the untoward effects of high-tech home care. Research findings imply that technologically dependent clients, for the most part, perceived that they had quality in their lives.

The benefits of early discharge for clients with serious wound or postsurgical infections and replacement of hospital intravenous antibiotic therapy with intramuscular administration of antibiotics at home were explored by Rubinstein (1993). This treatment decreased hospital stays by 7 days and increased the quality of life for clients. In addition to these benefits, it was hypothesized that home settings were safer for clients because of decreased exposure to harmful organisms in the hospital.

The rapid movement of high technology into homes is exemplified in the preface of the second edition of *Home Care for the High-Risk Infant* (Ahmann, 1996). The author identified a number of new or modified technologies that had been implemented in pediatric home care since the first edition of the book 10 years earlier. These technologies included more portable respiratory equipment, pulse oximetry, tracheostomy speaking valves, and parenteral nutrition. In addition, she identified research findings and changes in client groups that have altered practice substantially over a decade. Insights from research included the long-term sequelae of pre-

maturity, effectiveness of developmental interventions, benefits of breastfeeding the preterm infant, and the challenges faced by and strengths of families in home care. Challenges that emerged included the increasing numbers of infants and children born and living with human immunodeficiency virus (HIV), the earlier discharges of children surviving with complex health care needs, and the imperative of providing culturally competent and family-centered care.

Long-Term Home Care

Long-term care is needed by many disabled and elderly individuals (Magilvy et al, 1992). Home care and nursing-home care are considered to be the two primary mechanisms for the provision of terminal care for clients with disabilities and the aged. These two approaches to care have been extensively compared by populations served, cost, effectiveness, and acceptability in a number of research studies. Findings across studies consistently demonstrate that home care may not always be less expensive than institutional care for clients needing 24-hour services, but that home care is less disruptive to individuals and families than long-term care in other settings (Dellasega, King, 1996; Miller et al, 1996). Moreover, the elderly desire to stay at home to maintain control of their daily lives and have their individual needs addressed (Krothe, 1997).

Cummings and Weaver (1991) summarized the literature published in the 1970s and 1980s on the cost-effectiveness of home care for the elderly. They concluded that the total cost of services did not change when home care was added, that hospital use and nursing home cost and use did not essentially change, and that mortality, functional status, and cognitive status findings were variable. However, satisfaction with home care remained high across studies; clients and caregivers consistently perceived home as being the most desirable and acceptable site for care.

Chappell (1994) critiqued the long-term home care research literature from systems and policy perspectives. She validated the notion that functional disability was a major predictor for the use of home care services, but she also suggested that larger structural factors, such as availability of services and referral and coordination patterns, also affected home care use. She concluded that the evidence did not support the assumption that home care is less costly or higher in quality than institutional care.

After a recent, comprehensive, rigorous review of 32 well-designed studies on community-based, long-term care programs including home care, adult day care, and coordinated packages of services, Weissert and Hedrick (1994) concluded the following:

1. Community-based, long-term care does not increase survival and does not enhance or slow the rate of deterioration in functional status.

2. Unmet needs are reduced in some studies, and client and caregiver life satisfaction is increased in a few studies. The higher life-satisfaction levels tend to diminish and disappear over time.

3. The use of hospital and nursing homes is decreased in some studies, but the amount of decrease is too small to outweigh the costs of the community services, resulting in an overall average rise in costs of about 13%.

The integration of home care benefits into capitated systems has been a recent concern. Weissert et al (1997a) reported on an evaluation of the first statewide capitated, long-term Medicaid program. They concluded that the capitated incentive enabled contractors to effectively assess needs for long-term care and allocate services using creative, cost-saving approaches, emphasizing home and community-based care. Similar findings were observed and conclusions made in a study comparing home health resource-use patterns between clients enrolled in health maintenance organizations and in fee-for-service plans (Adams, Kramer, 1996).

In their discussion of the data and values associated with long-term home care for the chronically ill, Weissert and Hedrick (1994) advised:

> Policy makers who wish to support expanded community-based long term care should be prepared to support it because some patients prefer it and experience improved life satisfaction from it. Whether cheaper ways to achieve the same improvements in life satisfaction are available has not been tested. However, the popularity of community-based long term care, despite its lack of cost-effectiveness, suggests that life satisfaction improvements and consumer preference may be the most appropriate rationales for offering it, if costs can be kept reasonable.

Care of Adults with Acute Health Problems

Home care, as an alternative to extended hospitalization for acute health problems, has demonstrated high acceptability and cost savings. Home care is commonly substituted for extended acute hospital care across many diagnoses and needs or as an alternative to hospitalization, and research findings have consistently demonstrated positive outcomes and high acceptability, quality, and safety for such replacement. Examples of such recent studies include use of home care as an effective alternative for recovery from hip fractures (Levi, 1997) and the management of exacerbations of chronic obstructive pulmonary disease (Gravil et al, 1998).

Maloney and Preston (1992) synthesized much of the recent research information about home care for cancer clients and presented very practical applications to nursing care. This article can serve as a model for research reviews and their applications to nursing care for specific client groups. McCorkle et al (1994) measured symptom distress, mental health status, enforced social dependency, and health perceptions in two groups of cancer clients. The first group received home care services ($n = 49$), and the other group did not receive home care services ($n = 11$). Data regarding dependent variables were obtained at discharge and at 3 months. Clients who received home care demonstrated significant improvement in mental status and social dependency. Clients who did not receive home care did not improve on any variable. Similarly, van Harteveld, Mistiaen, and Dukkers van Emden (1997) documented a number of unmet needs of cancer clients discharged from the hospital that were effectively addressed by home care nurses.

Most home care clients are effectively served and are discharged to independent self-care or to self-care assisted by family members (Helberg, 1993b). Whereas early research concern was focused on home care as a cost-effective and safe alternative to extended hospital lengths of stay, more recent research has examined readmission to hospital after previous early discharge to home care (Dennis et al, 1996; Weissert et al, 1997b). Research has been focused on the identification of the characteristics associated with unplanned readmissions and the identification of high-risk clients requiring special interventions to prevent initial premature discharge and unplanned readmissions (Anderson et al, 1996). Martens and Mellor (1997) studied the relationship between home care services and hospital readmission of clients with congestive heart failure. Results indicated that nursing services may be influential in preventing readmission during the 90 days after hospital discharge for this category of clients. The following characteristics seem to be associated with such readmissions: complications during the initial hospital stay and required assistance with medical decision-making, bathing, dressing, feeding, or toileting (Anderson et al, 1996; Redeker, Brassard, 1996).

Clients with Acquired Immunodeficiency Syndrome

Clients with acquired immunodeficiency syndrome (AIDS) constitute a growing group of home care clients with very complex and changing home care needs. To gain insights into the problems experienced by AIDS clients at home and their related nursing care needs, Hurley and Ungvarski (1995), conducted an exploratory field study of AIDS clients' problems identified on admission to home care and the resultant nursing diagnoses. The study provided insights into the multifaceted and multitudinous needs of these clients and provided a base for services planning and intervention research. Fleishman (1997) documented the formal and informal home care services used by people with AIDS in 10 U.S. studies. The study validated the needs of this client group for substantial amounts of home care services and identified correlates of higher and lower home care use. Functional limitations and fatigue were associated with high levels of service need and use.

Pessin et al (1993) explored the mental health needs of home care clients with AIDS and described how research can assist practitioners in devising appropriate services for this client group. The cooperation between the formal and informal sources of home care seems to be essential for enabling AIDS clients to remain at home (Bunch, 1998).

Home Care for People with Psychiatric Problems

Home care can be cost effective for selected psychiatric clients and their families (Hauenstein, 1996). An example of a recent effectiveness

demonstration was reported by Pigott and Trott (1993), who described the outcomes of a 24-hour in-home crises-intervention, triage, and treatment service in a large health maintenance organization. The integrated program prevented hospitalization in about 80% of clients and demonstrated an impressive record of relapse prevention. The authors concluded that, for the majority of psychiatric clients, intensive in-home crisis-intervention and treatment programs are more effective and cost-efficient than hospitalization. The study also demonstrated how a managed-care environment, with access to various alternatives to care, can use these alternatives creatively for the organization's and the clients' benefit.

Maternal and Child Populations

Maternal and child health populations have long been a special focus of home nursing services. Historically the purpose of maternal and child interventions has been health promotion of pregnant and postpartum women and their infants. The effectiveness of such services has been documented in various studies.

Home care for health promotion has been extended to high-risk maternal and child health populations. Rhoads, McNellis, and Kessel (1991) reported on a workshop on home monitoring of uterine activity in women at high risk for preterm births. The extant research in the field was reviewed by workshop participants. They concluded that evidence existed for effectiveness of home monitoring in conjunction with daily nursing support and quality obstetrical care for very high-risk women. The conference participants also concluded that research evidence did not yet show a distinction between the relative effectiveness of uterine monitoring and nursing care, which were characteristically provided together. Gupton, Heaman, and Ashcroft (1997) studied this same high-risk maternity population in an ethnographic study to describe the experience of prolonged bedrest and mechanisms of coping with it, including recommendations for professional intervention.

Zahr (1994) analyzed research findings comparing the effectiveness of home versus hospital-based interventions on services to disadvantaged families of premature infants. She observed that although hospital-based intervention programs were easier to implement and less expensive, home-based intervention programs had the potential to provide longer-term benefits, such as improving developmental outcomes and parenting behaviors. She recommended additional study of a broad array of outcome assessments with the infants, including social and language measures and parental characteristics that affect response to and effectiveness of interventions.

Barnes-Boyd, Norr, and Nacion (1996) reported on a home-visiting program designed to reduce preventable morbidity among socioeconomically disadvantaged infants born healthy. Study results were promising and demonstrated positive, though not statistically significant, results on postneonatal mortality. However the study also demonstrated the need for health promotion in the areas of home safety, skin care, and early identification and treatment of upper respiratory infections.

In the conclusion of a recent review of home health programs for children and families, the Council on Child and Adolescent Health of the American Academy of Pediatrics (1998) acknowledged that the evidence for home visitation programs was inconclusive. However, they concluded that the more successful programs contained the following elements:

1. Focus on high-risk and high-need families
2. Initiation of interventions from pregnancy through the second to fifth year of life
3. Duration and frequency of visits adjusted to family need and risk level
4. Active promotion of positive health behaviors and social support
5. A broad multiproblem focus to address the totality of family needs
6. Measures to reduce family stress
7. Use of nurses or well-trained paraprofessionals

Research Related to Care Givers

Caregiving has been a major focus of home care research. Malonebeach and Zarit (1991) discussed the issues in this important area of home care exploration and effectively argued that caregivers represent a diverse set of variables operating in dissimilar circumstances and that caregiver research has not adequately measured the tasks and burdens of caregiving. Therefore all conclusions of caregiving research must be cautiously applied.

Dillehay and Sandys (1990) reviewed the literature focused on caregiving to Alzheimer's clients. Their review documented the multifaceted psychological, social, and physical health implications of caregiving. Research on psychological effects included explorations into burden, stress, strain, subjective well-being, and the efficacy of social support. Conclusions in additional reviews of research on home caregiving for elderly people consistently supported the significance of this area of home care research, uniformly concluded that caregivers are at personal risk for various health problems, and pinpointed major unresolved measurement issues in this arena of research (Pruchno et al, 1990; Schulz, Visintainer, Williamson, 1990; Winslow, 1998).

At the conclusion of a comprehensive review of the caregiver research and other literature, Worcester (1990) concluded, "Although concepts related to family theory, burden, role theory, and social support networks were all useful to understanding and organizing certain aspects of caregiver difficulties, no one framework contains all the caregiver difficulties that need to be addressed." She categorized caregiving problems into four categories: (1) the tasks required by caregiving, (2) caregivers' physical and mental well-being, (3) the effect of caregiving on the caregiver's lifestyle, and (4) the effect of caregiving on the caregiver's social network. Williams et al (1996) noted that caregivers often had unrealistic expectations about the burden of caregiving and the time needed for recovery.

Caregiver stress has the potential for seriously affecting not only the health of the caregiver, but also that of the care receiver. Steinmetz (1990) reviewed the literature on elder abuse and tested the relationships between task-related dependency, stress, and likelihood of elder abuse. She documented a substantial amount of elder abuse in her sample and concluded that the caregiver's perception of the stresses resulting from providing specific tasks, rather than the actual level of tasks performed, appeared to be more strongly related to elder abuse.

The impact of caregiving for pediatric clients has similar, as well as unique, impacts on families as compared to caregiving provided to adult clients and the elderly. Fleming et al (1994) compared the caregiving impact on families with four categories of technology-dependent children.

The sample, including 848 caregivers of children aged 3 to 19 years, reported varying amounts of burden. Children who were ventilator dependent, who required intravenous therapy, and who had specific supportive devices were more of a social impact and caused more personal strain on the family than those whose vital functions were monitored only (e.g., apnea monitoring).

Ahmann (1992) reviewed the family impact of home apnea monitoring and discussed the applicability of findings for nurses in clinical practice. She noted that the literature supports the notion that there are changes in family adaptation in response to home monitoring over time and that families experienced a number of health and behavior problems. These problems have included depression, anxiety, sleeping difficulty, fatigue, and sibling rivalry. In addition, home monitoring has been documented to interfere with maternal and paternal professional role choices and obligations and with social roles and activities. Likewise, the work of monitoring has placed great strain on marriages, resulting in divorce and separation in some. Social isolation and difficulties in the performance of daily household activities were often experienced by mothers. In such families, prior family problems and low satisfaction with social support were found to be the most important risk factors related to poor family functioning in the context of apnea monitoring.

Patterson et al (1994) provide powerful insights into the positive and negative aspects of the partnership between professional and family caregivers for medically fragile children. In their study, 48 mothers and fathers provided data about their relationships with home health care nurses and home health aides. Despite the necessity of formal caregivers and a number of positive aspects related to professional assistance, formal caregivers can inadvertently increase stress in complex home care situations.

Given the complexity and variability of informal caregiving, its true costs are difficult to calculate. Sevick and Bradham (1997) studied the costs of caring for ventilator-assisted clients across the United States. The economic value of the caregiving effort was estimated by calculating opportunity cost, aggregated market value, and aggregated replacement cost. The resultant data indicated that when caregiving costs were taken into account, home care may not be the least expensive care alternative for this group of clients. The mixed formal and informal economies of care make financial comparisons among long-term care alternatives very complex, although such data are urgently needed for the formulation of family policies for long-term care (McKeever, 1996).

Dura and Kiecolt-Glaser (1990) cautioned the home care field about possible biases in respondent selection for caregiver research. These investigators compared the caregiver burden reflected by caregivers who were interviewed at home with those who were able to travel for interviews. A second study compared data between users of respite services with nonusers. The caregivers who were available for participation in studies, especially at locations away from home, reflected a lower level of caregiver burden than those not available for participation and those available only in their homes.

The research questions related to caregiving will continue to be important into the future. The results of in-progress measurement work will assist in sorting out the factors in caregiving responses (Fritz et al, 1997) and the cultural context of caregiving that affect caregiving patterns and responses (Cromwell et al, 1996; Gonzalez, 1997).

International Research

Just as in the United States, home care is an expanding health care service in other parts of the world, and consequently international interest in research home care is growing (Mouk, Cox, 1992). For example, Fauroux, Howard, and Muir (1994) conducted a study of home care practices for chronic respiratory clients in 13 European countries. The authors documented important differences among the countries in the home care of respiratory clients. The authors suggested that the differences could be a very useful, natural research experiment into the relative effectiveness of different approaches to client needs.

Davies (1994) presented a very comprehensive, data-based discussion of the rationale and outcomes of a major home and community care policy change in Great Britain. Before the initiation of a new policy, the research related to needs and issues in home and community care was reviewed and summarized, and the resultant policy was based on research findings. This research analysis demonstrated that an excessive share of resources were consumed by low-need recipients, that inconsistencies and biases in the allocation of services were rampant, and that home-based services had a low impact on admissions to institutions for long-term care. The new policy, established in 1989, proposed to match resources to needs and to transform community care in ways that enable the maximal possible independence of all people in their homes or homelike community settings. Planning strategies have focused on discouragement of the building of additional nursing homes, support for the development and expansion of housing alternatives, the shift of responsibility to local governments for designing and delivering services, development of methods for the identification of high-risk and high-need individuals to better target appropriate services, and the provision of incentives for various types of professional caregivers to coordinate their work.

Additional European countries have addressed issues associated with a rapidly growing elderly population by systems-design innovations in long-term care planning. Coleman (1995) described how long-term care policies were explored and changed in Sweden, Denmark, the Netherlands, and Great Britain. Research into needs and costs were used as bases to improve quality of care, control costs, and ensure efficient delivery of home care and community services.

Findings of studies in other countries are consistent with those from the United States in the quality of home care in the case of early hospital discharge for acute surgical problems (Kaag, Wijkel, de Jong, 1996) and psychiatric clients (Boomsma, Dingermans, Dassen, 1997). Home oxygen respiratory therapy has also been investigated by Kawakami (1996) in Japan. Data from the Japanese study indicated that home oxygen therapy prolongs life and also improves the quality of daily life.

Researchers in Northern Ireland (Boydell, 1996; Boydell, McAllister, 1994) are exploring methods by which client information can be shared among different professionals in different settings by use of a common computerized database. The prototype system will be initially tested with assessment, planning for care, and care delivery to elderly clients in home care.

Professional Home Care Providers

A substantial amount of recent research attention has targeted home care nurses, their client caseloads, their clinical reasoning, and their work (Benefield, 1996). Because of the nature of home care, most providers' encounters are not witnessed by other providers. Most of the field's information about the content and conduct of home visits is from client records. Given the relative invisibility of home care practice and the limitations of recordings, research has focused on the processes of learning to provide care in the home, standardized tools to capture the content and essence of the home visit, methods by which clients are selected for services, and the relationship between resource consumption and outcomes.

Nursing is becoming increasingly community based, and more nurses are including home care nursing responsibilities as part or all of their roles. Thus training for community-based nursing practice has been a research area (Murray, 1998). Ark and Nies (1996) surveyed home care nurses to identify the skills and knowledge most needed by home care nurses in an effort to prepare nurses for the transition from institution to community roles. In another qualitative study, Scannell et al (1993) surveyed pediatric home care nurses to devise a description of their roles. Respondents described their roles as solitary, ambiguous, and unprogrammed. A number of differences between pediatric nursing practiced in institutions and pediatric nursing practiced in homes were identified, mostly focusing on less nurse control in homes and greater need to work with families. Daley and Miller (1996) collected qualitative data from 21 home care nurses representing various stages of professional maturation and demonstrated that home care nursing expertise develops along a measurable continuum. Expert nurses are able to integrate physiological data with environmental and family data to provide complex nursing care.

O'Neill (1994) explored the influence of education and experience on clinical inference tasks and diagnostic problems relevant to home care through responses to standardized clinical vignettes. Education and experience influenced achievement of normatively correct responses. In a later study, O'Neill (1997) used record data to determine the types of inferences and decisions made by home care nurses. Two main types of decisions were noted in the recordings: autonomous decisions, with the subcategories of self-directed and consultative decisions, and collaborative decisions. More experienced nurses' records reflected more decisions, and they used autonomous decision-making more frequently than less experienced nurses. Fowler (1997) explored home health care nurses' thinking processes in planning care for chronically ill adults and developed a useful typology of thinking activities that could be used in future research on this topic.

Lemire and Austin (1996) interviewed six home care case managers, two of whom were nurses, to determine what factors influenced care decisions. Findings indicated that client and caregiver characteristics were most influential in care decisions and that the case managers were not comfortable with fiscal accountability. However, Adams, Johnson, and Moore (1996) documented that nurses' and clients' perceptions of clients' problems may vary considerably.

Dalton et al (1996) examined the results of an education program for home care nurses on pain management. Nurses' knowledge increased, and although some change was noted in client-care practices as reflected by recordings, substantial changes in client-care practices were not observed. The authors suggested that recordings may be incomplete and that some behaviors related to client-care practices may be slowly assimilated. Dellasega (1992) explored home care nurses' methods of assessing the mental status of elderly people. She determined that nurses most frequently relied on clients' orientation as the determinant of mental status. Herth (1995) surveyed 158 home care and hospice nurses to determine what interventions were used to foster hope in chronically ill and terminally ill clients. The most commonly used strategies by both groups of nurses were provision of comfort and pain relief.

Martin, Sheet, and Stegman (1993) examined the home nursing care provided to 2403 home care clients in four agencies in the Midwest and eastern United States. The report of this study is rich in its description of the health problems addressed by nurses in home care, the interventions applied, and client outcomes at the termination of services. The methods used to collect and classify data, including the Omaha System, provide a useful framework for future research focused on describing client populations. Cohen et al (1991) documented the nursing interventions provided by nurses in transitional follow-up nursing care to very low–birth weight infants. They applied the taxonomy of ambulatory care nursing and assessed that the taxonomy was very appropriate for the description of such activities.

Dineen et al (1992) surveyed a total of 37 public health and home care agencies in a midwestern state to determine what antepartum services were being provided to pregnant women. Services differed considerably between types of agencies, with public health agencies focusing services on high-risk, especially adolescent, women, and home care agencies focusing services on the monitoring of preterm labor.

The identification of factors affecting resource consumption, which would assist managers in planning services and estimating the total cost of an episode of services, is a long-standing topic of research in home care. Early research focused on client demographic variables and medical diagnoses. More recent nursing research has been focused on variables more directly relevant to client need. Hays (1992) investigated the influence of nursing intensity and nursing diagnoses on the consumption of nursing time. Using data from the records of 237 discharged clients, she determined that both nursing intensity and nursing diagnoses explained significant (10% to 26%) variances in direct hours of home nursing care consumed.

Productivity is an important resource dimension affecting costs directly and quality indirectly. Clearly, both practitioner and client variables affect productivity. To develop a taxonomy of provider-focused productivity concepts and areas as bases for measurement in research and practice, Benefield (1996) identified the following areas of productivity-measurement classification for individual home health care registered nurses: client and family management, practice management, knowledge and skill maintenance, communication, nursing process, written documentation, and home health care knowledge.

To gain insights into client-focused variables affecting productivity, Helberg (1993a) studied the contributions of sociodemographic factors, medical conditions, and nursing dependency compared with the nursing problems identified and nursing care provided to clients during home care nursing visits. Data relating to 438 clients were obtained through multiple sources, including client interviews, direct observation, and record abstraction. Data indicated that nursing dependency was the strongest predictor of the nursing problems of and nursing care provided to home care clients.

Damato et al (1993) explored the relationship between the amount of direct-care time and total time spent by clinical nurse specialists with the families of 39 very low–birth weight infants in the hospital and for 18 months after discharge and outcomes at discharge from care. The total amount of clinical nurse specialist time per infant per the 1½-year period was 27.3 hours. Significant, logical relationships were observed between nurse direct time and the number of acute-care visits and rehospitalizations, implying that nurses spent more time with high-need infants. However no relationship between time spent and infant outcomes was observed, implying that all infants, regardless of need, were able to have optimal outcomes at the conclusion of service.

Brooten et al (1996) investigated nursing time in a slightly different context, examining the effects of morbidity on the allocation of nursing time for discharge planning and home care to mothers who delivered by unplanned cesarean section. They concluded that time allocated to the client situation was more dictated by client needs than by the reimbursement available for the family and that the two-visit limitation for postpartum home visits may not be sufficient for this population. Similar findings were observed in a study by Leonard, Brust, and Sielaff (1991), who explored variability in the nursing hours received by 31 Minnesota families with technology-assisted children. They concluded that family needs and characteristics, rather than the child's medical condition, influenced the number of hours. This finding suggests the preeminence of psychosocial nursing interventions as a major resource-use determinant.

ETHICAL QUESTIONS FOR HOME CARE RESEARCH

The current tensions in the field of home care related to need, cost, and quality are replete with ethical issues and questions. Given that the home

is the preferred site of health care for most individuals needing long-term care or follow-up for treatments related to acute illnesses, should the home care system be prepared to provide home care regardless of costs? In the following statement, Chappell (1994) eloquently pinpointed the needed balance among objective research findings, subjective values, and ethics in home care decisions regarding the elderly: "Ultimately, however, decisions have to be made and they will rest on value judgments. Do we as a society want seniors to have the option of remaining at home in relative independence?" Arras and Dubler (1994) discussed the myriad ethical issues associated with high-tech home care. The issues raised in their article were summarized by the editors of the *Hastings Center Report,* and the key points relevant to home care research are broadly listed (Executive summary of project conclusions, 1994):

1. Home care can generate difficult "problems of meaning" relating to body image, family identity, and the meaning of "home."
2. Home care can place excessive burdens on family and friends charged with caring for clients.
3. Family caregivers are often ill-prepared to undertake the high-tech care of loved ones at home.
4. Home care is rarely organized into an efficient, coherent, and comprehensive package for clients and their caregivers, many of whom must assume the onerous tasks of their own care management without the requisite knowledge, skills, and connections.
5. The worst home is not necessarily better than the best hospital or institution.
6. The high-tech home care industry has produced many useful devices but has also reaped enormous profits through questionable sales practices and price markups in an essentially unregulated environment.
7. Some extremely expensive high-tech home care services are administered to a wide variety of home care clients, yet researchers have virtually no hard data, gained through careful outcome studies, of their efficacy or cost effectiveness over hospital care.

This listing is rich with a home care research agenda that can complement the other research areas presented earlier in this chapter.

FUTURE OF HOME CARE RESEARCH

In an effort to focus and guide the research in home care, researchers (Albrecht, 1992; Albrecht, Perry, 1992) explored research priorities with its practitioners via a Delphi-type survey. The results indicated that the following were the top-priority research categories cited by home care administrators and educators:

1. Outcomes of care
2. Cost of home care
3. Policy analysis and reimbursement
4. Client-classification systems
5. Uniform data set
6. Predictors of care and managed care
7. Coordination of care and managed care
8. Productivity
9. Documentation
10. Use of health care services
11. Health promotion and disease prevention in home care
12. Nursing interventions and processes

Cost-effective and cost-efficient use of home care resources will continue to be a major topic of home care research into the future because of predictable movement of more complex therapies into the home and because of the growth of the aged population. More needs to be known about the most appropriate clients for home care services and the most appropriate amounts and configurations of resources for addressing problems and needs (Forbes, Neufield, 1997, Williams, 1995).

The managed care environment will present new issues and new possibilities for innovative configuration of services and services settings and intervention studies. Studies exploring factors affecting the use and allocation of services (e.g., using intensity and diagnoses to predict resource consumption [Hays, 1992]) and the manner in which staff time is allocated (e.g., Hedtcke, MacQueen, Carr, 1992) will continue to be important in providing insights into components of cost and productivity.

Although cost-related variables will continue to be important, a new array of variables for measuring the quality and effects of home care and home care innovations need to be considered. Variables such as quality of life and satisfaction in various care situations, along with the costs of care, need to be explored (Forbes, Neufield, 1997). As new therapies and technologies are integrated into home care, descriptive studies of client and family responses and needs will be indicated as the bases for care planning and intervention research.

For people with disabilities and the elderly needing long-term care, only two primary options for long-term care have been available, with home care being preferred, in most cases, over institutionalization. Additional options for long-term care through alternative living arrangements might address the needs of the elderly while also maintaining costs. Although proposals for special housing arrangements for the elderly are not new (MacDonald, Remus, Laing, 1994), the health and health care possibilities of such arrangements have not been more than minimally explored.

Clients with Alzheimer's disease have unique home care issues. Recent research may provide insights into behavioral approaches for the management of this problem (Montgomery, 1996; Radebaugh, Buckholtz, Khachaturian, 1996; Riesberg, 1996).

A number of questions related to caregiver needs and the problems associated with caregiving were identified in this chapter, and the references offer a wealth of insight into needed research about caregiving. Although the general needs of caregivers have been well documented, most care reimbursement plans do not directly pay for nursing services to caregivers. Clearly, exploration of interventions to alleviate caregiver symptoms and reduce stress are timely, as are policy changes to recognize the need for services to informal caregivers.

Although recent research and other examinations have shed light on the content of home visits and how nurses think about client information (Byrd, 1995; Greene, 1991), descriptors of nursing services need to be standardized within the profession. A number of taxonomies have been developed to describe client problems, nursing interventions, and the outcomes of services (Iowa Interventions Project, 1996; Iowa Outcomes Project, 1997; Martin, Leak, Aden, 1992). These developments and related research into their validation and application to home care are timely.

As homes become better equipped with computer technology, this technology is likely to become a powerful tool in the care of clients and may dramatically affect the activities of formal care providers (Maceratini, Rafanelli, Ricci, 1995). Computer use by nurses and clients will be a major focus of future research activity, both from the aspects of computer technology application, as well as the generation of data related to other questions (Alemi, Stephens, 1996; Wilson, Fulmer, 1998).

The continuing investigations of Shaughnessy et al (1997), which have served as a basis for the development of OASIS, will continue to provide insights and direction for research focused on care outcomes and quality.

The material in this chapter has aptly documented the importance of research to the field of home care and the richness of the home care field as a focus of research. New tools, such as advanced computer technology, the OASIS quality-evaluation data, and standardized nursing languages, will facilitate the quality of available home care data and access to data. Given the projected proliferation of home care data, dissemination activities in an evidence-based practice framework will become a research-related priority.

REFERENCES

Adams CE, Johnson JE, Moore JF: Patients' health problems: Differences in perceptions between home health patients and nurses, *Home Healthcare Nurse* 14:932-938, 1996.

Adams CE, Kramer S: Home health resource utilization: Health maintenance organization versus fee-for-service subscribers, *Journal of Nursing Administration* 26(2):20-27, 1996.

Adams CE et al: Using the outcome-based quality improvement model and OASIS to improve HMO patients' outcomes. Outcome Assessment and Information Set, *Home Healthcare Nurse* 15:395-401, 1998.

Agency for Health Care Policy and Research (AHCPR): *Clinical information* (on-line), 1999 http://www.ahcpr.gov/clinic/

Ahmann E: Family impact of home apnea monitoring: An overview of research and its clinical implications, *Pediatric Nursing* 18:611-616, 1992.

Ahmann E: *Home care for the high-risk infant,* Gaithersburg, Md, 1996, Aspen.

Albrecht M: Research priorities for home health nursing, Nursing & Health Care 13:538-541, 1992.

Albrecht MN, Perry KM: Home health care: Delineation of research priorities and formation of a national network group, *Clinical Nursing Research* 1:305-311, 1992.

Alemi F, Stephens RC: Computer services for patients. Description of systems and summary of findings, *Medical Care* 34(suppl 10):OS1-9, 1996.

American Academy of Pediatrics, Council on Child and Adolescent Health: The role of home-visitation programs in improving health outcomes for children and families, *Pediatrics* 101:486-489, 1998.

Anderson MA et al: Hospital readmission during home care: A pilot study, *Journal of Community Health Nursing* 13(1):1-12, 1996.

Ark PD, Nies M: Knowledge and skills of the home healthcare nurse, *Home Healthcare Nurse* 14:292-297, 1996.

Arras JD, Dubler NN: Bringing the hospital home: Ethical and social implications of high-tech home care, *Hastings Center Report* 24(5)(suppl):S19-S28, 1994.

Balding M: Practical research: An effective tool in home healthcare, *Home Healthcare Nurse* 15:509-511, 1997.

Balding M et al: *Home care: A research guide,* East Lansing, Mich, 1994, Michigan Foundation for Home Care.

Barkauskas VH: Home health care, *Annual Review of Nursing Research* 8:103-132, 1990.

Barnes-Boyd C, Norr KE, Nacion KW: Evaluation of an interagency home visiting program to reduce postneonatal mortality in disadvantaged communities, *Public Health Nursing* 13:201-208, 1996.

Benefield LE: Component analysis of productivity in home care RNs, *Public Health Nursing* 13:233-243, 1996.

Benefield LE: Research in home healthcare, *Home Healthcare Nurse* 15:871, 1997.

Boomsma J, Dingermans CA, Dassen TW: The nursing process in crisis-oriented psychiatric home care, *Journal of Psychiatric & Mental Health Nursing* 4:295-301, 1997.

Bowen P, LeDuc L: Alzheimer's Disease Research turned into reality, *Caring* 13(8):40-41, 1994.

Boydell L: European prototype for integrated care, *International Journal of Health Care Quality Assurance* 9(4):30-32, 1996.

Boydell L, McAllister B: European prototype for integrated care (EPIC), *Computer Methods and Programs in Biomedicine* 45(1-2):47-49, 1994.

Brooten D et al: Early discharge and home care after unplanned Cesarean birth: Nursing care time, *Journal of Obstetric, Gynecologic and Neonatal Nursing* 25:595-600, 1996.

Bunch EH: AIDS in Norway: A post hoc evaluation of an AIDS home care project, *Journal of Clinical Nursing* 7:183-187, 1998.

Byrd ME: A concept analysis of home visiting, *Public Health Nursing* 12(2):83-89, 1995.

Byrd ME: A typology of the potential outcomes of maternal-child home visits: A literature analysis, *Public Health Nursing* 14:3-11, 1997.

Chappell NL: Home care research: What does it tell us? *The Gerontologist* 34(1):116-120, 1994.

Chiu I, Shyu WC, Chen TR: A cost-effectiveness analysis of home care and community-based nursing homes for stroke patients and their families, *Journal of Advanced Nursing* 26:872-878, 1997.

Ciliska D et al: A systematic overview of the effectiveness of home visiting in a delivery strategy for public health nursing interventions, *Canadian Journal of Public Health* 87:193-198, 1996.

Clark LL: Incorporating OASIS into the Visiting Nurses Association, *Outcomes Management for Nursing Practice* 2(1):24-28, 1998.

Cohen SM et al: Taxonomic classification of transitional follow-up care nursing interventions and low birthweight infants, *Clinical Nursing Specialist* 5(1):31-36, 1991.

Coleman BJ: European models of long-term care in the home and community, *International Journal of Health Services* 25:455-474, 1995.

Cromwell SL et al: Uncovering the cultural context for quality of family caregiving for elders, *Western Journal of Nursing Research* 18:284-296, 1996.

Cummings JE, Weaver FM: Cost-effectiveness of home care, *Clinics in Geriatric Medicine* 7:865-874, 1991.

Daley BJ, Miller M: Defining home health care nursing: Implications for continuing nursing education, *Journal of Continuing Education in Nursing* 27:228-237, 1996.

Dalton JA et al: Changing the relationship among nurses' knowledge, self-reported, behavior, and documented behavior in pain management: Does education make a difference? *Journal of Pain and Symptom Management* 12:308-319, 1996.

Damato EG et al: The associate between CNS direct care time and total time and very low birth weight infant outcomes, *Clinical Nurse Specialist* 2(2):75-9, 1993.

Davies B: British home and community care: Research-based critiques and the challenge of the new policy, *Social Science and Medicine* 38:883-903, 1994.

Dellasega C: Home health nurses' assessments of cognition, *Applied Nursing Research* 5(3):127-133, 1992.

Dellasega C, King LE: The psychogeriatric nurse in home health care: Use of research to develop the role, *Clinical Nurse Specialist* 10(2):64-68, 1996.

Dennis LI et al: The relationship between hospital readmissions of Medicare beneficiaries with chronic illnesses and home care nursing interventions, *Home Healthcare Nurse* 14:303-309, 1996.

Dillehay RC, Sandys MR: Caregivers for Alzheimer's patients: What we are learning from the research, *International Journal of Aging and Human Development* 30:263-285, 1990.

Dineen K et al: Antepartum home-care services for high-risk women, *Journal of Obstetric, Gynecologic, and Neonatal Nursing* 21:121-125, 1992.

Dura JR, Kiecolt-Glaser JK: Sample bias in caregiving research, *Journal of Gerontology* 45(5):200-204, 1990.

Executive summary of project conclusions, *Hastings Center Report* 24(5)(suppl):S3, 1994.

Fauroux B, Howard P, Muir JF: Home treatment for chronic respiratory insufficiency: The situation in Europe in 1992, *European Respiratory Journal* 7:1721-1726, 1994.

Feinglass J, Slavensky R, Tang L: The intermittent claudication research study: Vascular outcomes research using home health nurses, *Journal of Vascular Nursing* 8(1):8-11, 1996.

Fleishman JA: Utilization of home care among people with HIV infection, *Health Services Research* 32:155-175, 1997.

Fleming J et al: Impact on the family of children who are technology dependent and cared for in the home, *Pediatric Nursing* 20:379-388, 1994.

Forbes DA, Neufeld A: Strategies to address the methodological challenges of client-satisfaction research in home care, *Canadian Journal of Nursing Research* 29(2):69-77, 1997.

Fowler LP: Clinical reasoning strategies used during care planning, *Clinical Nursing Research* 6:349-361, 1997.

Fritz CL et al: Correlation among three psychological scales used in research of caregivers for patients with Alzheimer's disease, *Psychological Reports* 80(1):67-80, 1997.

Gonzales EW: Resourcefulness, appraisals and coping efforts of family caregivers, *Issues in Mental Health Nursing* 18:209-227, 1997.

Gravil JH et al: Home treatment of exacerbations of chronic obstructive pulmonary disease by an acute respiratory assessment service, *The Lancet* 351(9119):1853-1855, 1998.

Greene JE: The relationship between nursing diagnostic reasoning and reimbursement in home health care. In Carroll-Johnson RM, ed: *Classification of nursing diagnoses: Proceedings of the ninth conference,* Philadelphia, 1991, Lippincott.

Gupton A, Heaman M, Ashcroft T: Bed rest from the perspective of the high-risk pregnant woman, *Journal of Obstetric, Gynecologic, and Neonatal Nursing* 26:423-430, 1997.

Harris MD: Nursing research in home health agencies, *Home Healthcare Nurse* 8(1):10-12, 1990.

Hays BJ: Nursing care requirements and resource consumption in home health care, *Nursing Research* 41(3):138-143, 1992.

Health Care Financing Administration (HCFA): *OASIS overview* (on-line), 1999 http://www/hcfa.gov/medicare/hsqb/oasis/hhoview.htm#A.

Hedtcke CS, MacQueen L, Carr A: How do home health nurses spend their time? *Journal of Nursing Administration* 22(1):18-22, 1992.

Hekelman FP et al: Clinical research in home care, *Journal of Nursing Administration* 22(1):29-32, 1992.

Helberg JL: Factors influencing home care nursing problems and nursing care, *Research in Nursing and Health* 16:363-370, 1993a.

Helberg JL: Patients' status at home care discharge, *Image* 25(2):93-99, 1993b.

Herth K: Engendering hope in the chronically and terminally ill: Nursing interventions, *American Journal of Hospice and Palliative Care* 12(5):31-39, 1995.

Hurley PM, Ungvarski PJ: Nursing research in HIV/AIDS home care. I. *Home Healthcare Nurse* 13(3):13-17+, 1995.

Iowa Interventions Project: *Nursing Interventions (NIC)*, ed 2, St Louis, 1996, Mosby.

Iowa Outcomes Project: *Nursing Outcomes Classification (NOC)*, St Louis, 1997, Mosby.

Jadad AR, Haynes RB: The Cochrane Collaboration—Advances and Challenges in improving evidence-based decision making, *Medical Decision Making* 18:2-9, 1998.

Kaag ME, Wijkel D, de Jong D: Primary health care replacing hospital care—the effect on quality of care, *International Journal for Quality in Health Care* 8:367-373, 1996.

Kawakami Y: Current status and research on chronic respiratory failure in Japan, *Internal Medicine* 35:436-442, 1996.

Kelly F et al: Developing a new method of record care at home for children with cancer: An example of research and practice collaboration in a regional paediatric oncology unit, *European Journal of Cancer Care* 5(1):26-31, 1996.

Krothe JS: Giving voice to elderly people: Community-based long-term care, *Public Health Nursing* 14:217-226, 1997.

Lemire AM, Austin CD: Care planning in home care: An exploratory study, *Journal of Case Management* 5(1):32-40, 1996.

Leonard BJ, Brust JD, Sielaff BH: Determinants of home care nursing hours for technology-assisted children, *Public Health Nursing* 8:239-244, 1991.

Levi SJ: Posthospital setting, resource utilization, and self-care outcome in older women with hip fracture, *Archives of Physical Medicine & Rehabilitation* 78:973-979, 1997.

MacDonald M, Remus G, Laing G: Research considerations: The link between housing and health in the elderly, *Journal of Gerontological Nursing* 20(7):5-10, 1994.

Maceratini R, Rafanelli M, Ricci FL: Virtual hospitalization: Reality or utopia? II. *Medinfo* 8:1482-1486, 1995.

Madigan EA: Evidence-based practice in home healthcare. A springboard for discussion, *Home Healthcare Nurse* 16:411-415, 1998.

Magilvy JK et al: Visions of rural aging: Use of photographic method in gerontological research, *Gerontologist* 32:253-257, 1992.

Malonebeach EE, Zarit SH: Current research issues in caregiving to the elderly, *International Journal of Aging and Human Development* 32:103-114, 1991.

Maloney CH, Preston F: An overview of home care for patients with cancer, *Oncology Nursing Forum* 19(1):75-80, 1992.

Martens KH, Mellor SD: A study of the relationship between home care services and hospital readmission of patients with congestive heart failure, *Home Healthcare Nurse* 15(2):123-129, 1997.

Martin K, Leak G, Aden C: The Omaha System. A research-based model for decision making, *Journal of Nursing Administration* 22(11):47-52, 1992.

Martin KS, Sheet NJ, Stegman MR: Home health clients: Characteristics, outcomes of care, and nursing interventions, *American Journal of Public Health* 83:1730-1734, 1993.

McCorkle R et al: The impact of posthospital home care on patients with cancer, *Research in Nursing and Health* 17:243-251, 1994.

McKeever P: The family: Long-term care research and policy formulation, *Nursing Inquiry* 3:200-206, 1996.

McWilliam CL, Desai K, Greig B: Bridging town and gown: Building research partnerships between community-based professional providers and academia, *Journal of Professional Nursing* 13:307-315, 1997.

Miller LL et al: Development of use and cost measures in a nursing intervention for family caregivers and frail elderly patients, *Research in Nursing & Health* 19:273-275, 1996.

Montgomery RJ: Next steps for social and behavioral research related to Alzheimer's disease, *International Psychogeriatrics* 8(suppl 1):103-107, 1996.

Mouk A, Cox C: Lessons to be learned. Home care in other countries, *Caring* 11(10):35-39, 1992.

Murray TA: From outside the walls: A qualitative study of nurses who recently changed from hospital-based practice to home health care nursing, *Journal of Continuing Education in Nursing* 29(2):55-60, 1998.

Navarra T, Ferrer M: *An insider's guide to home health care,* Thorofare, NJ, 1997, Slack.

O'Neill ES: Home health nurses' use of base rate information in diagnostic reasoning, *Advances in Nursing Science* 17(2):77-85, 1994.

O'Neill ES: Home care nurses' inferences and decisions, *Applied Nursing Research* 10(1):33-38, 1997.

Patterson JM et al: Caring for medically fragile children at home: The parent-professional relationship, *Journal of Pediatric Nursing* 9(2):98-106, 1994.

Pessin N et al: Integrating mental health and home care services for AIDS patients, *Caring* 12(5):30-34, 1993.

Pigott HE, Trott L: Translating research into practice: The implementation of an in-home crisis intervention triage and treatment service in the private sector, *American Journal of Medical Quality* 8(3):138-144, 1993.

Pruchno RA et al: Mental and physical health of caregiving spouses: Development of a causal model, *Journal of Gerontology* 45(5):192-199, 1990.

Radebaugh TS, Buckholtz N, Khachaturian Z: Behavioral approaches to the treatment of Alzheimer's disease: Research strategies, *International Psychogeriatrics* 8(suppl 1):7-12, 1996.

Raphael C, Angelicola J: The Center for Home Care Policy and Research, *Caring* 12(9):62-64, 1993.

Redeker NS, Brassard AB: Health patterns of cardiac surgery clients using home health care nursing services, *Public Health Nursing* 13:394-403, 1996.

Reisberg B: Behavioral intervention approaches to the treatment and management of Alzheimer's disease: A research agenda, *International Psychogeriatrics* 8(suppl 1):38-44, 1996.

Rhoads GG, McNellis DC, Kessel SS: Home monitoring of uterine contractility, *American Journal of Obstetrics and Gynecology* 165(1):2-6, 1991.

Rowland HS, Rowland BL: *Nursing administration handbook,* ed 4, Gaithersburg, Md, 1997, Aspen.

Rubinstein E: Cost implications of home care on serious infections, *Hospital Formulary* 28(1):46-50, 1993.

Salesberry PJ, Nickel JT, O'Connell M: AIDS research in the community: A case study in collaboration between researchers and clinicians, *Public Health Nursing* 8(3):201-207, 1991.

Scannell S et al: Negotiating nurse patient authority in pediatric home health care, *Journal of Pediatric Nursing* 8(2):70-78, 1993.

Schulz R, Visintainer P, Williamson GM: Psychiatric and physical morbidity effects of caregiving, *Journal of Gerontology* 45(5):181-191, 1990.

Sevick MA, Bradham DD: Economic value of caregiver effort in maintaining long-term ventilator-assisted individuals at home, *Heart & Lung* 26:148-157, 1997.

Shaughnessy PW et al: Outcomes across the care continuum. Home health care, *Medical Care* 35(suppl 11):NS115-23, 1997.

Smith CE: Technology and home care, *Annual Review of Nursing Research* 13:137-167, 1995.

Smith CE: Quality of life and caregiving in technological home care, *Annual Review of Nursing Research* 14:95-118, 1996.

Sperling RL: What's this OASIS anyway? Outcome and Assessment Information Set, *Home Healthcare Nurse* 15:373-374, 1998.

Steinmetz SK: Elder abuse by adult offspring: The relationship of actual vs. perceived dependency, *Journal of Health and Human Resources Administration* 12(4):434-463, 1990.

Stricklin ML, Hekelman FP: A model for integrating research into home care, *Caring* 10(3):39-43, 1991.

Suntken G et al: Implementation of a comprehensive skin care program across care settings using the AHCPR pressure ulcer prevention and treatment guidelines, *Ostomy Wound Management* 42(2):20-2, 24-6, 38-30, 1996.

Ungvarski PJ, Hurley PM: Nursing research in HIV/AIDS home care. II. *Home Healthcare Nurse* 13(4):9-13, 1995.

van Harteveld JT, Mistiaen PJ, Dukkers van Emden DM: Home visits by community nurses for cancer patients after discharge from hospital: An evaluation study of the continuity visit, *Cancer Nursing* 20:105-114, 1997.

Weissert WG, Hedrick SC: Lessons learned from research on effects of community-based long-term care, *Journal of the American Geriatrics Society* 42:348-353, 1994.

Weissert WG et al: Cost savings from home and community-based services: Arizona's capitated Medicaid long-term care program, *Journal of Health Politics, Policy & Law* 22:1329-1357, 1997a.

Weissert WG et al: Toward a strategy for reducing potentially avoidable hospital admissions among home care clients, *Medical Care Research & Review* 54:439-455, 1997b.

Williams JK: Measuring outcomes in home care: Current research and practice, *Home Health Care Services Quarterly* 15(3):3-30, 1995.

Williams MA et al: Family caregiving in cases of hip fracture, *Rehabilitation Nursing* 21:124-131, 1996.

Wilson R, Fulmer T: Home health nurses' initial experiences with wireless, pen-based computing, *Public Health Nursing* 15:225-232, 1998.

Winslow BW: Family caregiving and the use of formal community support services: A qualitative case study, *Issues in Mental Health Nursing* 19(1):11-27, 1998.

Worcester MI: Family coping: Caring for the elderly in home care, *Home Health Care Services Quarterly* 11(1-2):121-173, 1990.

Zahr L: An integrative research review of intervention studies with premature infants from disadvantaged backgrounds, *Maternal-Child Nursing Journal* 22(3):90-101, 1994.

ADDITIONAL READINGS

Humphrey CJ, Milone-Nuzzo P: *Orientation to home care nursing,* Gaithersburg, Md, 1996, Aspen.

Linne EB, ed: *Home care and managed care: Strategies for the future,* Chicago, 1995, American Hospital Publishing.

National Family Caregivers Association: *The resourceful caregiver: Helping family caregivers help themselves,* St Louis, 1996, Mosby.

Rief L, Martin KS: *Nurses and consumers: Partners in assuring quality care in the home,* Washington, DC, 1996, American Nurses.

Robbins DA: *Ethical and legal issues in home care and long term care: Challenges and solutions,* Gaithersburg, Md, 1996, Aspen.

Index

A

A, B, C, D, E framework. *See* Anthropometric, biochemical, clinical, dietary, and environmental (A, B, C, D, E) framework.
AAP. *See* American Academy of Pediatrics (AAP).
Abacavir sulfate, 478t
ABC, 478t
Access fee, definition of, 61
Accountable Health Plans (AHPs), definition of, 61
ACE. *See* Angiotensin-converting enzyme (ACE).
ACE inhibitors, 417, 448-449
ACOG. *See* American College of Obstetricians and Gynecologists (ACOG).
Acquired immunodeficiency syndrome (AIDS), 290
  HIV and. *See* HIV/AIDS.
  research in home care and, 546
Activities of daily living (ADLs)
  Alzheimer's disease and, 384-385
  elderly and, 252, 253
Activity levels, heart failure and, 427
Acute care, 3-13
Acute care facility, 4-6
Acute heath care problems, 545-546
Acute renal failure, 450-452
Acute tubular necrosis (ATN), 450, 451
AD. *See* Alzheimer's disease (AD).
Ad hoc interpreters
  cultural competency and, 199-200
  LEP and, 199-200
Adaptive equipment, occupational therapist and, 132
ADEAR Center. *See* Alzheimer's Disease Education and Resource (ADEAR) Center.
Adherence
  background and historical perspective of, 473
  definition of, 472-473
  factors influencing, 473-474
  heart failure management and, 420
  issues of, associated with HAART, HIV/AIDS and, 472-476
  scientific rationale for maintaining, 473
  strategies for home care nurses to facilitate, 474-476
Adherence outcomes, 473
ADLs. *See* Activities of daily living (ADLs).
Administration
  medication, 120-122, 121b
  of managed care services, 52-54
Administrative changes in reduction of stress, 516-517
Administrative styles, stress and, 506
Administrators, home care, 531
Adolescence, nutritional assessment in, 151-153

ADRD. *See* Alzheimer's disease and related disorders (ADRD).
Adult day care, 4-46
Adult foster care, 43-44
Adults
  enteral nutritional support for, 168-170, 169t-170t, 173f, 175f
  nutritional assessment in, 153-154, 153b
  older. *See* Elderly, home care of.
  outcome indicators of nutritional support for, 168-172
  parenteral nutritional support for, 170-172, 171t, 173f, 174f, 175f
Advanced practice nursing (APN), 519-534
  advanced-practice nursing in home care and, 519-520
  Alzheimer's disease and, 406
  barriers to implementation of, 526-528
  definition of, 519-524
  emerging roles in, 524-526
  implementation of, 531
  model of, 528-531
  rehabilitation, 135
Advanced practice rehabilitation nurse, 135
Adverse selection, definition of, 61
AFDC. *See* Aid to Families with Dependent Children (AFDC).
Affective objectives, 95-97
Age
  learning and, 94
  stress and, 507
Agency
  for Health Care Policy and Research (AHCPR), 417, 421, 540
  for Healthcare Research and Quality (AHRQ), 69, 540
Agenerase. *See* Amprenavir.
Aging
  and Dementia Center of New York University, 403
  common changes in, 257t-258t
  elderly home care and, 251-253
Agitation, Alzheimer's disease and, 393-395
AHCPR. *See* Agency for Health Care Policy and Research (AHCPR).
AHNA. *See* American Holistic Nurses Association (AHNA).
AHPs. *See* Accountable Health Plans (AHPs).
AHRQ. *See* Agency for Healthcare Research and Quality (AHRQ).
Aid to Families with Dependent Children (AFDC), 235
AIDS. *See* Acute heath care problems.
Airway clearance, ineffective, terminal care at home and, 291-292
Airway disease, 302t
Airway equipment and supplies, pulmonary compromise and, 319-320, 320f
Airway-pressure monitors, 322
Albrecht's nursing theory, 128b, 130

Page numbers followed by b indicate boxes; f, figures; and t, tables.

559